Gastroenterology: Diagnosis and Treatment

Gastroenterology: Diagnosis and Treatment

Edited by **Greg Callister**

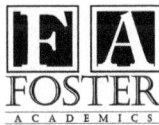

FA
FOSTER
ACADEMICS

New Jersey

Published by Foster Academics,
61 Van Reypen Street,
Jersey City, NJ 07306, USA
www.fosteracademics.com

Gastroenterology: Diagnosis and Treatment
Edited by Greg Callister

© 2016 Foster Academics

International Standard Book Number: 978-1-63242-464-8 (Hardback)

Contents

Permissions

List of Contributors

Preface

Gastroenterology is the branch of medicine that places its emphasis on the diagnosis and treatment of diseases related to digestive system and gastrointestinal tract. It studies the function and diseases of pancreas, esophagus, stomach, gallbladder, bile ducts, liver, small intestine, colon and rectum. It includes the treatment of diseases such as peptic ulcer disease, colitis, gallbladder and biliary tract disease, nutritional problems, colon polyps, gastrointestinal cancer, jaundice, cirrhosis of the liver, gastroesophageal reflux (heartburn), pancreatitis, Irritable Bowel Syndrome (IBS), etc. This book unravels the recent studies in the field of gastroenterology. The objective of this text is to give a comprehensive overview of the different areas of gastroenterology. The ever growing need for advanced medication and treatment is the reason that has fueled the research in this field in recent times. This book is a resource guide for experts as well as students.

Significant researches are present in this book. Intensive efforts have been employed by authors to make this book an outstanding discourse. This book contains the enlightening chapters which have been written on the basis of significant researches done by the experts.

Finally, I would also like to thank all the members involved in this book for being a team and meeting all the deadlines for the submission of their respective works. I would also like to thank my friends and family for being supportive in my efforts.

Editor

Transitioning to highly effective therapies for the treatment of chronic hepatitis C virus infection: A policy statement and implementation guideline

Daniel J Smyth MD FRCPC[1,3], Duncan Webster MD FRCPC[1,3], Lisa Barrett MD PhD FRCPC[2,3], Mark MacMillan MD FRCPC[1,3], Lisa McKnight MD FRCPC[1,3], Frank Schweiger MD FRCPC[1,3]

DJ Smyth, D Webster, L Barrett, M MacMillan, L McKnight, F Schweiger. Transitioning to highly effective therapies for the treatment of chronic hepatitis C virus infection: A policy statement and implementation guideline. Can J Gastroenterol Hepatol 2014;28(10):529-534.

Chronic hepatitis C virus (HCV) infection increases all-cause mortality, rates of cirrhosis, hepatocellular carcinoma, liver transplantation and overall health care utilization. Morbidity and mortality disproportionately affect individuals born between 1945 and 1975. The recent development of well-tolerated and highly effective therapies for chronic HCV infection represents a unique opportunity to dramatically reduce rates of HCV-related complications and their costs. Critical to the introduction of such therapies will be well-designed provincial programming to ensure immediate treatment access to individuals at highest risk for complication, and well-defined strategies to address the global treatment needs of traditionally high-risk and marginalized populations. HCV practitioners in New Brunswick created a provincial strategy that stratifies treatment according to those at highest need, measures clinical impact, and creates evaluation strategies to demonstrate the significant direct and indirect cost savings anticipated with curative treatments.

Key Words: *Direct-acting antiviral; Guideline; HCV; Policy; Treatment*

La transition vers des thérapies hautement efficaces pour traiter l'infection par le virus de l'hépatite C chronique : document de principes et directives de mise en œuvre

L'infection par le virus de l'hépatite C (VHC) chronique accroît la mortalité toutes causes confondues, les taux de cirrhose, de carcinome hépatocellulaire et de greffe du foie, ainsi que l'utilisation générale des soins de santé. La morbidité et la mortalité touchent de manière disproportionnée les personnes nées entre 1945 et 1965. La récente mise au point de thérapies bien tolérées et hautement efficaces contre l'infection à VHC chronique se veut une occasion unique de réduire considérablement le taux de complications et les coûts liés à cette infection. Pour adopter de telles thérapies, il est essentiel de prévoir des programmes provinciaux bien conçus qui assureront un accès immédiat aux personnes les plus vulnérables aux complications, ainsi que des stratégies bien définies pour répondre aux besoins thérapeutiques globaux des populations habituellement à haut risque et marginalisées. Les praticiens du VHC au Nouveau-Brunswick ont créé une stratégie provinciale qui stratifie le traitement en fonction des personnes les plus vulnérables, qui en mesure les répercussions cliniques et qui démontre les économies directes et indirectes importantes anticipées grâce aux traitements curatifs.

Chronic hepatitis C virus (HCV) infection significantly increases all-cause mortality and is a leading cause of hepatocellular carcinoma (HCC), liver transplantation and overall utilization of health care resources (1-3). Over the past decades, morbidity and mortality related to chronic HCV infection has continued to increase, particularly among persons infected between 1945 and 1975 (baby boomers) (4). Age-standardized incidence rates of HCC are rising in Canada, and this is largely attributable to chronic HCV infection (5,6). In contrast to other chronic viral infections, including hepatitis B and HIV, mortality related to HCV continues to increase, and now exceeds that of HIV (7). Without access to appropriate therapy, rates of cirrhosis, HCC and death related to chronic HCV infection will continue to increase (8).

The burden of chronic HCV infection is currently disproportionately affecting baby boomers, who have generally been infected for several decades and are at highest risk for HCV liver-related complications (9). Chronic HCV infection is also associated with other medical problems beyond the liver, including insulin resistance and diabetes, renal disease and, rarely, hematological malignancies (10,11). Highly concerning are data suggesting that the majority of chronically infected patients are unaware of their diagnosis, and the absence of symptoms in many patients makes targeted screening programs essential (12). Birth cohort-directed screening programs in these patients have been shown to be both cost effective and to reduce rates of chronic liver disease and HCC (9). Incident infections are now primarily concentrated in those engaging in high-risk activities, including intravenous drug use (13), and dedicated programming to minimize high-risk behaviours is essential for a successful comprehensive strategy.

Treatment and subsequent cure of chronic HCV infection reduces the risk of liver failure and HCC, and significantly decreases all-cause mortality (14-16). Treatment of chronic HCV infection currently requires the use of pegylated interferon for up to 48 weeks depending on the viral genotype and response to initial treatment (17). Side effects associated with interferon use are very often debilitating, and include flu-like symptoms, psychiatric complications, endocrinopathies, exacerbation of autoimmune conditions, cytopenias, and severe or life threatening complications (18). The introduction of the novel agents boceprevir and telaprevir allowed the interferon treatment course to be shortened by one-half in certain patient populations, and has increased sustained virological response (SVR) rates to 66% and 79% in treatment-naive patients (19,20). Despite these improvements, tolerance of prolonged interferon courses remains challenging and compromises patient adherence to therapy, resulting in significant health care expenditure to manage adverse effects.

We are currently witnessing the introduction of highly effective interferon-free treatment regimens (21). The era of new therapies will create a unique opportunity to offer high clinical cure rates, reduce

[1]Horizon Health Network, New Brunswick; [2]Capital Health; [3]Dalhousie University, Halifax, Nova Scotia
Correspondence and reprints: Dr Daniel J Smyth, Department of Medicine, Dalhousie University, 135 MacBeath Avenue, Moncton, New Brunswick E1C 6Z8. e-mail dr.daniel.smyth@horizonnb.ca

hepatic and nonhepatic medical complications, and also increase access to therapy in traditionally marginalized high-risk populations. Patient demand for these highly effective therapies will undoubtedly be intense, and payers – both public and private – will require structured programming to ensure stratified access to appropriate treatment. The current policy addresses the need for appropriate screening strategies, referral and treatment stratification processes, engagement and optimization of marginalized populations and, finally, data collection to evaluate epidemiological, clinical and cost effectiveness.

Understanding the impact of chronic HCV infection will dramatically improve our ability to build and deliver necessary programs for provincial HCV therapy, and target program resources and treatment plans to areas of highest impact. This strategy aims to significantly improve the HCV clinical paradigm in New Brunswick, and the comprehensive prospective approach may act as a benchmark for other provinces to implement similar strategies in their own areas.

METHODS

All HCV practitioners in New Brunswick were approached for participation in the project. A provincial advisory meeting was held on February 1, 2014 in Rothesay, New Brunswick, with the intention of identifying required resources and creating an optimal care model to facilitate access to and reimbursement of curative HCV treatments in the province.

Breakout sessions focussed discussion on multiple areas including provincial epidemiology, screening, treatment stratification, patient referral and follow-up, and a model of care that recognizes the limited resources currently available. Recommended programming was designed to be implemented in a phased and prioritized fashion, with strategies most likely to be budget neutral and cost effective taking precedence. Implementation tactics were developed for all strategic recommendations.

Following the meeting, subcommittees drafted policy sections related to screening, stratification, treatment, education and prevention, and program evaluation. A consensus document was circulated to all participating members for review before finalization of the following statement.

Implementation proposal

While there are reasonable data on the number of infected patients and the economic burden of HCV at the national and international level, the same cannot be said of the New Brunswick HCV landscape. HCV infection is a reportable disease in New Brunswick; however, there is currently no comprehensive provincial strategy for screening or monitoring HCV seroprevalence and new incident cases, especially in high-risk populations.

SCREENING BIRTH COHORT 1945 TO 1975 POPULATION

HCV is currently the leading cause of liver cirrhosis, HCC and liver transplantation (1,2). Advanced liver disease caused by HCV is on the rise, particularly in the birth cohort of 1945 to 1975, who are frequently unaware of their diagnosis (9,12). This results in significant health care expenditure to manage complications. The cost for an individual liver transplant in Organisation for Economic Co-operation and Development countries is approximately $103,548. This does not include long-term follow-up and antirejection medication costs (22). Other complications are also costly. The five-year net cost estimates for newly diagnosed HCC patients in Ontario alone are $106.4 million (23).

To identify these individuals and treat them before complications occur, a screening program for the 1945 to 1975 birth cohort is recommended (24). The Canadian Liver Foundation has issued a position statement advocating for birth-cohort screening in Canada. Screening of the birth cohort born between 1945 and 1975, coupled with a strategy for follow-up treatment and education, is the best method to identify and provide care to affected people in Canada (24,25). New guidelines issued by the Centers for Disease Control and Prevention

(Georgia, USA) suggest that all baby boomers (1945 to 1975) be screened for HCV (26).

Strategic recommendation

It is recommended that New Brunswick expand existing HCV screening to include one-time birth cohort screening of individuals born between 1945 and 1975.

Implementation tactics

Tactic 1   A budget impact analysis with incremental cost estimates of birth cohort screening will be provided to the Department of Health and associated laboratories within the Regional Health Authorities.

Tactic 2   A primary health education program on birth cohort screening will be developed and implemented, including pathways for subsequent referral.

Tactic 3   The screening role of catchment centres such as emergency rooms and addiction services (eg, methadone clinics, correctional services) will be evaluated.

Tactic 4   Public health education and awareness of the value of HCV screening will be promoted.

SCREENING: HIGH-RISK POPULATIONS

Within New Brunswick, cohorts with a high prevalence of HCV infection and at highest risk for new incident HCV infection include users of illicit drugs (IDUs), intravenous drug users (IVDUs), homeless individuals and the incarcerated population. Among IVDU, 50% to 80% become infected after one year of intravenous drug use and close to 100% are infected within eight years. This is due to sharing needles, syringes and other injection equipment, and is associated with at least 70% to 80% of newly acquired HCV cases in Canada (27,28). It is estimated that each infected IVDU is likely to infect approximately 20 people, on average, and one-half of these transmissions will take place within two years of the index infection (29). Little is currently known about the prevalence of HCV in New Brunswick IDU and IVDU populations; however, rates are likely very high. In fact, it is known that 42.14% of 298 opioid-dependent individuals at a New Brunswick methadone maintenance clinic are HCV positive (30).

There are multiple groups at high risk for HCV infection. Homeless individuals have been identified as being at greater risk for infection with blood-borne viruses than the general population (31). Within the correctional system, a projected 30% of the 14,900 inmates now housed in Canadian federal prisons are infected with HCV (32). It is highly likely that the same issues exist within the provincial corrections system. Certain minority ethnic groups are likely to have acquired HCV infection before immigration to this country. The Public Health Agency of Canada reports that Canadian Aboriginal people are approximately five times more likely than non-Aboriginal people to be infected with viral hepatitis (33). It is also known that in Nova Scotia, there are higher rates of infectious disease among the community members of the largest First Nations community compared with the general population of Cape Breton and Nova Scotia (34). It is unclear whether the First Nations of New Brunswick also have a disproportionate HCV-associated burden of illness.

Targeted screening of these high-risk groups will be essential to identify and treat those at high risk for hepatic adverse events, and to engage persons in critical harm reduction measures necessary to impact incident cases.

Strategic recommendation

It is recommended that the province of New Brunswick leverage, improve and expand existing provincial screening and related programs among at-risk populations.

Implementation tactics

Tactic 1	A coordinated patient intake and referral process will be developed and implemented by existing screening programs, addiction services and methadone clinics.
Tactic 2	Addiction services and methadone clinics will be mandated to screen for HCV.
Tactic 3	HCV at-risk population screening will be promoted to primary health care providers, regional public health offices, correctional services and emergency departments.
Tactic 4	Expansion into under-serviced areas will take place to offer and promote screening for HCV and other blood-borne diseases to those who attend harm reduction services.
Tactic 5	Public health education on the importance of screening at-risk populations will occur.
Tactic 6	Guidelines will be developed for HCV screening and harm reduction measures in individuals from high-risk endemic countries, First Nations communities and prisons.

TREATMENT STRATIFICATION: RECOMMENDED PATIENT STRATIFICATION BIRTH COHORT

In light of their excellent tolerance and high cure rates, interferon-free direct-acting antiviral (DAA) treatments will be in high demand by patient groups; however, the up-front direct pharmaceutical cost is significant. It is essential that a utilization management plan is established to ensure prioritization of those most in need and likely to benefit. These criteria, established by provincial HCV experts, will ensure maximal clinical and cost impact. Measureable cost savings in the birth cohort patients provided with curative HCV therapy are anticipated, particularly related to reduced hepatic adverse events. When direct and indirect costs savings are considered, the incremental costs associated with novel HCV therapies are anticipated to be minimal.

Strategic recommendation
A directed, multiphased treatment and patient stratification strategy is essential to ensure those at highest risk of immediate complication receive prioritized treatment. This approach minimizes up-front expenditure by deferring costs and maximizing potential cost savings.

Implementation tactics

Tactic 1	Implement patient stratification as a phased multiyear approach as outlined below. Prioritizing patients based on their current medical condition and stage of fibrosis.
Stratification model	**Phase 1 (short-term, years 1–2, highest risk of hepatic adverse event or complication):** Fibrosis documented at F3/F4; Extrahepatic manifestations of chronic HCV infection; HIV positive; or At discretion of HCV expert.
	Phase 2 (years 3–5, incorporates lower-risk patients who are at low risk for reinfection): Fibrosis documented at F2/F3/F4; Extrahepatic manifestations of chronic HCV infection; Patient with HCV infection >10 years; or At discretion of HCV expert.
	Phase 3 (year >5, incorporates most patients): All remaining patients at discretion of HCV expert.
Tactic 2	Following identification of chronic HCV infected patients, it is recommended to adopt and improve the existing referral plan directed to specialists at the HCV collaborative care clinics for program enrollment, assessment and treatment.
Tactic 3	Expansion of HCV collaborative care clinics to serve rural populations.

STRATIFICATION: HIGH-RISK POPULATIONS

There are several cohorts at increased risk for HCV infection. These cohorts include the baby boomers, IDU and IVDU populations, homeless persons, incarcerated populations, certain minority ethnic groups and First Nations communities. Recognizing the high risks for reinfection and incident infection in IVU and IVDU populations, this strategy suggests initial treatment in these populations to have maximal impact on individual and public health levels.

Despite international recommendations to treat HCV in the setting of injection and intravenous drug use, there are significant barriers to treating these cohorts, particularly with traditional interferon-containing regimens (35-37). These include concerns around the chaotic lifestyle of IDUs and IVDUs, lack of fixed address, social isolation, poor adherence to treatment, difficulties in the management of the psychiatric side-effects of treatment and risk of reinfection after HCV eradication.

Treating these cohorts in a strategic fashion will contribute to a significant reduction in the prevalence of HCV infection and new incident cases, thus reducing the associated clinical and social burden of the disease within the province. To address these barriers and to successfully contact, manage and treat these patients, a multidisciplinary approach is mandatory with a highly personalized approach to patient care (38). This is best achieved in a coordinated multidisciplinary clinic environment with interprofessional health care. This model of care is utilized at a pilot clinic in Saint John (New Brunswick), operated by the Centre for Research, Education, and Clinical Care of At-Risk Populations (RECAP), and will be an excellent site to test implementation of the multipronged strategy developed by the working group.

RECAP model of care
A New Brunswick medical model for managing IDU and IVDU cohorts had been established and evaluated (39). Within this model, which employed an interprofessional approach to care, there has been great success with treating HCV in this difficult-to-treat population. In accordance with the established WHO patient treatment pathway (40), this model ensures that each patient within at-risk cohorts is provided with an individualized approach to management based on individual circumstances. Following screening, diagnosis and disease staging, patients may be initiated on HCV treatment depending on defined dynamic and static clinical parameters. Patients who are active users of illicit drugs are stabilized before HCV treatment, and individuals meeting criteria for opioid abuse and/or dependence are actively engaged in methadone maintenance programs before starting HCV treatment. Social factors are addressed that will ensure treatment coverage and the ability for close follow-up and communication throughout the course of therapy. After optimization of clinical, mental and social status, and with consideration to other comorbidities, it is determined whether the patient is a candidate for HCV treatment. With the advent and availability of interferon-free treatment regimens, the safe and successful treatment of HCV within this cohort will be more easily attainable. It is anticipated that this will allow for a significant decrease in new incident cases of HCV within the province.

Strategic recommendation
At-risk patients require access to a multidisciplinary care model that addresses medical, psychiatric and addiction comorbidities, allowing patients to move toward HCV therapy. Multidisciplinary and interprofessional clinics for the management of HCV-positive and at-risk IDU and IVDU cohorts should be developed, supported, evaluated and promoted.

RECAP patient stratification model

Tactic 1	Implement patient stratification as a phased multiyear approach. Prioritize patients based on their medical condition, stage of fibrosis and patient readiness for treatment.

RECAP patient stratification model – CONTINUED

Stratification model	Phase 1 (short-term, year 1–5), highest risk of adverse event or complication:
	Fibrosis documented at F3/F4;
	Stable on methadone maintenance therapy if indicated;
	Fixed address and adherence to clinic follow-up for three months;
	Extrahepatic manifestation of HCV infection;
	HIV positive; or
	At the discretion of provincial HCV specialist.
	Phase 2 (year >5): All patients eligible at discretion of HCV specialist, providing:
	Stable on methadone maintenance therapy if indicated; and/or
	Fixed address and adherence to clinic follow up for three months or more.
Tactic 2	Expand the RECAP program and model of care in needed locations across New Brunswick.
Tactic 3	Following successful HCV treatment, patients must be retained in substance abuse treatment programs with a focus on harm-reduction to avoid reinfection.
Tactic 4	Ongoing long-term management must also be provided to those patients not currently suitable for treatment, and clinical pathways must be developed to assist them in working toward treatment suitability.
Tactic 5	Aligned collaboration of addiction and mental health services with the medical model of care in the RECAP program.
Tactic 6	Improved access to methadone maintenance therapy within the provincial corrections system, and improve access to methadone prescribers following release.
Tactic 7	Close analysis of HCV treatment outcomes and follow-up is critical in this difficult-to-treat population. To decrease new incident cases, the role of treating even the unstable active addict may be considered in light of program evaluation and trends in HCV prevalence and incidence within specific communities.

TREATMENT

Adherence to traditional interferon-based treatment regimens is often poor, and high indirect costs include employee absence and disability leave to complete therapy. Cost estimates of the current treatment often fail to take into account the significant economic losses resulting from work cessation, disability claims, physician visits, laboratory testing and emergency room visits, among other indirect costs. This does not begin to account for the significant impact these therapies have on quality of life measures. Clearly, the direct drug costs of interferon are small compared with the actual, real-life cost of completing complex and onerous interferon-based therapy.

In clinical trials, interferon-free DAA therapies demonstrate SVR rates ranging from 96% to 100% (where SVR is equivalent to viral eradication and cure) (41,42). Treatment-naive patients, patients who have previously failed treatment, and those traditionally difficult to treat including patients with cirrhosis and HIV are almost universally cured with these therapies (43,44). Concomitant use of these treatments in opiate-dependent patients with concomitant methadone use has been studied within the clinical trials, all with high SVR rates.

With the new regimens, treatment will be easier and adherence will be greatly improved. These new therapies represent a significant upgrade from existing therapies currently already covered by the New Brunswick Provincial Drug Plan. Current therapies will quickly become obsolete due to lower SVR rates and diminished cost effectiveness. The combined screening program and high SVR rates of new therapies will likely lead to reduced HCV incidence and provide significant health economic impact for the treating provinces. It is

suggested that incremental direct costs related to new treatments in this context will not be significant when compared with traditional interferon-based therapies when direct and indirect cost savings are comprehensively measured. Antiviral treatment will represent just one component of a global and personalized treatment strategy designed to optimize risk factors and medical comorbidities and also to reduce the likelihood of reinfection.

Strategic recommendation

Expedited access to interferon-free DAA therapies as part of the New Brunswick HCV Strategy for both public and private payers in the context of a comprehensive provincial strategy.

Implementation tactics

Tactic 1	Expedited approval of treatments in the Common Drug Review and subsequent Pan-Canadian Purchasing Alliance.
Tactic 2	Immediate approval and access to treatment reimbursement on the New Brunswick Provincial Drug Plan for DAA treatments (as made available to market).
Tactic 3	Immediate approval and access to treatment and reimbursement on private insurance plans offered in New Brunswick (payers).
Tactic 4	Evaluate economic and health outcomes of the New Brunswick HCV Strategy. Measure and evaluate treatment adherence, quality of life, patient success, direct medical savings and indirect cost savings.
Tactic 5	The use of Fibroscan (Echosens, France) or FibroTest (LabCorp, USA) technology and other clinical parameters will assist treating physicians in the allocation of limited resources to those who will benefit the most early in the treatment strategy, recognizing that others will need to be treated in the future.

EDUCATION AND PREVENTION

Public education is essential in identifying undiagnosed cases of HCV infection in New Brunswick and reducing new cases of HCV infection. Health care practitioners include physicians, nurse practitioners, registered nurses, emergency room staff, pharmacists, support staff and health care trainees. Target patient cohorts for educational initiatives include known HCV-positive individuals, those born from 1945 to 1975, IDU, incarcerated individuals, immigrants from countries of high HCV endemicity, First Nations communities, and those who received blood products in Canada before 1990. To ensure effectiveness of this screening strategy, all stakeholders in the province, including the Department of Health and Public Health, must collaborate with regard to an educational initiative for these target populations. Key agencies that should participate in this strategy include specialist treatment services, public health, general practitioners, associated community agencies and correctional services. Provision of information will increase awareness of HCV and will have a subsequent impact on service demand. This must be anticipated and capacity issues addressed through a patient stratification strategy.

The Public Health Agency of Canada is expected to release its review of the Canadian Liver Foundation recommendations in the near future. Currently, it advocates for screening based on risk factors (45). Risk factors include engaging in high-risk behaviours, history of potential exposures to HCV, and clinical signs or symptoms of active disease. For this 'at-risk' group, education is incredibly important to diagnose cases and to prevent new infections. The prevention of new cases is largely through the reduction of transmission of infection from those who are already infected.

The education, prevention and communication approaches completed to date are of value. However, the levels of provision can be described as reactive and patchy rather than strategic and comprehensive. This approach to education and prevention services can lead to a situation where the information provided to those at risk is inconsistent and not necessarily based on the latest available evidence. Competency-based standards for training in health promotion do not currently exist in each province for general health promotion or for training in issues relevant to IDU. In addition, there is little to no awareness among health care workers and the general population of the recent Canadian Liver Foundation recommendation for HCV screening among all individuals born between 1945 and 1975.

With regard to IDU and IVDU at-risk populations, a number of agencies within each province are involved in current education, prevention and communication initiatives. Agencies in New Brunswick include, but are not limited to, AIDS Saint John, AIDS New Brunswick, the Atlantic Interdisciplinary Research Network and the Canadian Liver Foundation. Individuals may also receive education around prevention through health care providers at infectious diseases clinics and gastroenterology clinics as well as through public health and addiction services. Education services provided through community advocacy groups are underfunded and there is currently only a modest focus on HCV education through local voluntary providers. Services are targeted at IVDUs and are generally provided on an ad hoc basis. Brief educational interventions are provided to those at risk of HCV within the formal health care setting.

Strategic recommendation
A broad public education campaign is required to inform the target populations and, importantly, the 1945 to 1975 birth cohort that HCV screening is recommended regardless of other risk factors. The health care community must also be informed of this recommendation.

Implementation tactics

Tactic 1	Review existing materials and provide up-to-date accurate and consistent information to all affected by HCV. Specific information will be required by different groups.
	The HCV information needs of service providers include:
	Information pertaining to disease prevalence and incidence, transmission risks, screening & diagnostic tests, treatment options, treatment benefits and risks
	The communication materials and channels include: CMEs and information packages
	The information needs of patients diagnosed with HCV include:
	Disease characteristics, prognosis, treatment options, treatment benefits and risks, complementary therapies and the means to accessing services
	The communication materials and channels include: brochures, posters in all public health access points including pharmacies.
	The information needs of high-risk populations such as IVDUs include:
	Risk factors, eliminating/minimizing risk, accessing preventative services, disease characteristics, testing for HCV, treatment benefits and risks. French and English material should be used
	The communication materials and channels include: Brochures, posters in all public health access points including pharmacies and community based programs.
Tactic 2	Methods of disseminating and providing information and education to different target groups should be evaluated and the most effective approach used. The accuracy of scientific information should be agreed upon and presented in an appropriate format.
Tactic 3	Adopt prevention and education initiatives targeting IVDUs.
Tactic 4	Include competency based training modules on harm reduction for all those working with IDUs in a community setting. Modules should be guided by national standards in health promotion.

PROGRAM EVALUATION

Measuring therapeutic efficacy and associated health care and societal cost savings are essential to the introduction of novel hepatitis C treatments. Following informed consent, referred patients will be registered in a provincial database that will collect comprehensive baseline demographic and epidemiological information. Detailed evaluation of comorbidities (medical history, substance abuse history and high-risk behaviours) will be completed and analysis used to guide risk-reduction strategies. The program will establish the efficacy of the implemented risk reduction measures, beginning with the Saint John RECAP clinic.

Data will be gathered and maintained through an integrated patient-centred health information system with an embedded program management platform. Data collected in provincial HCV clinics will be linked to Medicare billing records, and established provincial databases containing valuable indicators including laboratory testing and diagnostic imaging. Longitudinal outcome measures, including emergency room visits, hospitalizations and deaths, will be assessed. The database will establish the safety and efficacy of new therapies in New Brunswick patients, and also evaluate cost savings associated with their use, particularly savings related to a reduction of hepatic adverse events (liver decompensation, HCC and transplantation) and also savings related to reduced usage of health care resources when compared with traditional treatment. Reduced costs related to adverse event management are anticipated, which will offset costs related to the introduction of newer treatment modalities. Side effects from interferon-based therapies also have significant impacts on a patient's ability to work and quality of life, and measureable cost savings related to the improved tolerability of novel agents are anticipated.

The development of the provincial HCV database and proposed evaluation metrics will generate needed clinical outcomes data and health service utilization data. The inclusive patient capture, knowledge generation and translational medicine aspect of this program make it distinctly different from several other nascent programs around the country: potentially all DAA-treated patient data for the province are captured. Understanding the impact of chronic HCV infection will dramatically improve the ability to build and deliver necessary programs for HCV therapy in New Brunswick, and target program resources and treatment plans to areas of highest impact. This proposal will greatly improve the New Brunswick HCV clinical situation; however, the comprehensive approach may also act as a benchmark for other provinces that will need to implement similar strategies in their own regions.

Strategic recommendation
Measuring therapeutic efficacy and associated health care and societal cost savings are essential to the introduction of novel hepatitis C treatments.

Implementation tactics

Tactic 1	A prospective provincial database will establish the safety and efficacy of new therapies in New Brunswick, and also evaluate cost savings associated with their use, particularly savings related to a reduction of hepatic adverse events (including liver decompensation, HCC and transplantation) and also savings related to reduced usage of health care resources when compared to treatment with traditional interferon-based regimens.
Tactic 2	The database will establish the efficacy of the implemented risk reduction measures, beginning with the Saint John RECAP pilot clinic. Detailed evaluation of comorbidities will be completed and used to guide future risk reduction strategies.
Tactic 3	Indirect cost savings including those related to employee absence and quality of life will be measured.

CONCLUSION

The introduction of curative therapies for HCV represents a unique opportunity to significantly improve HCV-related morbidity and mortality in those who are traditionally marginalized and at high risk.

Utilization management is essential in this context to ensure treatment prioritization to highest-risk patients and to ensure clinical and cost effectiveness. New Brunswick practitioners recognized our unique ability to engage all treating HCV practitioners in the province in the formulation of a comprehensive provincial strategy. Many of the most affected populations in the province are directly applicable to those in other cities and towns across Canada and the United States. We believe the comprehensive program approach developed for New Brunswick patients can act as a benchmark for other provinces to implement similar strategies in a rational, timely manner that can improve HCV care across Canada.

DISCLOSURES: Support for the provincial advisory meeting was provided by Abbvie. The above manuscript was prepared independently by participants following the meeting.

REFERENCES

1. Lee MH, Yang HI, Lu SN, et al. Chronic hepatitis C virus infection increases mortality from hepatic and extrahepatic diseases: A community-based long-term prospective study. J Infect Dis 2012;206:469-77.
2. O'Leary JG, Lepe R, Davis GL. Indications for liver transplantation. Gastroenterology 2008;134:1764-76.
3. Moorman AC, Gordon SC, Rupp LB, et al. Baseline characteristics and mortality among people in care for chronic viral hepatitis: The chronic hepatitis cohort study. Clin Infect Dis 2013;56:40-50.
4. Armstrong GL, Wasley A, Simard EP, et al. The prevalence of hepatitis C virus infection in the United States, 1999 through 2002. Ann Intern Med 2006;144:705-14.
5. Canada, Public Health Agency. Canadian Cancer Statistics, 2013. <www.phac-aspc.gc.ca/publicat/cdic-mcbc/33-3/ar-11-eng.php> (Accessed May 1, 2014).
6. El-Serag HB. Epidemiology of hepatocellular carcinoma in USA. Hepatol Res 2007;7(Suppl 2):S88-94.
7. Ly KN, Xing J, Klevens RM, et al. The increasing burden of mortality from viral hepatitis in the United States between 1999 and 2007. Ann Intern Med 2012;156:271-8.
8. Rein DB, Wittenborn JS, Weinbaum CM, et al. Forecasting the morbidity and mortality associated with prevalent cases of pre-cirrhotic chronic hepatitis C in the United States. Dig Liver Dis 2011;43:66-72.
9. Rein DB, Smith BD, Wittenborn JS, et al. The cost-effectiveness of birth-cohort screening for hepatitis C antibody in U.S. primary care settings. Ann Intern Med 2012;156:263-70.
10. Jacobson IM, Cacoub P, Dal Maso L, et al. Manifestations of chronic hepatitis C virus infection beyond the liver. Clin Gastroenterol Hepatol 2010;8:1017-29.
11. Arrese M, Riquelme A, Soza A. Insulin resistance, hepatic steatosis and hepatitis C: A complex relationship with relevant clinical implications. Ann Hepatol 2010;9(Suppl):112-8.
12. Brady KA, Weiner M, Turner BJ. Undiagnosed hepatitis C on the general medicine and trauma services of two urban hospitals. J Infect 2009;59:62-9.
13. Centers for Disease Control and Prevention. Hepatitis C virus infection among adolescents and young adults: Massachusetts, 2002-2009. MMWR Morb Mortal Wkly Rep 2011;60:537-41.
14. Morgan TR, Ghany MG, Kim HY, et al. Outcome of sustained virological responders with histologically advanced chronic hepatitis C. Hepatology 2010;52:833-44.
15. Singal AG, Volk ML, Jensen D, et al. A sustained viral response is associated with reduced liver-related morbidity and mortality in patients with hepatitis C virus. Clin Gastroenterol Hepatol 2010;8:280-8, 288 e1.
16. Backus LI, Boothroyd DB, Phillips,BR, et al. A sustained virologic response reduces risk of all-cause mortality in patients with hepatitis C. Clin Gastroenterol Hepatol 2011;9:509-516 e1.
17. Myers RP, Ramji A, Bilodeau M, et al. An update on the management of hepatitis C: Consensus guidelines from the Canadian Association for the Study of the Liver. Can J Gastroenterol 2012;26:359-75.
18. Dusheiko G. Side effects of alpha interferon in chronic hepatitis C. Hepatology 1997;26(3 Suppl 1):112S-121S.
19. Poordad F, McCone J, Bacon BR, et al. Boceprevir for untreated chronic HCV genotype 1 infection. N Engl J Med 2011;364:1195-206.
20. Jacobson IM, McHutchison JG, Dusheiko G, et al. Telaprevir for previously untreated chronic hepatitis C virus infection. N Engl J Med 2011;364:2405-16.
21. Liang TJ, Ghany MG. Current and future therapies for hepatitis C virus infection. N Engl J Med 2013;368:1907-17.
22. Neff GW, Duncan CW, Schiff ER. The current economic burden of cirrhosis. Gastroenterol Hepatol (N Y) 2011;7:661-71.
23. Thein HH, Isaranuwatchai W, Campetelli,MA, et al. Health care costs associated with hepatocellular carcinoma: A population-based study. Hepatology 2013;58:1375-84.
24. Shah HA, Heathcote J, Feld JJ. A Canadian screening program for hepatitis C: Is now the time? CMAJ 2013;185:1325-8.
25. Canadian Liver Foundation, 2013. Hepatitis C testing. <www.liver.ca/support-liver-foundation/advocate/clf-position-statements/hepatitis_C_testing.aspx> (Accessed May 1, 2014).
26. Smith BD, Morgan RL, Beckett GA, et al. Recommendations for the identification of chronic hepatitis C virus infection among persons born during 1945-1965. MMWR Recomm Rep 2012;61:1-32.
27. Canadian Liver Foundation. Hepatitis C: Medical information update. Can J Public Health 2000;91:S4-S9.
28. Davis GL, Rodrigue JR. Treatment of chronic hepatitis C in active drug users. N Engl J Med 2001;345:215-7.
29. Magiorkinis G, Sypsa V, Magiorkinis E, et al. Integrating phylodynamics and epidemiology to estimate transmission diversity in viral epidemics. PLoS Comput Biol 2013;9:e1002876.
30. Manzer D, Materniak S, Murugesan A, Webster D. Infectious Diseases Diagnosis, Treatment and Prevention in the Setting of a Medical Model for Methadone Maintenance Therapy. Interprofessional Health Research Day. Saint John, New Brunswick, March 23, 2012.
31. Tompkins CN, Wright NM, Jones L. Impact of a positive hepatitis C diagnosis on homeless injecting drug users: A qualitative study. Br J Gen Pract 2005;55:263-8.
32. Webster PC. Prison puzzle: Treating hepatitis C. CMAJ 2012;184:1017-8.
33. Adelson N. The embodiment of inequity: Health disparities in aboriginal Canada. Can J Public Health 2005;96(Suppl 2):S45-61.
34. Webster D, Weerasinghe S, Stevens P. Morbidity and mortality rates in a Nova Scotia First Nations Community, 1996-1999. Can J Public Health 2004;95:369-74.
35. Edlin BR, Kresina TF, Raymond DB, et al. Overcoming barriers to prevention, care, and treatment of hepatitis C in illicit drug users. Clin Infect Dis 2005;40(Suppl 5):S276-85.
36. Zanini B, Lanzini A. Antiviral treatment for chronic hepatitis C in illicit drug users: A systematic review. Antivir Ther 2009;14:467-79.
37. Almasio PL, Babudieri S, Barbarini G, et al. Recommendations for the prevention, diagnosis, and treatment of chronic hepatitis B and C in special population groups (migrants, intravenous drug users and prison inmates). Dig Liver Dis 2011;43:589-95.
38. Zanini B, Benini F, Pigozzi MG, et al. Addicts with chronic hepatitis C: Difficult to reach, manage or treat? World J Gastroenterol 2013;19:8011-9.
39. Christie TK, Murugesan A, Manzer D, O'Shaughnessey MV, Webster D. Evaluation of a low threshold/high tolerance methadone maintenance treatment clinic in Saint John, New Brunswick, Canada: One year retention rate and illicit drug use. J Addict 2013:753409.
40. World Health Organization. Guidelines for the screening, care and treatment of persons with hepatitis C infection. April 2014. <www.who.int/hiv/pub/hepatitis/hepatitis-c-guidelines/en/> (Accessed May 1, 2014).
41. Kowdley KV, Gordon SC, Reddy KR, et al. Ledipasvir and sofosbuvir for 8 or 12 weeks for chronic HCV without cirrhosis. N Engl J Med 2014;370:1879-88.
42. Jordan JF, Kowdley, KV, Coakley E, et al, Phase 3 placebo-controlled study of interferon-free, 12-wwek regimen of ABT-450/r/ABT-267, ABT-333 and ribavirin in 631 treatment-naive patients with Hepatitis C virus genotype 1. 49th Annual Meeting of the European Association for the Study of the Liver. London, United Kingdon, April 11, 2014.
43. Afdhal N, Reddy KR, Nelson DR, et al. Ledipasvir and sofosbuvir for previously treated HCV genotype 1 infection. N Engl J Med 2014;370:1483-93.
44. Zeuzam S, Jacobson IM, Baykal T, et al. SAPPHIRE_II: Phase 3 placebo-controlled study of interferon-free, 12-week regimen of ABT-450/r/ABT-267, ABT-333, and ribavirin in 394 treatment-experienced adults with hepatitis C genotype 1. 49th Annual Meeting of the European Association for the Study of the Liver. London, United Kingdon, April 11, 2014.
45. Pinette G, Coc JJ, Heathcote J, et al. Public Health Agency of Canada, 2009. Primary care management of chronic hepatitis C: Professional desk reference. Ottawa, Ontario. <www.phac-aspc.gc.ca/hepc/archive-eng.php#a2009> (Accessed May 1, 2014).

2

Burden of disease and cost of chronic hepatitis C virus infection in Canada

Robert P Myers MD MSc[1], Mel Krajden MD[2], Marc Bilodeau MD[3], Kelly Kaita MD[4], Paul Marotta MD[5], Kevork Peltekian MD[6], Alnoor Ramji MD[7], Chris Estes MPH[8], Homie Razavi PhD[8], Morris Sherman MD[9]

RP Myers, M Krajden, M Bilodeau, et al. Burden of disease and cost of chronic hepatitis C virus infection in Canada. Can J Gastroenterol Hepatol 2014;28(5):243-250.

BACKGROUND: Chronic infection with hepatitis C virus (HCV) is a major cause of cirrhosis, hepatocellular carcinoma and liver transplantation.

OBJECTIVE: To estimate the burden of HCV-related disease and costs from a Canadian perspective.

METHODS: Using a system dynamic framework, the authors quantified the HCV-infected population, disease progression and costs in Canada between 1950 and 2035. Specifically, 36 hypothetical, age- and sex-defined cohorts were tracked to define HCV prevalence, complications and direct medical costs (excluding the cost of antivirals). Model assumptions and costs were extracted from the literature with an emphasis on Canadian data. No incremental increase in antiviral treatment over current levels was assumed, despite the future availability of potent antivirals.

RESULTS: The estimated prevalence of viremic hepatitis C cases peaked in 2003 at 260,000 individuals (uncertainty interval 192,460 to 319,880), reached 251,990 (uncertainty interval 177,890 to 314,800) by 2013 and is expected to decline to 188,190 (uncertainty interval 124,330 to 247,200) in 2035. However, the prevalence of advanced liver disease is increasing. The peak annual number of patients with compensated cirrhosis (n=36,210), decompensated cirrhosis (n=3380), hepatocellular carcinoma (n=2220) and liver-related deaths (n=1880) are expected to occur between 2031 and 2035. During this interval, an estimated 32,460 HCV-infected individuals will die of liver-related causes. Total health care costs associated with HCV (excluding treatment) are expected to increase by 60% from 2013 until the peak in 2032, with the majority attributable to cirrhosis and its complications (81% in 2032 versus 56% in 2013). The lifetime cost for an individual with HCV infection in 2013 was estimated to be $64,694.

CONCLUSIONS: Although the prevalence of HCV in Canada is decreasing, cases of advanced liver disease and health care costs continue to rise. These results will facilitate disease forecasting, resource planning and the development of rational management strategies for HCV in Canada.

Key Words: Cirrhosis; Hepatitis C; Hepatocellular carcinoma; Mortality; Outcomes; Treatment

Le fardeau et le coût de l'infection chronique par le virus de l'hépatite C au Canada

HISTORIQUE : L'infection chronique par le virus de l'hépatite C (VHC) est une cause importante de cirrhose, de carcinome hépatocellulaire et de transplantation hépatique.

OBJECTIF : Évaluer le fardeau et le coût des maladies liées au VIH dans une perspective canadienne.

MÉTHODOLOGIE : Dans un cadre dynamique, les auteurs ont quantifié la population infectée par le VHC, ainsi que l'évolution et le coût de la maladie au Canada entre 1950 et 2035. Plus précisément, 36 cohortes hypothétiques, définies en fonction de l'âge et du sexe, ont été suivies pour définir la prévalence, les complications et les coûts médicaux directs (à l'exception du coût des antiviraux) du VHC. Les hypothèses et les coûts des modèles ont été tirés des publications, particulièrement celles d'origine canadienne. Aucune augmentation incrémentielle du traitement aux antiviraux n'a été présumée par rapport aux taux actuels, malgré l'accessibilité potentielle à de futurs antiviraux.

RÉSULTATS : La prévalence estimative des cas d'hépatite C virémique a atteint un sommet en 2003, avec 260 000 individus (intervalle d'incertitude de 192 460 à 319 880). Elle a atteint 251 990 (intervalle d'incertitude de 177 890 à 314 800) en 2013 et devrait reculer à 188 190 (intervalle d'incertitude de 124 330 à 247 200) en 2035. Cependant, la prévalence de maladie hépatique avancée augmente. Le nombre annuel maximal de patients ayant une cirrhose compensée (n=36 210), une cirrhose décompensée (n=3 380), un carcinome hépatocellulaire (n=2 220) et décédés à cause de problèmes hépatiques (n=1 880) devrait être atteint entre 2031 et 2035. Pendant cet intervalle, on estime que 32 460 personnes infectées par le VHC mourront d'une cause liée à un problème hépatique. Les coûts de santé totaux associés au VHC (à l'exclusion du traitement) devraient augmenter de 60 % entre 2013 et le sommet de 2032, en majorité à cause de la cirrhose et de ses complications (81 % en 2032, par rapport à 56 % en 2013). En 2013, le coût à vie d'une personne atteinte d'une infection par le VHC était évalué à 64 694 $.

CONCLUSIONS : Même si la prévalence de VHC diminue au Canada, les cas de maladie hépatique avancée et les coûts des soins continuent d'augmenter. Ces résultats contribueront à la prévision des maladies, à la planification des ressources et à l'élaboration de stratégies rationnelles de prise en charge du VHC au Canada.

Chronic hepatitis C virus (HCV) infection is an important public health problem, with an estimated 170 million prevalent cases, three to four million newly infected cases annually and a mean seroprevalence of approximately 3% worldwide (1). Although the prevalence of HCV in Canada is unknown, the Public Health Agency of Canada (PHAC) has reported that 0.96% of the population was anti-HCV positive in 2011 (2). Whereas the peak prevalence is in young and middle-age (30 to 59 years) individuals, the peak age for incident or acute hepatitis C, which mainly results from injection drug use (IDU) (3), is approximately 20 years younger (4).

Modelling studies and anecdotal reports suggest that the burden of HCV in Canada is increasing (3,5). For example, PHAC estimated that cases of HCV-related end-stage liver disease, hepatocellular carcinoma (HCC), liver transplantation and deaths would increase by approximately 20% to 80% between 1997 and 2027 (3). However, the results of this and other modelling studies may underestimate the true

[1]Liver Unit, Division of Gastroenterology and Hepatology, Department of Medicine, University of Calgary, Calgary, Alberta; [2]BC Centre for Disease Control, Vancouver, British Columbia; [3]University of Montreal, Montreal, Quebec; [4]University of Manitoba, Winnipeg, Manitoba; [5]Western University, London, Ontario; [6]Dalhousie University, Halifax, Nova Scotia; [7]University of British Columbia, Vancouver, British Columbia; [8]Center for Disease Analysis, Louisville, Colorado, USA; [9]University of Toronto, Toronto, Ontario

Correspondence: Dr Robert P Myers, Liver Unit, University of Calgary, 6D22, Teaching, Research and Wellness Building, 3280 Hospital Drive Northwest, Calgary, Alberta T2N 4Z6. e-mail rpmyers@ucalgary.ca

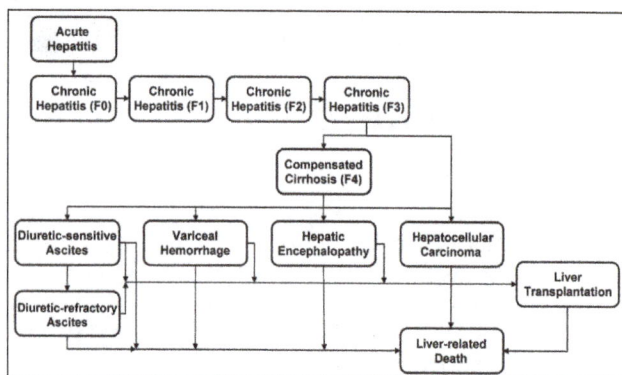

Figure 1) *Schematic of hepatitis C disease progression model*

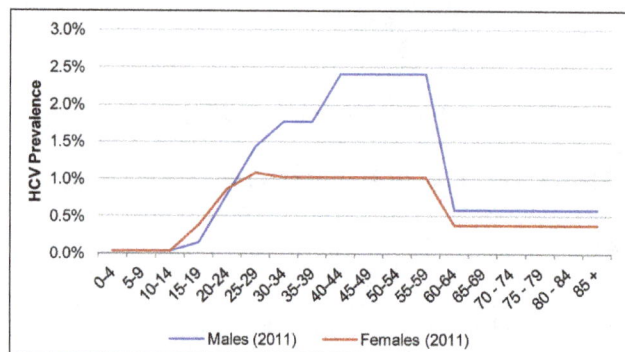

Figure 2) *Age and sex distribution of anti-hepatitis C virus (HCV)-positive cases in Canada, 2011*

TABLE 1
Model inputs and 2013 estimates

	Historical	Year	2013 Estimate
Anti-HCV+ cases*	329,760	2011	322,480
	(209,530–460,280)		
Anti-HCV prevalence*	0.9 (0.6–1.3)		0.7%
Total viremic cases*	253,910	2011	248,310
	(161,340–354,420)		
Viremic prevalence, %	0.7 (0.5–1.0)		0.5
Proportion viremic, %	77.0		77.0
Diagnosed, viremic cases	176,400	2013	176,400
Proportion of viremic cases diagnosed, %	70		70
Annual number of newly diagnosed cases, n	7640	2011	7640
New infections			5570
New infection rate, per 100,000			15.9
Treated cases, annually, n (%)			3600 (1.4)
HCV risk factors			
Active IDUs with HCV, n			54,630
Proportion of prevalent cases due to active IDU, %			22
Number of previously transfused cases with HCV			27,310
Proportion of prevalent cases due to previous blood transfusion, %			11
HCV genotype, %			
1a			36.5
1b			21.5
1 (other)			6.1
2			14.1
3			20.2
4			0.3
5			0
6			0
Other			1.3

Data presented as % (uncertainty interval). HCV Hepatitis C virus; IDU Injection drug use

burden of HCV. According to administrative data from Calgary, Alberta, liver-related hospitalizations, hospital costs and mortality rose fourfold between 1994 and 2004 (6). This apparent discrepancy between modelled and actual outcomes may relate, in part, to study methodology. Typically, Markov models have been used in which a homogenous cohort of HCV-infected individuals is introduced and the model is used to track their progression over time. However, the predictability of these models is highly sensitive to the number of age and

sex cohorts used due to differences in HCV incidence and mortality (among other factors) across the cohorts (7). In the current study, we aimed to create a disease progression model that was more refined. Specifically, we modelled 36 age- and sex-defined cohorts to provide maximum flexibility in changing inputs (eg, incidence, treatment and cure rate, and mortality). Our objective was to describe the future burden of disease and cost of HCV infection in Canada, assuming there is no incremental increase in treatment as the result of new therapies. Although more effective and better tolerated antivirals are on the horizon, our goal was to gain a better understanding of baseline estimates before the widespread use of these newer agents. Future analyses will model the impact of different management strategies aimed at reducing disease burden and costs (eg, increased treatment uptake, improved cure rates and enhanced case identification).

METHODS
System dynamic model
As previously described (8), a system dynamic modelling framework was used to construct a model in Excel (Microsoft Corporation, USA) to quantify the HCV-infected population, disease progression and associated costs in Canada from 1950 to 2035. The model was constructed for sensitivity and Monte Carlo analysis using Crystal Ball, an Excel add-in by Oracle (USA), and beta-PERT distributions were used for all uncertain inputs. A systematic review of the literature was conducted to identify studies reporting relevant Canadian data for incorporation into the model. Indexed articles were found by searching PubMed and Embase, and through consultation with Canadian HCV experts. Ranges were used to capture uncertainty in inputs with wider ranges implying greater uncertainty.

Progression from acute HCV infection through disease states encompassing all fibrosis stages and sequelae of chronic HCV infection was modelled as shown in Figure 1. The total numbers of cases at each disease stage were tracked according to age cohorts and sex. Thirty-six five-year age cohorts were used through 84 years of age; individuals ≥85 years of age were treated as one cohort. Each year, one-fifth of the population in each age group, except for ≥85 years, was moved to the next age cohort to simulate aging after accounting for mortality (see below). Background Canadian population data, obtained from the United Nations population database (9), were organized according to sex, five-year age groups and year (1950 to 2035).

HCV prevalent population
For anti-HCV prevalence, the rate reported by PHAC for 2011 (0.96% [uncertainty interval 0.61% to 1.34%]) was used (Table 1) (2). The age and sex distribution of the prevalent population was based on notification data from PHAC (10) (Figure 2). An estimated 77% of these cases were assumed to be viremic (11), with a genotype distribution based on data collected from Canadian patients between 1998 and 2004 (Table 1) (12). Viremic prevalence in 2011 was estimated to be 0.74% (uncertainty interval 0.47% to 1.0%).

There was considerable variation in the reported data regarding the proportion of infected patients diagnosed with HCV and the number aware of their infection. PHAC estimated that 79% of HCV-positive individuals were diagnosed in 2007 (3), while national household surveys conducted from 2007 to 2011 found that 30% of anti-HCV-positive individuals were aware of their infection (13). Based on expert consensus, it was estimated that 70% of the infected population was diagnosed in 2013. The newly diagnosed population was estimated based on the number of notifications from the most recent year of data reported by PHAC (2011): there were 9923 notifications (10) and 77% were assumed to be viremic (11). It was estimated that 176,400 viremic individuals were diagnosed in Canada in 2013 and 7641 viremic individuals were newly diagnosed.

New HCV cases
The number of PHAC-reported HCV case notifications peaked in 1998 at 19,379 (14). In the model, the annual magnitude of new cases, including the age and sex distribution of these cases, was back calculated to reach the estimated prevalent population value in 2011 (2), using Frontline Solver for Excel. Proportional changes in incidence according to year were derived from historical incidence estimates from a PHAC analysis (3). In 2013, 5570 new HCV cases were estimated to have occurred.

Antiviral treatment
The state of HCV care in Canada generally involves treatment of individuals with at least moderate (stage 2 to 4) liver fibrosis. In the model, it was assumed that all treated patients were between 18 and 64 years of age and had at least moderate fibrosis, and that 60% of all patients were medically eligible or willing to undergo antiviral therapy. According to the literature (15,16), approximately 40% to 60% of HCV patients are eligible for treatment. The definition of eligibility included contraindications to antiviral therapies (eg, severe cardiorespiratory disease or uncontrolled psychiatric conditions) as well as patient preference.

The historical treated population from 2001 to 2003 was estimated to be 5000 cases annually. During this period, sustained virological response (SVR) rates of 30% (genotype 1 [G1]), 66% (G2 and G3) and 40% (G4) were applied assuming the standard of care for all genotypes included interferon and ribavirin therapy. The treated population in 2004 to 2012 was calculated based on data for standard units of peginterferon sold in Canada as reported by IMS Health (17), with multipliers to account for under-reporting and compliance/persistence (85%). In this calculation, the Canadian genotype distribution (12) was used to estimate the average number of weeks of treatment per patient. SVR rates were the same as during 2001 to 2003, except for G1, for which SVR rate increased to 40% with the use of peginterferon-based therapy. Beginning in 2013, it was estimated that 3600 cases were treated annually. Historically, more patients were treated but deferral of treatment has recently increased due to the prospect of more effective therapies. It was assumed that SVR rates for patients with G1 would increase to 60% with triple therapy including a first-generation protease inhibitor (boceprevir or telaprevir) (18). Although second-generation, direct-acting antivirals with higher rates of treatment success were approved in Canada in late 2013, a status quo model was assumed, with no incremental increase in treatment as the result of these new therapies. Similarly, the higher SVR rates and costs of these therapies were specifically excluded to establish a baseline for future comparisons. This approach, however, will lead to higher projections of advanced liver disease compared with the real world.

Transition probabilities
Age- and sex-specific transition probabilities were used to progress patients annually through each disease state, as described previously (8). A spontaneous HCV clearance rate of 23% among new cases was assumed (19). For cases without spontaneous clearance, disease progression was simulated by multiplying the total number of cases at a particular stage of the disease by a progression rate to the next stages. The rates were gathered from previous studies (8,20-27) or calculated (Table 2).

Liver transplantation and mortality
The historical number of liver transplants completed annually in Canada was available through the Canadian transplant registry (28), along with the percentage of transplants attributable to chronic HCV infection (29). In 2011, there were 482 liver transplants performed in Canada. Of these, 33% were estimated to be HCV-related. Data from United States sources were used to estimate mortality among liver transplant recipients (30,31). Estimates of future liver transplants do not consider organ availability and include all cases progressing to liver transplant eligibility.

Background mortality rates according to year, age group and sex were extracted from the Berkeley Human Mortality database (32) and excess mortality related to IDU and transfusion were estimated. Specifically, a standardized mortality ratio (SMR) of 10.0 (uncertainty interval 9.5 to 29.9) for individuals between 15 and 44 years of age was applied for the population infected via active IDU (33-38) (an estimated 22% of the prevalent population) (3). In 2007, it was estimated that 11.0% of the prevalent population was infected through transfusion (3) and that this will decline to 0% by 2030. For these individuals, an SMR of 2.1 (uncertainty interval 1.3 to 17.6) was applied for all age groups (39).

Costs
To quantify costs associated with chronic HCV infection, cost data collected through Canadian studies were applied (Table 3) (40-42). The health care costs among noncirrhotic patients (F0 to F3 fibrosis) were adjusted for the proportion not under care, which varied from 39% (F0) to 24% (F3). Historical cost data were inflated through 2013 using the health care component of the Canadian consumer price index (43), and no future inflation was assumed. The range of low and high costs were calculated based on the ratios between base and high/low costs from United States data (8), except where Canadian data were available. The estimated future lifetime cost of an HCV-infected male 35 to 39 years of age in 2013 was calculated by introducing 100 viremic incident cases in 2013 in each disease state and using the model to track the progression of these cases and costs over time. The annual health care costs for all sequelae and all years were summed and divided by 100 to calculate the estimated individual lifetime cost.

RESULTS
Prevalence of chronic hepatitis C and complications
According to the model, the prevalence of HCV in Canada peaked in 2003 at 260,000 viremic individuals (Figure 3). In 2013, a total of 251,990 (uncertainty interval 177,890 to 314,800) viremic cases was estimated, with the highest number of cases in the 40- to 54-year age groups (Figure 4). By 2035, the chronically infected population is projected to decrease to 188,190 (uncertainty interval 124,330 to 247,200) cases, a 25% decline from the peak in 2003. However, cases of compensated and decompensated cirrhosis are expected to peak in 2031 at 36,210 and 3380 cases, respectively (Figure 5A). The number of individuals with HCC caused by HCV infection will increase to 2220 cases in 2035 before starting to decline. HCV-related mortality will peak in 2034, when annual liver-related deaths are estimated to reach 1880 cases. Between 2013 and 2035, the authors estimate that 32,460 HCV-infected individuals will die of liver-related causes (mean age at death, 67.8 years). In 2013, 8.7% of the chronically infected population is expected to experience cirrhosis or more advanced HCV-related sequelae, whereas this proportion will increase to 23% by 2035 (Figure 5B). Compared with 2013, cases of compensated cirrhosis, decompensated cirrhosis, HCC and liver-related deaths are expected to increase 89%, 80%, 205% and 160%, respectively, by 2035.

TABLE 2
Hepatitis C disease progression rates used in the model

Back-calculated progression rates: Males

	Age cohort, years																		
	0–4	5–9	10–14	15–19	20–24	25–29	30–34	35–39	40–44	45–49	50–54	55–59	60–64	65–69	70–74	75–79	80–84	≥85
F0 to F1	5.3	5.3	6.4	6.4	5.2	5.2	3.8	3.8	13.9	13.9	17.1	17.1	19.4	19.4	21.8	21.8	17.9	17.9
F1 to F2	3.8	3.8	4.7	4.7	3.8	3.8	2.7	2.7	10.1	10.1	12.4	12.4	14.1	14.1	15.8	15.8	13.0	13.0
F2 to F3	5.4	5.4	6.6	6.6	5.3	5.3	3.9	3.9	14.3	14.3	17.5	17.5	19.9	19.9	22.4	22.4	18.3	18.3
F3 to cirrhosis	0.0	0.0	0.8	0.8	2.5	2.5	5.7	5.7	8.8	8.8	4.8	4.8	9.9	9.9	19.1	19.1	19.1	19.1
F3 to HCC	0.0	0.0	0.0	0.0	0.0	0.0	0.0	0.0	0.1	0.1	0.1	0.1	0.2	0.2	0.3	0.3	0.3	0.3
Cirrhosis to HCC	0.3	0.3	0.3	0.3	0.3	0.3	0.5	0.5	0.9	0.9	1.4	1.4	2.4	2.4	3.9	3.9	3.9	3.9

Back-calculated progression rates: Females

	Age cohort, years																		
	0–4	5–9	10–14	15–19	20–24	25–29	30–34	35–39	40–44	45–49	50–54	55–59	60–64	65–69	70–74	75–79	80–84	≥85
F0 to F1	4.4	4.4	5.4	5.4	4.3	4.3	3.1	3.1	11.6	11.6	14.3	14.3	16.2	16.2	18.2	18.2	14.9	14.9
F1 to F2	3.2	3.2	3.9	3.9	3.1	3.1	2.3	2.3	8.4	8.4	10.4	10.4	11.7	11.7	13.2	13.2	10.8	10.8
F2 to F3	4.5	4.5	5.5	5.5	4.4	4.4	3.2	3.2	11.9	11.9	14.6	14.6	16.6	16.6	18.6	18.6	15.3	15.3
F3 to cirrhosis	0.0	0.0	0.6	0.6	2.1	2.1	4.7	4.7	7.4	7.4	4.0	4.0	8.3	8.3	15.9	15.9	15.9	15.9
F3 to HCC	0.0	0.0	0.0	0.0	0.0	0.0	0.0	0.0	0.0	0.0	0.1	0.1	0.1	0.1	0.2	0.2	0.2	0.2
Cirrhosis to HCC	0.3	0.3	0.3	0.3	0.3	0.3	0.4	0.4	0.7	0.7	1.2	1.2	2.0	2.0	3.3	3.3	3.3	3.3

Data presented as %. F Fibrosis stage; HCC Hepatocellular carcinoma

Disease progression	Reported progression rates, % (uncertainty interval)	Reference(s)
Diuretic-sensitive ascites to diuretic refractory ascites	6.7 (4.0–9.4)	8,20–27
Diuretic-sensitive ascites to liver-related death	11.0 (7.7–14.3)	8,20–27
Variceal hemorrhage to liver-related death (first year)	40.0 (33.4–46.6)	8,20–27
Variceal hemorrhage to liver-related death (subsequent years)	13.0 (8.5–17.5)	8,20–27
Hepatic encephalopathy to liver-related death (first year)	68.0 (65.9–70.1)	8,20–27
Hepatic encephalopathy to liver-related death (subsequent years)	40.0 (37.8–42.2)	8,20–27
Diuretic-refractory ascites to liver-related death	33.0 (28.0–38.0)	8,20–27
Hepatocellular carcinoma to liver-related death (first year)	70.7 (43–77.0)	26,58
Hepatocellular carcinoma to liver-related death (subsequent years)	16.2 (11–23.0)	58
Liver transplant to liver-related death (first year)	33.1–10.7 (2.8–0.4)	30,31
Liver transplant to liver-related death (subsequent years)	3.9–4.8 (7.6–1.0)	30,31

TABLE 3
Incremental costs of hepatitis C virus infection according to disease stage used in the model

Disease stage	Annual cost, $CAD	Reference	Range, $CAD	Reference(s)
Hepatitis C virus (F0 to F3)	383	40	215–551	8
Compensated cirrhosis (F4)	808	40	545–1,070	8
Diuretic-sensitive ascites	5,632	40	506–5,979	8
Diuretic-refractory ascites	16,762	40	15,731–17,793	8
Variceal hemorrhage (first year)	20,096	40	18,860–21,332	8
Variceal hemorrhage (subsequent years)	20,096	40	3,689–21,332	8
Hepatic encephalopathy (first year)	8,790	40	1,614–9,331	8
Hepatic encephalopathy (subsequent years)	8,790	40	1,227–9,331	8
Hepatocellular carcinoma	16,049	59	14,404–17,694	8
Liver transplant (first year)	117,284	42	63,664–170,905	40,42
Liver transplant (subsequent years)	40,164	40	32,819–47,509	8

F Fibrosis stage

Costs associated with chronic hepatitis C

Total cost is projected to increase by 60% from $161.4 million (uncertainty interval $85.4 million to $251.5 million) in 2013 to $258.4 million (uncertainty interval $121.4 million to $394.6 million) at the peak in 2032. In 2013, the authors estimated that 56% of total costs were attributable to cirrhosis and more advanced liver disease. By 2032, this proportion is expected to rise to 81%. The majority of peak cost will be attributable to cases of decompensated cirrhosis, including those who undergo liver transplantation (55% in 2032 versus 39% in 2013), compensated cirrhosis (12% versus 10%) and HCC (14% versus 7%). For a hypothetical male 35 to 39 years of age with HCV infection in 2013, the estimated lifetime cost is $64,694 in 2013

Canadian dollars. However, the estimated lifetime costs of HCV vary substantially according to disease state (Table 4). Specifically, lifetime future costs ranged from $51,946 for a patient with no fibrosis (F0) in 2013 up to $327,608 for a patient requiring liver transplantation in 2013. Of note, the future lifetime cost for prevalent HCC cases ($42,376) was estimated to be relatively low due to a high mortality rate from progressive liver-related disease in those infected.

DISCUSSION

Using a novel modelling approach, we have demonstrated that the prevalence of HCV infection in Canada will decrease, while the burden of advanced liver disease and associated costs will continue to

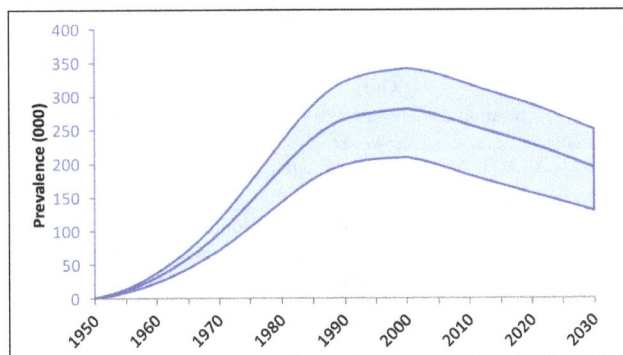

Figure 3) *Total number of viremic hepatitis C cases (with uncertainty intervals) according to year, 1950 to 2035*

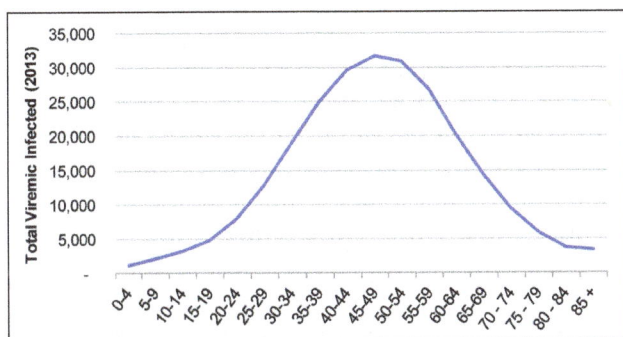

Figure 4) *Total number of viremic hepatitis C cases cases according to age, 2013*

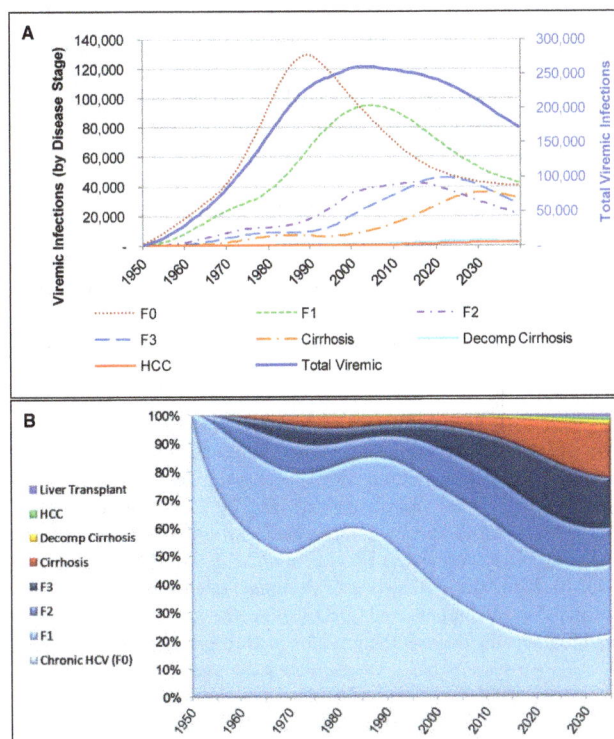

Figure 5) A *Number of viremic hepatitis C (HCV) cases, in total and according to disease stage.* **B** *Proportion of all viremic HCV cases according to disease stage, 1950 to 2035. Decomp Decompensated; F Fibrosis stage; HCC Hepatocellular carcinoma*

TABLE 4
Estimated future lifetime cost according to disease state for men 35 to 39 years of age with hepatitis C virus infection in 2013

	Cost in 2013, $CAD
Chronic hepatitis C virus infection (F0)	51,946
F1	62,184
F2	79,926
F3	100,589
Compensated cirrhosis (F4)	133,575
Diuretic-sensitive ascites	196,770
Diuretic-refractory ascites	139,330
Variceal hemorrhage	189,398
Hepatic encephalopathy	133,505
Hepatocellular carcinoma	42,376
Liver transplant	327,608

F Fibrosis stage

grow over the next 20 years. Already, there is evidence in Ontario that the disease burden from HCV exceeds that of all other infectious diseases (44); these data are likely generalizable to the remainder of the country. Our analysis predicted that HCV prevalence in Canada peaked in 2003 at 260,000 viremic cases and affected 251,990 individuals in 2013. At current levels of antiviral treatment utilization and efficacy, the prevalence in Canada is expected to decline to 188,190 cases by 2035. Although this 28% decline compared with the peak is encouraging, it is partly attributable to HCV-related mortality. We project that without increased treatment access and uptake, approximately 32,500 HCV-infected individuals will die of liver-related causes between 2013 and 2035. Moreover, premature mortality attributable to HCV infection is substantial, as emphasized by the disparity in the mean age at death of the cohort (68 years) compared with average life expectancy in Canada (81 years) (32).

The results of our analysis also show that >70% of the infected population in Canada was born between 1944 and 1978 (Figure 4). This figure is relevant given recent recommendations by the Canadian Liver Foundation advocating one time, birth-cohort screening for HCV among Canadians born between 1945 and 1975 (45,46). Based on our analysis, this approach would identify the majority of HCV-infected cases in Canada, including those most likely to develop liver-related complications. Birth-cohort HCV screening has also been recommended by the Centers for Disease Control and Prevention (Georgia, USA) based on data showing that 75% of prevalent cases in the United States were born between 1945 and 1965. To date, the uptake and impact of these recommendations have not been confirmed.

As shown in Figure 5A, the proportion of patients with advanced HCV-related liver disease will increase between 2013 and 2035. This phenomenon is due to aging of the infected population and resultant liver fibrosis progression. The incidence of decompensated cirrhosis, HCC and liver transplantation are expected to peak between 2031 and 2035. Figure 5B, which illustrates the proportions of the prevalent

HCV population within each disease state, is informative. First, most individuals with HCV (>75%) at any given point in time have non-cirrhotic disease (ie, stage 0 to 3 fibrosis). This represents an ideal opportunity to intervene with antiviral therapy to prevent progression to more advanced stages when treatment becomes less effective and less well tolerated, at least with interferon-based treatments. Second, a smaller proportion of the population will progress to develop HCC (<1% of prevalent cases). Third, nearly 23% of the chronically infected population is expected to experience cirrhosis or more advanced HCV-related sequelae in 2035 compared with only 9% in 2013. These increases (80% for decompensated cirrhosis, 205% for HCC and 160% for liver-related mortality) are substantially greater than those projected by Remis (3) between 2012 and 2027 (−1.2% for decompensated cirrhosis, 4.8% for HCC and 14.8% for liver-related mortality) (3). Similarly, our projected number of cases with HCV-related complications in 2035 are significantly higher. For example, in 2027, Remis (3) estimated 483 cases of decompensated cirrhosis (versus 3250 in our study), 325 cases of HCC (versus 1910 in our study) and 613 liver-related deaths (versus 1665 in our study). Finally, we estimate that approximately 35,000 individuals will have compensated, HCV-related cirrhosis in 2035. If left undiagnosed and/or untreated, these patients face a significant risk of death due to complications of HCV in the coming years.

We estimated that the total health care costs associated with chronic HCV infection in Canada will increase by 60% between 2013 and the peak in 2032. A key observation was that peak health care costs lag behind peak prevalence by nearly three decades due to the time required for infected cases to progress to more advanced disease stages, which are more costly to manage. In that regard, the majority of estimated costs (approximately 56%) were attributable to the treatment of HCV-related cirrhosis and its complications. In 2013, decompensated cirrhosis accounted for 39% of estimated costs (including those attributable to transplantation), and by 2032 it accounted for 55%. This was followed by compensated cirrhosis (10% of 2013 and 12% of 2032 total cost) and HCC (7% of 2013 and 14% of 2032 total cost). In 2013, the prevalence of decompensated cirrhosis was one-seventh that of compensated cirrhosis, but the annual cost was four-times higher, emphasizing the need for early diagnosis and treatment.

On a per-patient basis, we estimated the average lifetime cost of HCV to be $64,694, much higher than a recent United States report describing an average cost of $19,660 per patient in 2002 to 2010 (47). Not surprisingly, the estimated lifetime cost of an individual infected with HCV varied substantially depending on disease stage (Table 4), with the highest per-patient costs attributable to liver transplantation (approximately $328,000). Previous analyses of cost according to the age at HCV infection have also demonstrated a link between life expectancy and health care costs (8). Individuals infected in the 1950s were expected to have lower lifetime costs due to lower life expectancy and medical costs, while newly infected individuals are expected to cost the health care system more due to their longer life expectancy and higher medical costs. This highlights the importance of efforts aimed at preventing acute HCV infections (eg, by providing harm reduction, safer injection facilities or potentially using treatment of active injection drug users to prevent onward HCV transmission) (48,49) as a means of limiting future health care expenditures.

A strength of the present analysis was the availability of national estimates for HCV prevalence in Canada. However, these data have limitations, particularly with respect to the number of diagnosed cases that have been reported to the PHAC Notifiable Disease Surveillance System. Diagnosed cases may be double-counted and high-risk groups may be under-represented, which could underestimate both the prevalence as well as proportion of undiagnosed individuals in Canada (45). In an attempt to address this uncertainty, the Canadian Health Measures Survey, a stratified serosurvey of viral hepatitis across Canada, recently reported an HCV seroprevalence of 0.5% with 30.5% of individuals being aware of their infection (13). However, this survey undersampled high-risk communities including injection drug users, prisoners, the homeless and Aboriginals. Due to this limitation, the Canadian Liver Foundation has recommended a national study of HCV prevalence that adequately samples these communities (4).

The present model has several limitations. The model does not consider the potential for continued disease progression in cases cured of HCV infection based on current treatments. Some individuals with advanced liver disease are at risk for progressive liver disease after achieving SVR, albeit at a slower rate (50,51). The potential contribution of extrahepatic manifestations of HCV infection on all-cause mortality was also not included in the model, potentially leading to an underestimate of mortality among viremic cases (52). As a result, the projected numbers of decompensated cirrhosis and HCC may be overestimated. Finally, we have not addressed the costs of current antiviral therapies and testing costs, nor have we accounted for indirect medical costs such as reduced productivity and quality of life, which have a significant impact on individuals infected with HCV.

CONCLUSION

The present analysis demonstrated that overall HCV prevalence in Canada is decreasing; however, the prevalence of advanced liver disease and HCV-related costs will continue to increase as the infected population ages. These results will facilitate disease forecasting, resource planning and the development of rational management strategies for HCV in Canada. To reduce the future burden and costs of chronic hepatitis C, there is an urgent need to enhance case identification and optimize the utilization of antiviral therapies. Provincial organizations and the Canadian Liver Foundation have identified these strategies, especially among high-risk populations, as important priorities (53-57). Hopefully, higher rates of diagnosis during early disease stages, coupled with new treatment regimens with higher SVR rates and improved tolerability, will help stem the imminent tide of HCV-related morbidity and mortality.

DISCLOSURES: This study was supported by an unrestricted grant from Gilead Sciences Canada, manufacturers of antiviral therapies for HCV. The sponsor had no input into the design, conduct or analysis of this study, drafting of the manuscript, nor the decision to submit the manuscript for publication. Robert Myers has received research support, consulting, and/or speaking fees from Gilead, Merck, Roche, Vertex, Janssen, Boehringer-Ingelheim, Idenix, Abbvie and GlaxoSmithKline. Mel Krajden has received research support from Roche, Siemens, Hologic (Gen-Probe), Merck, and Boehringer-Ingelheim. Marc Bilodeau has received research support, consulting, and/or speaking fees from Gilead, Merck, Novartis, Vertex, GlaxoSmithKline, Synageva, Astellas and Bayer. Kelly Kaita has received consulting and/or speaking fees from Gilead, Merck, Roche, Vertex, Bristol-Myers Squibb, Boehringer-Ingelheim, Janssen and Abbvie. Paul Marotta has research support, consulting, and/or speaking fees from Gilead, Merck, Vertex, Boehringer-Ingelheim, Astellas, Abbvie and Novartis. Alnoor Ramji has received research support, consulting, and/or speaking fees from Gilead, Merck, Roche, Vertex, Janssen, Boehringer-Ingelheim, Novartis, Abbvie, Bristol-Myers Squibb and GlaxoSmithKline. Morris Sherman has received consulting and/or speaking fees from Gilead, Vertex, Merck, Janssen, Abbvie and Boehringer-Ingelheim. Homie Razavi and Chris Estes are employees of the Center for Disease Analysis (CDA).

REFERENCES

1. Mohd Hanafiah K, Groeger J, Flaxman AD, Wiersma ST. Global epidemiology of hepatitis C virus infection: New estimates of age-specific antibody to HCV seroprevalence. Hepatology 2013;57:1333-42.
2. Trubnikov M. Developing estimates of prevalent and undiagnosed HCV infection in Canada in 2011. <www youtube com/watch?v=2 34ru9AFA6U&list=PLy0zwf7_pKrXSh9bx6XxznPv65S44nN6q&n oredirect=1 2014> (Accessed February 9, 2014).
3. Remis RS. Modelling the incidence and prevalence of hepatitis C infection and its sequelae in Canada, 2007: Final report. Community Acquired Infections Division, Centre for Communicable Diseases and Infection Control, Public Health Agency of Canada 2009. <http://epe.lac-bac.gc.ca/100/200/301/phac-aspc/modeling_hepatis_c_infection-e/HP40-39-2009E.pdf> (Accessed February 9, 2014).
4. Canadian Liver Foundation. Liver disease in Canada – a crisis in the making. <www liver ca/support-liver-foundation/advocate/Liver_Disease_in_Canada_Report aspx 2013> (Accessed February 9, 2014).
5. Zou S, Tepper M, El Saadany S. Prediction of hepatitis C burden in Canada. Can J Gastroenterol 2000;14:575-80.
6. Myers RP, Liu M, Shaheen AA. The burden of hepatitis C virus infection is growing: A Canadian population-based study of hospitalizations from 1994 to 2004. Can J Gastroenterol 2008;22:381-7.
7. Kershenobich D, Razavi HA, Cooper CL, et al. Applying a system approach to forecast the total hepatitis C virus-infected population size: Model validation using US data. Liver Int 2011;31(Suppl 2):4-17.

8. Razavi H, Elkhoury AC, Elbasha E, et al. Chronic hepatitis C virus (HCV) disease burden and cost in the United States. Hepatology 2013;57:2164-70.

9. United Nations Dept of Economic and Social Affairs.Population Division (2011). World population prospects: The 2010 revision, Volume I: Comprehensive tables. ST/ESA/SER.A/313.2011 <http://esa.un.org/wpp/Documentation/pdf/WPP2010_Volume-I_Comprehensive-Tables.pdf> (Accessed February 9, 2014).

10. Public Health Agency of Canada. Hepatitis C in Canada: 2005-2010 surveillance report. 2012 <www.phac-aspc.gc.ca/sti-its-surv-epi/hepc/surv-eng.php> (Accessed February 9, 2014).

11. Seeff LB. Natural history of chronic hepatitis C. Hepatology 2002;36:S35-S46.

12. Antonishyn NA, Ast VM, McDonald RR, et al. Rapid genotyping of hepatitis C virus by primer-specific extension analysis. J Clin Microbiol 2005;43:5158-63.

13. Statistics Canada. Seroprevalence of hepatitis B and C virus infections: Results from the 2007 to 2009 and 2009 to 2011 Canadian Health Measures Survey. Nov 20 2013 <www.statcan.gc.ca/pub/82-003-x/2013011/article/11876-eng.htm> (Accessed February 9, 2014).

14. Public Health Agency of Canada. Notifiable Diseases Online.2005 1991-2004 <http://dsol-smed.hc-sc.gc.ca/dsol-smed/ndis/c_inda-eng.php> (Accessed February 9, 2014).

15. Evon DM, Verma A, Dougherty KA, et al. High deferral rates and poorer treatment outcomes for HCV patients with psychiatric and substance use comorbidities. Dig Dis Sci 2007;52:3251-8.

16. Morrill JA, Shrestha M, Grant RW. Barriers to the treatment of hepatitis C. Patient, provider, and system factors. J Gen Intern Med 2005;20:754-8.

17. IMS Health. IMS Health MIDAS Data. IMS Health Jan 1 2013 <www.imshealth.com/portal/site/ims/menuitem.edb2b81823f67dab41d84b903208c22a/?vgnextoid=4475e3de7e390310VgnVCM1000007f8c2ca2RCRD> (Accessed February 9, 2014).

18. Myers RP, Ramji A, Bilodeau M, Wong S, Feld JJ. An update on the management of hepatitis C: Consensus guidelines from the Canadian Association for the Study of the Liver. Can J Gastroenterol 2012;26:359-75.

19. Seeff LB, Hollinger FB, Alter HJ, et al. Long-term mortality and morbidity of transfusion-associated non-A, non-B, and type C hepatitis: A National Heart, Lung, and Blood Institute collaborative study. Hepatology 2001;33:455-63.

20. Deuffic-Burban S, Deltenre P, Buti M, et al. Predicted effects of treatment for HCV infection vary among European countries. Gastroenterology 2012;143:974-85.

21. Alter MJ, Margolis HS, Krawczynski K, et al. The natural history of community-acquired hepatitis C in the United States. The Sentinel Counties Chronic non-A, non-B Hepatitis Study Team. N Engl J Med 1992;327:1899-905.

22. Thomas DL, Seeff LB. Natural history of hepatitis C. Clin Liver Dis 2005;9:383-98.

23. Villano SA, Vlahov D, Nelson KE, Cohn S, Thomas DL. Persistence of viremia and the importance of long-term follow-up after acute hepatitis C infection. Hepatology 1999;29:908-14.

24. Thein HH, Yi Q, Dore GJ, Krahn MD. Estimation of stage-specific fibrosis progression rates in chronic hepatitis C virus infection: A meta-analysis and meta-regression. Hepatology 2008;48:418-31.

25. Bennett WG, Inoue Y, Beck JR, Wong JB, Pauker SG, Davis GL. Estimates of the cost-effectiveness of a single course of interferon-alpha 2b in patients with histologically mild chronic hepatitis C. Ann Intern Med 1997;127:855-65.

26. Bernfort L, Sennfalt K, Reichard O. Cost effectiveness of peginterferon alfa-2b in combination with ribavirin as initial treatment for chronic hepatitis C in Sweden. Scand J Infect Dis 2006;38:497-505.

27. Younossi ZM, Singer ME, McHutchison JG, Shermock KM. Cost effectiveness of interferon alpha2b combined with ribavirin for the treatment of chronic hepatitis C. Hepatology 1999;30:1318-24.

28. Canadian Institute for Health Information. e-Statistics report on transplant, waiting list and donor statistics. 2012 <www.cihi.ca/CIHI-ext-portal/internet/en/document/types+of+care/specialized+services/organ+replacements/report_stats2012> (Accessed February 9, 2014).

29. Canadian Institute for Health Information. Canadian organ replacement register annual report: Treatment of end-stage organ failure in Canada, 2001 to 2010. 2011.

30. Organ Procurement and Transplantation Network (OPTN). 2009 OPTN/SRTR annual report 1999-2008: Table 9.15a. Unadjusted patient survival by year of transplant at 3 months, 1 year, 3 years, 5 years and 10 years, deceased donor liver transplants. 2009 Annual report of the U S Organ Procurement and Transplantation Network and the Scientific Registry of Transplant Recipients: Transplant data 1999-2008 2009 <www.ustransplant.org/annual_reports/current/915a_li.htm> (Accessed February 9, 2014).

31. Organ Procurement and Transplantation Network (OPTN). National Data. Health Resources and Services Administration, U.S. Department of Health & Human Services; 2013.

32. University of California, Berkeley, Mack Planck Institute for Demographic Research. Human Mortality Database. <www.mortality.org> (Accessed February 9, 2014).

33. Engstrom A, Adamsson C, Allebeck P, Rydberg U. Mortality in patients with substance abuse: A follow-up in Stockholm County, 1973-1984. Int J Addict 1991;26:91-106.

34. Frischer M, Goldberg D, Rahman M, Berney L. Mortality and survival among a cohort of drug injectors in Glasgow, 1982-1994. Addiction 1997;92:419-27.

35. Hickman M, Carnwath Z, Madden P, et al. Drug-related mortality and fatal overdose risk: Pilot cohort study of heroin users recruited from specialist drug treatment sites in London. J Urban Health 2003;80:274-87.

36. Oppenheimer E, Tobutt C, Taylor C, Andrew T. Death and survival in a cohort of heroin addicts from London clinics: A 22-year follow-up study. Addiction 1994;89:1299-308.

37. Perucci CA, Davoli M, Rapiti E, Abeni DD, Forastiere F. Mortality of intravenous drug users in Rome: A cohort study. Am J Public Health 1991;81:1307-10.

38. Bjornaas MA, Bekken AS, Ojlert A, et al. A 20-year prospective study of mortality and causes of death among hospitalized opioid addicts in Oslo. BMC Psychiatry 2008;8:8.

39. Kamper-Jorgensen M, Ahlgren M, Rostgaard K, et al. Survival after blood transfusion. Transfusion 2008;48:2577-84.

40. El Saadany S, Coyle D, Giulivi A, Afzal M. Economic burden of hepatitis C in Canada and the potential impact of prevention. Results from a disease model. Eur J Health Econ 2005;6:159-65.

41. Thein HH, Isaranuwatchai W, Campitelli MA, et al. Health care costs associated with hepatocellular carcinoma: A population-based study. Hepatology 2013;58:1375-84.

42. Taylor MC, Greig PD, Detsky AS, McLeod RS, Abdoh A, Krahn MD. Factors associated with the high cost of liver transplantation in adults. Can J Surg 2002;45:425-34.

43. Statistics Canada. Consumer Price Index, health and personal care (Canada). <www.statcan.gc.ca/tables-tableaux/sum-som/l01/cst01/econ161a-eng.htm> (Accessed February 9, 2014).

44. Kwong JC, Crowcroft NS, Campitelli MA, et al. Ontario Burden of Infectious Disease Study (ONBOIDS): An OAHPP/ICES Report. Toronto, CA: Ontario Agency for Health Protection and Promotion; Institute for Clinical Evaluative Sciences; 2010.

45. Shah HA, Heathcote J, Feld JJ. A Canadian screening program for hepatitis C: Is now the time? CMAJ 2013;185:1325-8.

46. Canadian Liver Foundation. Hepatitis C Testing. 2012 <www.liver.ca/support-liver-foundation/advocate/clf-position-statements/hepatitis_C_testing.aspx> (Accessed February 9, 2014).

47. McAdam-Marx C, McGarry LJ, Hane CA, Biskupiak J, Deniz B, Brixner DI. All-cause and incremental per patient per year cost associated with chronic hepatitis C virus and associated liver complications in the United States: A managed care perspective. J Manag Care Pharm 2011;17:531-46.

48. Bayoumi AM, Zaric GS. The cost-effectiveness of Vancouver's supervised injection facility. CMAJ 2008;179:1143-51.

49. Hellard M, Doyle JS, Sacks-Davis R, Thompson AJ, McBryde E. Eradication of hepatitis C infection: The importance of targeting people who inject drugs. Hepatology 2014;59:366-9.

50. Aleman S, Rahbin N, Weiland O, et al. A risk for hepatocellular carcinoma persists long-term after sustained virologic response in patients with hepatitis C-associated liver cirrhosis. Clin Infect Dis 2013;57:230-6.

51. Singal AG, Volk ML, Jensen D, Di Bisceglie AM, Schoenfeld PS. A sustained viral response is associated with reduced liver-related morbidity and mortality in patients with hepatitis C virus. Clin Gastroenterol Hepatol 2010;8:280-8.

52. Yu A, Spinelli JJ, Cook DA, Buxton JA, Krajden M. Mortality among British Columbians testing for hepatitis C antibody. BMC Public Health 2013;13:291.

53. A proposed strategy to address hepatitis C in Ontario 2009-2014. Ontario Hepatitis C Task Force; 2009.

54. British Columbia Ministry of Health. Healthy Pathways Forward: A Strategic Integrated Approach to Viral Hepatitis in BC. 2007.

55. Government of Alberta, Alberta Health and Wellness -Community and Population Health Division. Alberta Sexually Transmitted Infections and Blood Borne Pathogens Strategy and Action Plan: 2011-2016. 2011.

56. Santé et Services Sociaux Quebec. [Quebec's strategy to fight against HIV and AIDS, HCV and sexually transmitted infections] Stratégie québécoise de lutte contre l'infection par le VIH et le sida, l'infection par le VHC et les infections transmissibles sexuellement: Orientations 2003-2009. 2004.

57. Canadian Liver Foundation. Eliminating Hepatitis C in Canada. 2013 <www.liver.ca/support-liver-foundation/advocate/clf-position-statements/Eliminating_hep_C_in_Canada.aspx> (Accessed February 9, 2014).

58. Ries LAG, Young GL, Keel GE, Eisner MP, Lin, YD Horner, MJ. SEER survival monograph: Cancer survival among adults: U.S. SEER program, 1988-2001, patient and tumor characteristics National Cancer Institute, SEER Program; 2007. NIH Pub. No. 07-6215.

59. Thein HH, Isaranuwatchai W, Campitelli MA, et al. Health care costs associated with hepatocellular carcinoma: A population-based study. Hepatology 2013;58:1375-84.

3

Care of the liver transplant patient

Mamatha Bhat MD FRCPC[1], Said A Al-Busafi MD FRCPC[1,2], Marc Deschênes MD FRCPC[1], Peter Ghali MD FRCPC[1]

M Bhat, SA Al-Busafi, M Deschênes, P Ghali. Care of the liver transplant patient. Can J Gastroenterol Hepatol 2014;28(4):213-219.

OBJECTIVE: To provide an approach to the care of liver transplant (LT) patients, a growing patient population with unique needs.
METHODS: A literature search of PubMed for guidelines and review articles using the keywords "liver transplantation", "long term complications" and "medical management" was conducted, resulting in 77 articles.
RESULTS: As a result of being on immunosuppression, LT recipients are at increased risk of infections and must be screened regularly for metabolic complications and malignancies.
DISCUSSION: Although immunosuppression is key to maintaining allograft health after transplantation, it comes with its own set of medical issues to follow. Physicians following LT recipients must be aware of the greater risk for hypertension, diabetes, dyslipidemia, renal failure, metabolic bone disease and malignancies in these patients, all of whom require regular monitoring and screening. Vaccination, quality of life, sexual function and pregnancy must be specifically addressed in transplant patients.

Key Words: *Liver transplant; Long-term complications; Medical management*

Les soins du greffé du foie

OBJECTIF : Proposer une approche aux soins des greffés du foie, une population croissante de patients aux besoins uniques.
MÉTHODOLOGIE : Les auteurs ont effectué une recherche dans les publications de PubMed et en ont extrait 77 lignes directrices et articles d'analyse à l'aide des mots-clés *liver transplantation, long term complications* et *medical management*.
RÉSULTATS : Parce qu'ils prennent des immunosuppresseurs, les greffés du foie sont plus vulnérables aux infections et doivent subir un dépistage régulier de complications métaboliques et de cancer.
EXPOSÉ : Même si l'immunosuppression est essentielle pour maintenir la santé de l'allogreffe après la transplantation, elle entraîne ses propres problèmes médicaux, qu'il faut garder à l'œil. Les médecins qui suivent des greffés du foie doivent savoir que ces patients sont plus vulnérables à l'hypertension, au diabète, à la dyslipidémie, à l'insuffisance rénale, aux maladies métaboliques osseuses et aux cancers, qui exigent tous une surveillance et un dépistage réguliers. Il faut absolument parler aux greffés de vaccination, de qualité de vie, de fonction sexuelle et de grossesse.

Since the 1960s, LT has offered a new lease on life to many patients with end-stage liver disease (ESLD) and acute liver failure (1). Survival after transplantation has continued to improve over time, with fine-tuned immunosuppression, postoperative care and management of infections. In 2011, 485 LTs were performed in Canada, with 4419 performed over the 10-year period between 2002 and 2011 (2). The one-year survival rate is as high as 85%, while 10-year survival rates approach 65% (3). The longer-term survival of LT recipients means that gastroenterologists and primary care physicians are caring for these patients concurrently with transplant specialists. The management of this patient population is both unique and complex. The gastroenterologist must be aware of the specialized needs of LT recipients, and be able to recognize and optimally manage key complications. In the present article, we provide an overview of issues pertinent to the management of LT recipients, principally based on consensus recommendations in the literature.

INFORMATION SOURCES

The PubMed database was searched using the keywords "liver transplantation", "long term complications" and "medical management", resulting in 77 review articles and guidelines. The Canadian Organ Replacement Register report was a source of information for LT in the Canadian context (2). The Cochrane collaboration website was consulted using the search term "liver transplantation". There were systematic reviews on infectious prophylaxis and quality of life after LT (Level I evidence). The recommendations in the present review are,

therefore, based on data from retrospective studies, case series (Level II) or expert consensus guidelines (Level III).

ESLD is the indication for 92% of LTs, with hepatitis C and alcoholic cirrhosis being the most common etiologies. Fulminant liver failure, mostly due to acetaminophen poisoning, autoimmune hepatitis or viral etiologies, was the indication for 4% of LTs. LT can be curative for hepatocellular carcinoma (HCC), and was the indication for 15.3% of LTs between 2002 and 2011 in Canada (2). Advanced, uncorrectable cardiopulmonary disease is an absolute contraindication to transplantation, while age, per se, is not.

IMMUNOSUPPRESSION

Following LT, immunosuppressants are started and the recipient is monitored closely to prevent organ rejection. Calcineurin inhibitors (CNIs), antimetabolites and corticosteroids are the main categories of available immunosuppressants (Table 1). Most LT centres in Canada choose to administer a combination of low-dose tacrolimus and mycophenolate mofetil (MMF) with or without concomitant glucocorticoids (4). Satisfactory immunosuppression can be achieved with monotherapy in many patients beyond six to 12 months post-transplantation, usually with a CNI alone.

EARLY COMPLICATIONS

Liver graft dysfunction is a serious complication that can result in loss of the donor organ. The most common presentation is an asymptomatic elevation of liver enzyme levels (Figures 1 and 2). Causes of early

[1]*Division of Gastroenterology and Hepatology, Department of Medicine, McGill University Health Centre, Montreal, Canada;* [2]*Division of Gastroenterology, Sultan Qaboos University, Oman*
Correspondence: Dr Mamatha Bhat, 687 Pine Avenue West, Montreal, Quebec H3A 1A1. e-mail mamatha.bhat@mcgill.ca

TABLE 1
Liver transplant medications, adverse effects and monitoring parameters

Immunosuppressant	Mechanism of action	Adverse effects	Monitoring parameters
Prednisone	Inhibits leukocyte, macrophage and T cell activity Decrease cytokines, prostaglandins and leukotrienes	Hyperglycemia, hypertension, dyslipidemia, infectious risk, osteoporosis	Blood pressure measurement Monitor glucose, lipids profiles, regular bone mineral density scan
Tacrolimus	Calcineurin inhibitor, prevents T cell activation	Renal failure, diabetes, hypertension, neuropathy, dyslipidemia	Blood pressure measurement, monitor glucose, lipids profiles, renal function, magnesium level, drug level
Cyclosporine	Calcineurin inhibitor, prevents T cell activation	Renal failure, diabetes, hypertension, neuropathy, dyslipidemia, hirsutism	Blood pressure measurement, monitor glucose, lipids profiles, renal function, magnesium level, drug level
Mycophenolate mofetil	Inhibits T cell and B cell proliferation	Bone marrow suppression with cytopenias, gastrointestinal side effects	CBC, liver and renal profile, contraindicated in pregnancy (fetal malformations, first trimester fetal loss)
Azathioprine	Purine analogue, impedes DNA and RNA synthesis	Bone marrow suppression with cytopenias, pancreatitis	CBC, thiopurine methyltransferase, liver profile
Sirolimus (rapamycin)	mTOR inhibitor	Hepatic artery thrombosis, impair wound healing, interstitial lung disease, edema, cytopenias, hyperlipidemia, proteinuria	CBC, lipid profile, liver profile, contraindicated in pregnancy due to teratogenicity

CBC Complete blood count; mTOR Mammalian target of rapamycin

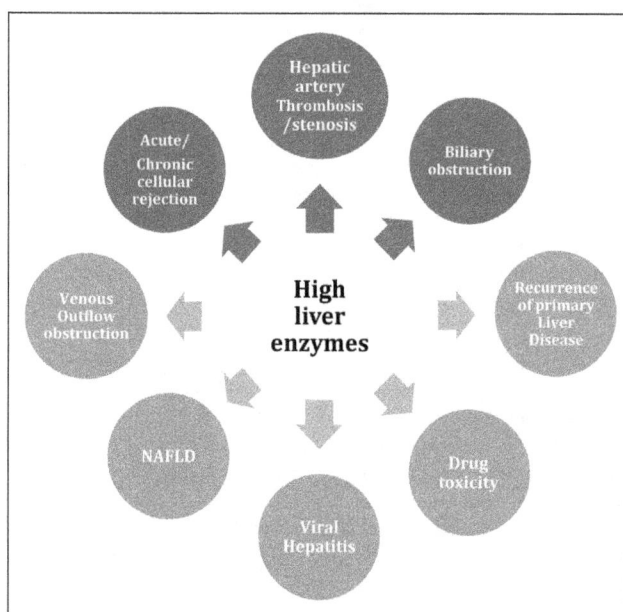

Figure 1) *Differential diagnosis of high liver enzyme levels in patients with liver transplant (darker circles indicate early post-liver transplant complications). NAFLD Nonalcoholic fatty liver disease*

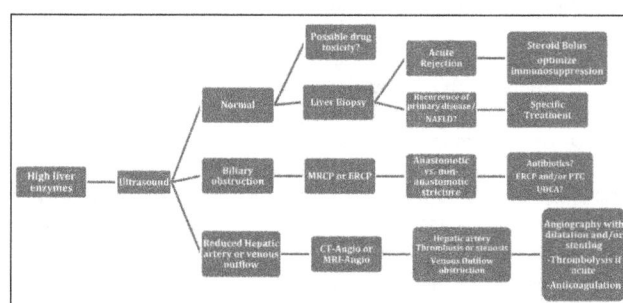

Figure 2) *Suggested diagnostic algorithm for liver transplant recipients with high liver enzyme levels. Angio Angiography; CT Computed tomography; ERCP Endoscopic retrograde cholangiopancreatography; MRCP Magnetic resonance cholangiopancreatography; MRI Magnetic resonance imaging; NAFLD Nonalcoholic fatty liver disease; PTC Percutaneous transhepatic cholangiography; UDCA Ursodeoxycholic acid*

liver allograft dysfunction are listed in Table 2, with acute cellular rejection being the most common. Salvage of the organ depends on accurate diagnosis and prompt treatment.

Post-transplant infections may develop in up to 20% of LT recipients during the first month after transplantation. Prophylaxis against infections is, therefore, routinely given to patients for at least six months after LT. A Cochrane review has proven the benefit of fluconazole as an antifungal agent in LT (5), and that of antivirals to prevent cytomegalovirus infection in all organ transplants (6). Trimethoprim-sulfamethoxazole is also given to prevent *Pneumocystis jirovecii* infection.

Recurrent disease following LT
Recurrent disease after LT is a concern, particularly when the indication for transplant was hepatitis C virus (HCV) infection or liver malignancies. Details regarding incidence, diagnosis and management are presented in Table 3. HCV infection recurs in virtually all patients in the long term, with development of cirrhosis in 30% of patients

over five years after LT (7). Protease inhibitors, such as boceprevir or telaprevir, have been used in combination with pegylated interferon and ribavirin in recent years, with sustained virological response of up to 51% at 12 weeks in the LT population with genotype 1 HCV infection (8). Next-generation protease inhibitors promise to improve on these outcomes even further (9). However, this has required a difficult balancing act with CNIs, given that they are all metabolized by the same cytochrome p450 3A4 enzyme. With the advent of polymerase inhibitors, such as sofosbuvir, with excellent cure rates and no drug-drug interactions with CNIs, treatment of HCV infection in the future will be significantly more easily managed both pre- and post-LT (10).

In the early years of LT, transplantation for hepatitis B virus (HBV) infection was regarded with trepidation. However, since the advent of hepatitis B immunoglobulin and nucleoside/nucleotide analogues, recurrence of disease has not been an issue (11). Future developments are likely to include the incorporation of more effective nucleoside/nucleotide analogues as prophylaxis against recurrence. This will enable us to forego the use of hepatitis B immunoglobulin, especially given that it is a pooled product that carries risk of virus transmission.

With HCC and cholangiocarcinoma, there are concerns for recurrent disease, especially if bulky disease is present on the explant (12). Furthermore, many groups are 'pushing the envelope' with acceptance of HCCs beyond the Milan criteria. Reducing recurrence may include switching to mammalian target of rapamycin (mTOR) inhibitor-based (ie, sirolimus) (13) or neoadjuvant therapies such as sorafenib (14).

TABLE 2
Causes of early liver allograft dysfunction: Incidence, risk factors, diagnosis and management

Cause	Incidence	Risk factors	Diagnosis	Management
Primary nonfunction	5.8%	Donor age, severity of illness in recipient	Graft loss, death within first 14 days after LT	Retransplantation
Acute cellular rejection	30% to 50% of LT recipients	Inadequate immunosuppression	Liver biopsy	Steroid bolus
		Treatment with immune-activating drugs (eg, interferon in HCV infection)		Conversion to tacrolimus-based regimen
		History of autoimmune liver disease		Thymoglobulin
		Patient noncompliance		
Chronic rejection	15% with cyclosporine and 5% with tacrolimus based regimens	LT for primary sclerosing cholangitis or primary biliary cirrhosis and CMV infection	Liver biopsy	Increase CNI levels or add sirolimus
				Retransplantation (approximately 15%)
HAT and stenosis	5% to 10% of LT recipients	Technical difficulties	Doppler ultrasound MRI or CT angiography	Thrombectomy, surgical repair, retransplantation in the case of HAT, stenting or balloon dilation of the artery for hepatic artery stenosis
Biliary complications (bile leaks and strictures)	5% to 15% (15% to 30% in living donor LT)	Prolonged organ ischemia, HAT, donor organs obtained after cardiac death, CMV infection, immunological rejection, and recurrence of primary sclerosing cholangitis	Ultrasound, MRCP, ERCP, liver biopsy	Percutaneous drainage, percutaneous transhepatic cholangiogram, biliary endoscopy, surgery or retransplantation
CMV infection	25% to 85%, typically occurs 1 to 4 months post-LT	Donor or recipient is CMV positive before LT	CMV PCR and/or CMV antigenemia or tissue samples (intestines or liver)	Prophylaxis with valganciclovir and treatment with ganciclovir
		Over immunosuppression		
		Noncompliance with prophylaxis		

Adapted from references 54 and 55. CMV Cytomegalovirus; CNI Calcineurin inhibitor; CT Computed tomography; ERCP Endoscopic retrograde cholangiopancreatography; HAT Hepatic artery thrombosis; HCV Hepatitis C virus; LT Liver transplantation; MRCP Magnetic resonance cholangiopancreatography; MRI Magnetic resonace imaging; PCR Polymerase chain reaction

TABLE 3
Diagnosis, prevention and management of recurrent liver diseases post-liver transplantation (LT)

Disease	Probability of recurrence (reference)	Diagnosis	Prevention	Management
HCV infection	60% to 90% (3)	HCV PCR; liver biopsy	Pre-LT ribavirin + peginterferon + protease Inhibitors; pre-LT polymerase inhibitor + ribavirin	Ribavirin + peginterferon + protease Inhibitors; pre-LT polymerase inhibitor + ribavirin; retransplantation
HBV infection	<10% (4)	HBsAg and HBV DNA PCR; liver biopsy	HBIg plus Nucleoside or nucleotide analogues	Nucleoside or nucleotide analogues; retransplantation rare
Nonalcoholic fatty liver disease	4% to 33% (5)	Ultrasound; liver biopsy	Lifestyle modifications; treatment of risk factors; Steroid-free immunosuppression	Lifestyle modifications; treatment of risk factors; retransplantation
Alcoholic liver disease	<5% (6)	History; measurement of ethanol level	Six months of abstinence before LT; assessment by addiction psychiatry; support group	Hospitalization (detoxification, withdrawal)
Hemochromatosis	0% (7)	Measurement of ferritin levels and transferrin saturation; liver biopsy	Regular phlebotomy	Regular phlebotomy
Hepatocellular carcinoma	Up to 12.9% with sirolimus, up to 38.7% with CNIs	Ultrasound every 6 months	Sirolimus for high-risk lesions (retrospective data) (8)	Resection; locoregional therapy (eg, TACE and RFA, sorafenib)
Cholangiocarcinoma	Five-year recurrence-free survival 70% (9)	Ultrasound and/or CT and/or MRCP/MRI	Possibly mTOR inhibitors (no evidence for this)	Resection, radiation, chemotherapy
Autoimmune hepatitis	20% to 42% (10)	Liver biopsy	Consider dual immunosuppression	Glucocorticoids ± azathioprine or MMF
Primary biliary cirrhosis	16% (11)	GGT; AP and bilirubin levels; liver biopsy	–	UDCA; retransplantation
Primary sclerosing cholangitis	17% (11)	GGT; AP and bilirubin levels; MRCP and/or ERCP and/or PTC; liver biopsy	–	Bile duct dilation; retransplantation

Data adapted from reference 54. AFP Alpha-fetoprotein; AP Alkaline phosphatase; CNI Calcineurin inhibitors; CT Computed tomography; ERCP Endoscopic retrograde cholangiopancreatography; GGT Gamma glutamyl transferase; HBIg Hepatitis B immunoglobulin; HBsAg Hepatitis B surface antigen; HBV Hepatitis B virus; MMF Mycophenolate mofetil; MRCP Magnetic resonance cholangiopancreatography; MRI Magnetic resonance imaging; mTOR Mammalian target of rapamycin; PCR Polymerase chain reaction; PTC Percutaneous transhepatic cholangiography; RFA Radiofrequency ablation; TACE Transarterial chemoembolization; TIPS Transjugular intrahepatic portosystemic shunt; UDCA Ursodeoxycholic acid

Over the years, it has come to be recognized that cryptogenic cirrhosis represents burnt-out nonalcoholic steatohepatitis (NASH). The incidence of NASH following LT is on the rise, and can be compounded by the metabolic syndrome to which LT recipients are susceptible (15). Recurrent NASH should be managed by treating the underlying metabolic syndrome.

TABLE 4
Antihypertensive agents used in liver transplantation

Antihypertensive agent	Benefits	Adverse effects
Calcium channel blockers, dihydropyridine class (eg, nifedipine) (first-line)	Decrease CNI-induced vasoconstriction	Headache, reflux tachycardia, edema, interact with CNIs
Beta-blockers	Decrease CNI-induced headache, decreased left ventricular hypertrophy	Impotence, bronchospasm, interact with CNIs
Angiotensin converting enzyme inhibitors and Angiotensin receptor blockers	Renal-sparing effects in diabetics, decreased CNI-induced vasoconstriction	Renal insufficiency and hyperkalemia (more with combination with CNIs)
Centrally acting alpha-2-agonists (eg, clonidine)	Decreases CNI-induced renal vasoconstriction	Sedation and depression

CNI Calcineurin inhibitor

TABLE 5
Hypoglycemic agents used in liver transplantation

Hypoglycemic agent	Target population	Advantage(s)	Disadvantages
Sulfonylureas	Recent-onset NODAT	Low cost, rapid onset of action	Weight gain, hypoglycemia
Metformin	Metabolic syndrome	No weight gain, lower risk of hypoglycemia	GI side effects, lactic acidosis (in CKD)
Thiazolidinediones	Metabolic syndrome	Lower risk of hypoglycemia	Weight gain, liver toxicity (rare)

Adapted from reference 23. CKD Chronic kidney disease; GI Gastrointestinal; NODAT New-onset diabetes after transplantation

TABLE 6
Risk factors for the development of renal dysfunction in liver transplantation

Pretransplant factors	Post-transplant factors
Female sex	Postoperative acute kidney injury and liver allograft dysfunction
Older age at transplant	
Pre-existing chronic kidney disease	Nephrotoxic drugs including calcineurin inhibitors
Hypertension	
Diabetes	Hypertension
Coronary artery disease	Diabetes
Hepatitis C virus infection	

Adapted from reference 60

Recurrent alcoholism has been reported in up to 20% of patients transplanted for alcoholic liver disease, with resultant decrease in long-term survival (16). However, the lower risk of recurrent disease is prompting an ethical discussion of appropriate selection of patients for LT. Many factors come into play such as the shortage of organs, optimal organ utilization and ensuring the best possible outcome for recipients. Currently, there is interest in studying and formalizing the indications for LT across Canada.

Metabolic complications following LT
Hypertension occurs in up to 70% of patients within the first year post-transplant secondary to CNI and corticosteroid use (17). Evidence-based information regarding optimal antihypertensive pharmacotherapy in LT is limited, although the effect of hypertension on renal function is particularly important. Based on expert opinion, the goal of antihypertensive therapy should be a blood pressure of 140/90 mmHg, or 130/80 mmHg in individuals with additional risk factors for atherosclerotic cardiovascular disease (18). The dihydropyridine class of long-acting calcium channel blockers, including nifedipine and amlodipine, are the first-line antihypertensives because they minimally interact with CNIs (Table 4). Beyond one year after LT, patients may benefit from the use of angiotensin-converting enzyme inhibitors or angiotensin receptor blockers, particularly those who are diabetic or have proteinuria (19).

New-onset diabetes after transplantation (NODAT) occurs in up to 26% of patients at one year (20). There is a strong association between insulin resistance and diabetes with HCV infection, with up to one-half of HCV-positive LT recipients developing NODAT (21). It is associated with increased cardiovascular morbidity and mortality, development of renal dysfunction, a higher incidence of fatal infections, more rejections and impaired graft survival (22). Screening for NODAT should begin in the immediate post-LT period with regular fasting blood glucose monitoring. As discussed above, treatment goals are similar to those of diabetes in general: prevention of complications such as renal failure, neuropathy, retinopathy, cardiovascular and cerebrovascular disease.

Treatment includes limiting caloric intake, appropriate diet/exercise with weight loss, and initiation of pharmacological agents for treatment of diabetes (Table 5) (23). In addition to steroid withdrawal and reducing CNI dose, switching from tacrolimus to cyclosporine (a less diabetogenic agent) is often effective (24).

Dyslipidemia affects up to 43% of patients after LT, and occurs particularly due to CNI use. Sirolimus is associated with an even higher risk of dyslipidemia than CNIs, although this has not translated into an increased incidence of cardiovascular events (25). Lipid profile screening every six months is recommended. Statins are safe and effective in controlling hyperlipidemia without impacting CNI levels (26). Concern regarding hepatotoxicity should not prevent their use, and routine monitoring should be observed. Statin-induced myalgia or myopathy was shown to affect 8.6% of patients in a retrospective study (27), although it was mild and disappeared with discontinuation of the statin.

Nutritional status is often compromised in patients with ESLD. Following LT, an improved sense of well-being, along with prednisone treatment, contributes to overeating and development of obesity. One cohort study showed that approximately 20% of nonobese transplant recipients became obese over a two-year follow-up period (28,29). Patients transplanted for NASH tend to develop recurrent hepatic steatosis after LT with weight gain (30). Treatment of obesity involves a balanced diet, aerobic exercise and considering altering immunosuppressive medications, including steroid withdrawal.

Low bone mineral density occurs in up to 70% of patients with liver disease (31). The use of steroids and CNIs can further precipitate decline in bone mass after LT, reaching a plateau six months postoperatively. Transplant recipients should be screened for metabolic bone disease with dual energy x-ray absorptiometry scan every two years. Preventive strategies, such as physical activity and smoking cessation, should be encouraged. Daily supplementation with 1500 mg of calcium and 800 IU of vitamin D should be given to all patients, along with bisphosphonates and testosterone replacement in hypoandrogenic states as needed.

Renal complications after LT
Chronic kidney disease (CKD), defined as a glomerular filtration rate (GFR) <30 mL/min/1.73 m^2 body surface area, occurs in up to 90% of LT recipients and is multifactorial in etiology (Table 6) (32). The incidence of renal dysfunction has especially increased with the

TABLE 7
Recommended screening intervals for malignancies for liver transplant patients

Malignancy	Recommended examination (screening interval, if applicable)
Breast cancer	Annual mammography starting at 50 years of age (similar to general population)
Cervical cancer	Pelvic examination and Pap smear (similar to general population)
Colon cancer	Colonoscopy every 5 to 10 years if no history of colonic neoplasia, every 3 to 5 years with history of neoplasia, yearly in ulcerative colitis patients
Esophageal cancer	EGD in patients with Barrett's esophagus and those at high risk for esophageal cancer (smokers and those transplanted for EtOH cirrhosis)
Lung cancer	Chest x-ray every 1 to 2 years in smokers and those transplanted for EtOH cirrhosis
Oropharyngeal cancer	Otolaryngological examination every 1 to 3 years in smokers and those transplanted for EtOH cirrhosis
Prostate cancer	Digital rectal examination and prostate-specific antigen
Skin cancer	Annual skin examination

EGD Esophagogastroduodenoscopy; EtOH Ethanol

adoption of the Model for End-stage Liver Disease score to prioritize patients for LT, with a 15% higher risk of post-LT end-stage renal disease (33,34). Based on prospective cohort data, CKD is associated with a 4.5 times greater probability of death versus patients with normal renal function, and a 2% to 5% per year risk of requiring dialysis (35). CNIs cause vasoconstriction of the renal afferent arterioles, resulting in decreased renal perfusion. Renal failure due to CNIs may be reversible with dose reduction or medication withdrawal (10,11).

Patients may be switched to the mTOR inhibitors sirolimus and everolimus for immunosuppression to preserve kidney function in the long term after LT. These patients should be screened for development of proteinuria, although its long-term impact on renal function is unclear (36).

Biliary complications

Biliary complications after LT usually occur as a result of impaired vascular supply at some time point during the patient's postoperative course (37). Bile leaks are the most common, affecting up to 30% of LT recipients in the early postoperative period. Stricturing at the biliary anastomosis may occur in the long term, which can be reversed with dilation and stenting via endoscopic retrograde cholangiopancreatography (ERCP). In patients who develop hepatic artery thrombosis or have other risk factors with a significant impact on hepatic arterial flow, ischemic cholangiopathy may result in the long term. This condition is often complicated by recurrent cholangitis, and can be treated with antibiotics and stenting, although retransplantation is often indicated. Some patients may have Roux-en-Y anatomy following LT, especially those transplanted for primary sclerosing cholangitis, which will render ERCP more technically challenging (this technical difficulty is due to the length of the Roux limb, which may be circumvented by performing ERCP assisted by double-balloon technique at certain Canadian centres with this expertise).

SCREENING FOR MALIGNANCIES AFTER TRANSPLANT

Transplant patients are at higher risk for developing malignancies because immunosuppression curtails the cancer-sensing function of the immune system (38). Improving patient survival has resulted in exposure to immunosuppression for an extended period; consequently, nonskin malignancies arise in up to 16% of recipients and represent a common cause of late deaths. This is especially true in patients with concurrent smoking and alcohol use, who should undergo annual endoscopy, laryngoscopy and chest-x-ray, as described in Table 7. Skin cancers are up to 100 times more common among LT recipients compared with the general population (25). Transplant recipients should avoid excessive sun exposure, apply sunscreen regularly and undergo a thorough dermatological examination annually. Post-transplant lymphoproliferative disorder (PTLD) is associated with Epstein-Barr virus infection in 90% of cases and occurs in up to 2% of LT patients within the first year (39). Overall, PTLD has been known to affect up to 2.8% of adult and up to 15% of pediatric LT recipients (40). This generally presents as fevers, night sweats, weight loss and malaise, with or without lymphadenopathy. PTLD is managed through reduction of immunosuppression, rituximab or chemotherapy. Colonoscopy for colorectal cancer screening should be performed every five years, and annually if patient has a diagnosis of primary sclerosing cholangitis with ulcerative colitis. All other malignancies are screened as per recommendations for the general population.

PREVENTIVE CARE, QUALITY OF LIFE, SEXUALITY AND PREGNANCY

Potential LT recipients should ideally receive all necessary vaccinations before transplant because immunosuppressants significantly suppress T cell function and increase risk for infection (41). Live-attenuated vaccines carry a potential risk of shedding live virus, although studies have confirmed that these can be safely given to transplant patients (42,43). Any administration of live-attenuated vaccines such as varicella, Bacillus Calmette-Guérin, measles-mumps-rubella, polio, typhoid, yellow fever and rotavirus, should be performed only in consultation with the transplant centre. Only the following vaccines may be safely administered to both LT recipients and their household contacts: hepatitis A, hepatitis B, inactivated influenza, meningococcal, pneumococcal, tetanus, diphtheria, *Haemophilus influenzae* type b, pertussis and human papilloma virus.

Transplant recipients who smoke should be counselled regarding smoking cessation because the adverse effects of tobacco are possibly heightened. Studies have shown that LT recipients who smoke are at increased risk for all-cause mortality and vascular events (coronary artery disease, stroke and hepatic artery thrombosis, which can lead to graft loss). Nicotine replacement therapy and medications, such as bupropion, can safely be offered. Cannabis should be discouraged because it is known to worsen hepatic steatosis and fibrosis in chronic liver disease patients (44,45). Proper dental hygiene and regular check-ups are essential because excess oral bacteria in the presence of immunosuppression can lead to development of serious infections such as infective endocarditis. Antibiotic prophylaxis is not required in the transplant patient population, even in the context of dental procedures, unless an underlying cardiac condition predisposing to endocarditis is present.

ESLD causes significant disability, to the point of being unable to perform activities of daily living. LT enables the return of most patients to the workforce, which greatly enhances daily activities, physical health, health-related quality of life, sexual function and psychosocial well-being (46). Recipients may not have a health-related quality of life equivalent to that of the general population because many are readmitted to hospital for complications such as impaired wound healing and infections. However, resources, such as a dedicated transplant nurse, an exercise program and psychosocial support, can help improve perception of health and quality of life (47).

The availability of psychological support is important because reactive depression can occur due to difficulty coping with post-transplant life. Occupational counselling should be offered if a patient is experiencing difficulties in returning to the workforce. A Canadian transplant centre determined that 57% of their patients surviving a minimum of nine months had returned to employment (48).

A majority of patients with ESLD lose sexual function and fertility (49). With LT, sexual function returns to normal in >90% of recipients (50). Erectile dysfunction may be treated with standard medications. Fertility could return at any time after transplantation; therefore, contraception should be used on resumption of sexual activity. Ideally, pregnancy should be delayed beyond the one-year mark after LT. The use of MMF in pregnant mothers has been associated with birth defects and miscarriages. MMF should either be avoided among women of reproductive age or should be discontinued at least six weeks before a planned conception. A live birth rate >70% with favourable maternal and fetal outcomes has been documented in the American National Transplantation Pregnancy Registry (51). During pregnancy, hypertension is a complication encountered in up to 45% of transplant recipients (49). An increase in plasma protein levels that bind cyclosporine and tacrolimus can lead to subtherapeutic levels. Pregnancy is, therefore, associated with a 10% risk of organ rejection and requires more frequent monitoring of immunosuppressant levels to maintain the therapeutic range (52). Prematurity and low birth weight are the most common fetal complications, occurring in 10% to 55% of pregnancies (53). Overall, the long-term outcomes of most babies exposed to immunosuppressants in utero is favourable, with normal development (51).

CONCLUSION

The care of LT recipients has evolved, with excellent survival rates following LT. Gastroenterologists and primary care physicians in the community often follow LT recipients in conjunction with the LT physician, and it is important to be aware of the unique medical needs and complications associated with long-term immunosuppression. Such comprehensive care will ensure that the LT recipient benefits from optimal health and quality of life.

DISCLOSURES: The authors have no financial disclosures or conflicts of interest to declare.

REFERENCES

1. McGuire B, Rosenthal P, Brown C, et al. Long term management of the liver transplant patient: Recommendations for the primary care doctor. Am J Transpl 2009;9:1988-2003.
2. Register COR. 2013 Canadian Organ Replacement Register (CORR) report-Treatment of end-stage organ failure report, 2002 to 2011, 2013.
3. Roberts MS, Angus DC, Bryce CL, Valenta Z, Weissfeld L. Survival after liver transplantation in the United States: A disease specific analysis of the UNOS database. Liver Transpl 2004;10:886-97.
4. Meier-Kriesche HU, Li S, Gruessner RW, et al. Immunosuppression: Evolution in practice and trends, 1994-2004. Am J Transpl 2006;6(5 Pt 2):1111-31.
5. Playford E, Webster A, Sorell T, Craig J. Antifungal agents for preventing fungal infections in solid organ transplant recipients. Cochrane Database Syst Rev (Online) 2004(3):CD004291.
6. Hodson E, Craig J, Strippoli G, Webster A. Antiviral medications for preventing cytomegalovirus disease in solid organ transplant recipients. Cochrane Database Syst Rev (Online) 2008(2):CD003774.
7. Berenguer M, Prieto M, Rayon JM, et al. Natural history of clinically compensated hepatitis C virus-related graft cirrhosis after liver transplantation. Hepatology 2000;32(4 Pt 1):852-8.
8. Coilly A, Roche B, Dumortier J, et al. Safety and efficacy of protease inhibitors to treat hepatitis C after liver transplantation: A multicenter experience. J Hepatol 2014;60:78-86.
9. Zeuzem S, Berg T, Gane E, et al. Simeprevir Increases Rate of Sustained Virologic Response Among Treatment-Experienced Patients With HCV Genotype-1 Infection: A Phase IIb Trial. Gastroenterology November 2013 (E-pub ahead of print).
10. Charlton MR, Gane EJ, Manns MP, et al. Sofosbuvir and Ribavirin for the Treatment of Established Recurrent Hepatitis C Infection After Liver Transplantation: Preliminary results of a prospective, multicenter study. 64th Annual Meeting of the American Association for the Study of Liver Diseases (AASLD 2013). Washington, DC, November 1 to 5, 2013. Abstract LB-2.
11. Fung J, Chan SC, Cheung C, et al. Oral nucleoside/nucleotide analogs without hepatitis B immune globulin after liver transplantation for hepatitis B. Am J Gastroenterol 2013;108:942-8.
12. Darwish Murad S, Kim WR, et al. Predictors of pretransplant dropout and posttransplant recurrence in patients with perihilar cholangiocarcinoma. Hepatology 2012;56:972-81.
13. Menon KV, Hakeem AR, Heaton ND. Meta-analysis: Recurrence and survival following the use of sirolimus in liver transplantation for hepatocellular carcinoma. Aliment Pharmacol Ther 2013;37:411-9.
14. Mancuso A, Mazzarelli C, Perricone G, Zavaglia C. Sorafenib efficacy for treatment of HCC recurrence after liver transplantation is an open issue. J Hepatol November 2013 (E-pub ahead of print).
15. Patil DT, Yerian LM. Evolution of nonalcoholic fatty liver disease recurrence after liver transplantation. Liver Transpl 2012;18:1147-53.
16. Pfitzmann R, Schwenzer J, Rayes N, Seehofer D, Neuhaus R, Nussler NC. Long-term survival and predictors of relapse after orthotopic liver transplantation for alcoholic liver disease. Liver Transpl 2007;13:197-205.
17. Sheiner PA, Magliocca JF, Bodian CA, et al. Long-term medical complications in patients surviving > or = 5 years after liver transplant. Transplantation 2000;69:781-9.
18. Munoz SJ, Elgenaidi H. Cardiovascular risk factors after liver transplantation. Liver Transpl 2005(11 Suppl 2):S52-6.
19. Najeed SA, Saghir S, Hein B, et al. Management of hypertension in liver transplant patients. Int J Cardiol 2011;152:4-6.
20. Navasa M, Bustamante J, Marroni C, et al. Diabetes mellitus after liver transplantation: Prevalence and predictive factors. J Hepatol 1996;25:64-71.
21. Gane EJ. Diabetes mellitus following liver transplantation in patients with hepatitis C virus: Risks and consequences. Am J Transpl 2012;12:531-8.
22. Moon JI, Barbeito R, Faradji RN, Gaynor JJ, Tzakis AG. Negative impact of new-onset diabetes mellitus on patient and graft survival after liver transplantation: Long-term follow up. Transplantation 2006;82:1625-8.
23. Davidson JA, Wilkinson A. New-onset diabetes after transplantation 2003 International Consensus Guidelines: An endocrinologist's view. Diabetes Care 2004;27:805-12.
24. Yoshida EM, Lilly LB, Marotta PJ, Mason AL, Bilodeau M, Vaillancourt M. Canadian national retrospective chart review comparing the long term effect of cyclosporine vs. tacrolimus on clinical outcomes in patients with post-liver transplantation hepatitis C virus infection. Ann Hepatol 2013;12:282-93.
25. Chinnakotla S, Davis GL, Vasani S, et al. Impact of sirolimus on the recurrence of hepatocellular carcinoma after liver transplantation. Liver Transpl 2009;15:1834-42.
26. Gazi IF, Liberopoulos EN, Athyros VG, Elisaf M, Mikhailidis DP. Statins and solid organ transplantation. Curr Pharm Des 2006;12:4771-83.
27. Martin JE, Cavanaugh TM, Trumbull L, et al. Incidence of adverse events with HMG-CoA reductase inhibitors in liver transplant patients. Clin Transpl 2008;22:113-9.
28. Everhart JE, Lombardero M, Lake JR, Wiesner RH, Zetterman RK, Hoofnagle JH. Weight change and obesity after liver transplantation: Incidence and risk factors. Liver Transpl Surg 1998;4:285-96.
29. Canzanello VJ, Schwartz L, Taler SJ, et al. Evolution of cardiovascular risk after liver transplantation: A comparison of cyclosporine A and tacrolimus (FK506). Liver Transpl Surg 1997;3:1-9.
30. Contos MJ, Cales W, Sterling RK, et al. Development of nonalcoholic fatty liver disease after orthotopic liver transplantation for cryptogenic cirrhosis. Liver Transpl 2001;7:363-73.
31. Neuhaus R, Lohmann R, Platz KP, et al. Treatment of osteoporosis after liver transplantation. Transplant Proc 1995;27:1226-7.
32. K/DOQI clinical practice guidelines for chronic kidney disease: Evaluation, classification, and stratification. Am J Kidney Dis 2002;39(2 Suppl 1):S1-266.
33. Sharma P, Schaubel DE, Guidinger MK, Goodrich NP, Ojo AO, Merion RM. Impact of MELD-based allocation on end-stage renal disease after liver transplantation. Am J Transpl 2011;11:2372-8.

34. Myers RP, Shaheen AA, Aspinall AI, Quinn RR, Burak KW. Gender, renal function, and outcomes on the liver transplant waiting list: Assessment of revised MELD including estimated glomerular filtration rate. J Hepatol 2011;54:462-70.

35. Ojo AO. Scope of the problem and impact on outcomes. Liver Transpl 2009;15(Suppl 2):S1.

36. Letavernier E, Pe'raldi MN, Pariente A, Morelon E, Legendre C. Proteinuria following a switch from calcineurin inhibitors to sirolimus. Transplantation 2005;80:1198-203.

37. Seehofer D, Eurich D, Veltzke-Schlieker W, Neuhaus P. Biliary complications after liver transplantation: Old problems and new challenges. Am J Transpl 2013;13:253-65.

38. Ulrich C, Schmook T, Sachse MM, Sterry W, Stockfleth E. Comparative epidemiology and pathogenic factors for nonmelanoma skin cancer in organ transplant patients. Dermatol Surg 2004;30(4p2):622-27.

39. Nalesnik MA, Starzl TE. Epstein-Barr virus, infectious mononucleosis, and posttransplant lymphoproliferative disorders. Transpl Sci 1994;4:61.

40. Taylor AL, Marcus R, Bradley JA. Post-transplant lymphoproliferative disorders (PTLD) after solid organ transplantation. Crit Rev Oncol Hematol 2005;56:155-67.

41. Zeldin GA, Maygers J, Klein A, Thuluvath PJ. Vaccination, screening for malignancy, and health maintenance of the liver transplant recipient. J Clin Gastroenterol 2001;32:148.

42. Kano H, Mizuta K, Sakakihara Y, et al. Efficacy and safety of immunization for pre-and post-liver transplant children. Transplantation 2002;74:543.

43. Khan S, Erlichman J, Rand EB. Live virus immunization after orthotopic liver transplantation. Pediatr Transpl 2006;10:78-82.

44. Missiha SB, Ostrowski M, Heathcote EJ. Disease progression in chronic hepatitis C: Modifiable and nonmodifiable factors. Gastroenterology 2008;134:1699-714.

45. Hézode C, Roudot Thoraval F, et al. Daily cannabis smoking as a risk factor for progression of fibrosis in chronic hepatitis C. Hepatology 2005;42:63-71.

46. Saab S, Wiese C, Ibrahim AB, et al. Employment and quality of life in liver transplant recipients. Liver Transpl 2007;13:1330-8.

47. Hunt CM, Tart JS, Dowdy E, Bute BP, Williams DM, Clavien PA. Effect of orthotopic liver transplantation on employment and health status. Liver Transpl 1996;2:148-53.

48. Adams PC, Ghent CN, Grant DR, Wall WJ. Employment after liver transplantation. Hepatology 1995;21:140-44.

49. Armenti VT, Herrine SK, Radomski JS, Moritz MJ. Pregnancy after liver transplantation. Liver Transpl 2000;6:671-85.

50. Ho JK, Ko HH, Schaeffer DF, et al. Sexual health after orthotopic liver transplantation. Liver Transpl 2006;12:1478-84.

51. Coscia LA, Constantinescu S, Moritz MJ, et al. Report from the National Transplantation Pregnancy Registry (NTPR): Outcomes of pregnancy after transplantation. Clin Transpl 2008:89.

52. Cardonick E, Moritz M, Armenti V. Pregnancy in patients with organ transplantation: A review. Obstet Gynecological Survey 2004;59:214.

53. Nagy S, Bush MC, Berkowitz R, Fishbein TM, Gomez-Lobo V. Pregnancy outcome in liver transplant recipients. Obstet Gynecol 2003;102:121.

54. Benten D, Staufer K, Sterneck M. Orthotopic liver transplantation and what to do during follow-up: Recommendations for the practitioner. Nat Clin Pract Gastroenterol Hepatol 2009;6:23-36.

55. Johnson SR, Alexopoulos S, Curry M, Hanto DW. Primary nonfunction (PNF) in the MELD era: An SRTR database analysis. Am J Transpl 2007;7:1003-9.

56. Singal AK, Chaha KS, Rasheed K, Anand BS. Liver transplantation in alcoholic liver disease current status and controversies. World J Gastroenterol 2013;19:5953-63.

57. Crawford DH, Fletcher LM, Hubscher SG, et al. Patient and graft survival after liver transplantation for hereditary hemochromatosis: Implications for pathogenesis. Hepatology 2004;39:1655-62.

58. Molmenti EP, Netto GJ, Murray NG, et al. Incidence and recurrence of autoimmune/alloimmune hepatitis in liver transplant recipients. Liver Transpl 2002;8:519-26.

59. Gautam M, Cheruvattath R, Balan V. Recurrence of autoimmune liver disease after liver transplantation: A systematic review. Liver Transpl 2006;12:1813-24.

60. Ojo AO, Held PJ, Port FK, et al. Chronic renal failure after transplantation of a nonrenal organ. N Engl J Med 2003;319:931 40.

4

Adherence to guidelines: A national audit of the management of acute upper gastrointestinal bleeding. The REASON registry

Yidan Lu MD[1], Alan N Barkun MD MSc[1,2], Myriam Martel BSc[1]; and the REASON investigators

Y Lu, AN Barkun, M Martel; and the REASON investigators. Adherence to guidelines: A national audit of the management of acute upper gastrointestinal bleeding. The REASON registry. Can J Gastroenterol Hepatol 2014;28(9):495-501.

OBJECTIVES: To assess process of care in nonvariceal upper gastrointestinal bleeding (NVUGIB) using a national cohort, and to identify predictors of adherence to 'best practice' standards.
METHODS: Consecutive charts of patients hospitalized for acute upper gastrointestinal bleeding across 21 Canadian hospitals were reviewed. Data regarding initial presentation, endoscopic management and outcomes were collected. Results were compared with 'best practice' using established guidelines on NVUGIB. Adherence was quantified and independent predictors were evaluated using multivariable analysis.
RESULTS: Overall, 2020 patients (89.4% NVUGIB, variceal in 10.6%) were included (mean [± SD] age 66.3±16.4 years; 38.4% female). Endoscopy was performed in 1612 patients: 1533 with NVUGIB had endoscopic lesions (63.1% ulcers; high-risk stigmata in 47.8%). Early endoscopy was performed in 65.6% and an assistant was present in 83.5%. Only 64.5% of patients with high-risk stigmata received endoscopic hemostasis; 9.8% of patients exhibiting low-risk stigmata also did. Intravenous proton pump inhibitor was administered after endoscopic hemostasis in 95.7%. Rebleeding and mortality rates were 10.5% and 9.4%, respectively. Multivariable analysis revealed that low American Society of Anesthesiologists score patients had fewer assistants present during endoscopy (OR 0.63 [95% CI 0.48 to 0.83], a hemoglobin level <70 g/L predicted inappropriate high-dose intravenous proton pump inhibitor use in patients with low-risk stigmata, and endoscopies performed during regular hours were associated with longer delays from presentation (OR 0.33 [95% CI 0.24 to 0.47]).
CONCLUSION: There was variability between the process of care and 'best practice' in NVUGIB. Certain patient and situational characteristics may influence guideline adherence. Dissemination initiatives must identify and focus on such considerations to improve quality of care.

Key Words: Gastrointestinal hemorrhage; Guideline adherence; Peptic ulcer hemorrhage; Quality of health care

L'adhérence aux lignes directrices : une analyse nationale de la prise en charge des hémorragies digestives hautes aiguës. Le registre REASON

OBJECTIFS : Évaluer le processus des soins chez les patients présentant une hémorragies digestives hautes non variqueuses (HDHNV) au sein d'une cohorte nationale et déterminer la conformité à la 'bonne pratique'.
MÉTHODOLOGIE : Une analyse de dossiers consécutifs de patients hospitalisés en raison d'hémorragies digestives hautes aiguës au sein de 21 hôpitaux canadiens a été effectuée, incluant les données relatives à la présentation initiale, au traitement endoscopique et aux résultats. La conformité quant aux lignes directrices a été quantifiée et les prédicteurs indépendants ont été évalués via une analyse multivariable.
RÉSULTATS : Au total, 2 020 patients (89,4 % HDHNV, et 10,6 % de cas variqueux) ont participé (âge moyen [±ÉT] de 66,3±16,4 ans; 38,4 % de sexe féminin). Une endoscopie a été exécutée chez 1 612 patients : 1 533 de ceux ayant une HDHNV avaient une lésion endoscopique (63,1 % des ulcères; 47,8 % des stigmates à haut risque). Une endoscopie précoce a été effectuée chez 65,6 % des patients, en présence d'un assistant dans 83,5 % des cas. Seulement 64,5 % des patients ayant des stigmates à haut risque ont reçu une hémostase endoscopique, de même que 9,8 % des patients présentant des stigmates à faible risque. Après l'hémostase endoscopique, des inhibiteurs de la pompe à proton par voie intraveineuse ont été administrés chez 95,7 % des patients. Les taux de récidive de l'hémorragie et de mortalité s'élevaient à 10,5 % et 9,4 %, respectivement. L'analyse multivariable a révélé que moins d'assistants étaient présents pendant l'endoscopie chez les patients ayant un score faible selon l'*American Society of Anesthesiologists* (RC 0,63 [95 % IC 0,48 à 0,83], tandis qu'un taux d'hémoglobine inférieur à 70 g/L était prédictif de l'utilisation d'inhibiteurs de la pompe à protons intraveineux à haute dose chez les patients ayant des stigmates à faible risque, et que les endoscopies effectuées pendant les heures normales s'associaient à des délais plus longs suivant la présentation (RC 0,33 [95 % IC 0,24 à 0,47]).
CONCLUSION : On note une variabilité entre le processus des soins et les recommandations de 'bonne pratique' chez les patients avec une HDHNV. Certaines caractéristiques relatives aux patients ou à la situation clinique semblent influencer l'adhérence aux lignes directrices. Toute initiative de diffusion des lignes directrices doivent prendre en compte ces résultats afin d'améliorer la qualité des soins.

Upper gastrointestinal bleeding (UGIB) is associated with significant morbidity and mortality. The incidence of acute nonvariceal UGIB (NVUGIB) ranges from 50 to 150 cases per 100,000 adults per year (1), while mortality varies from 2.5% to 10% (1,2). A large bleeding registry from 1999 to 2002 (3) revealed significant practice variations in the management of NVUGIB across Canadian hospitals (4). Several consensus recommendations have since been developed, setting well-defined standards (5-7). However, wide practice variations among physicians continue to be reported (8). Such variability calls to assess the quality of care delivered in NVUGIB. The latter extends beyond the measurement of outcomes such as rebleeding and mortality, and includes the evaluation of the structure and delivery of care through process-based measures (9,10). Optimally, the process of care should be consistent with evidence-based 'best practice' (8).

The Registry of patients undergoing Endoscopic and/or Acid Suppression therapy and an Outcome analysis for upper gastrointestinal bleeding (REASON) recorded the 'real-life' hospital and physician practice managing acute UGIB across Canadian hospitals. The process of care was compared with 'best practice' recommendations available at the time, namely international NVUGIB consensus guidelines (5) published one year before the national cohort study. We present Canadian nationwide data regarding the structure, process and

Divisions of [1]Gastroenterology; [2]Epidemiology Biostatistics and Occupational Health, McGill University Health Centre, McGill University, Montreal, Quebec
Correspondence: Dr Alan Barkun, Division of Gastroenterology, The McGill University Health Centre, Montreal General Hospital Site, 1650 Cedar Avenue, Room D7-185, Montreal, Quebec H3G 1A4. e-mail alan.barkun@muhc.mcgill.ca

outcomes of care as measures of quality of care (10) in light of 'best practice' guidelines and assess the impact of the latter.

METHODS

REASON initiative and data collection

A retrospective chart review of unselected hospitalized patients with a diagnosis of UGIB was performed in 21 Canadian hospitals. One hundred charts per institution were reviewed, starting from January 2004 until a total of 2000 cases was reached. Data collection was performed using an electronic system. Data were audited for the first 10 patients at each site, and randomly thereafter in 10% to ensure standardization.

Patient population

All hospitalized patients at least 18 years of age with a primary or secondary discharge diagnosis of NVUGIB and variceal UGIB were identified using *International Classification of Diseases, Ninth and 10th Revision* (ICD-9 and ICD-10) codes via each hospital's electronic record database. Only hospitalized patients were included. Patients discharged from the emergency room or those transferred from another institution were excluded. Individuals already hospitalized for another reason, but who developed UGIB during their stay, were included. The performance of endoscopy was not an inclusion criterion.

Study variables

Structure and process of care: *initial presentation and endoscopic management:* Baseline data with patient demographics (age, sex, relevant medical history and medications) and institutional information (staffing and facility) were obtained. A description of the initial bleeding event was collected for all patients. The performance of endoscopy (if any), in addition to timing, endoscopic findings and hemostatic modality used (if any) were reported. The single most likely culprit lesion in the opinion of the endoscopist was recorded, although additional findings were also recorded if present. High-risk endoscopic stigmata (HRS) were defined as active bleeding with spurting or oozing, or findings of a nonbleeding visible vessel or adherent clot. Low-risk stigmata (LRS) were comprised of pigmented spots and clean-based ulcers. Furthermore, data regarding pharmacotherapy, blood transfusions and *Helicobacter pylori* testing were also collected.

Information was retrieved for all patients presenting with acute UGIB (variceal and nonvariceal source) if they met the above inclusion criteria. However, for patients who were diagnosed with bleeding due to portal hypertension at endoscopy, only preprocedure data are presented and information collected after endoscopy is omitted.

Outcomes: Rebleeding, recourse to angiography and surgery, length of stay and mortality were reported. Rebleeding was defined as overt hematemesis; passage of fresh blood per rectum; fall in hemoglobin concentration >20 g/L within any 24 h period after the first 24 h; shock (systolic blood pressure of ≤90 mmHg or a heart rate of ≥110 beats/min) in the presence of continuing melena; or fresh blood in the stomach and/or duodenum at repeat endoscopy when further bleeding was suspected (3,11,12). All outcome data were collected for a 30-day period following the initial bleeding event.

Best practice: *adherence to guidelines and its possible predictors:* Adherence to guidelines was determined using the most recent guidelines available at the time of data collection (5), which featured 20 recommendations pertaining to the management of NVUGIB. Each recommendation was reviewed in light of available data from REASON, and adherence rates were calculated using ratios and percentages, except when data were insufficient or missing from the registry. Data were compared with a similar cross-sectional study preceding the publication of the guidelines (4).

For selected recommendations, possible independent predictors of guideline adherence were assessed, including the patient's age (<60, 60 to 80 or >80 years of age), sex, pre-endoscopic Rockall score (0 to 2, or >2) and Blatchford scores (0 to 2, 3 to 11, or >11), American Society of Anesthesiologists (ASA) classification (1 to 2, 3, or 4 to 5), presenting hemoglobin level (<70 g/L) and time of endoscopy (regular hours defined as Monday to Friday from 08:00 to 17:00 versus after hours).

Data analysis

Categorical data were expressed as proportions and 95% CIs, and continuous data as means ± SD. Interquartile range (IQR) and median were also used when appropriate. Univariable analysis was performed using χ^2 or Wilcoxon-rank testing. Independent predictors of guideline adherence were identified using the best fitting multivariable logistic regression models that were clinically relevant; $P<0.05$ was considered to be statistically significant. All statistical analyses were performed using SAS version 9.2 (SAS Institute Inc, USA).

Ethics

Informed consent from individual patients was not deemed necessary because the study was considered to be an audit at all sites. The institutional review boards from all participating centres gave approval for the REASON data collection and analysis.

RESULTS

Structure of care: institutional and endoscopic facility data

Across the 21 hospitals, the mean number of endoscopists on staff was 11 per hospital (median nine; range three to 26). After-hours trained endoscopic support staff were available in 17 of 21 (81%) hospitals, of which 13 of 17 (76%) were available 24 h/day. Assistants were present to assist endoscopy in 83.5% of cases. Fewer than one-half (10 of 21 [48%]) of the hospitals had explicit written guidelines on intravenous proton pump inhibitor (IV PPI) use; a standardized critical care path for the management of patients with suspected UGIB existed in a similar proportion of institutions (11 of 21 [52%]).

Clips were accessible in all hospitals, followed by injection (20 of 21 [95%]); other devices included gold probe (17 of 21 [81%]), argon plasma coagulation (15 of 21 [71%]), heater probe (15 of 21 [71%]), and bipolar or multipolar electrocoagulation (13 of 21 [62%]).

Study population

Data from 2020 patients with UGIB were collected between January 2004 and May 2005. A total of 1805 (89.4%) patients presented with NVUGIB and 215 (10.6%) with variceal bleeding. The mean (± SD) age was 66.3±16.4 years, with a male predominance (1245 of 2020 [61.6%]). Nearly one-fifth (356 of 2020 [17.6%]) of all patients experienced the bleeding episode while already hospitalized for another reason. The mean Blatchford score was 9.1±4.1 (minimum = 0; maximum = 23), while the pre-endoscopic mean Rockall scores were 2.0±1.5 (minimum = 0; maximum = 7). The overall ASA score distribution was 80.2% ASA score 1 to 3, 19.8% ASA score 4 and 5.

Process of care

Initial management: Twenty-two percent (448 of 2020) of patients underwent nasogastric tube lavage: 38.4% (172 of 448) revealed coffee-ground material, 27.5% (123 of 448) bright red blood and 4.0% (18 of 448) bile. Only five of the 21 (24%) hospitals routinely obtained nasogastric tube aspirates for the majority of their patients. The mean presenting hemoglobin level was 98.0±27.8 g/L. Sixty-nine percent of patients received a blood transfusion, at a median time of 8.7 h (IQR 3.9 h to 24.0 h) from presentation, with the vast majority (74.9%) occurring in the first 24 h. Among those transfused, 16.8% had an initial hemoglobin level ≤70 g/L, 39.2% between 71 g/L and 100 g/L and 44.0% a level >100 g/L.

Overall, 68.2% (1113 of 1632) of patients presenting with acute NVUGIB received pre-endoscopic IV PPIs. These were administered at high dose with an 80 mg bolus, followed by 8 mg/h infusion in 54.5% (698 of 1281). Prokinetic use was not recorded.

Time to endoscopy: The median time to endoscopy was 17.7 h (IQR 6.1 h to 29.4 h). Patients with suspected variceal bleeding underwent endoscopy significantly earlier than individuals with suspected nonvariceal bleeding, with a median time to endoscopy of 12.4 h (IQR 4.5 h to 25.0 h) compared with 18.3 h (IQR 6.3 h to 30.0 h)

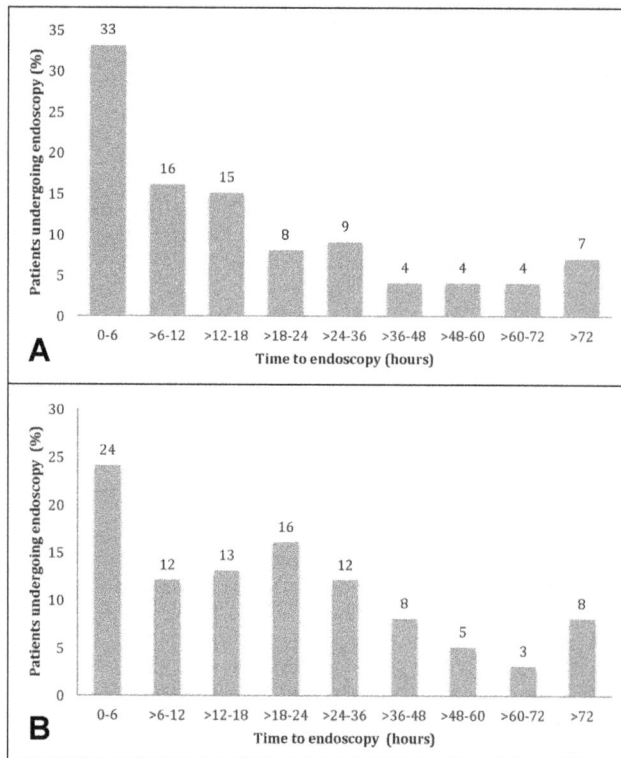

Figure 1) A *Time to endoscopy for patients with suspected variceal bleeding*. **B** *Time to endoscopy for patients with suspected nonvariceal bleeding*

for nonvariceal bleeding (P=0.0038). Overall, 65.6% of patients underwent endoscopy within 24 h. The distributions of time to endoscopy are shown in Figures 1A and 1B.

Endoscopic findings: Findings at endoscopy were recorded for both variceal and nonvariceal bleeding, although details pertaining to variceal bleeding will not be discussed further. A total of 89.4% (1805 of 2020) of patients were diagnosed with NVUGIB (Figure 2).

The etiologies of NVUGIB were distributed as follows: ulcers (967 of 1533 [63.1%]), erosions (341 of 1533 [22.2%]), esophagitis (313 of 1533 [20.4%]), Mallory-Weiss tear (113 of 1533 [7.4%]), malignancy (40 of 1533 [2.6%]), Dieulafoy lesion (35 of 1533 [2.3%]), gastric antral vascular ectasia syndrome (35 of 1533 [2.3%]) and esophageal strictures (34 of 1533 [2.2%]). More than one endoscopic diagnosis was possible for the same patient. Figure 3 illustrates the distribution of stigmata of recent hemorrhage in patients with nonvariceal bleeding, including ulcers and nonulcer lesions. While several diagnoses could be identified for the same patient, only the stigma from the lesion most likely to be the source of bleeding was recorded. Detailed documentation of endoscopic findings, more specifically, bleeding stigmata and description were unavailable in 30.1% (135 of 448) of cases. Excluding patients with no documentation of stigmata of recent bleeding, 71% had HRS.

Endoscopic therapy: Nearly two-thirds (64.5%) of patients with HRS from both ulcer and nonulcer bleeding received endoscopic hemostasis. Moreover, 9.8% of patients LRS were also treated with endoscopy (Table 1). Epinephrine injection was used as monotherapy in 23.8% of patients with high-risk ulcers and 20.7% of all high-risk lesions. The most common endoscopic modalities used for the management of HRS lesions were injection monotherapy (32.8%), combination therapy of injection and thermal (32.3%), followed by thermal monotherapy (14.5%) and clips (alone or in combination) (14.3%). A routine (preplanned) second-look endoscopy was performed in 9.0% (145 of 1612) of patients, while repeat endoscopy due to suspected rebleeding was performed in 56.7% (97 of 171).

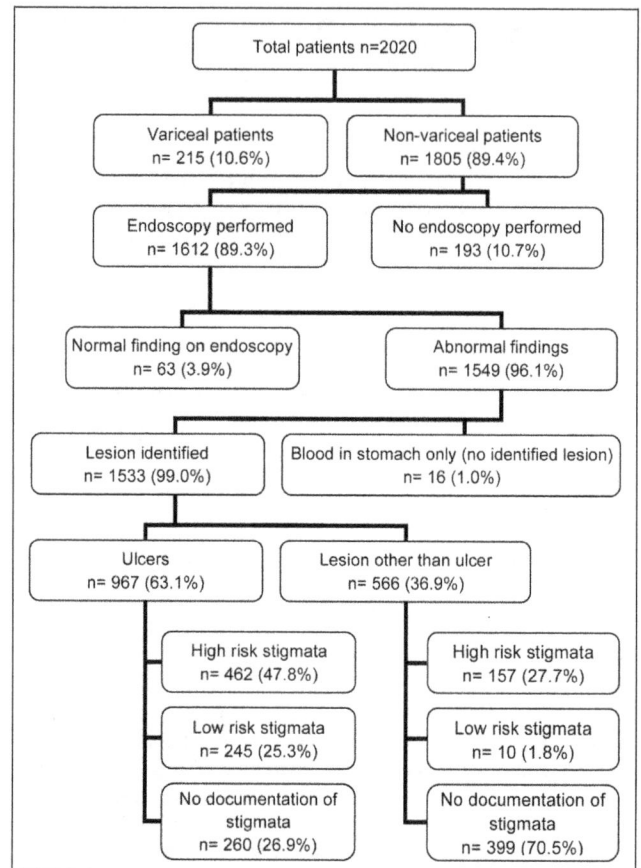

Figure 2) *Distribution of patients presenting with acute upper gastrointestinal bleeding according to endoscopic findings*

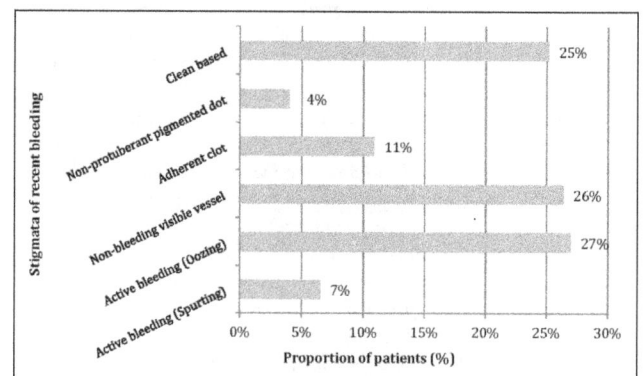

Figure 3) *Distribution of stigmata of recent bleeding in nonvariceal upper gastrointestinal (ulcer and nonulcer lesions). Data representing stigmata from the lesion most likely to be the source of bleeding are shown*

Pharmacotherapy: High-dose IV PPI (80 mg bolus followed by continuous infusion) was administered to 95.7% of patients with HRS after successful endoscopic hemostasis. Overall, 91.5% of patients with LRS received high-dose IV PPI after endoscopy, irrespective of endoscopic therapy.

H pylori testing and treatment: H pylori status was available on presentation for 10.8% of patients (7.5% positive, 3.3% negative). Thirty-six percent of patients with NVUGIB were further tested for H pylori during the course of their hospitalization, with eradication therapy initiated in 9.2% who tested positive. No data regarding the confirmation of eradication were available.

Outcomes: Rebleeding occurred in 10.5% (190 of 1805) of patients, with an overall mortality rate of 9.4% (169 of 1805). A small proportion

TABLE 1
Endoscopy and pharmacotherapy in ulcer and nonvariceal nonulcer upper gastrointestinal bleeding

| | Endoscopic hemostasis | | | | Post-endoscopic IV PPI* | | | | |
| | Total, n | Any endoscopic hemostasis, n | Epinephrine injection monotherapy, % | Combination therapy, % | Total, n† | High-dose postendoscopic IV PPI‡, % | Duration of IV PPI§, % | | |
Endoscopic findings							24 h	48 h	72 h
All ulcers¶	967	403	14.7	13.8	609	94.3	96.2	94.2	93.6
Ulcers (HRS and LRS)	707	348	17.0	17.3	453	94.3	96.3	94.2	93.7
HRS	462	323	23.8	25.5	296	96.0	97.7	96.2	95.8
LRS	245	25	4.1	1.6	157	91.1	93.3	90.0	89.2
Ulcers without documented stigmata	260	55	8.5	4.2	156	94.2	95.7	94.0	93.2
All NVNU lesions**	566	135	5.7	2.7	361	88.6			
NVNU lesions (HRS and LRS)	167	76	10.8	6.6	111	95.5			
HRS	157	76	11.5	7.0	103	95.2			
LRS	10	0	0.0	0.0	8	100.0			
NVNU without documented stigmata	399	59	3.5	1.0	250	85.6			
Total (ulcer and NVNU)	1533	538	11.4	9.7	970	92.2			
Total (HRS and LRS)	874	424	15.8	15.2	564	94.5			
Total HRS	619	399	20.7	20.8	399	95.7			
Total LRS	25	25	3.9	1.6	165	91.5			
Total without documented stigmata	659	114	5.5	2.3	406	88.9			

*Postendoscopic intravenous (IV) proton pump inhibitor (PPI) includes IV PPI therapy started after endoscopic therapy or continued if previous started pre-endoscopy; †Total number of patients who received postendoscopic PPI excluding those with missing information; ‡High-dose IV PPI defined as 80 mg IV bolus followed by 8 mg/h infusion started after endoscopic therapy or continued if started pre-endoscopy; §Data reported only for ulcer bleeding; ¶Includes ulcers with high-risk stigmata (HRS), ulcers with low-risk stigmata (LRS) and ulcers without documentation of stigmata; **Includes nonvariceal nonulcer (NVNU) lesions with HRS, NVNU lesions with LRS and NVNU lesions without documentation of stigmata

of patients (47 of 1805 [2.5%]) required surgery, while 1.2% (22 of 1805) required interventional radiology to control their bleeding. Of the patients who developed UGIB while hospitalized for another reason (n=356), rates of rebleeding, need for surgery and mortality were 14.4%, 1.4% and 21.9%, respectively. Length of hospital stay was, on average, six days. Patients with NVUGIB who were admitted to the intensive care unit were discharged to the floor after a median of 5.8±10.1 days.

Adherence to guidelines: The data from REASON were applicable to 13 of the 23 consensus recommendations (5) (Table 2). Comparing current adherence rates with data with a quantitative analysis of appropriateness in Canadian practice patterns performed before guidelines publication (4), higher adherence was noted in 67% (eight of 12) of the recommendations (Figure 4). Two recommendations showed arithmetically decreased adherence rates (two of 12 [17%]), namely the performance of early endoscopy within 24 h and endoscopic hemostatic therapy in HRS. Comparison was not performed for one recommendation due to the lack of preguideline values.

Predictors of adherence: *Predictors of recommended use of endoscopic resources:* Multivariable analysis revealed that the presence of qualified assistants during endoscopy occurred more frequently when endoscopy was performed during regular hours (OR 2.9 [95% CI 2.21 to 3.81]). In contrast, patients with low ASA classification (1 to 2) more often underwent endoscopy without assistance from support staff (OR 0.63 [95% CI 0.48 to 0.83]) (Table 3). Furthermore, the targeted delay of <24 h from presentation for early endoscopy was less likely to be met when an endoscopy was performed during regular hours (OR 0.33 [95% CI 0.24 to 0.47]). High Blatchford scores of 3 to 11 predicted the performance of endoscopic therapy in patients with HRS (OR 1.67 [95% CI 1.03 to 2.70]). No such predictors were identified to influence rates of endoscopic hemostasis in patients with LRS.

Predictors of recommended use of pharmacotherapy: The administration of high-dose IV PPI, which was not otherwise indicated in patients with LRS, was noted more frequently in patients with a presenting hemoglobin level <70 g/L (OR 6.84 [95% CI 1.97 to 23.76]). This practice was less often encountered in patients who were on

antithrombotic therapy (OR 0.39 [95% CI 0.20 to 0.79]). No significant factors impacting on the use of high-dose acid suppressant were identified among patients with HRS. Significant predictors of adherence to the different recommendations and their respective ORs and 95% CIs are listed in Table 3.

DISCUSSION

The assessment of quality of care in the management of patients with NVUGIB extends beyond the sole measurement of clinical outcomes, especially in view of high-level evidence now available to guide best practice. Process-based measures (9) were applied to REASON, a retrospective multicentre national registry of 2020 patients, to evaluate the quality of care in NVUGIB in Canada. Compared with data collected before the publication of consensus guidelines (4,5), REASON demonstrates an improved adherence across over one-half of the recommendations, the median adherence remains low (65.6%).

While the process of care is a dynamic exchange of events (8) and may preclude rigid application of guideline recommendations, adherence to guidelines remains an important surrogate of quality measurement. Such data for NVUGIB are scarce, with some reports suggesting marked differences in practice across countries (13) and suboptimal uptake of national guidelines (14). Predictors of adherence are poorly defined in the literature, even though some have been suggested as a result of a multifaceted randomized educational intervention for guideline dissemination (15). Inferential testing performed as part of the REASON data analysis shed some light on possible discrepancies between observed practice and existing guidelines. These are discussed below.

Areas where practice can be further improved include the implementation of a protocol to manage UGIB and access to adequate endoscopy assistance, even out-of-hours (recommendations 1 and 2). Interestingly, a low ASA class was associated with the absence of an assistant during endoscopy, independent of the time to endoscopy, suggesting a relaxing of standards for cases perceived to be less urgent or more stable.

Attention should be drawn to the use of appropriate resuscitation (recommendation 3) and transfusion thresholds because they impact

TABLE 2
Recommendation statements with associated adherence rates after guideline publication

	Recommendation statement (5)	Adherence, % (95% CI)
1	Hospitals should develop institution-specific protocols for multidisciplinary management, which should include access to an endoscopist with training in endoscopic hemostasis	52 (32.4–71.7)
2	Support staff trained to assist in endoscopy should be available for urgent endoscopy	83.5 (59.4–92.9)
3	Immediate evaluation and appropriate resuscitation are critical to proper management	N/A (–)
4	In selected patients, the placement of a nasogastric tube can be considered because the findings may have prognostic value	22 (20.4–24.0)
5A*	Clinical (nonendoscopic) stratification of patients into low- and high-risk categories for rebleeding and mortality is important for proper management. Available prognostic scales may be used to assist in decision making	N/A (–)
5B*	Early stratification of patients into low- and high-risk categories for rebleeding and mortality, based on clinical and endoscopic criteria, is important for proper management. Available prognostic scales may be used to assist in decision making	N/A (–)
6*	Early endoscopy (within the first 24 h) with risk classification by clinical and endoscopic criteria allows for safe and prompt discharge of patients classified as low risk; improves patient outcomes for patients classified as high risk and reduces resource use for patients classified as either low or high risk	65.6 (62.7–68.4)
7A	A finding of low-risk endoscopic stigmata (a clean-based ulcer or nonprotuberant pigmented dot in ulcer bed) is not an indication for endoscopic hemostatic therapy	90.2 (85.3–93.0)
7B*	Endoscopic hemostatic therapy is indicated for a patient with a clot in an ulcer bed, including targeted irrigation in an attempt at dislodgment, with appropriate treatment of the underlying lesion	N/A (–)
7C	A finding of high-risk endoscopic stigmata (active bleeding, nonbleeding visible vessel and/or adherent clot) in an indication for immediate endoscopic hemostatic therapy	64.5 (60.6–68.1)
8*	No single solution for endoscopic injection therapy is superior to another for hemostasis	N/A (–)
9	No single method of endoscopic thermal coaptive therapy is superior to another	N/A (–)
10*	Monotherapy, with injection or thermal coagulation, is an effective endoscopic hemostatic technique for high-risk stigmata; however, the combination is superior to either treatment alone	N/A (–)
11*	The placement of clips is a promising endoscopic hemostatic therapy for high-risk stigmata	14.3 (11.2–18.1)
12†	Routine second-look endoscopy is not recommended	91.0 (89.5–92.3)
13	In case of rebleeding, a second attempt at endoscopic therapy is generally recommended	56.7 (49.2–63.9)
14	Surgical consultation should be sought for patients who have failed endoscopic therapy	N/A (–)
15	H_2-receptor antagonists are not recommended in the management of patients with acute upper gastrointestinal bleeding	95.1 (94.1–96.0)
16	Somatostatin and octreotide are not recommended in the routine management of patients with acute nonvariceal upper gastrointestinal bleeding	100 (100)
17†	An intravenous bolus followed by continuous proton pump inhibitor infusion is effective in decreasing rebleeding in patients who have undergone successful endoscopic therapy	95.7 (93.2–97.4)
18*	In patients awaiting endoscopy, empirical therapy with a high-dose proton pump inhibitor should be considered	54.4 (51.8–57.2)
19	Patients considered at low risk for rebleeding after endoscopy can be fed within 24 h	N/A (–)
20*	Patients with upper gastrointestinal bleeding should be tested for Helicobacter pylori and receive eradication therapy if infection is present	N/A (–)

Recommendations that have been revised in the 2010 guidelines (7); †Statement updated from 2003 guidelines, but no change in the actual recommendation in the 2010 guidelines (7). N/A Not applicable

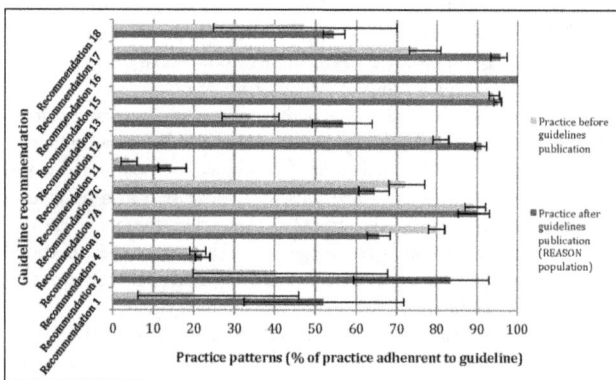

Figure 4) *Adherence to recommendations comparing practice before and after guidelines publication. *Guidelines in which collected data were insufficient to assess adherence are not included; **Data before guidelines publication were not available for recommendation 16. REASON Registry of patients undergoing Endoscopic and/or Acid Suppression therapy and an Outcome analysis for upper gastrointestinal bleediNg*

TABLE 3
Selected predictors of guideline adherence showing statistical significance

Recommendation with associated predictors of adherence	OR (95% CI)
Presence of assistants during endoscopy	
American Society of Anesthesiologists class 1 to 2	0.63 (0.48–0.83)
Endoscopy performed during regular hours*	2.9 (2.21–3.81)
Early endoscopy <24 h	
Endoscopy performed during regular hours*	0.33 (0.24–0.47)
Endoscopic therapy in patients with high-risk stigmata	
Blatchford score 3 to 11	1.67 (1.03–2.70)
High-dose IV PPI administration in patients with low-risk stigmata	
Presenting hemoglobin level <70 g/L	6.84 (1.97–23.76)
Use of antithrombotics	0.39 (0.20–0.79)

Regular hours endoscopy defined as Monday to Friday, 08:00 to 17:00. IV PPI Intravenous proton pump inhibitor

rebleeding and survival rates in UGIB (16). The mean initial hemoglobin value in REASON was 98.0±27.8 g/L, comparable with RUGBE (3) and the recent randomized control trial by Villanueva et al (16). Over the first 24 h, only 16.8% of those who received a transfusion had a presenting hemoglobin level ≤70 g/L. Of note, this proportion includes all patients, regardless of associated cardiovascular morbidity and hemodynamic status, a group excluded, in large part, by inclusion criteria in the large multisite Spanish trial (16).

The administration of IV PPIs before endoscopy is common (54.4%) even though their use is considered to be optional (recommendation 18) and no longer supported in recent United Kingdom guidelines (17) despite some clinical settings identified as possibly cost effective (18).

Overall, 65.6% of patients underwent early endoscopy within the recommended 24 h (recommendation 6). The point estimate is inferior to the 76% reported in RUGBE and European values ranging from 70% to 93% (13), while remaining superior to the 55% value reported in a true United Kingdom national bleeding audit (19). Additionally, longer delays (>24 h) to endoscopy were associated with the endoscopies being performed during regular hours. This suggests that some patients have their endoscopy postponed until regular working hours, even if this results in delays exceeding 24 h, perhaps because of limited out-of-hours support. Consistent with guidelines (20), patients with suspected variceal bleeding nevertheless underwent endoscopy significantly earlier, with a median of 12.4 h compared with 18.3 h for patients with NVUGIB (P=0.0038).

At endoscopy, even though lesions were identified in the great majority of cases after one or multiple endoscopies, a substantial proportion of endoscopy reports (26.9% for ulcers) failed to document the severity of the stigmata of recent bleeding. Such a high value is unsettling because this information is needed for adequate risk stratification into high- and low-risk categories, which in turn is crucial for appropriate endoscopic and pharmacological management (recommendation 5) Failure to record endoscopic stigmata was even more frequent (70.5%) among patients with nonvariceal, nonulcer bleeding, although both groups carry similar risk for unfavourable outcomes (21).

Patients exhibiting LRS do not require endoscopic therapy (recommendation 7A). Nonetheless, 9.8% of patients with LRS received endoscopic hemostasis in REASON, exceeding the 2.6% noted in an Italian prospective survey (22), although significantly inferior to a 24% endoscopic treatment rate for pigmented spots reported in the Clinical Outcomes Research Initiative database (23).

In contradistinction, although endoscopic hemostasis of lesions with HRS has clearly been shown to be associated with significant decreases in rebleeding, need for surgery and mortality (24) (recommendation 7C), adherence to such practice is suboptimal, with rates of 64.5% across all patients with NVUGIB and 69.9% among patients with ulcers. Reported rates of endoscopic treatment in high-risk patients in the literature range from 74% (3) to 85% (22,23). A French multicentre cohort proposes the lack of trained endoscopic assistance and out-of-hours endoscopy as possible factors for such practice (14).

The rate of injection monotherapy in REASON was 20.7%. This practice is not consistent with guidelines that rather suggest the added value of combination therapy (recommendation 10); it is, nonetheless, improved compared with the preguidelines value of 39% (3). Furthermore, IV PPI administration following successful endoscopy reached 95.7%, also superior to the previously reported 70.5% (recommendation 17). The only significant predictor of poor adherence in this regard was a low presenting hemoglobin level, which was associated with the use of high-dose IV PPI even in patients exhibiting LRS.

REASON did not record eradication rates, but reveals that H pylori testing (recommendation 20) was performed in only one-third of patients.

The REASON registry informs 'real life' practice in the management of UGIB, although it is limited by its retrospective nature. Our sampling excluded patients discharged from the emergency room,

although it includes patients already hospitalized who develop a secondary diagnosis of UGIB, a subset at higher risk for complications (25). Missing data inherent to retrospective chart analyses somewhat undermine the accuracy of the calculated guideline adherence rates, although our values remain within ranges reported in the literature. Furthermore, the selected predictors of guideline adherence evaluated in our multivariate analysis may not be exhaustive and should be interpreted as exploratory because objective data regarding such predictors are scarce.

The above observations identify both areas of discrepant clinical care and some possible reasons for poor adherence that may guide future guideline dissemination initiatives. However, the impact of such educational efforts is often only modest. In fact, recent national data obtained from a 48-site cluster randomized clinical trial show that a multifaceted educational intervention over a 12-month period to disseminate UGIB guidelines did not improve adherence (15). The issue of low guideline adherence is longstanding and complex involving attitude, knowledge, contextual and behavioural barriers (26,27). Alternatively, the development of quality indicators using a list of more context-specific detailed clinical scenarios (28) may further help clinicians to reconcile 'best practice' in 'real-life' settings.

CONCLUSION
The process-based measures from the REASON registry reveal variable adherence to 'best practice' in NVUGIB in Canada. Proper endoscopic documentation, and adequate use of appropriate pharmacological and endoscopic therapy are key elements that clinicians should target to improve quality of care in NVUGIB. Both patient- and process-related factors may predict guideline adherence, or its lack. More precise characterization of such variables can help identify both clinician and patient subgroups for interventions, enhancing clinical management.

GRANT SUPPORT: The REASON study was funded by an at-arms-length grant from Astra Zeneca Canada Inc for the data collection; they had no participation, nor input for the present article.

DISCLOSURES: The authors have no financial disclosures or conflicts of interest to declare.

AUTHOR CONTRIBUTIONS: Alan Barkun contributed to the conception, drafting and final approval of the work; Yidan Lu contributed to the conception, drafting and final approval of the work; Myriam Martel contributed to the conception, statistical analysis, drafting and final approval of the work; The REASON investigators contributed to the data collection of the REASON registry.

REASON INVESTIGATORS: David Armstrong, Alan Barkun, Raymond Bourdages, Marc Bradette, Ford Bursey, Naoki Chiba, Alan Cockeram, Gilbert Doummar, Carlo Fallone, James Gregor, Robert Hilsden, Gilles Jobin, Raymond Lahaie, Gaetano Morelli, Pardeep Nijhawan, Kenneth Render, Alaa Rostom, Gurpal Sandha, Thomas Sylwestrowicz, Sander Veldhuyzen van Zanten and Lawrence Worobetz.

REFERENCES
1. Hearnshaw SA, Logan RF, Lowe D, Travis SP, Murphy MF, Palmer KR. Use of endoscopy for management of acute upper gastrointestinal bleeding in the UK: Results of a nationwide audit. Gut 2010;59:1022-9.
2. Laine L, Yang H, Chang SC, Datto C. Trends for incidence of hospitalization and death due to GI complications in the United States from 2001 to 2009. Am J Gastroenterol 2012;107:1190-5.
3. Barkun A, Sabbah S, Enns R, et al. The Canadian Registry on Nonvariceal Upper Gastrointestinal Bleeding and Endoscopy (RUGBE): Endoscopic hemostasis and proton pump inhibition are associated with improved outcomes in a real-life setting. Am J Gastroenterol 2004;99:1238-46.

4. Bensoussan K, Fallone CA, Barkun AN, Martel M. A sampling of Canadian practice in managing nonvariceal upper gastrointestinal bleeding before recent guideline publication: Is there room for improvement? Can J Gastroenterol 2005;19:487-95.

5. Barkun A, Bardou M, Marshall JK. Consensus recommendations for managing patients with nonvariceal upper gastrointestinal bleeding. Ann Intern Med 2003;139:843-57.

6. British Society of Gastroenterology Endoscopy Committee. Non-variceal upper gastrointestinal haemorrhage: Guidelines. Gut 2002;(51 Suppl 4):iv1-6.

7. Barkun AN, Bardou M, Kuipers EJ, et al. International consensus recommendations on the management of patients with nonvariceal upper gastrointestinal bleeding. Ann Intern Med 2010;152:101-13.

8. Esrailian E, Gralnek IM, Jensen D, et al. Evaluating the process of care in nonvariceal upper gastrointestinal haemorrhage: A survey of expert vs. non-expert gastroenterologists. Aliment Pharmacol Ther 2008;28:1199-208.

9. Palmer RH. Process-based measures of quality: The need for detailed clinical data in large health care databases. Ann Intern Med 1997;127(8 Pt 2):733-8.

10. Donabedian A. The quality of care. How can it be assessed? JAMA 1988;260:1743-8.

11. Lau JY, Sung JJ, Lee KK, et al. Effect of intravenous omeprazole on recurrent bleeding after endoscopic treatment of bleeding peptic ulcers. N Engl J Med 2000;343:310-6.

12. Daneshmend TK, Hawkey CJ, Langman MJ, Logan RF, Long RG, Walt RP. Omeprazole versus placebo for acute upper gastrointestinal bleeding: Randomised double blind controlled trial. BMJ 1992;304:143-7.

13. Lanas A, Aabakken L, Fonseca J, et al. Variability in the management of nonvariceal upper gastrointestinal bleeding in Europe: An observational study. Adv Ther 2012;29:1026-36.

14. Zeitoun JD, Rosa-Hezode I, Chryssostalis A, et al. Epidemiology and adherence to guidelines on the management of bleeding peptic ulcer: A prospective multicenter observational study in 1140 patients. Clin Res Hepatol Gastroenterol 2012;36:227-34.

15. Barkun AN, Bhat M, Armstrong D, et al. Effectiveness of disseminating consensus management recommendations for ulcer bleeding: A cluster randomized trial. CMAJ 2013;185:E156-66.

16. Villanueva C, Colomo A, Bosch A, et al. Transfusion strategies for acute upper gastrointestinal bleeding. N Engl J Med 2013;368:11-21.

17. National Institute for Health and Clinical Excellence (NICE). Gastrointestinal bleeding: The management of acute upper gastrointestinal bleeding 2012 [updated June 2012; cited 2013 December 12]. <http://guidance.nice.org.uk/CG141> (Accessed April 3, 2014).

18. Barkun AN. Should every patient with suspected upper GI bleeding receive a proton pump inhibitor while awaiting endoscopy? Gastrointest Endosc 2008;67:1064-6.

19. Jairath V, Kahan BC, Logan RF, et al. Mortality from acute upper gastrointestinal bleeding in the United kingdom: Does it display a "weekend effect"? Am J Gastroenterol 2011;106:1621-8.

20. Garcia-Tsao G, Sanyal AJ, Grace ND, Carey WD; Practice Guidelines Committee of American Association for Study of Liver Disease, Practice Parameters Committee of American College of Gastroenterology. Prevention and management of gastroesophageal varices and variceal hemorrhage in cirrhosis. Am J Gastroenterol 2007;102:2086-102.

21. Marmo R, Del Piano M, Rotondano G, et al. Mortality from nonulcer bleeding is similar to that of ulcer bleeding in high-risk patients with nonvariceal hemorrhage: A prospective database study in Italy. Gastrointest Endosc 2012;75:263-72, 72 e1.

22. Loperfido S, Baldo V, Piovesana E, et al. Changing trends in acute upper-GI bleeding: A population-based study. Gastrointest Endosc 2009;70:212-24.

23. Enestvedt BK, Gralnek IM, Mattek N, Lieberman DA, Eisen GM. Endoscopic therapy for peptic ulcer hemorrhage: Practice variations in a multi-center U.S. consortium. Dig Dis Sci 2010;55:2568-76.

24. Cook DJ, Guyatt GH, Salena BJ, Laine LA. Endoscopic therapy for acute nonvariceal upper gastrointestinal hemorrhage: A meta-analysis. Gastroenterology 1992;102:139-48.

25. Muller T, Barkun AN, Martel M. Non-variceal upper GI bleeding in patients already hospitalized for another condition. Am J Gastroenterol 2009;104:330-9.

26. Cabana MD, Rand CS, Powe NR, et al. Why don't physicians follow clinical practice guidelines? A framework for improvement. JAMA 1999;282:1458-65.

27. Hayes SM, Murray S, Dupuis M, Dawes M, Hawes IA, Barkun AN. Barriers to the implementation of practice guidelines in managing patients with nonvariceal upper gastrointestinal bleeding: A qualitative approach. Can J Gastroenterol 2010;24:289-96.

28. Kanwal F, Barkun A, Gralnek IM, et al. Measuring quality of care in patients with nonvariceal upper gastrointestinal hemorrhage: Development of an explicit quality indicator set. Am J Gastroenterol 2010;105:1710-8.

5

Use of fecal occult blood testing in hospitalized patients: Results of an audit

Stephen Ip MD[1], AbdulRazaq AH Sokoro PhD[1,2,3], Lisa Kaita BN[4], Claudia Ruiz BA[4],
Elaine McIntyre RN[4], Harminder Singh MD MPH[1,5,6,7]

S Ip, AAH Sokoro, L Kaita, C Ruiz, E McIntyre, H Singh. Use of fecal occult blood testing in hospitalized patients: Results of an audit. Can J Gastroenterol Hepatol 2014;28(9):489-494.

BACKGROUND: The fecal occult blood test (FOBT), widely used as a colorectal cancer screening tool, continues to be used in hospitalized patients. However, the utility of this test for hospitalized patients is unclear.

OBJECTIVE: To assess FOBT use in a large urban regional health authority.

METHODS: Reports of all FOBTs performed between April 1, 2011 and March 30, 2012 from two academic and four community hospitals in Winnipeg (Manitoba) were extracted. Of 650 hospitalizations with a positive FOBT result and 1254 with a negative FOBT result, random samples of 230 and 97 charts, respectively, were reviewed. Information including demographics, admission diagnos(es), indication(s) for ordering the FOBT and clinical management was extracted.

RESULTS: Thirty-four percent (650 of 1904) of hospitalizations with an FOBT had a positive FOBT result. Family medicine physicians ordered approximately one-half of the reviewed FOBTs. The most common indication for ordering an FOBT was anemia. Of those with a positive FOBT, 66% did not undergo further gastrointestinal investigations. Of those with a positive FOBT and overt gastrointestinal bleeding and/or melena who underwent endoscopy, 60% had their endoscopy performed before the FOBT result being reported while 38% underwent their endoscopy ≥3 days after the stool sample was collected. There were minimal differences in clinical practices between academic and community hospitals.

CONCLUSIONS: The present study suggests that FOBT results in hospitalized patients may have little beneficial impact on clinical management. Hospital laboratories may be better served in directing resources to other tests.

Key Words: *Inpatients; Occult blood; Utilization*

La recherche de sang occulte dans les selles chez les patients hospitalisés : les résultats d'une vérification

HISTORIQUE : La recherche de sang occulte dans les selles (RSOS), généralisée comme outil de dépistage du cancer colorectal, continue d'être utilisée chez les patients hospitalisés, même si sa pertinence n'est pas claire dans cette population.

OBJECTIF : Évaluer la RSOS dans une grande régie régionale de la santé en milieu urbain.

MÉTHODOLOGIE : Les chercheurs ont extrait les rapports de toutes les RSOS effectuées entre le 1er avril 2011 et le 30 mars 2012 dans deux hôpitaux universitaires et quatre hôpitaux généraux de Winnipeg, au Manitoba. Sur les 650 hospitalisations dont le résultat de la RSOS était positif et 1 254 dont le résultat était négatif, ils ont analysé un échantillon aléatoire de 230 et 97 dossiers, respectivement. Ils en ont tiré les données démographiques, les diagnostics à l'admission, les indications pour demander une RSOS et la prise en charge clinique.

RÉSULTATS : Au total, 34 % des hospitalisés (650 sur 1 904) ayant subi une RSOS avaient obtenu des résultats positifs. Les médecins de famille avaient demandé environ la moitié des RSOS analysées. L'anémie était la principale indication. Chez les patients dont la RSOS était positive, 66 % n'avaient pas subi d'autres examens gastro-intestinaux. Parmi ceux dont la RSOS était positive, qui avaient des saignements gastro-intestinaux ou un méléna manifestes et avaient subi une endoscopie, 60 % l'avaient subie avant l'obtention des résultats de la RSOS, et 38 % au moins trois jours après la coproculture. Les pratiques cliniques différaient très peu entre les hôpitaux universitaires et les hôpitaux généraux.

CONCLUSIONS : D'après la présente étude, les résultats de la RSOS chez les patients hospitalisés auraient peu d'effets bénéfiques sur la prise en charge clinique. Les laboratoires des hôpitaux auraient avantage à orienter leurs ressources vers d'autres tests.

Although the fecal occult blood test (FOBT) was developed for use in the outpatient setting for colorectal cancer (CRC) screening, it continues to be used in hospitalized patients to detect gastrointestinal (GI) bleeding (GIB). However, several studies suggest that FOBT may have limited positive impact in hospitalized patients because it may not change management (ie, patients will undergo an endoscopy regardless of test results, such as those with obvious bleeding) or delay investigations while waiting for the result of the test (1-3). Inappropriate use of the FOBT can lead to unnecessary additional investigations (eg, colonoscopy), which carry their own risks and can limit the availability of such investigations for more appropriate indications.

Our health care region, the Winnipeg Regional Health Authority (WRHA), uses Hemoccult II Sensa (Beckman Coulter Inc, USA), a more sensitive version of the guaiac test. The utility of this test among hospitalized patients was not evaluated before its introduction.

Furthermore, data regarding FOBT use among hospitalized patients in Canada are also lacking.

The objectives of the present study were to assess indications for ordering FOBTs in hospitalized patients, determine the potential utility of its use in the hospital setting, and assess the current clinical practice and management of hospitalized patients with a positive FOBT according to Hemoccult II Sensa.

METHODS

Reports of all FOBTs performed between April 1, 2011 and March 30, 2012 from the laboratory databases of both the academic and all four community hospitals in Winnipeg, Manitoba (population 723,491 [4]) were extracted. A single regional health authority (WRHA) administers all hospitals in Winnipeg. All of the hospital laboratories in the WRHA exclusively use Hemoccult II Sensa.

[1]Department of Medicine; [2]Department of Pathology, University of Manitoba; [3]Diagnostic Services of Manitoba; [4]Winnipeg Regional Health Authority; [5]Department of Community Health Sciences, University of Manitoba; [6]Department of Hematology and Oncology, CancerCare Manitoba; [7]University of Manitoba IBD Clinical and Research Centre, Winnipeg, Manitoba
Correspondence: Dr Harminder Singh, Section of Gastroenterology, University of Manitoba, 805-715 McDermott Avenue, Winnipeg, Manitoba R3E 3P4. e-mail harminder.singh@med.umanitoba.ca

TABLE 1
Description of positive and negative fecal occult blood test patients

	Fecal occult blood test	
	Positive (n=230)	Negative (n=97)
Sex		
Male	111 (48)	47 (49)
Female	119 (52)	50 (51)
Age, years, median (interquartile range)	76 (67–85)	75 (65–85)
Admission site		
Academic hospitals	105 (46)	27 (28)
Community hospitals	125 (54)	70 (72)
Comorbidities*		
Heart disease	94 (41)	44 (45)
Chronic obstructive pulmonary disease	46 (20)	11 (11)
Dementia	40 (17)	13 (13)
Active malignancy	32 (14)	4 (4)
Liver disease	21 (9)	5 (5)
Documented family history of CRC	3 (1)	0 (0)
Documented digital rectal examination	46 (20)	5 (5)
Medications†		
Acetylsalicylic acid	78 (33)	36 (37)
Vitamin C	37 (16)	5 (5)
Warfarin	36 (16)	2 (1)
Clopidogrel	20 (9)	7 (7)
Selective serotonin reuptake inhibitor	15 (7)	10 (10)
Nonsteroidal anti-inflammatory drug(s)	13 (6)	5 (5)

*Data presented as n (%) unless otherwise indicated. *Some patients had more than one comorbidity; †Some patients were taking more than one medication. CRC Colorectal cancer*

Of the 650 admissions with at least one positive FOBT result in the study time period, a random sample of 230 (approximately 35%) was selected.

During the same time period, there were 1254 admissions with a negative FOBT (with no concomitant positive FOBT). For comparison with those with a positive FOBT, a random sample of 97 (approximately 8%) of the patients with negative FOBT was selected. The focus was on individuals with a positive FOBT. Of those with multiple positive FOBTs, information circa the first positive result was abstracted.

Information including demographics, admission service (eg, internal medicine [IM]), admission diagnos(es), indication(s) for ordering the FOBT, diet orders, medications that could affect FOBT and clinical management of the patients (including performance of rectal examination and/or GI endoscopy) was extracted by a trained experienced nurse auditor (LK) and/or an IM resident (SI). Laboratory data collected include hemoglobin (Hb) values, coagulation values and iron studies before stool specimen collection. The types of consultation service input (gastroenterology, surgery and hematology) sought were also gathered. If an endoscopy was performed, findings were recorded. The day on which the FOBT was reported (with respect to the day the stool specimen was collected) was recorded to determine the relative timing of initiating a consultation or investigations and the reporting of FOBT results.

Also assessed was whether investigations were delayed while potentially waiting for FOBT reporting (eg, ≥3 days after ordering of FOBT among individuals in whom investigations for overt GIB were indicated irrespective of FOBT results). The prevalence of significant findings on endoscopy (eg, mass, actively bleeding lesions, etc) were assessed among individuals with a positive FOBT result and determined whether there were other indications (eg, iron deficiency anemia [IDA]) that should have resulted in endoscopy in those with clinically significant findings irrespective of the FOBT results.

TABLE 2
Medical specialty of the physician ordering fecal occult blood test

	Fecal occult blood test	
Specialty	Positive (n=230)	Negative (n=97)
Family medicine	104 (45)	54 (56)
Internal medicine	43 (19)	19 (20)
Orthopedics	23 (10)	6 (6)
Intensive care	19 (8)	0 (0)
Psychiatry	8 (4)	5 (5)
General surgery	8 (4)	3 (3)
Nephrology	8 (4)	2 (2)
Cardiology	4 (2)	3 (3)
Neurosurgery	3 (1)	0 (0)
Cardiac surgery	2 (1)	1 (1)
Oncology	2 (1)	0 (0)
Gynecology	2 (1)	0 (0)
Respiratory medicine	2 (1)	0 (0)
Gastroenterology	1 (1)	1 (1)
Vascular surgery	1 (1)	0 (0)
Emergency medicine	0 (0)	1 (1)
Plastic surgery	0 (0)	1 (1)

Data presented as n (%)

Comparisons between the positive FOBT and negative FOBT groups were performed using Fisher's exact test using GraphPad Prism (GraphPad Inc, USA). Potential differences in FOBT ordering practices and clinical management among different admitting specialties, as well as differences between academic and community hospitals, were assessed. Statistical significance was set at P<0.05 (two-tailed).

The present study was approved by the Research Ethics Board of the University of Manitoba (Winnipeg, Manitoba).

RESULTS

Demographic characteristics

There were 1904 hospitalizations with ≥1 FOBT(s) performed; of these, 34% (n=650) had at least one positive FOBT result. Of 230 admitted patients with a positive FOBT whose charts were reviewed, approximately 50% were male and the median age was 76 years (interquartile range [IQR] 67 to 84 years) (Table 1). The negative FOBT group consisted of 97 patients (Table 1), of which 50% were male and the median age was 79 years (IQR 65 to 85 years). An equal proportion of positive FOBTs were from academic and community hospitals, but negative FOBTs were more commonly found in community hospitals (27% versus 78%). In both groups (positive and negative FOBTs), the most common documented comorbidities were heart disease, chronic obstructive pulmonary disease and dementia. One percent of those with a positive FOBT had a family history of CRC compared with none among those with a negative FOBT.

For both the positive and negative FOBT groups (Table 2), the most common subspecialty to order an FOBT was family medicine (FM) (45% versus 56%) followed by IM (19% versus 20%) and orthopedics (10% versus 6%), respectively (even though IM provide care for a higher proportion of admitted patients in the city than FM). The attending physicians themselves ordered the FOBTs for 44% of those with positive FOBT and 58% for those with negative FOBT; residents and physician extenders ordered the rest.

No patients received advice regarding dietary or medication restrictions before completing an FOBT.

Clinical features

The most common indication for ordering an FOBT was anemia (87% versus 85% for the positive and negative FOBT groups, respectively) (Table 3). A digital rectal examination was documented among only

TABLE 3
Indications* for ordering a fecal occult blood test (FOBT)

	FOBT		
	Positive[†]	Negative[‡]	
Indication	(n=226)	(n=87)	P
Anemia	196 (87)	74 (85)	0.72
Black stools	63 (28)	5 (6)	<0.01
Overt gastrointestinal bleeding	29 (13)	3 (4)	0.01
Upper gastrointestinal bleeding	15 (7)	1 (1)	0.05
Rectal bleeding	14 (6)	2 (2)	0.25
Gastrointestinal symptoms	39 (17)	12 (14)	0.86
Nonbloody diarrhea	23 (10)	6 (8)	0.51
Abdominal pain or distension	6 (4)	2 (2)	1.00
Weight loss or weakness	2 (1)	2 (2)	0.31
Nausea or vomiting	2 (1)	2 (2)	0.31
Dysphagia	2 (1)	0 (0)	1.00
Bloody diarrhea	3 (1)	1 (1)	1.00
Iron deficiency anemia	2 (1)	1 (1)	1.00
Colorectal cancer screening	1 (1)	1 (1)	0.46
Before initiating anticoagulation	1 (1)	1 (1)	0.46

*Data presented as n (%) unless otherwise indicted. *Some patients had more than one indication for ordering an FOBT; [†]Indication could not be determined in four cases; [‡]Indication could not be determined in 10 cases*

TABLE 4
Percentage of documented and abnormal* laboratory values

	Positive FOBT (n=230)		Negative FOBT (n=97)	
	Documented	Abnormal	Documented	Abnormal
Hb	199 (87)	177/199 (90)[†]	76 (78)	72/76 (95)
INR	108 (47)	63/108 (58)	32 (33)	18/32 (56)
Ferritin	65 (28)	4/65 (12)	44 (45)	6/44 (14)
Fe	77 (34)	45/77 (58)	37 (38)	24/37 (65)
TIBC	77 (34)	56/77 (73)	37 (38)	18/37 (49)

*Data presented as n (%) or n/n (%). *Abnormal refers to values outside the lower limits of normal (for age and sex) for hemoglobin (Hb), ferritin and iron (Fe). For international normalized ratio (INR), abnormal refers to values outside the higher limits of normal; [†]Percentage of abnormal laboratory values was calculated according to the number of documented laboratory values. FOBT Fecal occult blood test; TIBC Total iron binding capacity*

TABLE 5
Types and timeline of consultations sought

	Fecal occult blood test (FOBT)		
	Positive	Negative	
	(n=230)	(n=97)	P
Any consult	165 (72)	28 (29)	<0.01
Gastroenterology	108 (47)	18 (19)	<0.01
General surgery	37 (16)	5 (5)	0.01
Hematology	20 (4)	5 (5)	0.36
No consult	65 (28)	71 (71)	<0.01
Gastroenterology consult			
Before FOBT reporting	34/108 (32)*	5/18 (28)	1.00
After FOBT reporting	61/108 (57)	11/18 (61)	0.80
Could not be determined	13/108 (12)	2/18 (11)	1.00
General surgery consult			
Before FOBT reporting	14/37 (38)	2/5 (40)	1.00
After FOBT reporting	18/37 (49)	2/5 (40)	1.00
Could not be determined	5/37 (14)	1/5 (20)	0.56
Hematology consult			
Before FOBT reporting	11/20 (55)	3/5 (60)	1.00
After FOBT reporting	8/20 (40)	2/5 (40)	1.00
Could not be determined	1/20 (5)	0/5 (0)	1.00

*Data presented as n(%) or n/n (%) unless otherwise indicated. *Percentage calculated according to the total number of consults*

TABLE 6
Gastrointestinal endoscopies performed during hospitalization

	Fecal occult blood test		
	Positive (n=230)	Negative (n=97)	P
Endoscopy*	77 (33)	9 (9)	<0.01
Gastroscopy	68 (30)	6 (6)	<0.01
Colonoscopy	35 (15)	4 (4)	<0.01
Other[†]	1 (1)	1 (1)	0.51
No endoscopy	153 (67)	88 (91)	<0.01

*Data presented as n (%) unless otherwise indicated. *Patients may have undergone more than one endoscopy; [†]Includes capsule endoscopy and push enteroscopy*

20% with a positive FOBT compared with 5% among those with a negative FOBT (Table 1). Approximately one-half of patients were taking acetylsalicylic acid (Table 1).

Laboratory values
An Hb value was measured before ordering an FOBT in 87% of the positive FOBT group compared with 78% in the negative FOBT group (Table 4). An international normalized ratio was measured in 47% of positive FOBT group and in 33% of the negative FOBT group. A ferritin level was ordered in 28% of the positive FOBT group compared with 45% in the negative FOBT group. Iron saturation (ratio of serum iron to total iron binding capacity) was measured in 33% of the positive FOBT and 38% of the negative FOBT group. Approximately one-third (37%) of patients with a positive FOBT and 42% of patients with a negative FOBT had no iron studies (ferritin, iron or total iron binding capacity) ordered before stool specimen collection.

In both FOBT groups (Table 4), >90% of Hb values were lower than the normal range. International normalized ratio was elevated above the normal range in ≥50% in both groups. Ferritin level was abnormally low in approximately 15% of patients in both groups in whom it was measured.

FOBT reporting
Approximately 80% of FOBTs were reported three to four days after sample collection. Laboratory protocols dictate that any sample collected without adherence to test dietary requirements be incubated (on the inoculated card) at room temperature for three days to allow for degradation of nonheme peroxidase activity in the collected samples.

Types and timing of consultations
Among individuals with a positive FOBT, a consultation request to gastroenterology, general surgery or hematology service was more likely to be initiated compared with those with a negative FOBT (72% versus 29%: P<0.01) (Table 5). Up to 60% of all consultations were sought before a FOBT result was reported (Table 5).

Endoscopy types and findings
As expected, patients with a positive FOBT were more likely to receive an inpatient endoscopy compared with those with a negative FOBT (34% versus 9%; P<0.01) (Table 6). Among individuals with a positive FOBT who underwent endoscopy, 88% had a gastroscopy while 45% underwent a colonoscopy. The most common findings on gastroscopy were ulcer(s) (38%), normal findings (18%) and esophagitis (15%) (Table 7). The most common findings on colonoscopy were diverticular disease (32%), polyp(s) (29%) and normal findings (13%) (Table 7). Eight (3%) patients in the positive FOBT group and three (3%) in the negative FOBT group had recommendations for an outpatient endoscopy.

There were five documented masses within the positive FOBT group: four found on colonoscopy and one found on upper endoscopy.

TABLE 7
Endoscopic findings* among individuals who underwent one or more endoscopic evaluation(s), stratified according to positive and negative fecal occult blood test (FOBT)

	Positive FOBT	Negative FOBT
Gastroscopy†	76 (100)	8 (100)
Ulcer	29 (38)	3 (38)
Normal	14 (18)	3 (38)
Esophagitis	11 (15)	3 (38)
Gastritis	7 (9)	0 (0)
Stricture	3 (4)	0 (0)
Arteriovenous malformation	2 (3)	1 (13)
Polyp	1 (1)	1 (13)
Mass	1 (1)	0 (0)
Colonoscopy†	38 (100)	4 (100)
Diverticular disease	12 (32)	1 (25)
Polyp	11 (29)	1 (25)
Normal	5 (13)	0 (0)
Ulcer	5 (13)	0 (0)
Mass	4 (11)	0 (0)
Hemorrhoids	4 (11)	2 (50)
Inflammatory bowel disease	1 (3)	0 (0)

Data presented as n (%). *Some patients had more than one finding on endoscopy; †Some patients underwent more than one endoscopy during their admission

TABLE 8
Comparison among subspecialties for admissions with positive fecal occult blood test (FOBT)

	Subspecialty			
	FM (n=103)	IM (n=42)	Other* (n=81)	P
Indication(s)†				
Anemia	91 (88)	37 (88)	68 (84)	0.66
Black stools	27 (26)	9 (21)	27 (33)	0.34
Overt GIB	5 (5)	7 (17)	17 (21)	<0.01
GI symptoms	19 (18)	8 (19)	12 (15)	0.80
Bloody diarrhea	1 (1)	1 (2)	1 (1)	0.76
Iron deficiency anemia	0 (0)	1 (2)	1 (1)	0.30
CRC screening	1 (1)	0 (0)	0 (0)	1.00
Before initiating anticoagulants	0 (0)	1 (2)	0 (0)	0.19
Consultations				
Gastroenterology	47 (45)	26 (61)	35 (42)	0.12
Surgery	6 (6)	3 (7)	28 (34)	<0.01
Consulting before reporting of FOBT result				
Gastroenterology	11/47 (23)	10/26 (39)	13/35 (37)	0.28
Surgery	1/6 (16)	1/3 (33)	12/28 (43)	0.61

Data presented as n (%) or n/n (%) unless otherwise indicated. *Includes surgical subspecialties; †Some patients had more than one indication for ordering an FOBT. CRC Colorectal cancer; FM Family medicine; GI Gastrointestinal; GIB GI bleeding; IM Internal medicine

All cases had IDA; one of these cases also had a family history of CRC. There were no other actively bleeding lesions.

Clinical management of the positive FOBT group
When the positive FOBT group was further examined, there were 86 patients with overt GIB and/or melena. Only 38 (44%) of these patients underwent endoscopy. Among this subgroup, nine (27%) had an endoscopy performed before the FOBT even being collected. All of these patients underwent gastroscopy while one patient had a colonoscopy as well. Of the remaining 29 patients, 14 (48%) underwent

TABLE 9
Comparison between academic and community hospitals for admissions with positive fecal occult blood test (FOBT)

	Hospital		
	Academic (n=79)	Community (n=147)	P
Indication(s)*			
Anemia	62 (78)	134 (91)	0.01
Black stools	25 (32)	38 (26)	0.44
Overt gastrointestinal bleeding	17 (22)	13 (9)	0.01
Gastrointestinal symptoms	17 (22)	22 (15)	0.27
Bloody diarrhea	1 (1)	2 (1)	1.00
Iron deficiency anemia	2 (3)	0 (0)	0.12
Colorectal cancer screening	1 (1)	0 (0)	0.35
Before initiating anticoagulants	1 (1)	0 (0)	0.35
Consultations			
Gastroenterology	49 (62)	59 (40)	0.01
Surgery	9 (19)	28 (19)	0.20
Consulting before reporting of FOBT result			
Gastroenterology	15/29 (52)	19/59 (32)	0.10
Surgery	2/9 (22)	12/28 (43)	0.43

Data presented as n (%) or n/n (%) unless otherwise indicated. *Some patients had more than one indication for ordering an FOBT

endoscopy before the reporting of FOBT results (11 gastroscopies, one colonoscopy and two both). Eleven patients (38%) underwent endoscopies ≥3 days after the FOBT had been collected (six gastroscopies, two colonoscopies and three both).

Comparisons among subspecialties for admissions with positive FOBT
When the indications for ordering an FOBT were compared among FM, IM and remaining subspecialties, the remaining subspecialties (which included surgical subspecialties) were more likely to order a FOBT for overt GIB and initiate a surgery consultation compared with FM and IM physicians (P<0.01 for both) (Table 8). No differences were found among subspecialties in initiating consults before the reporting of FOBT results.

Comparisons between academic and community hospitals for admissions with positive FOBT
Among community hospitals, an FOBT was more likely ordered for anemia but less likely for overt GIB (P=0.01 for both) (Table 9). A gastroenterology consultation was more likely to be initiated at an academic hospital compared with a community hospital (P=0.01). No differences were found in the timing of initiating consultations.

DISCUSSION
In an assessment of a city-wide practice of hospitalized patients within a single health authority, we found that the FOBT (Hemoccult II Sensa) was positive in approximately one-third of the cases for whom it was ordered. FOBT was most commonly ordered by FM physicians followed by IM physicians. The most common indication for ordering an FOBT was anemia. Fifteen percent of those in whom serum ferritin was ordered were documented to have IDA, which would have been an indication for endoscopy regardless of FOBT result. Two-thirds of those with positive FOBTs had no further GI investigations. Investigations were frequently completed before the reporting of results or unnecessarily delayed. Overall, our findings suggest that FOBT has limited beneficial effect on clinical management among hospitalized patients.

The very high positivity rate of FOBT observed in our study has several potential explanations: use of Hemoccult II Sensa, lack of dietary restrictions and use of FOBT among those with reported overt GIB. Hemoccult II Sensa is a version of a guaiac test that was developed to be more sensitive for blood but also has a higher false-positive rate (lower specificity) (5). As found in our study, dietary restrictions are usually not observed when FOBT is performed in the hospital setting. Although most of the traditional dietary restrictions are no longer considered necessary for the older guaiac FOBTs (6), the effect of disregarding dietary restrictions on Hemoccult II Sensa has not been well studied.

It is disappointing that a rectal examination, which could confirm the patient's history of overt GIB, was often not performed and, instead, an FOBT was ordered, presumably to corroborate the history of overt GIB. Furthermore, a standard policy within the WRHA is to not develop the FOBT for three days to ensure degradation of plant peroxidases in the collected specimens to decrease false-positive results (7). This test is, therefore, a poor choice to assess for overt GIB, for which results would be needed immediately. Even then, in our study, overt GIB was a common indication for ordering an FOBT. It was also surprising that an FOBT was often ordered for patients with anemia before obtaining other investigations such as serum iron or ferritin levels.

Anemia was the most common indication for ordering an FOBT in our study of hospitalized patients, which is similar to previous studies (1-3,8). There are often multiple causes of anemia among hospitalized patients including frequent blood draws and bone marrow suppression secondary to the active illness. Instead of delineating the etiology of a non-IDA, a positive FOBT could lead to colonoscopy even among individuals for whom CRC screening is not indicated due to their age or comorbidities and, thus, expose them unnecessarily to the low but definite risks of colonoscopy. Interestingly, all four patients in our study with CRC should have undergone a colonoscopy for IDA regardless of the FOBT result.

FM physicians accounted for >50% of FOBTs ordered for hospitalized patients in our study; however, we found minimal differences in clinical practices among other subspecialties as well as between academic and community hospitals. These findings corroborate our previous survey of WRHA physicians in which a higher proportion of FM physician respondents reported ordering FOBTs for hospitalized patients than other physicians (8). Further qualitative studies involving FM physicians are necessary. It is possible that a higher use of FOBT for symptomatic patients (regardless of whether hospitalized) by FM physicians may be due to perceived and/or real difficulties and delays in accessing GI endoscopy by FM physicians and resultant attempts to triage patients for timing of GI endoscopy with use of FOBT. However, use of FOBT for triaging symptomatic patients is controversial and, to the best of our knowledge, not recommended by any guidelines.

Although there are no previous reports of practices in Canadian hospitals, previous studies over the past decade from other jurisdictions have also shown limited benefits of FOBT use in hospitals. Sharma et al (1) conducted a retrospective chart review of 421 patients admitted to a medicine service across four teaching hospitals in the United States. They considered 70.5% of FOBTs to be ordered inappropriately including in patients with severe life-limiting comorbidities or while taking acetylsalicylic acid or nonsteroidal anti-inflammatory medications, and 17% had an FOBT performed despite active GIB. Moreover, even with a positive FOBT, only 41% were referred for endoscopy. In a second study, Friedman et al (2) examined the use of FOBT (both guaiac and immunochemical) among 330 admitted patients in three acute care hospitals in Australia. These investigators found that 62% of FOBTs were ordered for symptoms consistent with GIB and approximately 10% of FOBTs were ordered for anemia. They found that patient care was potentially adversely affected or delayed in 16% (54 patients) of all cases: 34 of these patients had endoscopy delayed despite overt GIB; and, because of a negative FOBT, another 10 patients did not undergo endoscopy even though they had clearly demonstrated overt GIB. In a more recent study, van Rijn et al (3) showed similar findings in 201 admitted patients across 15 hospitals in the Netherlands. Anemia (41%) was the most common reason for ordering an FOBT. Only 38% of those with a positive FOBT underwent further GI investigations.

Our study had several strengths. We were able to evaluate FOBT use in hospitalized patients in the entire city and evaluate potential differences among different admitting specialties as well as between academic and community hospitals. The diverse population allows for greater generalizability of our results. Furthermore, we were able to correlate the timing of FOBT reporting and clinical management, confirming a significant drawback of inpatient use of the FOBT with Hemoccult II Sensa.

A limitation of the present study was the retrospective collection of data. Some of the clinical data were incompletely recorded in the patient charts. We could not assess point-of-care (bedside) testing because there are no databases for such tests. Given the design of our study, we cannot generate any definitive conclusions whether limiting the use of FOBT or switching to a different FOBT, such as fecal immunochemical test would, in fact, alter clinical outcomes including length of stay, mortality or endoscopy utilization.

Future directions could include studies in which the availability of the current version of FOBT (Hemoccult II Sensa) in hospitals is restricted to predefined consensus indications or even altogether discontinued to determine whether clinically relevant outcomes are affected. Although the FOBT kit itself is inexpensive, there are associated costs with specimen collection, transportation, storage of the completed kit for three days and subjective visual reading of the test by a technician, as well as indirect costs of unnecessary consultations and/or endoscopies. Although some hospital laboratories in United Kingdom have reportedly stopped performing this test for hospitalized patients (9), to the best of our knowledge and, as suggested by our recent survey (8), FOBT continues to be widely available in North American hospitals. Continuing medical education of the appropriate use (primarily CRC screening) and numerous limitations of guaiac-based FOBT use in hospitalized patients is essential. Professional societies (gastroenterology, surgery, IM, clinical biochemistry and/or FM) should develop position statements/clinical practice guidelines on the use of FOBT for non-CRC screening indications. We believe, given the results of our study as well as other studies, hospitalized laboratory services may be better served in diverting resources for guaiac FOBTs to other, more useful services and tests.

CONCLUSIONS

In a study involving a large North American citywide practice of hospitalized patients, we found that the Hemoccult II Sensa FOBT was positive in a very high proportion of cases. FOBT was commonly ordered for patients with anemia. Investigations were frequently performed before the reporting of FOBTs or potentially unnecessarily delayed while waiting for test results. Two-thirds of positive FOBTs did not lead to GI investigations. The present study suggests that FOBT results in hospitalized patients may have little positive impact on clinical management and, therefore, hospital laboratory services should direct resources to other, more useful tests.

ACKNOWLEDGEMENTS: This study was supported by the WRHA Standards Committee and the Health Sciences Centre Medical Staff Fellows Fund.

DISCLOSURES: The authors have no conflict of interest to declare. Study funders had no influence on the conduct of the study or the manuscript. The opinions expressed are that of the authors and their endorsement by WRHA is neither intended nor should be inferred.

REFERENCES

1. Sharma VK, Komanduri S, Nayyar S, et al. An audit of the utility of in-patient fecal occult blood testing. Am J Gasternetol 2001;96:1256-60.
2. Friedman A, Chan A, Chin, LC, et al. Use and abuse of faecal occult blood tests in an acute hospital inpatient setting. Int Med J 2010;40:107-11.

3. Van Rijn, AF, Stroobants AK, Deutekom M, et al. Inappropriate use of the faecal occult blood test in a university hospital in the Netherlands. Eur J Gastroenterol Hepatol 2012;24:1266-9.

4. Government of Manitoba. Manitoba Health Population Report. Winnipeg, Manitoba, 2012. <www.gov.mb.ca/health/population/2012/pr2012.pdf> (Accessed May 19, 2014).

5. Whitlock EP, Lin JS, Liles E, et al. Screening for colorectal cancer: A targeted, updated systematic review for the U.S. Preventive Services Task Force. Ann Intern Med 2008;149:638-58.

6. Konrad G. Dietary interventions for fecal occult blood testing. Can Fam Physician 2010;56:229-38.

7. Sinatra MA, St John DJ, Young GP. Interference of plant peroxidases with guaiac-based fecal occult blood tests is avoidable. Clin Chem 1999;45:123-6.

8. Ip S, Sokoro AA, Buchel A, et al. Use of fecal occult blood test in hospitalized patients: Survey of physicians practicing in a large central Canadian health region and Canadian gastroenterologists. Can J Gastroenterol 2013;27:711-6.

9. Fraser C. Fecal occult blood test: Life savers or outdated colorectal screening tools? Clin Lab News 2011;37:8-10.

6

Colon capsule endoscopy: Detection of colonic polyps compared with conventional colonoscopy and visualization of extracolonic pathologies

Alexander F Hagel MD[1]*, Erwin Gäbele MD[2]*, Martin Raithel MD[1], Wolfgang H Hagel MD[1], Heinz Albrecht MD[1], Thomas M de Rossi MD[1], Christine Singer MD[3], Thomas Schneider MD[4], Markus F Neurath MD[1], Michael J Farnbacher MD[4]

AF Hagel, E Gäbele, M Raithel, et al. Colon capsule endoscopy: Detection of colonic polyps compared with conventional colonoscopy and visualization of extracolonic pathologies. Can J Gastroenterol Hepatol 2014;28(2):77-82.

BACKGROUND: Conventional colonoscopy (CC) is the gold standard for diagnostic examination of the colon. However, the overall acceptance of this procedure is low due to patient fears of complications or embarrassment. Colon capsule endoscopy (CCE) represents a minimally invasive, patient-friendly procedure that offers complete visualization of the entire intestine.

OBJECTIVE: To assess the PillCam Colon 2 (Given Imaging Ltd, Israel) capsule with regard to feasibility, sensitivity and specificity for the detection of colonic pathologies and additional recorded extracolonic findings.

METHODS: CCE was performed before CC in patients indicated for CC for known or suspected colonic disease. The results of both techniques were compared with regard to polyp detection. Additionally, bowel preparation and extracolonic pathologies were analyzed.

RESULTS: Twenty-four patients (mean age 51.1 years) were included in the analysis. Visualization of the colon was complete in 23 CCs and 17 CCEs. No adverse events or major technical failures occurred. CC detected 47 polyps and CCE detected 43 polyps of any size (per-finding sensitivity 90.9%, specificity 67.6%). The accuracy of CCE in detecting polyp carriers was 81.5% (per-patient analysis). On average, the colon was adequately cleansed in 90.1% of patients. CCE identified esophageal, gastric and small bowel pathologies in seven (24%), nine (38%) and 14 (58%) patients, respectively.

CONCLUSIONS: CCE proved to be technically feasible and safe. Acceptable sensitivity and moderate specificity levels in polyp detection were recorded. Bowel preparation was adequate in most patients. Because extracolonic pathologies were effectively visualized, new indications for the PillCam Colon 2 may be defined.

Key Words: *Cancer prevention; Capsule endoscopy; Colon; Colonoscopy; Colorectal cancer*

La vidéo-capsule endoscopique du côlon : la détection des polypes du côlon par rapport à la coloscopie classique et à la visualisation des pathologies extracoliques

HISTORIQUE : La coloscopie classique (CC) est la référence pour l'examen diagnostique du côlon. Cependant, l'acceptation globale de cette intervention est peu élevée en raison de la peur de complications ou de l'embarras. La vidéo-capsule endoscopique du côlon (VCEC) est une intervention peu invasive et facile à accepter pour le patient, qui permet de visualiser l'ensemble de l'intestin.

OBJECTIF : Évaluer la faisabilité, la sensibilité et la spécificité de la capsule *PillCam Colon 2* (Given Imaging Ltd, Israël) pour déceler les pathologies du côlon et saisir d'autres observations extracoliques.

MÉTHODOLOGIE : La VCEC a été effectuée avant la CC chez les patients devant effectuer une CC en raison d'une maladie colique connue ou présumée. Les chercheurs ont comparé les résultats des deux techniques pour déceler des polypes. De plus, ils ont analysé la préparation intestinale et les pathologies extracoliques.

RÉSULTATS : Vingt-quatre patients (âge moyen de 51,1 ans) ont participé à l'analyse. La visualisation du côlon était complète dans 23 CC et 17 VCEC. Aucun événement indésirable ou échec technique majeur ne s'est produit. La CC a permis de déceler 47 polypes et la VCEC, 43 polypes de toute dimension (sensibilité de 90,9 % par détection, spécificité de 67,6 %). La précision de la VCEC à déceler les porteurs de polypes s'établissait à 81,5 % (analyse par patient). En moyenne, le côlon était bien nettoyé chez 90,1 % des patients. La VCEC a permis de dépister des pathologies œsophagienne, gastrique et du grêle chez sept (24 %), neuf (38 %) et 14 (58 %) patients, respectivement.

CONCLUSIONS : La VCEC s'est révélée sécuritaire et faisable sur le plan technique. On a signalé un taux de sensibilité acceptable et de spécificité modérée dans la détection des polypes. La préparation intestinale était adéquate chez la plupart des patients. Puisque la visualisation des pathologies extracoliques était efficace, de nouvelles indications pourraient être définies pour la capsule *PillCam Colon 2*.

Colon cancer represents one of the most common malignancies, with an incidence of 15 to 45 per 100,000 per year (1). Consequent identification and removal of adenomatous polyps during colonoscopy has been shown to be highly effective in cancer prevention (2). However, the most important limiting factor of screening colonoscopy is the limited adherence by the screening population, which arises from its invasiveness, discomfort, embarrassment for the patient and the need for bowel preparation (3), resulting in lower screening rates compared with other screening programs (eg, breast and prostate cancer) (4).

Noninvasive diagnostic techniques, such as colon capsule endoscopy (CCE), have proven to be one alternative to increase uptake of endoscopic colorectal cancer (CRC) screening (5).

The PillCam Colon (Given Imaging Ltd, Israel) represented the first such noninvasive diagnostic tool for CRC screening. However, the diagnostic yield of its first-generation model introduced in 2006 was rather inadequate, with a sensitivity of 71% and specificity of 75% (6). Consequently, an improved second-generation model – PillCam Colon 2 – was developed. In two large multicentre studies, notably improved sensitivity rates of 85% to 89%, and specificity rates of 64% to 95% were reported in per-patient analyses (7,8).

The primary aim of our study was to evaluate the sensitivity of PillCam Colon 2 for the detection of colonic polyps compared with conventional colonoscopy (CC). As a secondary aim, all visualized extracolonic findings were recorded.

*Authors who contributed equally to the manuscript

[1]Department of Gastroenterology, University of Erlangen; [2]Department of Gastroenterology, Asklepios Clinic Burglengenfeld, Burglengenfeld; [3]Institute of Employment Research, Nuremberg; [4]Department of Gastroenterology, Clinical Centre Fuerth, Teaching Hospital of the University of Erlangen, Erlangen, Germany

Correspondence: Dr Michael J Farnbacher, Department of Gastroenterology, Clinical Centre Fuerth, Jakob-Henle-Str. 1, Fuerth 91058, Germany. e-mail farnbacher.denkes@t-online.de

TABLE 1
Colon cleansing regimen

Schedule	Intake
Day 1	
Evening	4 senna tablets
Day 2	
All day	Liquid diet
Afternoon	2 L PEG
Capsule examination day/day 3	
Early morning (05:00)	2 L PEG
09:00	Capsule ingestion
Capsule in small bowel	30 mL NaP and 1 L water
3 h after first boost (If no capsule egestion has occurred)	15 mL NaP and 0.5 L water
2 h after second boost (If no capsule egestion has occurred)	10 mg bisacodyl as suppository
Evening	2 L PEG
Colonoscopy examination day/day 4	
10:00	Colonoscopy

PEG Polyethylene glycol; NaP Sodium phosphate

METHODS

Second-generation CCE, which was used exclusively in the present study, has improved hardware and software compared with its predecessor. Both cameras have an increased angle of 172° (compared with 156° in the first generation) to enable nearly 360° coverage of the colon. Furthermore, the frame rate has been changed from a stable rate of 4 images/s to a variable rate of 4 images/s to 35 images/s depending on capsule propulsion. To increase battery life span, the first generation was inactive during the first 1 h 45 min of deployment, which resulted in missed examination of the cecum in a minority (9.8%) of cases (9). To prevent this possible disadvantage, second-generation CCE does not become completely inactive but only transmits 14 images/min while in the stomach and switches to the normal examination rate of 4 images/s to 35 images/s after automatic identification of the small bowel (SB). Alternatively, this automatically steered frame rate can be manually activated by the examiner at any time. The latter enables physicians to examine the entire intestine, if necessary; however, in this setting, automatic detection of the SB is disabled.

To facilitate capsule propulsion, reduce colonic transit times and, subsequently, increase the chance of complete capsule colonoscopies, additional doses of sodium phosphate boosters were administered after capsule ingestion. The appropriate moment for boost administration is indicated visually and acoustically by the data recorder of the capsule system after automatic detection of SB mucosa.

Because CC represents the gold standard for diagnosing colonic pathologies, all patients underwent this procedure the day after CCE.

Patient characteristics

Twenty-four patients who were scheduled to undergo CC for known or suspected colonic diseases were included in the present study. Indications included CRC screening, personal or family history of CRC or adenomatous polyps, with no previous colonoscopy within three years. Exclusion criteria were swallowing disorders, congestive heart failure, contraindication for the laxatives used in the study, pregnancy or implanted cardiac devices. All patients gave written consent to participate in the present study, which was conducted according to the Declaration of Helsinki. Approval of the institutional review board was obtained.

Cleansing and administration of CCE

A typical cleansing regimen was used (Table 1). In all cases, CCE was performed first, followed by CC the day after. During the day of CCE, two boosts (the second boost administered if no capsule egestion occurred) consisting of sodium phosphate were administered, followed by additional laxative (if no egestion occurred) to accelerate capsule propulsion and ensure adequate bowel preparation for endoscopy. This two-day regimen was scheduled to avoid any interference with CCE as described in previous studies (8).

Standardized video reading

The recorded CCE videos were interpreted by two investigators who are highly experienced with SB capsule endoscopy and specifically trained for CCE. Video recording was performed using the RAPID version 7 software (Given Imaging Ltd, Israel) and standardized using the following protocol. A combination of sharpness level (grade 3) and brightness level (grade 0) was used as a standard baseline to enhance all images (Quick Adjust settings). After defining the essential anatomical landmarks (first and last cecal images, hepatic and splenic flexures, first and last rectal images) the entire video was read in the normal mode using single-head viewing. Thumbnail images of all polyp findings were taken. Reading velocity in this 'cruise and capture' phase was 5 frames/s to 6 frames/s. If necessary, manual frame-by-frame viewing was performed. Then, the correct number of polyps was defined and confirmed in double-head viewing. Polyp size was measured using the polyp size estimation tool of the RAPID 7 software. If multiple frames showed the finding, the biggest diameter was adopted into the analysis.

Reading of extracolonic segments of capsule videos was performed by single-head viewing only. Viewing was routinely started with the green head. To assess the value of PillCam Colon 2 in presenting extracolonic findings, the esophageal transit time, as well as the durations of gastric and SB video sequences, were measured. Additionally, the visualization of anatomical landmarks (esophagogastric junction, pylorus, papilla of Vater and ileocecal valve) as well as esophageal, gastric and SB cleanliness using a four-point grading scale and, finally, pathological as well as physiological findings, were recorded.

To assess the quality of colon preparation, a previously described four-point grading scale (excellent, good, fair, poor) was used (9). Using this grading scale, fair and poor conditions represented inadequate cleansing not enabling complete evaluation of the colonic mucosa. Adequate preparation was recorded if cleanliness enabled the reader to detect polyps ≥5 mm in size, as suggested by Leighton and Rex (10).

CC was performed by experienced endoscopists in all cases. Colonoscopists were blinded to the capsule reader's results. In case of a CCE-reported finding missed during CC, the endoscopist was unblinded with respect to this finding only.

Statistical methods

Patient age, sex, colon cleanliness, adverse events, transit times and completeness of examinations were recorded. Matching of colonic polyps recorded in CCE and flexible colonoscopy was performed by comparison of size, location and morphology. Matching of the size was determined if the size measured in CC (visually compared with the open forceps or to the pathology report if snare polypectomy had been performed) was within 50% of its reference standard measure at CCE.

The primary end point of the study was the accuracy of CCE versus CC in identifying colorectal polyps. For this per-finding analysis, polyps were divided into three subgroups according to their size (<6 mm, 6 mm to 9 mm and ≥10 mm) or location (right, transverse, left colon). Polyps in CCE with corresponding polyps regarding size and/or location in CC were classified as true positive. Cases with no polyps at CCE and CC were classified as true negative. If CCE detected a polyp with no corresponding polyp at CC, this finding was classified as false positive for CCE. If CC detected a polyp that was not reported by CCE, this finding was classified as false negative for CCE.

As a secondary end point, a per-patient analysis was conducted to evaluate the accuracy of PillCam Colon 2 in identifying patients with any colonic polyps whatsoever. Patients without polyps at CC were classified as negative in the reference standard. A positive result was defined if CC detected ≥1 polyp of any size. CCE results were reported

TABLE 2
Patient characteristics

Age, years, mean (range)	51 (24–75)
Sex, male/female, n/n	14/10
Indications	**n (%)**
Colorectal cancer screening	–
Positive family history	5 (22)
No increased risk	8 (33)
Polyp surveillance	7 (29)
Suspected inflammatory bowel disease	2 (8)
Surveillance colonoscopy in ulcerative colitis	2 (8)

TABLE 3
Colonic polyps at colon capsule endoscopy (CCE) compared with conventional colonoscopy (CC) in the per-findings analysis

	CC, n	CCE, n	Sensitivity, %	Specificity, %
Polyp size, mm				
<6	16	20	100	83.3
6–9	17	14	72.2	90.9
≥10	11	9	75	100
Overall	44	43	80.0	93.7
Polyp location				
Right colon	12	12	75.0*	72.7
Transverse	10	9	90	100
Left colon	22	22	100	100
Overall	44	43	90.1	76.9

Polyps found at CCE were not identical to the polyps found at CC in every case (ie, not all polyps in the right colon detected in CCE could be verified using CC and vice versa). Therefore, the sensitivity was merely 75%, although 12 polyps could be detected using each modality

as positive if ≥1 polyp of any size was identified, otherwise they were reported as negative. Definitions for true/false-positive/negative results had been assessed analogous to the per-findings analysis.

Statistical analysis was performed using SPSS version 11.5.1 (IBM Corporation, USA) for Windows (Microsoft Corporation, USA). For normally distributed quantitative data, the summary statistics were the mean, SD and the range shown as mean (SD, range) within the given values. Non-normally distributed data are presented as median (interquartile range). Sensitivity and specificity with their exact 95% CIs as well as the negative predictive value (NPV) and positive predictive value (PPV) were calculated.

RESULTS
In total, 24 patients (14 male, 10 female) with an average age of 51 years (range 24 to 75 years) were included in the present study. Seven (29%) patients had undergone polypectomy in the past, five (22%) had a positive family history for CRC, eight (33%) underwent endoscopy for screening purposes, two (8%) experienced diarrhea for more than two weeks and two (8%) were scheduled for surveillance colonoscopy due to known ulcerative colitis (Table 2).

No technical difficulties that led to termination of the examinations occurred. All patients were able to swallow the capsule. The colon was reached in 23 of 24 CCEs. Twenty-three of 24 CCs were completed (including successful intubation of the ileum); one examination was terminated in the transverse colon due to unmanageable pain in the patient.

Colon capsule egestion rate
In 17 of 24 (71%) patients, CCE was completed by capsule egestion within the battery lifespan. Egestion rates were 10 of 17 (59%) within 6 h, 12 of 17 (71%) within 8 h, 14 of 17 (82%) within 10 h, 17 of 17 (100%) within >10 h postingestion. The mean (± SD) overall examination time for 17 completed CCEs was 07:05±03:49 h (range 02:17 h to 16:18 h). The passage time for the separate sections of the intestine were 00:58±01:02 h (00:06 h to 03:50 h) for the stomach, 01:46±01:36 h (00:20 h to 07:09 h) for the SB and 05:15±03:38 h (01:06 h to 14:13 h) for the colon. In seven of 24 patients, the colon was incompletely visualized, with a mean working time of 11:16±3:20 h (range 9:21 h to 17:49 h), which was longer than CCEs with completed colon visualization. Due to the battery's lifespan, six of seven examinations were terminated before egestion (one CCE during passage of the transverse colon and all others during passage of the sigmoid colon). In a one patient, the capsule remained in the stomach for nearly 4 h and did not reach the colon thereafter, albeit with an examination and capsule working time of almost 11 h (10:53 h). This particular case was excluded from further analyses.

Colon cleansing level
CCE bowel preparation was evaluated individually for the various segments (eg, cecum, ascendens, transversum, descending, sigmoid/rectum). Overall, bowel cleansing was categorized as adequate (good or excellent) in 90.1% of patients. The percentage of adequately cleansed patients varied depending on the segment (cecum 82.4%, ascending

colon 88.2%, transverse colon 94.1%, descending colon 93.3%, sigmoid/rectum 93.3%).

Adverse events
One patient reported headache during preparation for the CCE procedure. No other adverse events were recorded during the CCE and the CC endoscopies. However, temporary transmission failures, resulting in a partial loss of frames, were recorded in four (16.7%) early videos, with a mean duration of 23±13 min (range 7 min to 45 min) mainly (n=3 [75%]) after the capsule had already reached the rectum. In one patient, six gaps were found, two gaps were found in another and one gap was recorded in each of the remaining patients. After changing the standard sensor array placement, with one sensor on the patient's back above the right buttock, this problem was avoided in all subsequent procedures.

Colonic findings
CCE accuracy for detecting polyps (per-finding analysis): In six of 23 cases, both CC and CCE did not detect polyps (true negative). In the other 17 cases, 47 polyps were detected. Forty of 47 (85.1%) polyps were apparent in both examinations (true positive). Locations were: cecum (n=3), ascending (n=6), transverse (n=9), descending (n=8), sigmoid colon (n=10) and rectum (n=4). Four (8.5%) polyps were detected by CC but missed at CCE (false negative). These polyps had a size of 6 mm to 12 mm and were located in the transverse colon and the cecum. Three (6.4%) polyps were detected by CCE: size 3 mm and 7 mm, and 11 mm in the cecum or the ascending colon but not reconfirmed at CC (false positive). One of these three polyps (3 mm) was located in the cecum and could not be identified by CC even after unblinding of the endoscopist for this finding. However, three of the latter seven polyps were recorded in patients who had more than one polyp, which were all detected by both methods.

According to this per-finding analysis, CCE achieved an overall sensitivity of 90.9% (95% CI 85% to 100%) and a specificity of 67.6% (95% CI 36% to 98%) in the detection of any size polyp. Compared with CC, polyps were found by CCE with a PPV and NPV of 93.0% and 71.4%, respectively. When sensitivity and specificity levels were considered according to subgroup (eg, size and polyp location), the individual percentage varied significantly (Table 3).

CCE accuracy for identifying patients as polyp carriers (per-patient analysis): At CC, a total of 16 of 23 (69.6%) patients had ≥1 polyp of any size. At least one polyp was identified by CCE in 14 of 23 (60.8%) patients. In 13 (56.5%) patients, CCE-positive patients were reconfirmed by CC (true positive). In six (26.1%) patients, CCE and CC detected no polyp (true negative). In a single CCE-positive patient

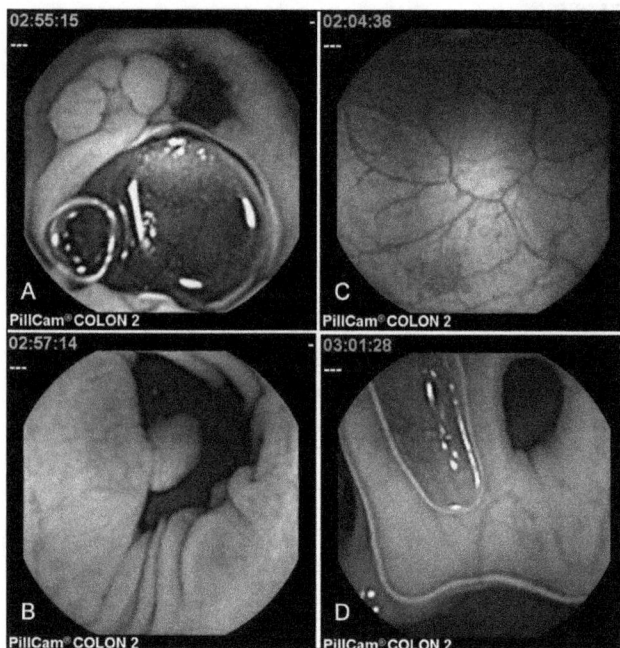

Figure 1) *Different colonic pathologies found in capsule endoscopy. Two colorectal polyps measuring 17 mm (**A**) and 10 mm (**B**), an angiodysplasia (**C**) and a diverticulum (**D**)*

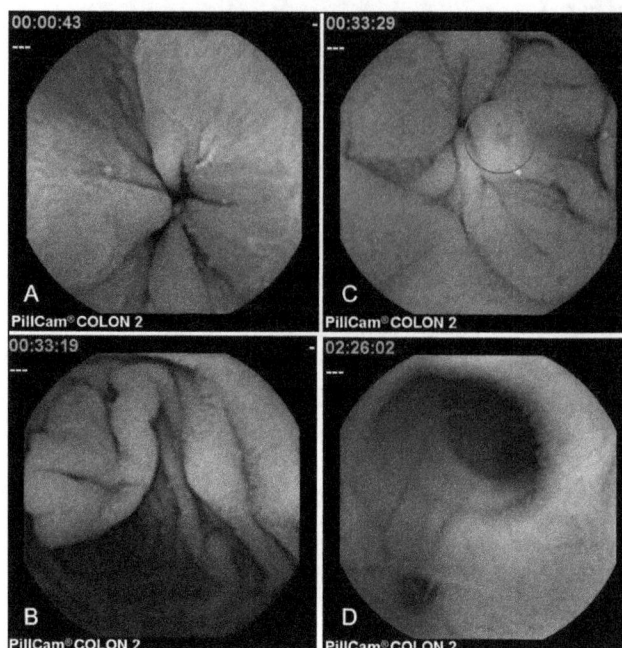

Figure 2) *Extracolonic landmarks and findings. Z-line (**A**); papilla of Vater (**B**); small bowel angiodysplasia (**C**); ileic diverticulum (**D**)*

(4.3%) no polyp was recorded at CC (false positive). In three (13.1%) CCE-negative patients, CC identified at least one polyp (false negative).

According to these data, in the per-patient analysis, CCE could identify patients with polyps regardless of the number or size with a sensitivity of 81.5% (95% CI 62% to 100%) and a specificity of 85.7% (95% CI 60% to 100%). The PPV of CCE with respect to identifying patients with colorectal polyps was 92.9%; the NPV was 67%.

Nonpolyp colonic findings

In addition to polyps (Figure 1A/B), CCE detected additional colonic lesions such as an angiodysplasia in the ascending colon (Figure 1C) as well as diverticulae (Figure 1D) in four patients (17%) and a severe inflammation due to ulcerative colitis in one patient each (4%). These lesions were reconfirmed by flexible colonoscopy in all cases.

Extracolonic findings

In 22 of 24 (92%) cases, CCE presented a median of 17 (range one to 685) frames of the esophagus. Only in two (8%) cases, esophageal transit was abrupt without recording any images. The Z line was visible in 19 of 24 patients (79%) in 4±3 (range one to 10) frames on average (Figure 2A). Excellent or good cleanliness of the esophagus and the Z line were recorded in 20 of 22 (91%) and 19 of 19 (100%), respectively. Cleanliness was reduced due to bubbles/saliva in only a minority of patients. Pathological findings, such as esophagitis (I°: n=4, IV°: n=1), suspected Barrett's esophagus (C0M1 according to the Prague classification) and varices (I° according to Sarin's classification) due to portal hypertension, were recorded in seven of 24 patients (29%).

The gastric video segment had a mean duration of 58 min. Due to the battery-saving sleep mode and automatic capsule activation after detection of SB mucosa, the pylorus was visible only in exceptional cases (four of 24 [17%]). Gastric cleanliness was limited in most cases (20 of 24 [84%]) due to saliva and bubbles. In nine of 24 (38%) patients, pathological findings, such as mucosal erythema, erosions and portal hypertensive gastropathy, were recorded.

The mean length of SB video was 1:46 h. Analogous to the pylorus, Vater's papilla (Figure 2B) was visible in the same four (17%) cases. SB cleanliness was adequate (excellent or good) in 20 of 24 cases (84%) and inadequate (moderate or poor) in four of 24 (16%) cases. In 14 of

24 (58%) patients, pathological findings, such as angiodysplasias (Figure 2C), erosions, ulcerations, strictures, diverticula orifices (Figure 2D) or polyps, were recorded within the SB (Table 4).

DISCUSSION

In the present study, colonic findings using PillCam Colon 2 CCE and flexible CC were compared. As a single-centre study, the present analysis offers the advantage of a limited number of physicians with expertise in capsule video reading and flexible colonoscopy. According to our data, CCE afforded good sensitivity and specificity (>81% and 85%, respectively) in identifying patients with polyps regardless of polyp size (per-patient analysis). These data are similar to previously published rates for sensitivity (89% and 88%) and specificity (76% and 89%) found in other studies involving the second-generation PillCam Colon for polyps ≥6 mm and ≥10 mm, respectively (7,8), showing a clear advantage over the first-generation model, which had sensitivity rates of between 60% and 72% (11). Apart from the improved angle of vision of the two lenses (from 156° to 172°), the increase in sensitivity may be very likely due to the increased and automatically steered variability of the frame rate according to the velocity of the capsule motion (12). Nine of the polyps were recorded in ≤5 images. These may have been missed using the lower frame rate of first-generation CCE. Another major factor influencing the rate of polyp detection is the level of bowel preparation (13). Similar to previous studies (7,8), our data show an adequate preparation in 90.1% of all evaluated segments. The overall egestion rate of 71% was slightly lower than in previous studies (7,8), which may be explained by the smaller number of patients included. In our patient cohort, cleansing was not as complete in patients with missing egestion. Therefore, slower peristalsis may have hampered both bowel preparation and capsule propulsion. The only adverse event recorded in our study was one patient who experienced headache during preparation for CCE. Overall, the standardized cleansing regimen, including sodium phosphate for capsule propulsion, proved to be safe and effective (14).

Additionally, we compared CCE and CC polyp-by-polyp with respect to size and location. This per-findings analysis showed a capsule sensitivity and specificity for polyp identification of 91.0% and 76.9%, respectively. The apparently suboptimal specificity of CCE mainly arises from the small number of true-negative capsule videos as a result of our

TABLE 4
Extracolonic capsule endoscopy findings

Intestine	Video length (range)	Presentation of anatomical landmarks, n (%)	Degree of cleanliness*	n (%)	Capsule findings	n (%)
Esophagus	58±138 min (0–685) frames	Z line: Yes: 19 (79) No: 5 (21)	I°	9 (38)	Esophagitis	5 (21)
			II°	11 (46)	Suspected Barrett's esophagus	1 (4)
			III°	4 (16)	Varices	1 (4)
			IV°	–		
Stomach	00:58±01:02 h (00:06 h – 03:50 h)	Pylorus: Yes: 4 (17) No: 20 (83)	I°	4 (16)	Mucosal erythema	3 (13)
			II°	17 (71)	Erosion	7 (29)
			III°	3 (13)	Portal hypertensive gastropathy	1 (4)
			IV°	–		
Small bowel	01:46±01:36 h (00:20h – 07:09 h)	Papilla of Vater: Yes: 4 (17) No: 20 (83)	I°	9 (38)	Angiodysplasia	5 (21)
			II°	11 (46)	Erosion	7 (29)
			III°	4 (16)	Diverticulae	3 (13)
			IV°	–	Stricture	1 (4)
					Polyp	1 (4)
					Lymphangiectasia	19 (79)
					Lymphatic hyperplasia	3 (13)
					Brunner's gland tumours	2 (8)

*I° = Excellent; II° = Good; III° = Moderate; IV° = Poor

polyp-enriched study population. In a screening population, a higher specificity for CCE might be expected. Additionally, false-positive findings in CCE hamper its specificity. However, as previously described, CC may be an imperfect reference standard, with reduced sensitivity especially for polyps <9 mm in size (15,16). In fact, it cannot be ruled out that false-positive findings at CCE were false-negative findings at CC. Further studies with different methodology (eg, unblinding colonoscopists) are necessary to evaluate the true specificity of CCE. However, even after unblinding, detection of polyps at CC previously identified at CCE cannot be expected in every case due to a limited flexibility and angular field of the endoscope as well as air insufflation, as occurred in one case in our series.

All CC-proven polyps missed during CCE were located either in the right or the transverse colon. A similar distribution of location of missed polyps was reported earlier by Spada et al (8). This result is especially frustrating because it confirms problems in detecting polyps and cancerous lesions in the right colon, similar to CC (17).

Three polyps detected at CC had been missed at CCE in patients with additional polyps identified by both techniques. Despite the lower per-findings sensitivity in these cases, the per-patient sensitivity was unaffected because CCE could, in fact, identify those patients as polyp carriers. Undoubtedly, this is an important secondary aim of CCE and its efficacy regarding this issue is highlighted by the notable PPV of CCE compared with flexible colonoscopy in the per-patient analysis. However, concerning CCE as a CRC screening tool, the NPV will be even more important. The limited NPV of CCE appears to challenge its value in this respect. However, NPV and PPV are highly affected by prevalence of findings and, similar to previous studies, our patient cohort was polyp enriched. Therefore, the low NPV may be the result of an under-represented CRC screening population among the study attendees and must be re-evaluated in future studies.

The cost effectiveness of CRC screening depends on three main criteria: adenoma detection rate; financial expenditure of the screening tool; and adherence to the screening program. The latter can be increased by CCE as previously published (5). Whether the high costs – depending on the national health care system – and the limited adenoma detection rate of CCE are compensated by the increased compliance to CRC screening has not, to date, been proven (18,19).

Apart from colonic polyps, several other colonic pathologies were recorded, such as ulcerative colitis, diverticulae or angiodysplasias, which were reconfirmed at CC in every case. Ulcerative colitis imaging of colonic mucosa by CCE has been previously evaluated (20); the lack of air insufflation and avoidance of the shear forces executed by the endoscope may reduce the risk of reinjury during evaluation of the mucosal healing under therapy.

CCE is also able to effectively visualize esophageal, gastric and SB pathologies. Similar to PillCam Eso (21), frames of the Z line were present in >90% of the videos despite a capsule administration in a sedentary position and without a specific ingestion protocol. Even cleansing was excellent, with little bubbles/saliva having no or only a minor negative effect on Z line images.

In contrast, due to the sleep mode, presentation of the pylorus was rare and, consequently, gastric appraisal was incomplete. Additionally, cleanliness was limited in most cases, and the lack of a steering device and air insufflation leads to a reduced ability to examine the entire gastric mucosa. Nevertheless, pathological findings, such as mucosal erythema, erosions and portal hypertensive gastropathy, were recorded in more than one-third of the patients. Therefore, once capsule steering (which has been investigated in recent studies [22]) becomes available, re-evaluation of gastric imaging using CCE may be warranted.

SB visualization was excellent and cleanliness was adequate in the majority (84%) of the patients. The ileocecal valve was visualized in all videos. If CCE was activated within the stomach, the papilla of Vater was visible in every case. Although inconsequential to our analysis, SB findings were recorded in more than one-half of the patients. The accuracy in visualizing frames of anatomical landmarks illustrates that doubling the number of optical devices and the movement-adapted frame rate of CCE optimizes visualization of SB mucosa. Therefore, with adequate cleansing and appropriate application protocols, indications for CCE may be expanded. It may be useful to evaluate the extent of Crohn disease to facilitate the classification of indeterminate colitis and, furthermore, in the screening of patients with familial adenomatous polyposis or Peutz-Jeghers syndrome.

Similar to virtual colonoscopy, CCE offers the benefit of earlier diagnosis of clinically significant extracolonic – yet gastrointestinal – lesions in a one-step assessment, possibly decreasing patients' morbidity or mortality. On the other hand, extracolonic gastrointestinal findings may also lead to additional diagnostic evaluation or intervention leading to patient anxiety, morbidity and increased health care costs, once again challenging the cost effectiveness of CCE (23,24). Therefore, further analyses will be necessary to evaluate the impact of CCE on extracolonic gastrointestinal pathologies.

SUMMARY

CCE is technically feasible and safe. The per-patient and per-finding analysis demonstrate a viable sensitivity and moderate specificity of the new generation of the PillCam Colon 2 in polyp detection compared with the current gold standard of flexible colonoscopy. However, the limited NPV as well as high cost of CCE challenge its application as a screening tool at present. Because extracolonic landmarks and findings are effectively visualized, indications for CCE may be extended, especially with respect to inflammatory bowel diseases and polyposis syndromes.

DISCLOSURES: The capsule endsocopes used in this study were supplied by Given Imaging, Israel. The work originated from the Department of Gastroenterology, University of Erlangen, Erlangen, Germany.

REFERENCES

1. International Agency for Research on Cancer. WHO and International Association of cancer registries. In: Parkin DM, Whelan SL, Ferlay J, Raymond L, Yung J, eds. Cancer Incidence in Five Continents. Lyon: IARC Scientific Publications, 1997.
2. Atkin WS, Edwards R, Kralj-Hans I, et al. UK Flexible Sigmoidoscopy Trial Investigators. Once-only flexible sigmoidoscopy screening in prevention of colorectal cancer: A multicentre randomised controlled trial. Lancet 2010;8:1624-33.
3. Knöpnadel J, Altenhofen L, Brenner G. Epidemiologic and health economic significance of colorectal cancers in Germany. Internist (Berl) 2003;44:268-74;276-7.
4. Lisi D, Hassan C, Crespi M, AMOD Study Group. Participation in colorectal cancer screening with FOBT and colonoscopy: An Italian, multicentre, randomized population study. Dig Liver Dis 2010;42:371-6.
5. Groth S, Krause H, Behrendt R, et al. Capsule colonoscopy increases uptake of colorectal cancer screening. BMC Gastroenterology 2012;12:80.
6. Spada C, Hassan C, Marmo R, et al. Meta-analysis shows colon capsule endoscopy is effective in detecting colorectal polyps. Clin Gastroenterol Hepatol 2010;8:516-22.
7. Eliakim R, Yassin K, Niv Y, et al. Prospective multicenter performance evaluation of the second-generation colon capsule compared with colonoscopy. Endoscopy 2009;41:1026-31.
8. Spada C, Hassan C, Munoz-Navas M, et al. Second-generation colon capsule endoscopy compared with colonoscopy. Gastrointest Endosc 2011;74:581-9.
9. Schoofs N, Devière J, Van Gossum A. PillCam Colon capsule endoscopy compared with colonoscopy for colorectal tumor diagnosis: A prospective pilot study. Endoscopy 2006;38:971-7.
10. Leighton JA, Rex DK. A grading scale to evaluate colon cleansing for the PillCam COLON capsule: A reliability study. Endoscopy 2011;43:123-7.
11. Riccioni ME, Urgesi R, Cianci R, Bizzotto A, Spada C, Costamagna G. Colon capsule endoscopy: Advantages, limitations and expectations. Which novelties? World J Gastrointest Endosc 2012;4:99-107.
12. Adler SN, Metzger YC. PillCam COLON capsule endoscopy: Recent advances and new insights. Therap Adv Gastroenterol 2011;4:265-8.
13. Van Gossum A, Munoz-Navas M, Fernandez-Urien I, et al. Capsule endoscopy versus colonoscopy for the detection of polyps and cancer. N Engl J Med 2009;361:264-70.
14. Sieg A. Capsule endoscopy compared with conventional colonoscopy for detection of colorectal neoplasms. World J Gastrointest Endosc 2011;3:81-5.
15. Hixon LJ, Fennerty MB, Sampliner RE, et al. Prospective blinded trial of the colonoscopic miss-rate of large colorectal polyps. Gastrointest Endosc 1991;37:125-7.
16. Rex DK, Cutler CS, Lemmel GT, et al. Colonoscopic miss rates of adenomas determined by back to back colonoscopies. Gastroenterology 1997;112:24-8.
17. Brenner H, Hoffmeister M, Arndt V, Stegmaier C, Altenhofen L, Haug U. Protection from right-and left-sided colorectal neoplasms after colonoscopy: Population-based study. J Natl Cancer Inst 2010;102:89-95.
18. Sonnenberg, A, Delcó F, Inadomi JM, Cost-effectiveness of colonoscopy in screening for colorectal Cancer. Ann Intern Med 2000;133:573-84.
19. Hassan C, Zullo A, Winn S, Morini S. Cost-effectiveness of capsule endoscopy in screening for colorectal cancer. Endoscopy 2008;40:414-21.
20. Sung J, Ho KY, Chiu HM, Ching J, Travis S, Peled R. The use of Pillcam Colon in assessing mucosal inflammation in ulcerative colitis: a multicenter study. Endoscopy 2012;44:754-8.
21. Gralnek IM, Adler SN, Yassin K, Koslowsky B, Metzger Y, Eliakim R. Detecting esophageal disease with second-generation capsule endoscopy: Initial evaluation of the PillCam ESO 2. Endoscopy 2008;40:275-9.
22. Capri F, Kastelein N, Talcott M, Pappone C. Magnetically controllable gastrointestinal steering of video capsules. IEEE Trans Biomed Eng 2011;58:231-4.
23. Yee J, Sadda S, Aslam R, Yeh B. Extracolonic findings at CT colonography. Gastrointest Endosc Clin N Am 2010;20:305-22.
24. Xiong T, McEvoy K, Morton DG, Halligan S, Lilford RJ. Resources and costs associated with incidental extracolonic findings from CT colonogaphy: A study in a symptomatic population. Br J Radiol 2006;79:948-61.

7

Small bowel obstruction following computed tomography and magnetic resonance enterography using psyllium seed husk as an oral contrast agent

Yingming Amy Chen MD[1], Patrick Cervini MD[2], Anish Kirpalani MD [1], Paraskevi A Vlachou MD[1], Samir C Grover MD MEd [3], Errol Colak MD[1]

YA Chen, P Cervini, A Kirpalani, PA Vlachou, SC Grover, E Colak. Small bowel obstruction following computed tomography and magnetic resonance enterography using psyllium seed husk as an oral contrast agent. Can J Gastroenterol Hepatol 2014;28(7):391-395.

The authors report a case series describing four patients who developed small bowel obstruction following the use of psyllium seed husk as an oral contrast agent for computed tomography or magnetic resonance enterography. Radiologists who oversee computed tomography and magnetic resonance enterography should be aware of this potential complication when using psyllium seed husk and other bulking agents, particularly when imaging patients with known or suspected small bowel strictures or active inflammation.

Key Words: *CT enterography; MR enterography; Oral contrast*

L'obstruction du grêle après une tomodensitométrie et une entérographie par résonance magnétique faisant appel à l'enveloppe de psyllium comme agent oral de contraste

Les auteurs rendent compte d'une série de cas de quatre patients qui ont présenté une obstruction du grêle après avoir consommé l'enveloppe de psyllium comme agent oral de contraste en vue d'une tomodensitométrie ou d'une entérographie par résonance magnétique. Les radiologues qui supervisent les tomodensitométries et les entérographies par résonance magnétique devraient connaître cette complication potentielle lorsqu'ils utilisent l'enveloppe de psyllium et les autres agents gonflants, notamment lorsque les patients qui se soumettent à l'imagerie présentent un rétrécissement connu ou présumé ou une inflammation active du grêle.

Computed tomography (CT) and magnetic resonance enterography (MRE) play an increasingly critical role in the diagnosis, assessment and management of patients with small bowel disease. CT and MRE have largely replaced fluoroscopic examinations, such as small bowel follow-through and enteroclysis, by providing accurate characterization of the bowel wall and visualization of disease beyond the bowel wall (1-3). Furthermore, CT enterography (CTE) and MRE provide a more comfortable patient experience by circumventing the need for nasojejunal intubation (4).

The diagnostic accuracy of CTE and MRE is predicated on adequate distension of the small bowel by oral contrast. Multiple oral contrast options are available, including psyllium seed husk, which is a nondigestible bulk fibre laxative. To date, there is no established consensus on the ideal oral contrast agent for CTE and MRE.

We report three cases of small bowel obstruction following CTE at Windsor Regional Hospital (Ouellette Campus, Windsor, Ontario) and one case following MRE at St Michael's Hospital (Toronto, Ontario) with psyllium seed husk (Metamucil, Proctor & Gamble, USA) as the oral contrast agent.

EXAMINATION PROTOCOL

CTE protocol

Patients were instructed to be nil per os from midnight and to arrive 1 h before the examination. Three doses of oral contrast were prepared by diluting 15 mL Metamucil in 450 mL of water. Patients were instructed to drink 450 mL of oral contrast 60 min, 40 min and 20 min before the examination.

MRE protocol

Patients were instructed to be on a clear liquid diet after 17:00 the day before the examination, to take an enema (Fleet, CB Fleet, USA) the morning of the examination, and to arrive 2 h before the examination. Patients were administered 10 mg metoclopramide orally before drinking the Metamucil solution to promote peristalsis. Metamucil at a dose of 1.6 g/kg was diluted in 2000 mL of water. Patients were instructed to drink 500 mL every 30 min. An additional 10 mg of metoclopramide was administered after drinking 1000 mL of oral contrast to ensure adequate transit of oral contrast into the small bowel.

Case 1

A 55-year-old woman underwent CTE for the assessment of Crohn disease. CT demonstrated active disease involving 20 cm of the distal ileum characterized by bowel wall thickening, mucosal hyperenhancement, mural stratification, significant luminal narrowing and mesenteric inflammation (Figure 1A). Approximately 6 h after CTE, she presented to the emergency department with diffuse abdominal pain. Abdominal radiographs performed 9 h after CTE demonstrated dilated small bowel with air-fluid levels (Figure 1B). The patient was admitted overnight for conservative treatment and discharged the next day following resolution of symptoms.

Case 2

An 88-year-old man underwent CTE to rule out a small bowel cause of anemia. No small bowel abnormalities were demonstrated by CTE. The patient developed progressively worsening abdominal pain in the

[1]Department of Medical Imaging, St Michael's Hospital, Toronto; [2]Department of Diagnostic Imaging, Windsor Regional Hospital – Ouellette Campus, Windsor; [3]Division of Gastroenterology, St Michael's Hospital, Toronto, Ontario

Correspondence: Dr Errol Colak, Department of Medical Imaging, St Michael's Hospital, 30 Bond Street, Toronto, Ontario M5B 1W8. e-mail colake@smh.ca

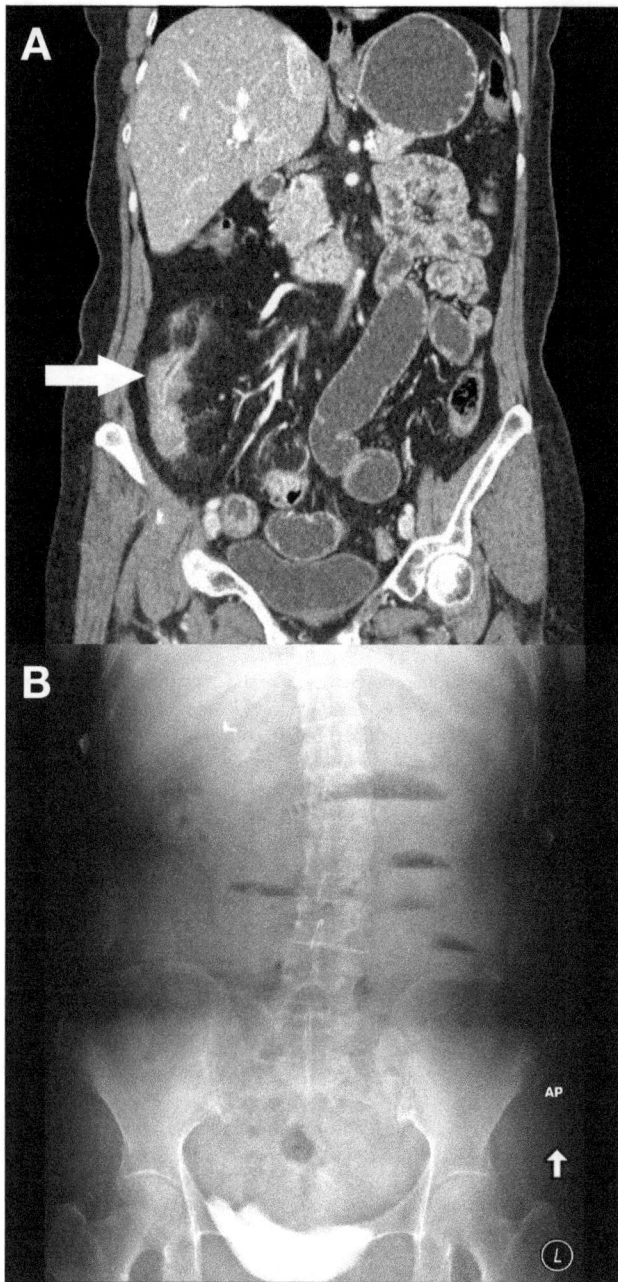

Figure 1) A *Coronal computed tomography enterography image demonstrating active inflammation of the terminal ileum (arrow). The upstream small bowel is filled with oral contrast.* B *Upright abdominal radiograph performed 9 h later demonstrating dilated small bowel with air-fluid levels consist with a small bowel obstruction*

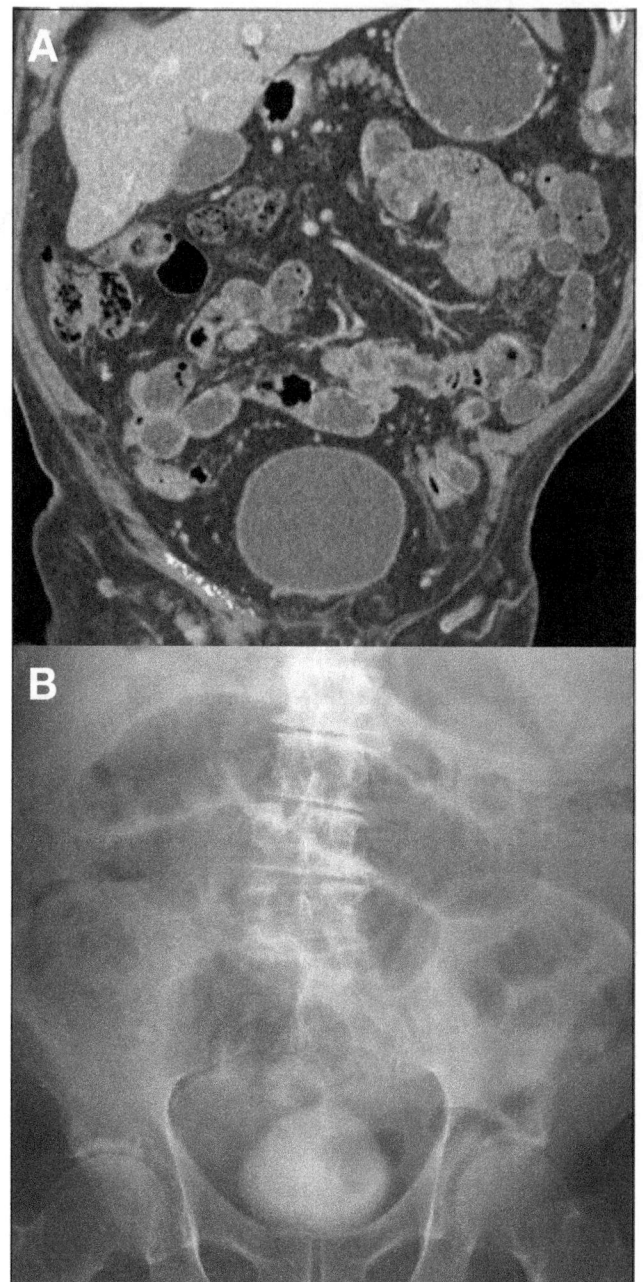

Figure 2) A *Coronal image from a normal computed tomography enterogram.* B *Supine abdominal radiograph performed the subsequent day demonstrating multiple distended loops of small bowel*

hours that followed the examination and returned to hospital the next morning. Abdominal radiographs were consistent with a small bowel obstruction (Figure 2). The patient improved with conservative management and his symptoms resolved by the next day.

Case 3

A 61-year-old woman with a presumed history of ulcerative colitis and remote total colectomy underwent CTE for symptoms of intermittent bowel obstruction. The patient was treated conservatively for a small bowel obstruction three weeks earlier. CTE revealed a right lower quadrant parastomal hernia with active inflammation of the immediately upstream small bowel (Figures 3A and 3B). The remainder of the small bowel was unremarkable. The patient presented 10 h later with

generalized abdominal pain and nausea. Repeat CT scan of the abdomen showed diffuse small bowel dilation with a transition point at the parastomal hernia (Figures 3C and 3D). The patient did not improve with conservative management and exploratory laparotomy was undertaken the next day. Multiple adhesions were found around the stoma that resulted in kinking of the adjacent bowel. An ischemic segment of bowel was resected and a new stoma was created. There were no perioperative complications and the patient was discharged in stable condition.

Case 4

A 51-year-old man with a history of Crohn disease and distal ileal resection underwent MRE that demonstrated a long segment of narrowing of the efferent limb of the side-to-side ileoileal anastomosis

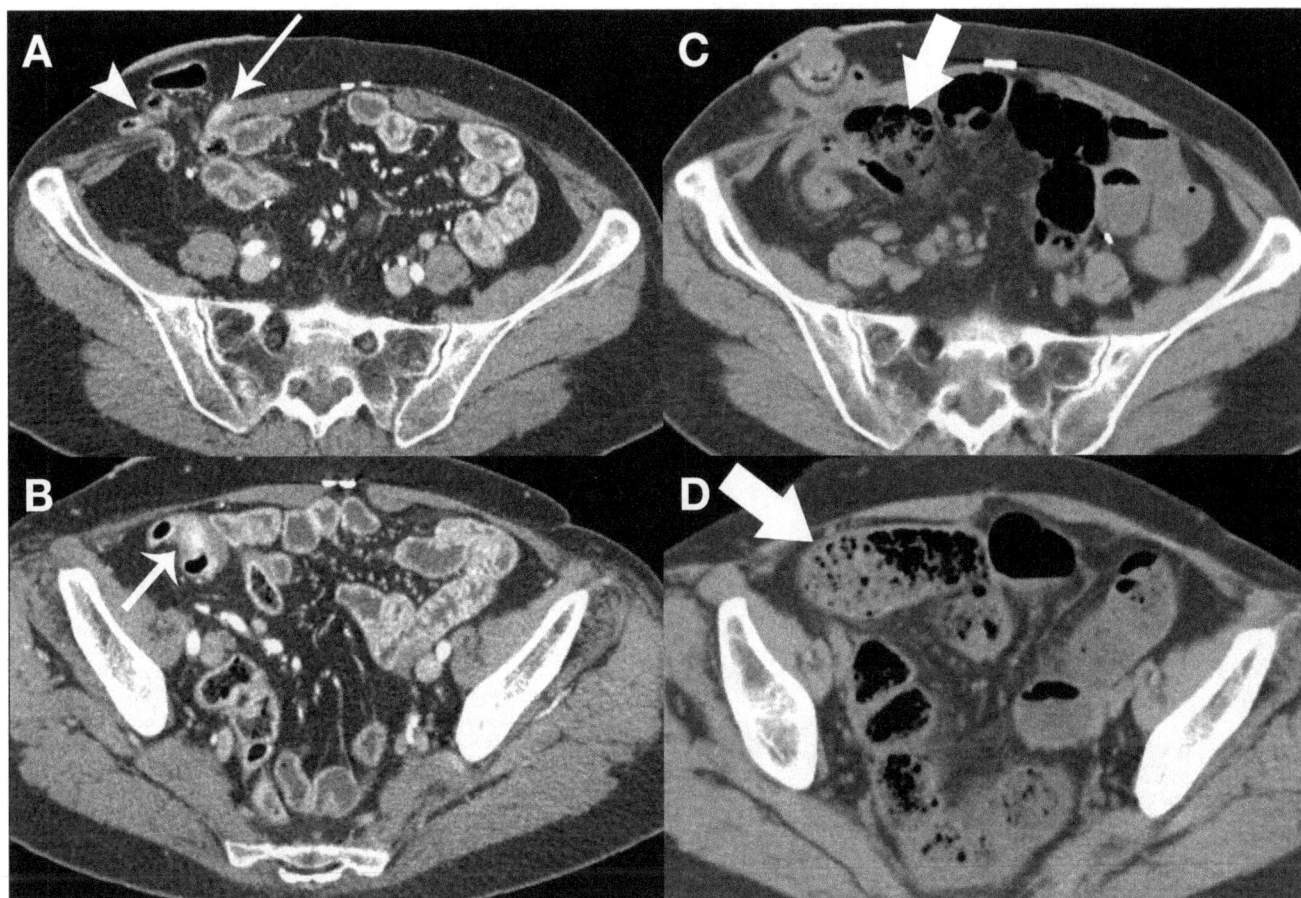

Figure 3) A *and* B *Axial computed tomography enterography images demonstrating a right lower quadrant parastomal hernia (arrowhead) with active inflammation of the immediately upstream small bowel (thin arrows).* C *and* D *Computed tomography scan performed 10 h later demonstrates diffuse small bowel dilation and fecalization of small bowel content (thick arrows) to the level of a transition point in the parastomal hernia*

(Figure 4A). There were no imaging features to suggest active small bowel inflammation. Approximately 12 h after the examination, the patient developed severe nausea and vomiting, diffuse abdominal pain and bloating. A CT scan of the abdomen demonstrated a high-grade small bowel obstruction with a transition point just beyond the site of the ileoileal anastomosis at the narrowed segment of the efferent limb (Figure 4B). He was managed conservatively by nasogastric intubation and bowel rest. His symptoms resolved completely by 48 h.

DISCUSSION

CTE and MRE have emerged as important investigations for small bowel disorders (2,3), and in influencing clinical management of Crohn disease (5,6). Established indications for CTE and MRE include staging and follow-up of inflammatory bowel disease and its complications, evaluation of obscure gastrointestinal bleeding and investigation of small bowel tumours (7). Emerging uses include evaluation of diffuse small bowel diseases, such as celiac disease (8) and vasculitis, as well as screening of strictures before capsule endoscopy (9). The added advantages of MRE include improved tissue contrast and lack of ionizing radiation, making it ideal for younger patients with inflammatory bowel disease who often require repeated cross-sectional imaging. Furthermore, MRE is capable of real-time functional imaging, which assesses small bowel peristaltic patterns in gastrointestinal motility disorders (10).

Bowel distension is essential for small bowel imaging because collapsed bowel may mimic or obscure small bowel pathology. To date, there is no established consensus on the ideal oral contrast agent for CTE and MRE. Multiple oral contrast agents are available, with the choice varying among institutions based on extent of bowel distension, uniformity of luminal opacification, availability, ease of use, cost and side-effect profile. CTE and MRE oral contrast agents are either hyperosmolar agents that prevent the absorption of water from the small bowel or bulking agents that result in small bowel distension.

The most commonly used oral agents are polyethylene glycol and low-density barium suspensions such as VoLumen (Bracco Diagnostics, USA) with mannitol, sorbitol, methylcellulose, locust bean gum and bulk fibre laxatives representing less commonly used options (11).

While VoLumen is a commonly used oral contrast agent in many jurisdictions, it has not been approved by Health Canada (the Canadian drug regulatory agency) for use as an oral contrast agent. We have anecdotally observed variable small bowel distension and gastrointestinal tract transit time when using polyethylene glycol as an oral contrast agent.

Psyllium seed husk products, including Metamucil, are commonly used bulking laxative and fibre supplement products. When mixed with water, psyllium can function as an oral contrast agent by forming a nondigestible hydrogel that absorbs water and subsequently distends the small bowel (12). It is relatively inexpensive, easy to prepare and administer, and well-tolerated by patients. Reported side effects are typically mild and include bloating, flatulence and diarrhea (13). The reported experience of other centres (12) supported its performance and safety as an oral contrast agent. Consequently, Metamucil was being used as the oral contrast agent for CTE at Windsor Regional Hospital (Ouellette Campus) and MRE at St Michael's Hospital.

Small bowel obstruction following use of psyllium is an uncommon occurrence. Only two cases of small bowel obstruction have been reported after CTE or MRE when using Metamucil or a psyllium-equivalent oral

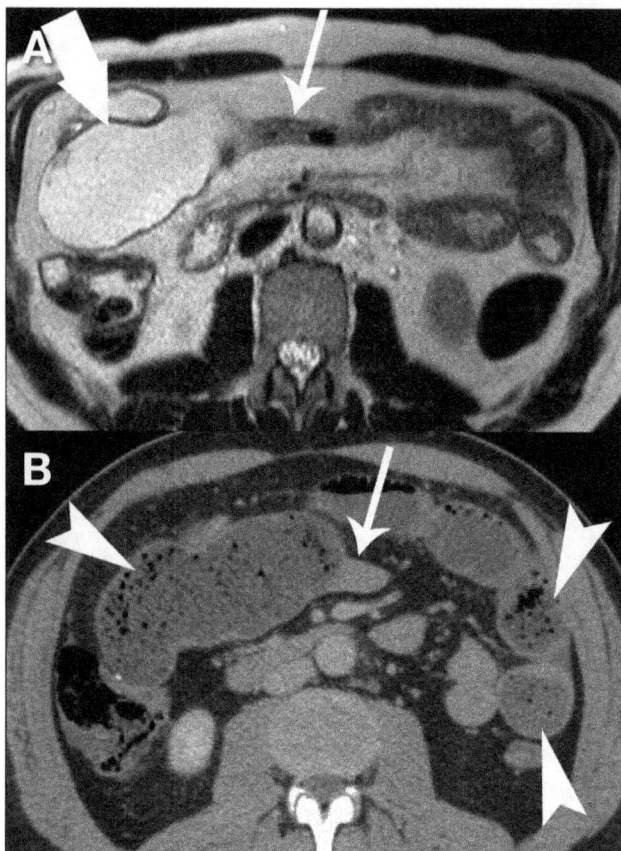

Figure 4) **A** *Axial T2-weighted magnetic resonance enterography image demonstrating a long segment of narrowing (thin arrow) distal to an ileoileal anastomosis (thick arrow) without evidence of active inflammation.* **B** *Computed tomography imaging performed 12 h later showing diffuse dilation of the small bowel with fecalization of bowel content (arrowheads) and a transition point at the narrowed segment of bowel demonstrated on magnetic resonance enterography (thin arrow)*

active inflammation. For centres that continue to use psyllium or other bulking agents, patients should be informed of the potential risk of obstruction and of symptoms that should prompt them to seek medical attention. Metamucil has been replaced by a 3% sorbitol solution for both CTE and MRE examinations at our institutions, with no negative impact on small bowel distension (25), patient acceptance and side effects, or departmental workflow.

CONCLUSION
We report a case series describing four patients who developed small bowel obstruction following the use of psyllium seed husk (Metamucil) as an oral contrast agent for CTE or MRE. Radiologists who oversee CTE and MRE examinations should be aware of the potential complication of Metamucil and other bulking agents, particularly when imaging patients with known or suspected small bowel strictures or active inflammation.

DISCLOSURES: The authors have no financial disclosures or conflicts of interest to declare.

contrast agent (14,15). The time course between psyllium ingestion to the development of small bowel obstruction was 12 h in one case and 'several days' in the other. Neither circumstances were well described nor had subsequent imaging available to confirm the obstruction. Several other trials evaluating the side effects of psyllium and other bulking agents on healthy individuals did not report any severe complications (4,11,12,15-18).

Psyllium bezoar causing small bowel obstruction has been reported in elderly populations that chronically use high concentrations of psyllium without adequate water consumption (19,20). Incidents of psyllium bezoar causing esophageal obstruction have also been described in patients who ingest dry psyllium preparations without adequate water (21-24).

We suspect that the presence of small bowel strictures represents a risk factor for obstruction following the use of psyllium as an oral contrast agent. The transition point of the small bowel obstruction in one of our patients occurred at an active segment of Crohn disease in which there was significant luminal narrowing. Transition points in two other patients occurred at a narrowed surgical anastomotic site and within a parastomal hernia. The Metamucil-water suspension may have formed a semisolid mucilaginous mass, causing intrinsic obstruction at these points with higher predisposition to obstruction due to narrowing.

As a result of our experience, we suggest that centres exercise caution when using psyllium or other bulking agents as an oral contrast agent in patients with known or suspected small bowel strictures or

REFERENCES
1. Bernstein CN, Greenberg H, Boult I, Chubey S, Leblanc C, Ryner L. A prospective comparison study of MRI versus small bowel follow-through in recurrent Crohn's disease. Am J Gastroenterol 2005;100:2493-502.
2. Hara AK, Leighton JA, Heigh RI, et al. Crohn disease of the small bowel: Preliminary comparison among CT enterography, capsule endoscopy, small-bowel follow-through, and ileoscopy. Radiology 2006;238:128-34.
3. Lee SS, Kim AY, Yang SK, et al. Crohn disease of the small bowel: Comparison of CT enterography, MR enterography, and small-bowel follow-through as diagnostic techniques. Radiology 2009;251:751-61.
4. Frokjaer JB, Larsen E, Steffensen E, Nielsen AH, Drewes AM. Magnetic resonance imaging of the small bowel in Crohn's disease. Scand J Gastroenterol 2005;40:832-42.
5. Ha CY, Kumar N, Raptis CA, Narra VR, Ciorba MA. Magnetic resonance enterography: Safe and effective imaging for stricturing Crohn's disease. Dig Dis Sci 2011;56:2906-13.
6. Messaris E, Chandolias N, Grand D, Pricolo V. Role of magnetic resonance enterography in the management of Crohn disease. Arch Surg 2010;145:471-5.
7. Masselli G, Gualdi G. CT and MR enterography in evaluating small bowel diseases: When to use which modality? Abdom Imaging 2013;38:249-59.
8. Tennyson CA, Semrad CE. Small bowel imaging in celiac disease. Gastrointest Endosc Clin N Am 2012;22:735-46.
9. Fork FT, Aabakken L. Capsule enteroscopy and radiology of the small intestine. Eur Radiol 2007;17:3103-11.
10. Amzallag-Bellenger E, Oudjit A, Ruiz A, Cadiot G, Soyer PA, Hoeffel CC. Effectiveness of MR enterography for the assessment of small-bowel diseases beyond Crohn disease. Radiographics 2012;32:1423-44.
11. Lauenstein TC, Schneemann H, Vogt FM, Herborn CU, Ruhm SG, Debatin JF. Optimization of oral contrast agents for MR imaging of the small bowel. Radiology 2003;228:279-83.
12. Patak MA, Froehlich JM, von Weymarn C, Ritz MA, Zollikofer CL, Wentz K. Non-invasive distension of the small bowel for magnetic-resonance imaging. Lancet 2001;358 987-8.
13. Singh B. Psyllium as therapeutic and drug delivery agent. Int J Pharm 2007;334:1-14.
14. Doerfler OC, Ruppert-Kohlmayr AJ, Reittner P, Hinterleitner T, Petritsch W, Szolar DH. Helical CT of the small bowel with an alternative oral contrast material in patients with Crohn disease. Abdom Imaging 2003;28:313-8.
15. Reittner P, Goritschnig T, Petritsch W, et al. Multiplanar spiral CT enterography in patients with Crohn's disease using a negative oral contrast material: Initial results of a noninvasive imaging approach. Eur Radiol 2002;12:2253-7.
16. Ajaj W, Goehde SC, Schneemann H, Ruehm SG, Debatin JF, Lauenstein TC. Oral contrast agents for small bowel MRI: Comparison of different additives to optimize bowel distension. Eur Radiol 2004;14:458-64.

Small bowel obstruction following computed tomography and magnetic resonance enterography using psyllium...

45

17. Froehlich JM, Daenzer M, von Weymarn C, Erturk SM, Zollikofer CL, Patak MA. Aperistaltic effect of hyoscine N-butylbromide versus glucagon on the small bowel assessed by magnetic resonance imaging. Eur Radiol 2009;19:1387-93.

18. Jensen MD, Nathan T, Kjeldsen J, Rafaelsen SR. Incidental findings at MRI-enterography in patients with suspected or known Crohn's disease. World J Gastroenterol 2010;16:76-82.

19. Fisher RE. Psyllium seeds: Intestinal Obstruction. Cal West Med 1938;48:190.

20. Frohna WJ. Metamucil bezoar: An unusual cause of small bowel obstruction. Am J Emerg Med 1992;10:393-5.

21. Herrle F, Peters T, Lang C, von Fluee M, Kern B, Peterli R. Bolus obstruction of pouch outlet by a granular bulk laxative after gastric banding. Obes Surg 2004;14:1022-4.

22. Perez-Piqueras J, Silva C, Jaqueti J, et al. Endoscopic diagnosis and treatment of an esophageal bezoar resulting from bulk laxative ingestion. Endoscopy 1994;26:710.

23. Sauerbruch T, Kuntzen O, Unger W. Agiolax bolus in the esophagus. Report of two cases. Endoscopy 1980;12:83-5.

24. Veronelli A, Ranieri R, Laneri M, et al. Gastric bezoars after adjustable gastric banding. Obes Surg 2004;14:796-7.

25. Saini S, Colak E, Anthwal S, Vlachou PA, Raikhlin A, Kirpalani A. Comparison of 3% sorbitol versus psyllium fibre as oral contrast agents in magnetic resonance enterography. Society of Abdominal Radiology 2014 Annual Scientific Meeting and Educational Course, Boca Raton, 2014.

8

Iron overload is rare in patients homozygous for the H63D mutation

Melissa Kelley MD, Nikhil Joshi MD, Yagang Xie MD, Mark Borgaonkar MD MSc

M Kelley, N Joshi, Y Xie, M Borgaonkar. Iron overload is rare in patients homozygous for the H63D mutation. Can J Gastroenterol Hepatol 2014;28(4):198-202.

BACKGROUND: Previous research has suggested that the H63D *HFE* mutation is associated with elevated iron indexes. However, the true penetrance of this mutation remains unclear.

OBJECTIVE: To assess the proportion of H63D homozygotes with laboratory abnormalities consistent with iron overload.

METHODS: The present study was a retrospective analysis of all individuals referred for *HFE* genotyping in Newfoundland and Labrador between 1999 and 2009, who were found to be homozygous for the H63D mutation. Using electronic health records, results of ferritin, transferrin saturation, aspartate aminotransferase and alanine aminotransferase testing performed closest to the time of genetic testing were recorded for each patient. Iron overload was classified using previously published definitions from the HealthIron study. SPSS version 17.0 (IBM Corporation, USA) was used for descriptive statistics and to compare means using one-way ANOVA.

RESULTS: Between 1999 and 2009, 170 individuals tested positive for H63D/H63D. At the time of genotyping, 28.8% had an elevated mean (± SD) ferritin level of 501±829 µg/L and 15.9% had an elevated transferrin saturation of 0.45±0.18. At genotyping, 94 individuals had sufficient data available to classify iron overload status. Only three (3.2%) had documented iron overload while the majority (85.1%) had no evidence of iron overload. Sixty individuals had follow-up data available and, of these, only four (6.7%) had documented iron overload, while 45 (75.0%) had no evidence of iron overload. Only one individual had evidence of iron overload-related disease at genotyping and at follow-up.

CONCLUSIONS: H63D homozygosity was associated with an elevated mean ferritin level, but only 6.7% had documented iron overload at follow-up. The penetrance of the H63D mutation appeared to be low.

Key Words: *Ferritin; Hemochromatosis; HFE*

La surcharge en fer est rare chez les patients homozygotes à la mutation H63D

HISTORIQUE : D'après des recherches passées, la mutation H63D *HFE* s'associe à des indices de fer élevés. Cependant, on n'en connaît pas la véritable pénétrance.

OBJECTIF : Évaluer la proportion d'homozygotes H63D ayant des anomalies de laboratoire compatibles avec une surcharge en fer.

MÉTHODOLOGIE : La présente étude était une analyse rétrospective de toutes les personnes aiguillées pour le génotypage du *HFE* à Terre-Neuve-et-Labrador entre 1999 et 2009, diagnostiquées comme homozygotes à la mutation H63D. Au moyen des dossiers de santé électroniques, les chercheurs ont compilé pour chaque patient les résultats des tests de ferritine, de saturation de la transferrine, d'aspartate aminotransférase et d'alanine aminotransférase effectués le plus près du moment du test génétique. Ils ont classé la surcharge en fer d'après les définitions déjà publiées dans l'étude HealthIron et utilisé le logiciel SPSS version 17.0 (IBM Corporation, États-Unis) pour compiler les statistiques descriptives et comparer les moyennes à l'aide de l'analyse de variance unidirectionnelle.

RÉSULTATS : Entre 1999 et 2009, 170 personnes ont obtenu des résultats positifs à la mutation H63D/H63D. Au moment du génotypage, 28,8 % présentaient un taux de ferritine moyen (± ÉT) élevé de 501±829 µg/L et 15,9 %, une saturation de la transferrine élevée de 0,45±0,18. Au génotypage, les chercheurs possédaient assez de données pour classer le statut de surcharge en fer de 94 personnes. Seulement trois (3,2 %) présentaient une surcharge en fer vérifiée, tandis que la majorité (85,1 %) n'en présentait aucune manifestation. Soixante personnes avaient des données de suivi, et de ce nombre, seulement quatre (6,7 %) avaient une surcharge en fer vérifiée, tandis que 45 (75,0 %) n'en présentaient aucune manifestation. Une seule personne avait des manifestations de maladie liée à une surcharge en fer à la fois au génotypage et au suivi.

CONCLUSIONS : L'homozygotie H63D s'associait à un taux de ferritine moyen élevé, mais seulement 6,7 % présentaient une surcharge en fer vérifiée au suivi. La pénétration de la mutation H63D semblait faible.

Hereditary hemochromatosis (HH) is one of the most common inherited conditions affecting individuals of Northern European descent. HH is inherited in an autosomal recessive pattern and is characterized by increased iron absorption and tissue deposition (1). This may cause organ damage including cirrhosis, diabetes, cardiomyopathy, arthropathy and impotence. However, the majority of patients are asymptomatic at the time of diagnosis (1).

In 1996, Feder et al (2) identified the candidate gene for HH (subsequently designated *HFE*), which encoded a major histocompatability complex class 1-like molecule that was involved in iron uptake. The two most common mutations are C282Y and H63D. The C282Y is a missense mutation, with a cysteine-to-tyrosine substitution at amino acid position 282. The C282Y mutation has been the most strongly implicated in the development of hemochromatosis. The H63D *HFE* mutation is a histidine-to-aspartic acid substitution at amino acid position 63. It has also been associated with hemochromatosis, but

to a lesser extent than C282Y; the overall clinical significance of this mutation remains unclear. Some postulate that it plays a role in the development of the disease but that the penetrance tends to be low (3-8). Some studies have suggested that the H63D mutation is simply a polymorphism and may not be of clinical significance when present without any other mutations (9-11).

If HH is recognized early in its course, phlebotomy therapy can prevent the complications of iron deposition. This has led to some discussion regarding screening individuals for HH because the condition meets many of the WHO criteria for population screening (1). However, the penetrance of the disease is variable and some studies have shown that even individuals homozygous for the C282Y mutation may not develop clinically overt disease (12).

In a previous study, we found that H63D homozygotes had a significantly higher transferrin saturation than the wild-type genotype. We also showed that the degree of transferrin saturation elevation was

Faculty of Medicine, Memorial University, St John's, Newfoundland and Labrador

Correspondence: Dr Melissa Kelley, Toronto Western Hospital, 399 Bathurst Street, 6B Fell Pavilion, Toronto, Ontario M5T 2S8.
E-mail melkelley08@gmail.com

TABLE 1
Iron overload categories*

Variable	Clinical finding or laboratory measure
Documented iron overload	At least one of the following:
	1. Increased iron content shown by hepatic iron staining 3 or 4, iron concentration >90 µmol/g or hepatic iron index >1.9, OR
	2. Serum ferritin >1000 µg/L at baseline with documented therapeutic venesection
Provisional iron overload	1. Elevated serum ferritin (>300 µg/L for men and postmenopausal women, >200 µg/L for premenopausal women), AND
	2. Elevated transferrin saturation (>55% for men and >45% for women).
	Either normal or elevated serum ferritin with normal transferrin saturation
Iron overload-related disease	Meet the criteria for documented iron overload plus at least one of the following:
	1. Hepatocellular carcinoma
	2. Cirrhosis or fibrosis on liver biopsy
	3. Tenderness or effusion of the second and third metocarpophalangeal joints
	4. Elevated aspartate aminotransferase (>45 IU/L) or alanine aminotransferase (>40 IU/L)
	5. Diagnosis by a physician owing to symptoms associated with hereditary hemochromatosis

*Data adapted from the HeathIron study (14)

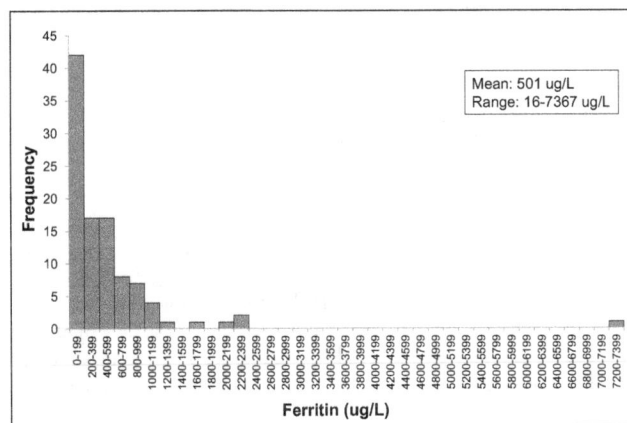

Figure 1) *Histogram of ferritin levels at the time of genotyping*

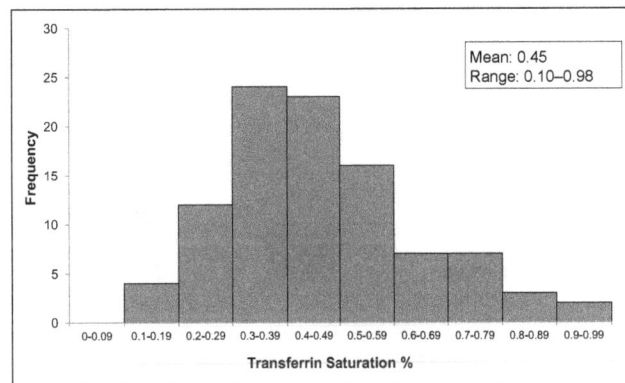

Figure 2) *Histogram of transferrin saturation levels at the time of genotyping*

comparable with C282Y homozygotes and compound heterozygotes. However, the clinical significance of these results could not be determined (13).

The purpose of the present study was to determine the penetrance of H63D homozygosity in a referred population in Newfoundland and Labrador by following a cohort of H63D homozygotes for evidence of iron overload.

METHODS

The present study was approved by the Research Ethics Board of Memorial University of Newfoundland (St Johns, Newfoundland and Labrador) before commencement. Subjects were from Newfoundland and Labrador, an island comprised predominantly of Caucasians of Irish and English descent. The present study was a retrospective analysis of all individuals referred for *HFE* genotyping in Newfoundland and Labrador from 1999 to 2009, who were identified to be homozygous for the *HFE* H63D mutation. The indication for genotyping was not stated on the requisition. There is only one laboratory in the province that performs genotyping for HFE, enabling the authors to identify every individual who tested positive for H63D homozygosity. During the study period, only the C282Y and H63D mutations were assessed.

Using electronic health records, age, sex, ferritin levels, serum iron, transferrin saturation, aspartate aminotransferase (AST) and alanine aminotransferase (ALT) levels closest to the time of genetic testing were recorded. To avoid including information from partially treated individuals, only bloodwork data obtained within six months of the genetic test were recorded. Measurement of transferrin saturation was not performed specifically in the fasting state. Follow-up laboratory values were recorded annually up to February 2011. Ferritin >335 µg/L, AST and ALT >37 IU/L and transferrin saturation >0.55 were considered to be abnormally elevated. Liver biopsy results and treatment

with phlebotomy were also documented if recorded in the electronic health record. Iron overload was classified using previously published definitions from the HealthIron study (14) (Table 1). Briefly, this system classifies patients into one of four iron overload categories, ranging from no evidence of iron overload to iron overload-related disease.

The data were summarized using descriptive statistics. Incidence and prevalence of iron-overload were calculated using the number of patients with complete data as the denominator. SPSS version 17.0 (IBM Corporation, USA) was used for descriptive statistics and to compare means using Student's t test or one-way ANOVA; P≤0.05 was considered to be statistically significant.

RESULTS

A total of 4138 individuals underwent *HFE* genotyping in Newfoundland and Labrador between 1999 and January 2009. There were 366 (8.8%) C282Y homozygotes, 170 (4.1%) H63D homozygotes, 758 (18.3%) C282Y heterozygotes, 858 (20.7%) H63D heterozygotes, 267 (6.4%) compound heterozygotes and 1719 (41.5%) wild type. Of the 170 H63D homozygotes, 116 (68.2%) were male and 54 (31.8%) were female. The mean age at the time of genotyping was 48.9 years. At the time of genotyping, 28.8% had an elevated ferritin level and 15.9% had an elevated transferrin saturation. The mean ferritin level was 501 µg/L (range 16 µg/L to 7367 µg/L) (Figure 1) and the mean transferrin saturation was 0.45 (range 0.10 to 0.98) (Figure 2). The mean AST level was 56 IU/L, ALT 72 IU/L, bilirubin 22.6 µmol/L, international normalized ratio 1.5 and albumin 40.7 g/L (Table 2).

The mean follow-up duration was 4.2±2.6 years. There was no significant increase in the mean ferritin level over time.

At the time of genotyping, the records of 94 individuals contained sufficient data to determine iron overload status (Figure 3). The

TABLE 2
Baseline characteristics

Characteristic	Mean (range)
Age at genotyping, years	48.9 (17–77)
Ferritin, μg/L	501 (16–7367)
Transferrin saturation	0.45 (0.10–0.98)
Aspartate aminotransferase, IU/L	56.3 (14–992)
Alanine aminotransferase, IU/L	71.7 (12–1190)
Bilirubin, μmol/L	22.6 (3–223)
International normalized ratio	1.5 (0.87–10.0)
Albumin, g/L	40.7 (21–48)

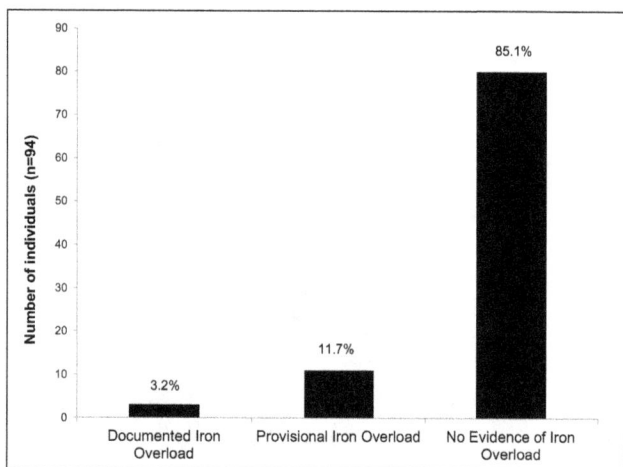

Figure 3) *Iron overload status at time of genotyping*

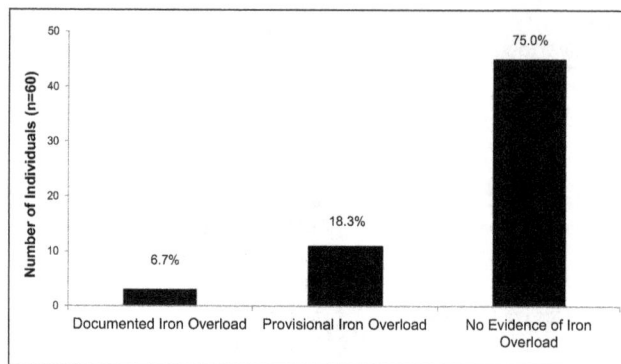

Figure 4) *Iron overload status at follow-up*

majority of H63D homozygotes (85.1%) had no evidence of iron overload. Three (3.2%) had documented iron overload, with one (1.1%) meeting criteria for iron overload-related disease. Eleven (11.7%) had provisional iron overload. Sixty individuals had follow-up data available and, of these, four (6.7%) had documented iron overload. Only one (1.7%) of these individuals met criteria for iron overload-related disease. Eleven (18.3%) had provisional iron overload and 45 (75.0%) had no evidence of iron overload (Figure 4).

Only one individual had iron overload-related disease, both at the time of genotyping and at follow-up. Clinical records noted excess alcohol consumption in that case. Two (3.3%) individuals progressed from no evidence of iron overload to provisional iron overload. There were two individuals without sufficient data for a baseline classification of iron status who did meet criteria for some degree of iron overload during follow-up. One met the criteria for documented iron overload and one met the criteria for provisional iron overload.

Eight individuals underwent phlebotomy after genotyping. The details of the frequency and duration of phlebotomy were not available. None of the six individuals for whom follow-up data were available showed progression of iron overload.

DISCUSSION

The results of the present study suggest a low penetrance of H63D homozyosity. Although serum ferritin levels were elevated at baseline, there was no significant increase in mean ferritin level for the cohort over time. Only three individuals met the criteria for iron overload at the time of genotyping and four at follow-up. Within this group, only one individual met the criteria for iron overload-related disease. That patient was documented to have abused alcohol, such that one cannot be certain whether iron overload was the primary cause of his liver disease. The majority of the individuals in our study showed no evidence of iron overload (85.1% at baseline and 75.0% at follow-up). Only two individuals demonstrated any progression of their iron overload status during the study (3.3%).

In a previous study involving this same population, we found that H63D homozygosity was associated with a significantly higher mean transferrin saturation when compared with the wild-type genotype (0.44±0.18 versus 0.34±0.17; P<0.01). In that study, 42.0% of H63D homozygotes had elevated ALT levels compared with 30.1% of C282Y heterozygotes (P=0.04) (15).

The results of the present study are consistent with other studies that have found the H63D mutation to be associated with elevated iron levels (3,7,9,10,13,16,17). Phatak et al (17) found that the H63D homozygotes had a significantly elevated mean transferrin saturation when compared with the wild-type genotype, but this was not above the upper limit of normal. Gochee et al (10) found that 15% of male H63D homozygotes and 12% of male H63D heterozygotes had an elevated transferrin saturation compared with only 5% in the wild-type genotype (P<0.01). Samarasena et al (13) conducted a study involving the Newfoundland and Labrador population and found that the H63D homozygotes had significantly elevated transferrin saturation compared with the wild-type genotype (0.51±0.21 versus 0.34±0.17; P<0.01). They also had an elevated mean ferritin level (920.3±1687.1 μg/L) but it was not statistically significant compared with the other genotypes (13). The Hemochromatosis and Iron Overload Screening (HEIRS) study (18) also found elevated ferritin levels and transferrin saturation to be more common among compound heterozygotes and H63D homozygotes when compared with the wild type, although the mean values were within the normal range.

Although the H63D homozygous mutation has been associated with elevated iron indexes, it is unclear whether these individuals require phlebotomy or whether they will progress to develop clinically significant iron overload. Several studies have suggested that H63D homozygosity has a much lower penetrance than C282Y homozygosity and are at a lower risk for developing clinically significant iron overload (4,11). Neghina et al (19) conducted a meta-analysis examining the association between the various HFE genotypes and iron overload. They found that in individuals with a clinical diagnosis of hemochromatosis, the C282Y homozygous genotype had a 100 times greater association with an elevated transferrin saturation (>55%) and elevated serum iron and serum ferritin when compared with H63D homozygotes. In cases for which hemochromatosis was documented by an elevated hepatic iron index and/or mobilizable iron by quantitative phlebotomy, C282Y homozygosity was 100 times more strongly associated with iron overload than H63D homozygosity (19).

Other studies have shown the H63D mutation to be associated with clinically significant iron overload. One study found that three of 61 individuals with a phenotypic diagnosis of hemochromatosis were homozygous for the H63D mutation (5). These patients had either a hepatic iron index >1.9 or mobilizable iron stores of >4 g. A study by Brissot et al (20) determined the HFE genotypes of 217 patients with a phenotypic diagnosis of hemochromatosis. The majority (96.3%) were homozygous for the C282Y mutation. Four individuals were compound heterozygotes, one was homozygous for the H63D mutation and one was heterozygous for the H63D mutation. Although the C282Y mutation was most frequently associated with hemochromatosis, they did find that the H63D mutation occurred more frequently in the hemochromatosis population when compared with the control group. However, not all of these patients underwent liver biopsies and, in some, the phenotypic diagnosis was based solely on the elevated transferrin saturation.

Aguilar-Martinez et al (21) conducted a study involving a population referred for *HFE* genotyping and found a wide variety of phenotypes among the H63D homozygotes, ranging from normal to severe iron overload. Within this population, 24% of H63D homozygotes had a hemochromatosis phenotype characterized by an elevated ferritin and transferrin saturation level plus either iron overload on liver biopsy or quantitative phlebotomy. This study suggests a significantly higher penetrance of the H63D mutation than what was shown in our population. This difference is likely due to the reason for genotyping. Aguilar-Martinez et al (21) included patients referred for testing with either a personal or family history of iron overload, including 12 individuals (24% of the study population) previously diagnosed with hemochromatosis. Therefore, one would expect to find a more severe phenotype in this cohort. In our cohort, the reason for referral was not documented. Family history and elevated iron studies would have been the reason for referral in a proportion of our cohort. Some of the H63D homozygotes in our cohort had elevated transaminase levels, which likely was the reason for investigation in some patients. This heterogeneity in patients sent for genotyping is likely the reason why our cohort demonstrated a broader spectrum of iron overload severity than reported by Aguilar-Martinez et al (21).

Some have postulated that H63D homozygotes who develop clinically significant iron overload may have another unidentified contributing mutation. One study examined H63D homozygotes with significantly elevated transferrin saturation and serum ferritin levels for mutations affecting other iron regulatory genes (22). The investigators screened specifically for 18 known *HFE*, *TFR2* and *FPN1* mutations and had complete sequencing of the *HAMP* gene. They were unsuccessful in finding any mutations affecting these genes in the 45 H63D homozygotes.

Some authors have proposed that environmental factors play a role in the variable penetrance of the hemochromatosis mutations. Aranda et al (16) found that iron intake, alcohol intake, tobacco habit and male sex were all positively associated with elevated iron studies in all *HFE* genotypes containing C282Y or H63D and in S65C homozygotes. It has also been postulated that another process affecting the liver may actually be contributing to the increase in iron load. Bacon et al (11) measured the hepatic iron concentration of 132 patients with liver disease. Five of these were homozygous for H63D and there was no significant difference in the hepatic iron concentration or the hepatic index compared with the wild-type genotype. All five patients received a diagnosis of conditions other than hemochromatosis causing their liver disease (11).

The distribution of genotypes in our cohort does differ from a population-based study of hemochromatosis. The HEIRS study (18) examined a primary care population of 99,711 individuals. Within the Caucasian population of this group, 0.44% were homozygous for the C282Y mutation and 2.4% were homozygous for the H63D mutation (18). The individuals in our study were referred by a health professional for *HFE* genotyping and were, therefore, not a true population-based sample. The distribution of C282Y (8.8%) and H63D homozygotes (4.1%) present in our population was closer to the referred population studied by Aguilar-Martinez et al (21), which consisted of 18.4% C282Y homozygotes and 6.2% H63D homozygotes.

The present study had several strengths. It was a large cohort followed for a long duration of time. Although the study was retrospective in nature, the data collection had been performed prospectively and provided us with ample data on a subset of patients.

There were, however, some limitations to the present study. It was retrospective in design and, therefore, was limited to the data that could be obtained from the electronic health records. Although we had the genotyping results from all individuals in the province, access to the primary health record (including clinical letters, additional laboratory tests, imaging and pathology results) was limited to only a subset of patients in the Eastern Health region. Consequently, only partial (or no) baseline and follow-up data were available for 69.4% of patients. We do not believe that the reason for incomplete data for some patients would bias the findings to affect the validity of our results. We were unable to obtain clinical information, such as alcohol consumption, for most individuals. However, for 30% of patients, we did have sufficient baseline and follow-up data to assess the natural history of H63D homozygosity. The duration of follow-up was limited by the health records themselves and when genotyping became available in this region. It is possible that if patients were followed for a longer duration, the results would be different.

The indication for genotyping was unknown for all patients in the cohort. Although we did find that the H63D homozygous mutation was associated with significantly elevated ferritin levels, it is possible that this was the reason the individuals underwent genotyping, which would bias these results.

CONCLUSION

The H63D homozygous mutation was associated with elevated iron indexes. Despite this, the incidence of documented iron overload was low (6.7% at follow-up) and only one individual met the criteria for iron overload-related disease. The results of our study indicate that although the H63D mutation may be related to alterations in iron indexes and transaminase levels, the penetrance of this mutation in causing iron overload-related disease is low.

REFERENCES

1. Bacon BR. Hemochromatosis: Diagnosis and management. Gastroenterology 2001;120:718-25.
2. Feder J, Gnirke A, Thomas A, et al. A novel MHC class I-like gene is mutated in patients with hereditary haemochromatosis. Nat Genet 1996;13:399-408.
3. Matas M, Guix P, Castro JA, et al. Prevalence of *HFE* C282Y and H63D in Jewish populations and clinical implications of H63D homozygosity. Clin Genet 2006;69:155-62.
4. Burke W, Imperatore G, McDonnell SM, Baron RC, Khoury MJ. Contribution of different *HFE* genotypes to iron overload disease: A pooled analysis. Gene Med 2000;2:271-7.
5. Sham RL, Ou CY, Cappuccio J, et al. Correlation between genotype and phenotype in hereditary hemochromatosis: Analysis of 61 cases. Blood Cells Mol Dis 1997;23:314-20.
6. Fairbanks VF, Brandhagen DJ, Thibodeau SN, Snow K, Wollan PC. H63D is an haemachromatosis associated allele. Gut 1998;43:441-4.
7. Pedersen P, Milman N. Genetic screening for *HFE* hemochromatosis in 6,020 Danish men: Penetrance of C282Y, H63D, and S65C variants. Ann Hematol 2009;88:775-84.
8. Beutler E. The significance of the 187G (H63D) mutation in hemochromatosis. Am J Hum Genet 1997;61:762-4.
9. Jackson HA, Carter K, Darke C, et al. *HFE* mutations, iron deficiency and overload in 10,500 blood donors. Br J Haematol 2001;114:474-84.
10. Gochee PA, Powell LW, Cullen DJ, et al. A population-based study of the biochemical and clinical expression of the H63D hemochromatosis mutation. Gastroenterology 2002;122:646-51.
11. Bacon BR, Olynyk JK, Brunt EM, Britton RS, Wolff RK. *HFE* genotypes in hemochromatosis and other liver diseases. Ann Intern Med 1999;130:1018-9.
12. Andersen RV, Tybjaerg-Hansen A, Appleyard M, Birgens H, Nordestgaard BG. Hemochromatosis mutations in the general population: Iron overload progression rate. Blood 2004;103:2914-9.
13. Samarasena J, Winsor W, Lush R, et al. Individuals homozygous for the H63D mutation have significantly elevated iron indexes. Dig Dis Sci 2006;51:803-7.
14. Allen KJ, Gurrin LC, Constantine CC, et al. Iron overload-related disease in *HFE* hereditary hemochromatosis. N Engl J Med 2008;358:221-30.

15. Kelley M, Joshi N, Xie Y, Borgaonkar M. Hemochromatosis gene mutations in Newfoundland and their association with iron indices and transaminase levels. Gut 2010;59:A313.

16. Aranda N, Viteri FE, Montserrat C, Arija V. Effects of C282Y, H63D, and S65C *HFE* gene mutations, diet, and life-style factors on iron status in a general Mediterranean population from Tarragona, Spain. Ann Hematol 2010;89:767-73.

17. Phatak PD, Ryan DH, Cappuccio J, et al. Prevalence and penetrance of HFE mutations in 4865 unselected primary care patients. Blood Cells Mol Dis 2002;29:41-7.

18. Adams PC, Reboussin DM, Barton JC, et al. Hemochromatosis and iron-overload screening in a racially diverse population. N Engl J Med 2005;352:1769-78.

19. Neghina AM, Anghel A. Hemochromatosis genotypes and risk of iron overload – a meta-analysis. Ann Epidemiol 2011;21:1-14.

20. Brissot P, Moirand R, Jouanolle AM, et al. A genotypic study of 217 unrelated probands diagnosed as "genetic hemochromatosis" on "classical" phenotypic criteria. J Hepatol 1999;30:588-93.

21. Aguilar-Martinez P, Bismuth M, Picot MC, et al. Variable phenotypic presentation of iron overload in H63D homozygotes: Are genetic modifiers the cause? Gut 2001;48:836-42.

22. Diego C de, Opazo S, Murga MJ, Martínez-Castro P. H63D homozygotes with hyperferritinaemia: Is this genotype, the primary cause of iron overload? Eur J Haematol 2007;78:66-71.

9

The 3rd Canadian Symposium on Hepatitis C Virus: Expanding care in the interferon-free era

Sonya A MacParland PhD[1], Marc Bilodeau MD[2], Jason Grebely PhD[3], Julie Bruneau MD[4], Curtis Cooper MD[5], Marina Klein MD[6], Selena M Sagan PhD[7], Norma Choucha[2], Louise Balfour PhD[5], Frank Bialystok PhD[1], Mel Krajden MD[8,9], Jennifer Raven PhD[10], Eve Roberts MD[1], Rodney Russell PhD[11], Michael Houghton PhD[12], D Lorne Tyrrell MD PhD[12], Jordan J Feld MD[1]; on behalf of the National CIHR Research Training Program in Hepatitis C

SA MacParland, M Bilodeau, J Grebely, et al. The 3rd Canadian Symposium on Hepatitis C Virus: Expanding care in the interferon-free era. Can J Gastroenterol Hepatol 2014;28(9): 481-487.

Hepatitis C virus (HCV) currently infects approximately 250,000 individuals in Canada and causes more years of life lost than any other infectious disease in the country. In August 2011, new therapies were approved by Health Canada that have achieved higher response rates among those treated, but are poorly tolerated. By 2014/2015, short-course, well-tolerated treatments with cure rates >95% will be available. However, treatment uptake is poor due to structural, financial, geographical, cultural and social barriers. As such, 'Barriers to access to HCV care in Canada' is a crucial topic that must be addressed to decrease HCV disease burden and potentially eliminate HCV in Canada. Understanding how to better care for HCV-infected individuals requires integration across multiple disciplines including researchers, clinical services and policy makers to address the major populations affected by HCV including people who inject drugs, baby boomers, immigrants and Aboriginal and/or First Nations people. In 2012, the National CIHR Research Training Program in Hepatitis C organized the 1st Canadian Symposium on Hepatitis C Virus (CSHCV) in Montreal, Quebec. The 2nd CSHCV was held in 2013 in Victoria, British Columbia. Both symposia were highly successful, attracting leading international faculty with excellent attendance leading to dialogue and knowledge translation among attendees of diverse backgrounds. The current article summarizes the 3rd CSHCV, held February 2014, in Toronto, Ontario.

Key Words: *Biomedical; Clinical; Epidemiology; Hepatitis C; Public health; Social sciences*

Le 3ᵉ symposium canadien sur le virus de l'hépatite C : élargir les soins en cette ère de traitement sans interféron

Le virus de l'hépatite C (VHC), qui infecte environ 250 000 personnes au Canada, est responsable de plus d'années de vie perdues que toute autre maladie infectieuse au pays. En août 2011, Santé Canada a approuvé de nouvelles thérapies, dont les taux de réponse sont plus élevés chez les patients traités, mais qui sont mal tolérées. En 2014-2015, des traitements de courte durée, mais bien tolérés, assurant un taux de guérison de plus de 95 %, seront mis en marché. Cependant, la participation au traitement est faible, en raison d'obstacles structurels, financiers, géographiques, culturels et sociaux. C'est pourquoi les obstacles à l'accès aux soins du VHC au Canada constituent un sujet essentiel, qu'il faut aborder pour réduire le fardeau du VHC et peut-être éliminer le virus au Canada. Pour comprendre comment mieux soigner les personnes infectées par le VHC, il faut parvenir à intégrer de multiples disciplines, y compris les chercheurs, les services cliniques et les décideurs, afin de répondre aux besoins des principales populations atteintes du VHC, incluant les utilisateurs de drogues injectables, les baby-boomers, les immigrants et les personnes autochtones ou des Premières nations. En 2012, la Subvention nationale de formation des IRSC sur l'hépatite C a organisé le 1ᵉʳ symposium canadien sur le virus de l'hépatite C à Montréal, au Québec. Le 2ᵉ a eu lieu à Victoria, en Colombie-Britannique, en 2013. Ces deux symposiums ont obtenu un franc succès, car ils ont attiré des conférenciers internationaux réputés et suscité une excellente participation, ce qui a favorisé le dialogue et le partage de connaissances entre congressistes provenant de divers horizons. Le présent article résume le 3ᵉ symposium, qui s'est déroulé en février 2014 à Toronto, en Ontario.

In 2013, it was estimated that there were >250,000 Canadians with chronic hepatitis C virus (HCV) infection (1). HCV infection causes progressive liver injury, and approximately 15% to 25% will develop cirrhosis, end-stage liver disease and liver cancer over a 30-year follow-up period (2). In August 2011, two protease inhibitors approved by Health Canada have led to higher response rates among treated individuals. In December 2013, Health Canada approved the first polymerase inhibitor (sofosbuvir) and a new protease inhibitor with milder side effects than the first-generation inhibitors (simeprevir). These recent advances ensure that by 2014/2015, more effective and less toxic therapies will be available, leading to higher cure rates than ever before with shortened courses of therapy. However, treatment uptake is poor across the country, with <2% (n=3600) of the total population with chronic HCV treated in 2013 (1). Treatment uptake is limited by structural, financial, geographical, cultural and social barriers. In 2013, the lifetime cost for an individual infected with HCV was estimated to be $64,694 (1). To maximize the impact of the highly effective therapies that have recently been developed, it will be critical to improve treatment access, which can only be achieved by addressing the barriers to access to HCV care in Canada, with the goal to reduce disease burden and, ultimately, eliminate HCV infection from Canada.

Extending care to HCV-infected individuals requires a coordinated effort by clinicians, nurses, researchers and policy makers, and requires consideration of the unique needs of specific Canadian populations affected by HCV including people who inject drugs (PWID) and

[1]*University of Toronto, Toronto, Ontario;* [2]*Liver Unit, Department of Medicine, Université de Montréal, Montréal, Québec;* [3]*The Kirby Institute, UNSW Australia, Sydney, Australia;* [4]*Department of Family Medicine, Université de Montréal, Montréal, Québec;* [5]*Division of Infectious Diseases, University of Ottawa, Ottawa, Ontario;* [6]*Division of Infectious Diseases;* [7]*Department of Microbiology & Immunology, McGill University, Montreal, Quebec;* [8]*British Columbia Centre for Disease Control;* [9]*University of British Columbia, Vancouver, British Columbia;* [10]*Canadian Institutes of Health Research – Institute of Infection and Immunity, Ottawa, Ontario;* [11]*Division of Biomedical Sciences, Memorial University of Newfoundland, St John's, Newfoundland & Labrador;* [12]*Li Ka Shing Institute of Virology, University of Alberta, Edmonton, Alberta*

Correspondence and reprints: Dr Sonya MacParland, University of Toronto, 1 Kings College Circle, Toronto, Ontario M5S 3K5. e-mail sonyamacparland@gmail.com

HCV-infected Aboriginal persons, with both groups being identified by the Public Health Agency of Canada (PHAC) as being at increased risk for new HCV infections (3,4). In February 2012, the Canadian Institutes of Health Research (CIHR)-based National CIHR Research Training Program in Hepatitis C (NCRTP-HepC) organized the 1st Canadian Symposium on Hepatitis C Virus (CSHCV) in Montreal, Quebec. The 2nd CSHCV was held in March 2013 in Victoria, British Columbia (5). These symposia were well attended and attracted leading international experts, leading to dialogue and knowledge translation among attendees of diverse backgrounds. The current article summarizes the 3rd CSHCV, held February 2014, in Toronto, Ontario, where new Canadian and international HCV research findings were presented. It also gives an overview of the multidisciplinary discussions centred on improving access to care for HCV-infected Canadians. Specifically discussed were the challenges of delivering care to special populations of HCV-infected persons. Also highlighted was the need for a Canadian HCV action plan that would guide the provision of prevention, care and treatment for all Canadians infected with or at risk for acquiring HCV. The absence of such a plan remains a major obstacle that limits the marshalling of resources needed for HCV-infected Canadians to benefit from these potent, curative antivirals.

THE NCRTP-HepC

The NCRTP-HepC is a CIHR-supported Strategic Training Initiative in Health Research that was first funded in 2003 (www.ncrtp-hepc.ca/). The NCRTP-HepC is a partnership funded by public groups including the CIHR, PHAC and the Canadian Liver Foundation, and which receives private funding from both industry and community organizations. The main goal of the NCRTP-HepC is to build translational HCV research capacity, and to prevent, care and treat HCV with the desire to eliminate HCV disease in Canada within the next 10 to 15 years. The training program uses the knowledge of 35 leading researchers from universities across Canada, who act as mentors for the trainees and who advance Canadian HCV research. The NCRTP-HepC is interdisciplinary, with members representing diverse research backgrounds, including social and behavioural sciences, epidemiology and public health, clinical and biomedical sciences. Since 2003, the NCRTP-HepC has supported 71 trainees (11 MSc, 35 PhD, thee MD and 22 postdoctoral) and 45 summer students. This has significantly enhanced Canadian HCV research capacity, knowledge translation and interdisciplinary collaboration.

The NCRTP-HepC is a leader in facilitating HCV research in Canada (5). In response to feedback from the 1st and 2nd CSHCV, and questionnaires completed by community groups including the Canadian Liver Foundation's 'Living with Liver Diseases' support group and the Toronto Community Hepatitis C Program, the specific aims of the 3rd CSHCV were:

1. To facilitate transdisciplinary knowledge exchange and collaborations among Canadian trainees, established researchers, health care practitioners, health policy makers and community-based groups working in the field of HCV.

2. To discuss approaches that would lead to increased treatment uptake across the country with a focus on expanding care and access to difficult-to-reach populations with the ultimate goal of eliminating HCV in Canada.

3. To implement, plan and deliver knowledge exchange and dissemination of symposium findings to support practice change, community awareness, harm reduction and policy development.

4. To implement a long-term plan for sustaining an annual CSHCV.

THE 3rd CSHCV

Providing better care for HCV-infected individuals requires integration between researchers and policy makers across multiple disciplines. The theme of the 3rd CSHCV was "Expanding care for HCV-infected Individuals" and the program was divided into four sessions focusing on biomedical sciences, clinical sciences, social sciences, and epidemiology and public health. The primary audience included Canadian investigators, research trainees (including MSc, PhD and postdoctoral fellows), health care practitioners, policy makers, industry representatives and members of the affected community. The sessions, summarized below, consisted of an international plenary speaker, a Canadian speaker and peer-reviewed original oral abstracts.

Biomedical sciences

Advances in drug discovery and development have led to the approval of the first generation of direct-acting antivirals (DAAs) for the treatment of HCV (1,6). Triple therapy with first-generation protease inhibitors significantly improved sustained virological response rates compared with pegylated interferon (IFN) alpha-2a and ribavirin alone. However, first-generation protease inhibitors are associated with additional side effects and complicated regimens. This has made treatment more successful but more difficult than previous standard therapy with pegylated-IFN/ribavirin (6). At the end of 2013, Health Canada approved the second-wave protease inhibitor (simeprevir) and, most significantly, the first nucleotide inhibitor of the viral polymerase (sofosbuvir). These developments will pave the way for increased availability of IFN-free anti-HCV drug regimens for Canadians infected with HCV.

Although IFN will largely be replaced by IFN-free DAA oral regimens in the near future, IFN-based therapies may still have a role due to the prohibitively high cost of the new treatments. Hence, strategies to predict or enhance the success rate of IFN-based therapies will remain relevant for patient selection and, furthermore, understanding how IFN acts will still be of importance given its central role in the innate antiviral immune response. Dr Markus Heim (University Hospital Basel, Switzerland), a world leader on IFN as an antiviral, presented data from his laboratory on IFN responsiveness and discussed the future role of IFN in a world of highly effective DAAs (7). He suggested that most countries will develop algorithms to ensure that DAAs are used to treat individuals in greatest need but perhaps not all patients. If new treatments continue to be very expensive, he projected that IFN-based regimens will still have an important role, particularly for those who are likely to respond to therapy. Thus, it is critical that we gain a better understanding of why some, but not all, patients clear chronic HCV infections with IFN-based therapy.

While there have been great advances in our understanding of the innate immune response to HCV infection, it remains unclear why some patients have a relatively high level of baseline activation of IFN-responsive genes whereas others have minimal or no activation of these genes despite persistent HCV infection (8). The baseline expression of IFN-responsive genes is the strongest predictor of treatment outcome with IFN-based therapy (9). The gene expression pattern in a given individual is at least partially genetically determined, with strong associations with variants near the IFN lambda-3 (IFNλ3) gene (formerly known IL-28B), as well as with the recently identified IFNλ4 (10-15). Patients with the treatment-unfavourable variants tend to have activated IFN systems before receiving treatment and tend to be refractory to further stimulation with IFN. Overcoming IFN refractoriness by combining DAAs with IFN, using alternative dosing strategies or other IFNs, such as IFNλ, could enhance IFN responsiveness, allowing for shorter, more effective treatments that may be an acceptable alternative to cost-prohibitive IFN-free DAA regimens.

In addition to its association with treatment outcome, the IFNλ3 polymorphism is also associated with spontaneous resolution of acute HCV infection (15,16). Dr Naglaa Shoukry (Université de Montréal, Montreal, Quebec) discussed recent work that indicated increases in IFNλ3 in plasma occurring in acute HCV infection correlated with natural killer cell markers and degranulation (17). Natural killer cellular degranulation also correlates with the magnitude of the HCV-specific T cell responses, suggesting crosstalk between innate and adaptive immunity in acute HCV infection (18). A pilot transcriptome analysis of peripheral blood mononuclear cells from acute HCV patients of the Montreal Acute Hepatitis C Cohort (HEPCO) using RNA sequencing will hopefully shed some light on this important interaction (17). Preliminary results indicate differential expression of numerous genes, many of which function in innate and adaptive immunity. A robust induction of IFN-stimulated gene expression was demonstrated during acute HCV and, surprisingly, despite spontaneous clearance of the virus, peripheral blood mononuclear cells from resolver patients continued to demonstrate altered expression of immune genes for >1 year after clearance. Future studies will correlate parameters of HCV disease progression and compare these findings with data from patients infected with other viruses, vaccine studies and in vitro models. This will provide further insight into the interplay between innate and adaptive immunity on the outcome of HCV infection.

Clinical sciences

Access to care and treatment for marginalized and remotely located patients living with HCV is a critical issue along the cascade of care. Dr Sanjeev Arora, Director of Project ECHO (Extension for Community Healthcare Outcomes) at the University of New Mexico (Albuquerque, USA), described the objectives, structure, operation, successes and obstacles encountered with this innovative program (19). The mission of Project ECHO is to develop capacity to safely and effectively treat chronic, common and complex diseases in rural and underserved areas, and to monitor the outcomes of these treatments (20). HCV lends itself well to this model of care. Expert interdisciplinary specialist teams are linked with primary care clinicians via tele-ECHO clinics (21). Experts comanage patient cases and impart their expertise by way of mentorship, guidance, feedback and didactic education. In the case of HCV, primary care physicians retain responsibility for patient management, with the ultimate goal of developing independent expertise allowing them to manage future patients and become 'local experts' for their peers, thereby reducing travel costs, wait times and improving health care quality (21). HCV care and expertise has been dramatically expanded to remote regions and marginalized populations including prisoners who historically had never received HCV treatment in New Mexico. Evaluation of this care model demonstrates health care provider and patient satisfaction, as well as cure rates that are as good, if not better, than those achieved within an academic setting. This approach to HCV care appears to be ideal for Canada but will require a willingness to demonopolize specialist knowledge, and to task shift from services traditionally provided by physicians to other health care providers, as well as convincing public payers that investing in this type of care delivery system is cost-effective and sustainable.

In an extension of this topic, Drs Curtis Cooper and Julie Bruneau engaged in a lively and humorous debate entitled "Treatment should be strictly delivered by specialists rather than by primary care practitioners in the community" (22). Dr Cooper was given the difficult task of representing the 'pro' side and presenting arguments in favour of specialists strictly providing HCV care (when in fact he supported a broader approach of primary care physician involvement). Quoting *Hamlet* as well as research on HIV and oncology care, Dr Cooper argued that specialists were more likely to initiate treatment and choose appropriate regimens when facing complex conditions. He also pointed out that general practitioners may lack training, expertise and experience to treat specific conditions for which treatment evolves rapidly, such as with HIV and cancer survivorship (23,24). He suggested that, similar to HIV and cancer, HCV treatment is quite complex and management by specialists may be required.

On the 'con' side, Dr Bruneau pointed out that, to reduce HCV morbidity and mortality, we must first and foremost substantially increase treatment uptake among those who are infected. Currently, <10% of all infected people have access to treatment (25). Conceding that patients with severe liver conditions or multiple comorbidities should be treated in specialized academic settings with skilled and experienced specialists, she stressed the importance of having primary care physicians engaged in treating HCV-infected individuals. Not only are primary care physicians qualified to treat HCV, they can provide testing, counselling, and treat other medical conditions that often coexist with HCV, such as addiction and psychiatric disorders, ultimately improving the overall health outcomes (21). In the end, both debaters amicably concluded that HCV treatment should be widely available to patients according to best practices via the collaboration of primary care physicians and specialists in the best-adapted environment to meet individualized needs.

In further discussion regarding access to care, there was an emphasis on the population of HIV/HCV coinfected individuals. This group is a key population in Canada at risk for accelerated disease progression, and which faces multiple barriers in access to care and successful HCV treatment. Based on information generated from the Canadian Co-Infection Cohort, Dr Marina Klein (McGill University, Montreal, Quebec) described the current characteristics of HIV/HCV coinfected individuals in Canada, as well as the modifiable risk factors and interventions that could improve health outcomes (26). From 2003 to 2013, this population had a standardized mortality rate that was >12-fold that of the Canadian population (27). This is driven primarily by end-stage liver disease, drug overdose and malignancy. Use of current IFN-based HCV antiviral and HIV antiretroviral therapies reduces this risk for the individual but not at the general population level. Although HCV antiviral therapy initiation rates are higher than in other cohorts, females, Aboriginals and those with a history of crack/cocaine use were less likely to initiate treatment. HCV antiviral initiation rates differed considerably among the 18 sites contributing data to this cohort, suggesting that standardizing HCV care in coinfection should be prioritized. The value of enhanced access to HCV antiviral therapy was also discussed. Benefits include improved patient quality of life scores and reduced health care utilization following achievement of a sustained virological response. However, the multiple socioeconomic barriers faced by the HIV-HCV coinfected population will need to be addressed to ensure maximum benefit.

Social and behavioral sciences

In Canada, the majority of new and existing cases of HCV occur among PWID, either currently or in the past (1,28). Dr Jason Grebely (University of New South Wales, Australia), discussed a community-based study of PWID in Vancouver (British Columbia) documenting that HCV treatment uptake was only 2% per year in 2010 (29), despite universal access to health care. Treatment among PWID has added benefits, including the potential to reduce HCV transmission. Treatment as prevention has the potential to markedly reduce incidence and, ultimately, prevalence across the country (25,30). Clearly, strategies are needed to enhance HCV treatment uptake, particularly among PWID.

Barriers to HCV treatment are multifactorial and include issues of access to therapy and barriers at the level of the patient, practitioner and the health care system (31-33). Dr Carla Treloar (University of New South Wales, Australia), explored how stigma, social exclusion, symbolic violence and trust could be better understood and used to develop more effective therapeutic encounters to address barriers to HCV care, particularly among PWID (34). Drawing from social theory and research from a number of qualitative studies with clients and practitioners (35-39), she suggested some pragmatic strategies of how practitioners could develop inclusive, nondiscriminatory, trust-building HCV services to enhance HCV assessment and treatment.

In addition to enhancing engagement to HCV care and treatment, strategies to enhance responses to HCV therapy are also needed. Dr Louise Balfour (University of Ottawa, Ottawa, Ontario), highlighted the importance of adherence to HCV therapy (40). Specifically, Dr Balfour emphasized the important role that psychologists can play in helping to address barriers to care at the level of the patient, and helping to better prepare HCV patients for therapy, which may lead to improved adherence and, ultimately, improved outcomes in HCV therapy (41). Adherence will be particularly important with the new oral DAA regimens given the very high costs of failed therapy. Adherence strategies are particularly important for PWID or individuals with serious mental health issues (42).

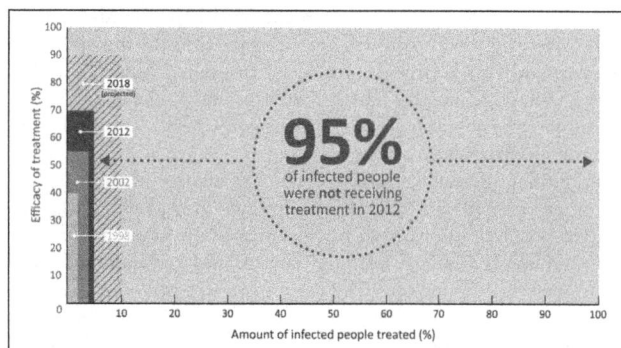

Figure 1) *The disparity between potential hepatitis C virus (HCV) treatment efficacy and projected HCV treatment effectiveness. High efficacy of HCV treatment is projected over five to 10 years. Sustained virological response (SVR) has increased from 40% with interferon (IFN) and ribavirin (RBV) in 1998, 55% with pegylated-IFN (PEG-IFN) and RBV in 2002, approximately 70% in the era of PEG-IFN, RBV, and a protease inhibitor in 2012 (genotype 1 only; patients with HCV genotype 2 or 3 will still have an SVR of approximately 80% with PEG-IFN-RBV) and IFN-free regimens are anticipated to be available by 2018, with an expected SVR of 90%. However, the global effects of new treatments are negligible without expanded access given the low treatment uptake among individuals with HCV infection (57-59). Reproduced with permission from reference 25*

One collaborative community-based group model of care that has been incredibly successful for treating a highly marginalized population was presented by Dr Jeff Powis from the Toronto Community Hep C program (43). This model has demonstrated that PWID can be engaged in HCV treatment (44) and treatment responses resemble those observed in clinical trials, despite the presence of multiple comorbidities (44,45).

The impressive advances in the development of DAA-based therapy, particularly IFN-free regimens, provide the potential to cure HCV infection in the vast majority of treated individuals. However, as shown in Figure 1, there is a considerable disparity between the potential treatment efficacy (>90%) and the current HCV treatment effectiveness (<10%), given that <10% of people have been treated in most countries, including Canada. Unless the proportion of individuals screened, assessed and treated for HCV infection is substantially increased, these anticipated therapeutic advances will have limited impact at the population level (46).

Epidemiology and public health
More than one-half of all existing HCV infections are estimated to be in current or former PWID (2,25). HCV treatment uptake in this population is low overall, and is especially low among current PWID (47-49). Barriers to HCV treatment are multifactorial and include issues of access to therapy and barriers at the level of the patient, practitioner and the health care system (25). Active drug use and mental health problems are often key factors affecting HCV treatment decision by both patients and providers (25). Some of these barriers are associated with medication side effects, factors that affect therapy adherence and concerns regarding reinfection. However, there is ample evidence that, with appropriate care and support, PWID can be effectively treated for HCV, with international guidelines recommending HCV treatment for PWID on a case-by-case basis (25,50). Dr Kim Page (University of San Francisco, California, USA), discussed HCV 'treatment cascade' in PWID and individuals with substance use and mental health issues, how these issues impact care delivery and reviewed strategies that may impact successful delivery of care in this population (51). She spoke of the 'incredible shrinking patient'. After clinicians apply a series of criteria to exclude patients (eg, AUDIT score for alcohol use, depression scores, laboratory criteria and active

injection drug use) as few as 4% of patients are deemed eligible for current HCV treatments. Dr Page described the UFO "You Find Out" study, which provides an opportunity for PWID younger than 30 years of age in San Francisco to undergo testing and learn if they are infected with HCV or HIV. The UFO model was presented as an example of a successful HCV education and prevention program, demonstrating how integration of harm reduction, outreach, testing, education and onsite primary care can engage and care for young injection drug users.

Another significant at-risk population with a high prevalence of HCV and low treatment uptake is the First Nations community (52). Dr Kathy Pouteau (Family Physician, Sioux Lookout and Kasabonika Lake First Nation, Ontario) shared her experiences and model for delivering HCV prevention and care to a remote Aboriginal community in Northern Ontario (53). First Nations communities in Northwestern Ontario have seen markedly increased rates of HCV infection. Risk factors for infection include injection drug use and, in 2009, the Chiefs of the Nishnawbe Aski Nation declared a state of emergency around prescription drug use in their communities. Dr Pouteau discussed the challenges, opportunities and collaborative response of health service providers and First Nations in rural and remote communities in the Sioux Lookout area. Barriers to HCV prevention, diagnosis and care in these communities include fragmented primary and public health systems, limited access to harm reduction programs, difficulties in confirming HCV diagnosis and accessing post-test counselling, limited access to HCV support and treatment, barriers due to intergenerational and personal trauma as well as ongoing inequities in social, economic and political determinants of health. These barriers are being addressed by health care providers in First Nations communities using a collaborative approach. This approach centres around five main priorities: building political advocacy and support; encouraging communication and collaboration with health services agencies; establishing meaningful partnerships based in First Nations communities (ie, opioid substitution programs); building First Nations HCV capacity, local 'expert' resources and tertiary partnerships; and promoting culturally safe and trusting relationships between health care providers and community members.

A critical player in the national response to HCV is PHAC. One of the challenges facing policy makers is the limitations in the comprehensiveness of HCV surveillance data in Canada, which makes it highly challenging to estimate the HCV disease burden. Dr Maxim Troubnikov from PHAC presented an updated model for determining estimates of the prevalent and undiagnosed HCV infections in Canada in 2011 (54). This model followed approaches used by the Center for Communicable Diseases and Infection Control (CCDIC) to estimate the 2011 HCV disease burden using the workbook and the back-calculation modelling methods. Using the workbook method, preliminary results, based on a Canadian population of 34,483,975, estimated that the anti-HCV+ prevalence for 2011 was 0.96% (95% CI 0.61 to 1.34), corresponding to 331,046 persons (95% CI 210,352 to 462,085 persons), while the chronic HCV prevalence was 0.71% (95% CI 0.45% to 0.99%), corresponding to 244,836 persons (95% CI 155,177 to 341,391 persons). It was further estimated that 44% of anti-HCV-positive persons were likely undiagnosed in 2011, although before having a final estimate, input from the back-calculation process and validation is required.

The second PHAC presentation, by Dr Margaret Gale-Rowe of the CCDIC, outlined the actions and the current federal response to HCV prevention and control (55). The current PHAC response includes HCV research collaboration and support, active disease surveillance and epidemiology, as well as the development of professional guidelines and resources for the management of HCV (56). Workshops and studies held by PHAC over the past year include discussion of birth cohort screening for HCV, a topic that was debated in the 2nd CSHCV (5). As a result, there is an interim statement that is under development on HCV screening based on the birth cohort approach in addition to current risk-based screening. Programs and partnerships that PHAC has fostered include promoting public and professional awareness campaigns including World Hepatitis Day and funding for the expansion of HCV knowledge including funding for the NCRTP-HepC and the Global Hepatitis C Technical Network. The current PHAC response to HCV was outlined and presently exists as part of an integrated response to sexually transmitted and blood borne infections including HIV, HCV and other infections. In the discussion period following these presentations, there was discussion about the need for a unified national strategy for hepatitis C in Canada. Although the PHAC representatives acknowledged the value of such an approach, no concrete plans to develop a national strategy currently exist.

OUTCOMES OF THE 3rd CSHCV

Although current treatments for HCV are effective, the severe side effect profile, prolonged duration, need for specialized support and the high cost, greatly limit treatment uptake. By 2014/2015, it is likely that all-oral, well-tolerated HCV treatment will be available with cure rates >95% in treated individuals. These new treatments will dramatically improve the ability to initiate treatment and cure those infected. However, translating these remarkable therapeutic improvements into tangible reductions in disease morbidity and mortality will require significant improvements in treatment uptake. With this in mind, the major focus on HCV in Canada will likely shift from the drug discovery to developing strategies to engage people into care and treatment. The 3rd CSHCV highlighted strategies that have proven effective in increasing treatment uptake internationally and nationally, with a focus on practical implementation of successful approaches in Canada.

The challenges of increasing HCV treatment uptake in Canada are structural, financial, geographical, cultural and social. It is time to develop achievable goals of treating the four major population groups in Canada that are most affected – PWID, baby boomers, immigrants and Aboriginal/First Nations people – so that HCV in Canada can be eliminated within the next 10 to 15 years. Among those at risk, PWID will require a specific focus for harm reduction to prevent reinfection. Without a screening program to identify those who remain undiagnosed, disease elimination will not be achieved. It will be critical to confirm whether the preliminary PHAC estimate that 44% of Canadians are unaware of their infection is correct. The key topic of discussion at this symposium was whether HCV care should be strictly provided by subspecialist clinicians or whether primary care physicians should treat HCV-infected individuals. The issues raised were the complexity of HCV treatment regimens in addition to the fact that, if all HCV-infected individuals were to be treated, there would not be a sufficient number of subspecialists to fill the need. The broad consensus was that a blended model of care, including many health care disciplines, will be required to maximize identification, treatment initiation and HCV cure. The notion of employing the ECHO model of telemedicine to reach geographically isolated areas was presented, a model that has been especially effective in providing HCV care in remote areas of the United States (21).

This symposium highlighted that given the unique challenges of the HCV epidemic and the imminent potential for curability, there is a clear need for national coordination of HCV prevention, care and treatment. National strategies have been adopted in countries, such as Australia, Scotland and the United States, which have resulted in improvements in HCV prevention, care and treatment (5). Canada needs a national strategy or action plan so that Canadians can also benefit from the imminent curability of HCV so that disease elimination within the next 10 to 15 years can become a realized dream.

ACKNOWLEDGEMENTS: National CIHR Research Training Program in Hepatitis C (NCRTP-HepC) Mentors – Marc Bilodeau (Program Director, Université de Montréal), Norma Choucha (Program Administrator, CRCHUM), Louise Balfour (University of Ottawa), Julie Bruneau (Université de Montréal), Gail Butt (University of British Columbia), Brian Conway (Vancouver Infectious Diseases Centre), Curtis Cooper (University of Ottawa), Aled Edwards (University of Toronto), Jordan Feld (University of Toronto), Benedikt Fischer (Simon Fraser University), Matthias Götte (McGill University), Jason Grebely (University of New South Wales), Michael Houghton (University of Alberta), Marina Klein (McGill University), Norman Kneteman (University of Alberta), Murray Krahn (University of Toronto), Mel Krajden (University of British Columbia), Gary Levy (University of Toronto), Qiang Liu (University of Saskatchewan), Ian McGilvray (University of Toronto), Thomas Michalak (Memorial University), Gerry Mugford (Memorial University), Rob Myers (University of Calgary), Mario Ostrowski (University of Toronto), Arnim Pause (McGill University), John Pezacki (University of Ottawa), Chris Richardson (Dalhousie University), Eve Roberts (University of Toronto), Rod Russell (Memorial University), Luis Schang (University of Alberta), Naglaa Shoukry (Université de Montréal), Nahum Sonenberg (McGill University), Hugo Soudeyns (Université de Montréal), Raymond Tellier (University of Toronto), Mark Tyndall (University of Ottawa), D Lorne Tyrrell (University of Alberta), and Joyce Wilson (University of Saskatchewan). Postdoctoral Trainees – Maude Boisvert (Université de Montréal), Marion Depla (Université de Montréal), Benoît Dupont (Université de Montréal), Maryam Ehteshami (Emory University), Moheshwarnath Issur (McGill University), Sonya MacParland (University of Toronto), Andrea Olmstead (University of British Columbia), Mohamed Sarhan (University of Alberta), Rick Siu (Dalhousie University) Nick van Buuren (Stanford University). PhD Trainees – Christopher Ablenas (McGill University), Annie Bernier (McGill University), Evan Cunningham (University of New South Wales), Thomas Fabre (Université de Montréal), Ahmed Fahmy (Université de Québec), Brett Hoffman (University of Saskatchewan), Anastasia Hyrina (University of British Columbia), Hassan Kofahi (Memorial University), Anupriya Kulkarni (McGill University), Nasheed Moqueet (McGill University), Neda Nasheri Ardakan (University of Ottawa), Ragunath Singaravelu (University of Ottawa), Patricia Thibault (University of Saskatchewan), Qi Wu (University of Saskatchewan). MSc Trainees – Adelina Artenie (McGill University), Svetlana Puzhko (McGill University), Sahar Saeed (McGill University), Nathan Taylor (Memorial University), Jason Wong (University of Alberta). Lay members – Frank Bialystok (University of Toronto), Andrew Cumming.

FUNDING: The NCRTP-HepC is funded by a Training Grant from the Canadian Institutes of Health Research (CIHR, grant number 63298). In addition, the NCRTP-HepC receives funding from AbbVie, Boehringer Ingelheim, Bristol Myers Squibb Canada Co., the Canadian Liver Foundation, Gilead, Merck, Novartis, Roche and Vertex. The 1st CSHCV (Grant number 264748), the 2nd CSHCV (grant number 290924) and the 3rd CSHCV (Grant number 309251) were supported by the CIHR. Additional funding for the 3rd CSHCV was provided by: AbbVie, Boehringer-Ingelheim, Bristol-Myers Squibb, Gilead, Janssen, Merck, Novartis, Roche and Vertex. SM is supported through a CIHR postdoctoral fellowship and was an NCRTP-HepC postdoctoral trainee. JG is supported through a National Health and Medical Research Council Career Development Fellowship. SMS was an Amgen Fellow of the Life Sciences Research Foundation (LSRF) and was an NCRTP-HepC postdoctoral trainee. The views expressed in this publication are those of the author(s) and do not reflect the position of the CIHR or PHAC.

REFERENCES

1. Myers RP, Krajden M, Bilodeau M, et al. Burden of disease and cost of chronic hepatitis C infection in Canada. Can J Gastroenterol Hepatol 2014;28:243-50.
2. Hajarizadeh B, Grebely J, Dore GJ. Epidemiology and natural history of HCV infection. Nat Rev Gastroenterol Hepatol 2013;10:553-62.
3. PHAC. Public Health Agency of Canada: Hepatitis C in Canada: 2005-2010 surveillance report. 2012. <www.phac-aspc.gc.ca/sti-its-survepi/hepc/surv-eng.php> (Accessed June 5, 2014).
4. Dinner K DT, Potts J, Sirna J, Wong T. Hepatitis C: A public health perspective and related implications for physicians. Royal College Outlook 2005;2:20-22.
5. Grebely J, Bilodeau M, Feld JJ, et al. The Second Canadian Symposium on Hepatitis C Virus: A call to action. Can J Gastroenterol 2013;27:627-32.

6. Muir AJ. The rapid evolution of treatment strategies for hepatitis C. Am J Gastroenterol 2014;109:628-35.

7. Heim M. The Role of the Innate Immune Response in HCV in the Era of Interferon-free Therapy. 3rd Canadian Symposium on Hepatitis C Virus Infection. Toronto, February 7, 2014:10. <www.ncrtp-hepc.ca/images/documents/Symposium2014/2014_01_23_symposium_program_and_abstract_book_final.pdf> (Accessed September 12, 2014).

8. Wieland S, Makowska Z, Campana B, et al. Simultaneous detection of hepatitis C virus and interferon stimulated gene expression in infected human liver. Hepatology 2014;59:2121-30.

9. McGilvray I, Feld JJ, Chen LM, et al. Hepatic cell-type specific gene expression better predicts HCV treatment outcome than IL28B genotype. Gastroenterology 2012;142:1122-31.

10. Ge D, Fellay J, Thompson AJ, et al. Genetic variation in IL28B predicts hepatitis C treatment-induced viral clearance. Nature 2009;461:399-401.

11. Rauch A, Kutalik Z, Descombes P, et al. Genetic variation in IL28B is associated with chronic hepatitis C and treatment failure: A genome-wide association study. Gastroenterology 2010;138:1338-45,45:e1-7.

12. Suppiah V, Moldovan M, Ahlenstiel G, et al. IL28B is associated with response to chronic hepatitis C interferon-alpha and ribavirin therapy. Nat Genet 2009;41:1100-4.

13. Tanaka Y, Nishida N, Sugiyama M, et al. Genome-wide association of IL28B with response to pegylated interferon-alpha and ribavirin therapy for chronic hepatitis C. Nat Genet 2009;41:1105-9.

14. Bibert S, Roger T, Calandra T, et al. IL28B expression depends on a novel TT/-G polymorphism which improves HCV clearance prediction. J Exp Med 2013;210:1109-16.

15. Prokunina-Olsson L, Muchmore B, Tang W, et al. A variant upstream of IFNL3 (IL28B) creating a new interferon gene IFNL4 is associated with impaired clearance of hepatitis C virus. Nat Genet 2013;45:164-71.

16. Thomas DL, Thio CL, Martin MP, et al. Genetic variation in IL28B and spontaneous clearance of hepatitis C virus. Nature 2009;461:798-801.

17. Shoukry N. Immune signatures during acute HCV. 3rd Canadian Symposium on Hepatitis C Virus Infection. Toronto, February 7, 2014:11. <www.ncrtp-hepc.ca/images/documents/Symposium2014/2014_01_23_symposium_program_and_abstract_book_final.pdf> (Accessed September 12, 2014).

18. Pelletier S, Drouin C, Bedard N, Khakoo SI, Bruneau J, Shoukry NH. Increased degranulation of natural killer cells during acute HCV correlates with the magnitude of virus-specific T cell responses. J Hepatol 2010;53:805-16.

19. Arora S. Project ECHO: A Model to Improve Care in Canada. 3rd Canadian Symposium on Hepatitis C Virus Infection. Toronto, February 7, 2014:8. <www.ncrtp-hepc.ca/images/documents/Symposium2014/2014_01_23_symposium_program_and_abstract_book_final.pdf> (Accessed September 12, 2014).

20. Arora S, Geppert CMA, Kalishman S, et al. Academic Health Center management of chronic diseases through knowledge networks: Project ECHO. Acad Med 2007;82:154-60.

21. Arora S, Kalishman S, Thornton K, et al. Expanding Access to Hepatitis C Virus Treatment-Extension for Community Healthcare Outcomes (ECHO) Project: Disruptive innovation in specialty care. Hepatology 2010;52:1124-33.

22. Bruneau J, Cooper C. Debate: Treatment should be strictly delivered by specialists rather than by primary care practitioners in the community. 3rd Canadian Symposium on Hepatitis C Virus Infection. Toronto, February 7, 2014:18. <www.ncrtp-hepc.ca/images/documents/Symposium2014/2014_01_23_symposium_program_and_abstract_book_final.pdf> (Accessed September 12, 2014).

23. Bober SL, Recklitis CJ, Campbell EG, et al. Caring for cancer survivors: A survey of primary care physicians. Cancer 2009;115:4409-18.

24. Kitahata MM, Koepsell TD, Deyo RA, Maxwell CL, Dodge WT, Wagner EH. Physicians' experience with the acquired immunodeficiency syndrome as a factor in patients' survival. N Engl J Med 1996;334:701-6.

25. Grebely J, Dore GJ. Can hepatitis C virus infection be eradicated in people who inject drugs? Antiviral Res 2014;104:62-72.

26. Klein MB, Rollet KC, Saeed S, et al. HIV and hepatitis C virus coinfection in Canada: Challenges and opportunities for reducing preventable morbidity and mortality. HIV Med 2013;14:10-20.

27. Klein M. The Canadian Co-infection Cohort Study: Building the Case for Increased Access to HCV Therapy for HIV-HCV Co-Infected Persons. 3rd Canadian Symposium on Hepatitis C Virus Infection. Toronto, February 7, 2014:9. <www.ncrtp-hepc.ca/images/documents/Symposium2014/2014_01_23_symposium_program_and_abstract_book_final.pdf> (Accessed September 12, 2014).

28. Remis R. Modelling the incidence and prevalence of hepatitis C infection and its sequelae in Canada, 2007. Final Report. Ottawa: Health Canada.

29. Alavi M, Raffa JD, Deans GD, et al. Continued low uptake of treatment for HCV in a large community-based cohort of inner city residents. J Hepatol 2013;58:S319-S20.

30. Grebely J, Matthews GV, Lloyd AR, Dore GJ. Elimination of hepatitis C virus infection among people who inject drugs through treatment as prevention: Feasibility and future requirements. Clin Infect Dis 2013;57:1014-20.

31. Grebely J, de Vlaming S, Duncan F, Viljoen M, Conway B. Current approaches to HCV infection in current and former injection drug users. J Addict Dis 2008 2008;27:25-35.

32. Grebely J, Oser M, Taylor LE, Dore GJ. Breaking down the barriers to hepatitis C virus (HCV) treatment among individuals with HCV/HIV coinfection: Action required at the system, provider, and patient levels. J Infect Dis 2013;207:S19-S25.

33. Grebely J, Tyndall MW. Management of HCV and HIV infections among people who inject drugs. Curr Opin HIV AIDS 2011;6:501-7.

34. Treloar C. Social issues in HCV. 3rd Canadian Symposium on Hepatitis C Virus Infection. Toronto, February 7, 2014:12. <www.ncrtp-hepc.ca/images/documents/Symposium2014/2014_01_23_symposium_program_and_abstract_book_final.pdf> (Accessed September 12, 2014).

35. Hopwood M, Treloar C, Bryant J. Hepatitis C and injecting-related discrimination in New South Wales, Australia. Drugs Educ Prev Policy 2006;13:61-75.

36. Rance J, Treloar C, ETHOS Study Group. 'Not just Methadone Tracy': Transformations in service-user identity following the introduction of hepatitis C treatment into Australian opiate substitution settings. Addiction 2014;109:452-9.

37. Treloar C, Rance J; on behalf of the ESG. How to build trustworthy hepatitis C services in an opioid treatment clinic? A qualitative study of clients and health workers in a co-located setting. Int J Drug Policy 2014;26:00014-0.

38. Treloar C, Newland J, Rance J, Hopwood M. Uptake and delivery of hepatitis C treatment in opiate substitution treatment: Perceptions of clients and health professionals. J Viral Hepat 2010;17:839-44.

39. Treloar C, Rance J, Grebely J, Dore GJ, ETHOS Study Group. Client and staff experiences of a co-located service for hepatitis C care in opioid substitution treatment settings in New South Wales, Australia. Drug Alcohol Dep 2013;133:529-34.

40. Lo Re V III, Teal V, Localio AR, Amorosa VK, Kaplan DE, Gross R. Relationship between adherence to hepatitis C virus therapy and virologic outcomes. Ann Internal Med 2011;155:353-46.

41. Balfour L. Bio-psycho-social framework for HCV care. 3rd Canadian Symposium on Hepatitis C Virus Infection. Toronto, February 7, 2014:13. <www.ncrtp-hepc.ca/images/documents/Symposium2014/2014_01_23_symposium_program_and_abstract_book_final.pdf> (Accessed September 12, 2014).

42. Mathes T, Antoine S-L, Pieper D. Factors influencing adherence in hepatitis-C infected patients: A systematic review. BMC Infect Dis 2014;14.

43. Powis J. Treating the "difficult to treat": A prospective evaluation of a community-based collaborative care, group support model of HCV treatment and education. 3rd Canadian Symposium on Hepatitis C Virus Infection. Toronto, February 7, 2014:25. <www.ncrtp-hepc.ca/images/documents/Symposium2014/2014_01_23_symposium_program_and_abstract_book_final.pdf> (Accessed September 12, 2014).

44. Charlebois A, Lee L, Cooper E, Mason K, Powis J. Factors associated with HCV antiviral treatment uptake among participants of a community-based HCV programme for marginalized patients. J Viral Hepat 2012;19:836-42.

45. Sockalingam S, Blank D, Banga CA, Mason K, Dodd Z, Powis J. A novel program for treating patients with trimorbidity: Hepatitis C, serious mental illness, and active substance use. Eur J Gastroenterol Hepatol 2013;25:1377-84.

46. Dore GJ. The changing therapeutic landscape for hepatitis C. Med J Australia 2012;196:629-32.
47. Grebely J, Raffa JD, Lai C, et al. Low uptake of treatment for hepatitis C virus infection in a large community-based study of inner city residents. J Viral Hepat 2009;16:352-8.
48. Mehta SH, Genberg BL, Astemborski J, et al. Limited uptake of hepatitis C treatment among injection drug users. J Commun Health 2008;33:126-33.
49. Iversen J, Grebely J, Topp L, Wand H, Dore G, Maher L. Uptake of hepatitis C treatment among people who inject drugs attending needle and syringe programs in Australia, 1999-2011. J Viral Hepat 2014;21:198-207.
50. Robaeys G, Grebely J, Mauss S, et al. Recommendations for the management of hepatitis C virus infection among people who inject drugs. Clin Infect Dis 2013;57:S129-S37.
51. Page K. Delivering Care to PWID & Those with Substance/Mental Health Issues. 3rd Canadian Symposium on Hepatitis C Virus Infection. Toronto, February 7, 2014:16. <www.ncrtp-hepc.ca/images/documents/Symposium2014/2014_01_23_symposium_program_and_abstract_book_final.pdf> (Accessed September 12, 2014).
52. PHAC. Summary: Estimates of HIV Prevalence and Incidence in Canada, 2011. 2012 <www.phac-aspc.gc.ca/aids-sida/publication/index-eng.php#er> (Accessed June 25, 2014).
53. Pouteau K. Barriers to HCV Care for Remote First Nations in North Western Ontario. 3rd Canadian Symposium on Hepatitis C Virus Infection. Toronto, February 7, 2014:17. <www.ncrtp-hepc.ca/images/documents/Symposium2014/2014_01_23_symposium_program_and_abstract_book_final.pdf> (Accessed September 12, 2014).
54. Troubnikov M. Developing Estimates of the Prevalent and Undiagnosed HCV Infections in Canada in 2011. 3rd Canadian Symposium on Hepatitis C Virus Infection. Toronto, February 7, 2014:14. <www.ncrtp-hepc.ca/images/documents/Symposium2014/2014_01_23_symposium_program_and_abstract_book_final.pdf> (Accessed September 12, 2014).
55. Gale-Rowe M. The Public Health Agency of Canada Actions in Hepatitis C Prevention and Control. 3rd Canadian Symposium on Hepatitis C Virus Infection. Toronto, February 7, 2014:15. <www.ncrtp-hepc.ca/images/documents/Symposium2014/2014_01_23_symposium_program_and_abstract_book_final.pdf> (Accessed September 12, 2014).
56. Pinette GD CJ, Heathcote J, Moore L, Adamowski K, Riehl G. Primary Care Management of Chronic Hepatitis C – Professional Desk Reference 2009.
57. NCHECR. Epidemiological and economic impact of potential increased hepatitis C treatment uptake in Australia: National Centre in HIV Epidemiology and Clinical Research, The University of New South Wales, 2010.
58. Lettmeier B, Muehlberger N, Schwarzer R, et al. Market uptake of new antiviral drugs for the treatment of hepatitis C. J Hepatol 2008;49:528-36.
59. Volk ML, Tocco R, Saini S, Lok AS. Public health impact of antiviral therapy for hepatitis C in the United States. Hepatology 2009;50:1750-5.

10

Efficacy and safety of, and patient satisfaction with, colonoscopic-administered fecal microbiota transplantation in relapsing and refractory community- and hospital-acquired *Clostridium difficile* infection

Muhammad Ali Khan MD[1]*, Aijaz Ahmed Sofi MD[2]*, Usman Ahmad MD[2], Osama Alaradi MD[2], Abdur Rahman Khan MD[1], Tariq Hammad MD[1], Jennifer Pratt RN[2], Thomas Sodeman MD[2], William Sodeman MD[2], Sehrish Kamal MD[1], Ali Nawras MD[2]

MA Khan, AA Sofi, U Ahmad, et al. Efficacy and safety of, and patient satisfaction with, colonoscopic-administered fecal microbiota transplantation in relapsing and refractory community- and hospital-acquired *Clostridium difficile* infection. Can J Gastroenterol Hepatol 2014;28(8):434-438.

OBJECTIVE: To report the efficacy and safety of, and patient satisfaction with, colonoscopic fecal microbiota transplantation (FMT) for community- and hospital-acquired *Clostridium difficile* infection (CDI).
METHODS: A retrospective medical records review of patients who underwent FMT between July 1, 2012 and August 31, 2013 was conducted. A total of 22 FMTs were performed on 20 patients via colonoscopy. The patients were divided into 'community-acquired' and 'hospital-acquired' CDI. Telephone surveys were conducted to determine procedure outcome and patient satisfaction. Primary cure rate was defined as resolution of diarrhea without recurrence within three months of FMT, whereas secondary cure rate described patients who experienced resolution of diarrhea and return of normal bowel function after a second course of FMT.
RESULTS: Nine patients met the criteria for community-acquired CDI whereas 11 were categorized as hospital-acquired CDI. A female predominance in the community-acquired group (88.89% [eight of nine]) was found (P=0.048). The primary cure rate was 100% (nine of nine) and 81.8% (nine of 11 patients) in community- and hospital-acquired CDI groups, respectively (P=0.189). Two patients in the hospital-acquired group had to undergo a repeat FMT for persistent symptomatic infection; the secondary cure rate was 100%. During the six-month follow-up, all patients were extremely satisfied with the procedure and no complications or adverse events were reported.
CONCLUSION: FMT was a highly successful and very acceptable treatment modality for treating both community- and hospital-acquired CDI.

Key Words: Clostridium difficile *infection; Community-acquired; Fecal microbiota transplantation; Hospital-acquired*

L'efficacité et l'innocuité de la transplantation de microbiote fécal par coloscopie et la satisfaction des patients à cet égard en cas d'infection à *Clostridium difficile* récurrente ou réfractaire d'origine nosocomiale ou non nosocomiale

OBJECTIF : Rendre compte de l'efficacité et de l'innocuité de la transplantation de microbiote fécal (TMF) par coloscopie et la satisfaction des patients à cet égard en cas d'infection à *Clostridium difficile* (ICD) d'origine nosocomiale ou non nosocomiale.
MÉTHODOLOGIE : Les chercheurs ont effectué une analyse rétrospective des dossiers médicaux des patients qui ont subi une TMF entre le 1er juillet 2012 et le 21 août 2013. Au total, 22 TMF par coloscopie ont été effectuées chez 20 patients, divisés en ICD « d'origine non nosocomiale » et « d'origine nosocomiale ». Des sondages téléphoniques ont été effectués pour déterminer le résultat de l'intervention et la satisfaction des patients. Le taux de guérison primaire était défini comme la résolution de la diarrhée sans récurrence dans les trois mois suivant la TMF, tandis que le taux de guérison secondaire incluait les patients dont la diarrhée se résorbait et la fonction intestinale reprenait après une deuxième TMF.
RÉSULTATS : Neuf patients respectaient les critères d'ICD d'origine non nosocomiale et 11, ceux d'origine nosocomiale. Il y avait prédominance de femmes dans le groupe d'infection d'origine non nosocomiale (88,89 % [huit sur neuf]) (P=0,048). Le taux de guérison primaire s'élevait à 100 % (neuf sur neuf) et à 81,8 % (neuf sur 11) dans les groupes d'origine non nosocomiale et nosocomiale, respectivement (P=0,189). Deux patients du groupe d'ICD d'origine nosocomiale ont dû subir une deuxième TMF en raison d'une infection symptomatique persistante, mais le taux de guérison secondaire s'élevait à 100 %. Pendant la période de suivi de six mois, tous les patients étaient extrêmement satisfaits de l'intervention. Aucune complication et aucun effet secondaire n'ont été déclarés.
CONCLUSION : La TMF était une modalité thérapeutique très acceptable et fructueuse des ICD d'origine nosocomiale et non nosocomiale.

*C*lostridium difficile infection (CDI) was initially believed to be a nosocomial infection associated with the use of antibiotics. However, recent epidemiological studies have shown CDI to be an increasingly common cause of community-acquired infectious diarrhea. Additionally, the conventional risk factors associated with CDI, such as old age, comorbid conditions and previous use of antibiotics, are less common in cases acquired outside of hospital settings (1). As a result of these observations, the Infectious Diseases Society of America proposed a classification of CDI as 'community-acquired' if symptoms occur in the community or within 48 h of admission to a hospital, after no hospitalization in the past 12 weeks. The term 'hospital-acquired' CDI was used if onset of symptoms occured >48 h after admission to or <4 weeks after discharge from a health care facility; or indeterminate if symptom onset occurs in the community between four and 12 weeks after discharge from a hospital (2). Further studies assessing the outcome of treatment showed that

*Authors who contributed equally to the manuscript
[1]Department of Internal Medicine; [2]Department of Internal Medicine, Division of Gastroenterology, University of Toledo Medical Center, Toledo, Ohio, USA
Correspondence: Dr Ali Nawras, Department of Internal Medicine, Division of Gastroenterology, University of Toledo Medical Center, 3000 Arlington Avenue, Ruppert Health Center, Room 007 C, Toledo, Ohio 43614, USA. e-mail ali.nawras@utoledo.edu or aijazasofi@yahoo.co.uk

community-acquired CDI can be associated with complications and poor outcome including recurrence (3).

The majority of CDI cases are effectively treated with oral metronidazole or vancomycin. However, the overall risk of relapse after conventional therapy can range from 20% to 30% (4). One recent study (3) reported a recurrence rate of 28% in community-acquired CDI. Following one relapse, the risk of additional relapses can be as high as 65% (5). These recurrences are treated with prolonged courses of vancomycin or fidoxomicin with some success. In recent years, there has been a great deal of enthusiasm for fecal microbiota transplantation (FMT) for the treatment of patients with recurrent CDI. Multiple systematic reviews and one recent controlled study have shown FMT to be a highly effective method of treatment for recurrent CDI (5,6). Currently, data regarding the treatment outcome of FMT in community-acquired versus hospital-acquired CDI are lacking. We began performing FMT in patients with CDI at our institution in July 2012. In the present study, we attempted to investigate the efficacy and safety of, and patient satisfaction with, colonoscopic methods of delivery of FMT. In addition, we evaluated the difference in patient demographics, charactersitics and treatment outcome with FMT in patients with community-acquired and hospital-acquired recurrent CDI.

METHODS

Patients
A retrospective medical record review of all patients who underwent FMT for CDI at the authors' institution between July 1, 2012 and August 31, 2013 was performed. Patients who underwent FMT <6 months before data gathering were excluded. Patients were divided into two categories – community-acquired and hospital-acquired CDI – as per the definitions provided by the Infectious Diseases Society of America (2). The data collected on baseline characteristics in both groups were divided into the following categories: patient characteristics, index infections, antibiotic courses for CDI and donor relationship. As a part of the protocol followed at the authors' institution, clinical outcome following FMT was obtained during follow-up outpatient visit or by contact via telephone. Telephone surveys were conducted later, as part of the present study, to determine procedure outcome and patient satisfaction. Time between FMT and telephone survey ranged between six and 18 months' duration. The telephone survey is presented in Appendix 1.

Donor screening and FMT protocol
Suitable stool donors were individuals who had not undergone antibiotic therapy for any cause for three months before stool donation and who did not have any active gastrointestinal symptoms such as diarrhea, constipation, abdominal pain, bloating, nausea or vomiting. Stool and serum tests (Table 1) were performed in all potential donors unless the donor was a spouse or significant other, in which case only stool screening tests were performed.

All FMT procedures were performed via colonoscopic route. Patients were advised to discontinue antibiotic treatment 48 h before the procedure. Colonic lavage (ingestion of 4 L of polyethylene glycol solution) was given to all patients the day before the procedure. Donors were given standard stool collection kits; stool samples were obtained within 30 min before performing FMT. Fifty grams of donor stool was mixed with 200 mL of normal saline in a blender until liquefied to milkshake consistency and was then aspirated into a 60 mL syringe and injected via the biopsy channel of the colonoscope into the cecum and ascending colon.

The primary cure rate was defined as resolution of diarrhea without recurrence of symptoms (as documented during the follow-up) within three months of FMT, whereas the secondary cure rate highlighted patients with resolution of diarrhea and return of normal bowel function after a second course of FMT. Treatment failure was defined as recurrence of diarrhea (≥3 loose stools) with positive *C difficile* polymerase chain reaction stool test.

The present study was approved by the University of Toledo Institutional Review Board (Toledo, Ohio, USA).

TABLE 1
Donor screening

Stool tests
• *Clostridium difficile* toxin polymerase chain reaction
• Bacterial culture (enteric pathogens)
• Ova and parasites
• Cryptosporidium antigen
• Microspora

Serum tests
• Hepatitis A immunoglobulin (Ig) M
• Hepatitis B surface antigen
• Hepatitis B core antibodies (IgM and IgG)
• Hepatitis C antibody
• HIV 1 and 2 antibodies
• Human T lymphotropic virus antibody
• *Helicobacter pylori* antibody
Rapid plasma reagin or syphillis enzyme immunoassay

Statistical analysis
Continuous variables were expressed as mean ± SD and qualitative data were expressed as percentages. Differences between groups were evaluated using unpaired *t* tests; P<0.05 was considered to be statistically significant. The effect of FMT was evaluated in terms of diarrhea, abdominal pain, nausea and fatigue between the hospital- and community-acquired CDI groups before and after FMT. Statistical analysis was performed using SPSS version 20.0 (IBM Corporation, USA).

RESULTS
A total of 22 FMT procedures were performed on 20 patients via colonoscopic route, of which only three were performed in an inpatient setting. Of the 20 patients included in the study, nine met the criteria for community-acquired CDI and 11 were categorized as hospital-acquired CDI. Patient demographic data are summarized in Table 2. Baseline characteristics revealed a female predominance in the community-acquired group (Table 2). There was no difference in the mean age, duration of CDI before FMT and use of proton-pump inhibitors between community-acquired and hospital-acquired CDI (Table 1). Fluoroquinolone was the most common previously used antibiotic in hospital-acquired CDI (55%) compared with community-acquired CDI patients, in whom clindamycin (33%) and β-lactam antibiotics (44%) were commonly used before the onset of symptoms.

Pre- and post-FMT data analysis
Four symptom outcomes were evaluated in the present study: diarrhea, abdominal pain, nausea and fatigue. Table 3 highlights the aforementioned clinical features of pre- and post-FMT. The mean number of days for return of normal bowel function was similar in community-acquired (4.5 days) and hospital-acquired (4.45 days) groups (P=0.328). Prophylactic oral metronidazole was given concomitantly to any patient in either group who had to use antibiotic for any infection other than CDI. In the community-acquired CDI group, the primary cure rate was 100%. There were no relapses of CDI following FMT in any of the patients during the six-month follow-up. During the six-month post-FMT follow-up, three patients used antibiotics for infections other than CDI. On the other hand, in the hospital-acquired group, the primary cure rate was 82%. A repeat FMT procedure was performed in two (18%) nonresponders in this group. One experienced persistent diarrhea and developed toxic megacolon; a repeat colonoscopy with FMT was performed seven days after the initial one, following which his diarrhea resolved over the next three days. The second patient had a history of microscopic colitis and her diarrhea (CDI) recurred after using amoxicillin and clavulanic acid for a dental procedure, despite being on prophylactic metronidazole, and stools for *C difficile* were positive according to polymerase chain reaction. FMT was repeated 78 days after the initial FMT and the diarrhea

TABLE 2
Demographics and characteristics in community- and hospital-acquired *Clostridium difficile* infection (CDI)

| Demographic or characteristic | CDI | | |
	Community acquired (n=9 [45%])	Hospital acquired (n=11 [55%])	P
Age, years, mean ± SD	64±10.26	68.27±17.88	0.361
Female sex	8 (88.9)	5 (45.5)	0.048
Duration of symptoms, months, median	7	5	0.169
Index infection			
Pneumonia	0 (0)	4 (36)	
Urinary tract infection	3 (33)	5 (45)	
Cellulitis	3 (33)	0 (0)	
Dental infection	2 (22)	0 (0)	
Osteomyelitis	0 (0)	1 (9)	
Sepsis	0 (0)	1 (9)	
No infection	1 (11)	0 (0)	
PPI and H_2 blocker use	6 (67)	7 (64)	0.647
Episodes of CDI, n, mean	5.6	4.6	0.175
Courses of metronidazole before FMT, n			
1	1 (11)	0 (0)	1.0
2	1 (11)	6 (55)	0.26
3	7 (78)	5 (45)	0.15
Courses of vancomycin before FMT, n			
1	2 (22)	0 (0)	1.0
2	5 (55)	7 (64)	0.108
3	2 (22)	2 (18)	0.214
Pulsed therapy	0 (0)	2 (18)	1.0
Fidaxomicin	3 (33)	6 (55)	0.355
Donor relationship			
Spouse or partner	2 (22)	3 (27)	0.8
First-degree relative	7 (78)	7 (64)	0.5
Nonrelative	0 (0)	1 (9)	0.36

Data presented as n (%) unless otherwise indicated. FMT Fecal microbiota transplantation; PPI Proton pump inhibitor

TABLE 3
Comparison of clinical features between community-acquired and hospital-acquired *Clostridium difficile* infection (CDI), both pre- and post-fecal microbiota transplantation (FMT)

| Symptoms (pre- and post FMT) | CDI | |
	Community acquired	Hospital acquired
Mild diarrhea (3–6/day)		
Pre-FMT	1	0
3 days post-FMT	2	0
3 months post-FMT	0	1
6 months post-FMT	0	0
Moderate diarrhea (7–10/day)		
Pre-FMT	4	4
3 days post-FMT	0	1
3 months post-FMT	0	0
6 months post-FMT	0	0
Severe diarrhea (>10/day)		
Pre-FMT	1	5
3 days post-FMT	0	0
3 months post-FMT	0	0
6 months post-FMT	0	0
Fatigue		
Pre-FMT	9	6
3 days post-FMT	9	4
3 months post-FMT	0	0
6 months post-FMT	0	0
Nausea		
Pre-FMT	3	5
3 days post-FMT	0	2
3 months post-FMT	0	0
6 months post-FMT	0	0
Abdominal pain		
Pre-FMT	2	5
3 days post-FMT	0	3
3 months post-FMT	0	0
6 months post-FMT	0	0

Data presented as n

resolved within two days. The patient did not report recurrence of symptoms during the six-month follow-up after second FMT. The secondary cure rate was 100%. There was no association between donor relationship and the treatment outcome.

Overall, 16 of 20 (80%) patients preferred stool donation from a relative. During the post-FMT survey, all patients indicated that they would recommend FMT to other patients with recurrent CDI.

DISCUSSION

CDI is no longer considered to be exclusively a nosocomial infection. Recent studies have shown that community-acquired CDI can be associated with severe outcomes (3). Therefore, it is imperative to understand the differences in treatment outcome between hospital-acquired and community-acquired CDI. In the present study, we observed a cure rate of 100% with FMT during a follow-up of six months in patients with community-acquired CDI compared with only 82% with hospital-acquired CDI. Symptom resolution following FMT was similar in community-acquired and hospital-acquired CDI. There were no relapses during the six-month follow-up in community-acquired CDI group.

In the present study, we also found a predominance of females in community-acquired CDI, which is supported by some earlier studies (7). Close contact with children <2 years of age has been identified as a risk factor for community-acquired CDI (8). A few other studies have shown infants to be carriers for several toxicogenic and nontoxicogenic strains of C *difficile* (9). Although infants are believed to be

protected from the infection due to lack of receptors for C *difficile* in the immature colon (10), the same does not hold true for mothers who are frequently exposed to infant stools during diaper change. Therefore, this may explain the high incidence of community-acquired CDI in women.

Primary cure rates with FMT were slightly better, although they did not reach statistical significance in community- compared with hospital-acquired CDI in the present study (Table 4). An explanation for this observation needs to be explored in future studies. Among other yet unknown factors, the presence of other comorbid factors in the hospital-acquired group may be contributory to the slightly lower response observed in the present study. Additionally, infection relapse after successful FMT occurred in hospital-acquired CDI group following exposure to antibiotics in two of three patients compared with zero of three patients in community-acquired CDI. More data are needed to confirm these potential differences in the treatment outcomes between community-acquired and hospital-acquired CDI.

Limitations to the present study were its small sample size, retrospective nature and, therefore, potential for bias. There is a need for controlled studies to examine the differences in short- and long-term outcome of treatment with FMT in patients with community-acquired and hospital-acquired CDI.

TABLE 4
Comparison of clinical outcomes post-fecal microbiota transplantation (FMT)

Clinical outcomes post-FMT	*Clostridium difficile* infection (CDI)		
	Community-acquired (n=9)	Hospital-acquired (n=11)	P
Primary cure rate	9 (100)	9 (81.8)	0.189
Secondary cure rate	N/A	2 (100)	
Relapsed or unresolved CDI	0 (0)	2 (18.2)	
Antibiotic use post-FMT for infection other than CDI	3 (33)	3 (27)	

Data presented as n (%) unless otherwise indicated

The efficacy of FMT for treatment of recurrent community-acquired CDI is similar to hospital-acquired CDI.

DISCLOSURES: The authors have no financial disclosures or conflicts of interest to declare.

APPENDIX I

Questionnaire

Patient's date of birth: _____.

Gender: _____.

Questions pertaining to period before undergoing fecal microbiota transplant.

Q1. What was the time duration between diagnosis of C *diff* (*Clostridium difficile*) and FMT?

A1. (months)

Q2. When you were first diagnosed with C *diff*, had you taken any antibiotic for any other infection?

A2. Yes / No

Q3. If yes, what was the name of antibiotic and what was the infection?

A3. _____.

Q4. Before FMT how was your C *diff* treated? Please name antibiotics and number of courses.

A4. _____.

Q5. Were you taking any acid suppressive medication like PPI or H$_2$ inhibitors?

A5. Yes / No

Q6. What was the severity of diarrhea? (Select one)

A6. (i) ≤3 stools per day
(ii) 4–6 stools per day
(iii) 7–10 stools per day
(iv) >10 stools per day

Q7. Did you have abdominal pain during C *diff* infection?

A7. Yes / No

Q8. Did you have nausea during C *diff*?

A8. Yes / No

Q9. Did you have fatigue during C *diff* infection?

A9. Yes / No

Questions pertaining to fecal transplant and immediate follow-up (3 days)

Q1. Was the fecal donor related to you? (Select one)

A1. (i) Spouse / partner
(ii) First-degree relative (parent, child)
(iii) Nonrelative

Q2. What was the number of days for normal bowel function to return post FMT?

A2. _____.

Q3. What was the severity of diarrhea 3 days post FMT? (Select one)

A3. (i) ≤3 stools per day
(ii) 4–6 stools per day
(iii) 7–10 stools per day
(iv) >10 stools per day

Q4. If you had abdominal pain prior to FMT, did you continue to have it 3 days after FMT?

A4. Yes / No

Q5. If you had nausea prior to FMT, did you continue to have it 3 days after FMT?

A5. Yes / No

Q6. If you had fatigue prior to FMT, did you continue to have it 3 days after FMT?

A6. Yes / No

Questions pertaining to 3-month follow-up.

Q1. What was the number of bowel movements per day during 3 months following FMT?

A1. (i) ≤3 stools per day
(ii) 4–6 stools per day
(iii) 7–10 stools per day
(iv) >10 stools per day

Q2. Within the 3 months following FMT, have you had any abdominal pain requiring physician/ER visit?

A2. Yes / No

Q3. Within the last 3 months following FMT, have you had any nausea requiring a physician/ER visit?

A3. Yes / No

Q4. Within the last 3 months following FMT, have you had any fatigue requiring a physician/ ER visit?

A4. Yes / No

Q5. Within the 3 months following FMT, did you experience any episodes of diarrhea requiring physician/ER visit or treatment for C *diff* (metronidazole/oral vancomycin/fidaxomicin)?

A5. Yes / No

Q6. Did you use any antibiotics for any other infection during this period? (Name infection and antibiotic)

A6. _____.

Questions pertaining to 6-month follow-up.

Q1. What was the number of bowel movements per day during 6 months following FMT?

A1. (i) ≤3 stools per day
(ii) 4–6 stools per day
(iii) 7–10 stools per day
(iv) >10 stools per day

Q2. Within the last 6 months following FMT, have you had any abdominal pain requiring physician/ER visit?

A2. Yes / No

Q3. Within the last 6 months following FMT, have you had any nausea requiring a physician/ER visit?

A3. Yes / No

Q4. Within the last 6 months following FMT, have you had any fatigue requiring a physician/ER visit?

A4. Yes / No

Q5. Within the 6 months following FMT, did you experience any episodes of diarrhea requiring physician/ER visit or treatment for C *diff* (metronidazole/oral vancomycin/fidaxomicin)?

A5. Yes / No

Q6. Did you use any antibiotics for any other infection during this period? (Name infection and antibiotic)

A6. _____.

Q7. How satisfied were you with the results of the procedure? (Select one)

A7. Extremely satisfied / satisfactory / dissatisfied

Q8. This procedure can be done by a number of routes via NG tube, colonoscopy or retention enemas, out of these three which would you have preferred? (We explained all the three procedures)

A8. _____.

Q9. Would you recommend this procedure to a family member or friend having CDI?

A9. Yes / No

REFERENCES

1. Khanna S, Pardi DS, Aronson SL, et al. The epidemiology of community-acquired *Clostridium difficile* infection: A population-based study. Am J Gastroenterol 2012;107:89-95.

2. McDonald LC, Coignard B, Dubberke E, et al. Recommendations for surveillance of *Clostridium difficile*-associated disease. Infect Control Hosp Epidemiol 2007;28:140-5.

3. Khanna S, Pardi DS, Aronson SL, Kammer PP, Baddour LM. Outcomes in community-acquired *Clostridium difficile* infection. Aliment Pharmacol Ther 2012;35:613-8.

4. Louie TJ, Miller MA, Mullane KM, et al. Fidaxomicin versus vancomycin for *Clostridium difficile* infection. N Engl J Med 2011;364:422-31.

5. van Nood E, Vrieze A, Nieuwdorp M, et al. Duodenal infusion of donor feces for recurrent *Clostridium difficile*. N Engl J Med 2013;368:407-15.

6. Sofi AA, Silverman AL, Khuder S, Garborg K, Westerink JM, Nawras A. Relationship of symptom duration and fecal bacteriotherapy in *Clostridium difficile* infection-pooled data analysis and a systematic review. Scand J Gastroenterol 2013;48:266-73.

7. Leffler DA, Lamont JT. Editorial: Not so nosocomial anymore: The growing threat of community-acquired *Clostridium difficile*. Am J Gastroenterol 2012;107:96-8.

8. Wilcox MH, Mooney L, Bendall R, Settle CD, Fawley WN. A case-control study of community-associated *Clostridium difficile* infection. J Antimicrob Chemother 2008;62:388-96.

9. Rousseau C, Lemee L, Le Monnier A, Poilane I, Pons JL, Collignon A. Prevalence and diversity of *Clostridium difficile* strains in infants. J Med Microbiol 2011;60(Pt 8):1112-8.

10. Leffler DA, Lamont JT. Treatment of *Clostridium difficile*-associated disease. Gastroenterology 2009;136:1899-912.

Third-generation cephalosporin-resistant spontaneous bacterial peritonitis: A single-centre experience and summary of existing studies

Jennifer Chaulk MD[1], Michelle Carbonneau NP MN RN[1], Hina Qamar MD[1], Adam Keough BSc[1], Hsiu-Ju Chang MSc[1], Mang Ma MD FRCPC[1], Deepali Kumar MD MSc FRCPC[2], Puneeta Tandon MD MSc FRCPC[1]

J Chaulk, M Carbonneau, H Qamar, et al. Third-generation cephalosporin-resistant spontaneous bacterial peritonitis: A single-centre experience and summary of existing studies. Can J Gastroenterol Hepatol 2014;28(2):83-88.

BACKGROUND: Spontaneous bacterial peritonitis (SBP) is the most prevalent bacterial infection in patients with cirrhosis. Although studies from Europe have reported significant rates of resistance to third-generation cephalosporins, there are limited SBP-specific data from centres in North America.

OBJECTIVE: To evaluate the prevalence of, predictors for and clinical impact of third-generation cephalosporin-resistant SBP at a Canadian tertiary care centre, and to summarize the data in the context of the existing literature.

METHODS: SBP patients treated with both antibiotics and albumin therapy at a Canadian tertiary care hospital between 2003 and 2011 were retrospectively identified. Multivariate logistic regression was used to determine independent predictors of third-generation cephalosporin resistance and mortality.

RESULTS: In 192 patients, 25% of infections were nosocomial. Forty per cent (77 of 192) of infections were culture positive; of these, 19% (15 of 77) were resistant to third-generation cephalosporins. The prevalence of cephalosporin resistance was 8% with community-acquired infections, 17% with health care-associated infections and 41% with nosocomial acquisition. Nosocomial acquisition of infection was the only predictor of resistance to third-generation cephalosporins (OR 4.0 [95% CI 1.04 to 15.2]). Thirty-day mortality censored for liver transplantation was 27% (50 of 184). In the 77 culture-positive patients, resistance to third-generation cephalosporins (OR 5.3 [1.3 to 22]) and the Model for End-stage Live Disease score (OR 1.14 [1.04 to 1.24]) were independent predictors of 30-day mortality.

CONCLUSIONS: Third-generation cephalosporin-resistant SBP is a common diagnosis and has an effect on clinical outcomes. In an attempt to reduce the mortality associated with resistance to empirical therapy, high-risk subgroups should receive broader empirical antibiotic coverage.

Key Words: Antibiotic resistance; Cirrhosis; Infection; Nosocomial

Une péritonite bactérienne spontanée résistante aux céphalosporines de troisième génération : l'expérience d'un seul centre et le sommaire des études

HISTORIQUE : La péritonite bactérienne spontanée (PBS) est l'infection bactérienne la plus prévalente chez les patients atteints d'une cirrhose. Même si des études menées en Europe ont fait état de taux significatifs de résistance aux céphalosporines de troisième génération, les données propres à la PBS provenant de centres nord-américains sont limitées.

OBJECTIF : Évaluer la prévalence, les prédicteurs et les conséquences cliniques de la PBS résistante aux céphalosporines de troisième génération dans un centre de santé canadien et résumer les données compte tenu des publications sur le sujet.

MÉTHODOLOGIE : Les chercheurs ont fait la recension rétrospective des patients ayant une PBS traités à la fois par des antibiotiques et de l'albumine dans un hôpital canadien de soins tertiaires entre 2003 et 2011. Ils ont utilisé la régression logistique multivariée pour déterminer les prédicteurs indépendants de résistance aux céphalosporines de troisième génération et la mortalité.

RÉSULTATS : Chez 192 patients, 25 % des infections étaient d'origine nosocomiale. Quarante pour cent (77 cas sur 192) des infections étaient confirmée par culture; de ce nombre, 19 % (15 cas sur 77) étaient résistants aux céphalosporines de troisième génération. La prévalence de résistance à la céphalosporine s'élevait à 8 % des infections d'origine communautaire, à 17 % des infections associées aux soins de santé et à 41 % des infections d'origine nosocomiale. L'origine nosocomiale de l'infection était le seul prédicteur de la résistance aux céphalosporines de troisième génération (RRR 4,0 [95 % IC 1,04 à 15,2]). La mortalité dans les 30 jours expurgée des transplantations hépatiques s'élevait à 27 % (50 cas sur 184). Chez les 77 patients dont l'infection était confirmée par culture, la résistance aux céphalosporines de troisième génération (RRR 5,3 [1,3 à 22]) et le score du modèle d'insuffisance hépatique terminale (RRR 1,14 [1,04 à 1,24]) étaient des prédicteurs indépendants de mortalité dans les 30 jours.

CONCLUSIONS : La PBS résistante aux céphalosporines de troisième génération est un diagnostic courant qui a un effet sur les issues cliniques. Dans une tentative pour réduire la mortalité associée à la résistance à un traitement empirique, les sous-groupes à haut risque devraient recevoir un antibiotique empirique à plus large spectre.

Spontaneous bacterial peritonitis (SBP) is the most prevalent bacterial infection in patients with cirrhosis (1,2) and is diagnosed in one-quarter of cirrhotic patients hospitalized with bacterial infections (2). Existing guidelines recommend third-generation cephalosporins as the empirical therapy of choice in SBP (3,4). Studies from Europe (predominantly Spain) and Asia have challenged this recommendation based on subgroups of patients with high rates of third-generation cephalosporin-resistant infection (2,5-8), and data showing that inappropriate empirical antibiotic therapy is associated with increased morbidity and mortality (2,9). The majority of the existing antibiotic resistance data are from Spain, a country well recognized to have disproportionately high rates of antibiotic resistance (10-14). Before globalizing our local recommendations to broaden empirical antibiotic coverage in high-risk SBP subgroups, we aimed to evaluate the prevalence and predictors of third-generation cephalosporin resistance in SBP patients from our local tertiary care centre, and to interpret these data in the context of the existing literature.

METHODS

Patients and study design
The present analysis was a retrospective cohort study including patients with cirrhosis diagnosed with SBP between February 2003 and May 2011.

[1]*Division of Gastroenterology, Department of Medicine;* [2]*Division of Infectious Diseases, Department of Medicine, University of Alberta, Edmonton, Alberta*
Correspondence: Dr Puneeta Tandon, Division of Gastroenterology, Department of Medicine, University of Alberta, 130 University Campus, Edmonton, Alberta T6G 2X8. e-mail ptandon@ualberta.ca

Local ethics approval was obtained for retrospective data collection. Adult patients with cirrhosis (as determined by compatible radiology, laboratory markers and clinical presentation), a diagnosis of SBP, and treatment with both antibiotics and intravenous albumin therapy if criteria for high-risk were met (serum creatinine ≥88.4 µmol/L or serum bilirubin ≥68.1 µmol/L) (3,4), were included. To avoid an over-representation of a single patient's demographic characteristics, only a single episode of SBP was included per patient. Due to the retrospective nature of the study, the type of antibiotics and dose of albumin given were at the discretion of the treating physician. Patients were excluded if they had undergone a previous liver transplant, or had secondary peritonitis, a malignant ascites or HIV infection. Due to the difficulties in identifying cases of SBP according to *International Classification of Diseases* codes, two sources to identify cases of SBP were used. First, local health records provided information on all paracenteses in which patients had a >24 h stay in the hospital (n=2094). This enabled identification of patients who were diagnosed with SBP and then admitted after an outpatient paracentesis, and also those who were diagnosed with SBP in hospital. Second, the local hospital laboratory provided details of patients who had fluid polymorphonuclear cell counts ≥250 cells/mm³ (n=642). All of these records were manually searched and cross-referenced, with removal of duplicate patients as well as patients not meeting inclusion and exclusion criteria. Many samples were removed because they were not ascites fluid (ie, joint aspirations), were ascites fluid but did not meet inclusion criteria (ie, secondary bacterial peritonitis, post-transplant ascites, malignant ascites) or because patients had not received albumin therapy. Patients were followed for 30 days after the diagnosis of SBP to determine outcomes.

Definitions

Spontaneous bacterial peritonitis was defined as an ascitic fluid cell count ≥250 cells/mm³, independent of culture results. Both culture-positive and culture-negative patients were included. Patients with ascitic fluid cultures positive for skin contaminants, such as coagulase-negative staphylococci, *Bacillus* species, *Propionibacterium* or *Corynebacterium* (7), were considered to be culture negative. Individuals with negative ascitic fluid cultures but positive blood cultures were considered to be culture positive (6). The site of SBP acquisition was characterized into one of three groups based on accepted definitions (2): community-acquired infection when the diagnosis was made within 48 h of hospitalization in patients not meeting criteria for health care-associated infection; health care-associated infection when the diagnosis was made within 48 h of hospitalization in patients who had contact with the health care system in the preceding 90 days (lived in a nursing home, on chronic hemodialysis or admitted to hospital for at least two days); and nosocomial infection – when the diagnosis was made after >48 h of hospitalization. Organisms were deemed to be resistant to third-generation cephalosporins if this class of antibiotics was known to be ineffective for therapy (ie, *Enterococcus*), or if the organisms were resistant or had intermediate susceptibility on sensitivity testing. Broad-spectrum antibiotics were considered to be those with activity against both Gram-positive and Gram-negative organisms (ie, cephalosporins, carbapenems, piperacillin/tazobactam). Renal insufficiency was defined as a creatinine level >132 µmol/L at any time from diagnosis to and including day 7 postdiagnosis. This value was chosen because it represents the threshold for a diagnosis of hepatorenal syndrome (3,4) and has been the most commonly used value for defining acute kidney injury in previous studies evaluating SBP prognosis (15).

Statistical analysis

Patient characteristics were analyzed using descriptive statistics. Univariate and multivariate logistic regression analysis were used to determine independent predictors of third-generation cephalosporin resistance and 30-day mortality. Variables with P<0.10 on univariate analysis were entered into the multivariable model. The results of the univariate and multivariate models were reported as OR and 95% CIs.

RESULTS

Patients and infection acquisition

A total of 192 patients met the criteria for study inclusion. The median age was 54 years (interquartile range 48 to 63 years) and 66% were male. The majority (76%) had either alcohol or hepatitis C virus infection as the etiology of cirrhosis. The median Model for End-stage Liver Diseases (MELD) score at presentation was 20 (interquartile range 16 to 26). Sites of SBP infection were divided into nosocomial (25%), health care associated (37.5%) and community acquired (37.5%). Twenty-eight per cent (54 of 192) of patients had exposure to antibiotics within the 30 days before the diagnosis of SBP and, of these, 56% (30 of 54) were receiving fluoroquinolone (FQ) prophylaxis for SBP. The remaining baseline characteristics are presented in Table 1.

Microbiology and patterns of antibiotic resistance

Culture-positive infections were present in 77 of 192 (40%) patients. Of these infections, 44 (57%) were with Gram-positive bacteria and 15 (19%) were resistant to third-generation cephalosporins (intrinsic or acquired resistance). The prevalence of antibiotic resistance increased from 8% (two of 25) in community-acquired infections to 17% (six of 35) in health care-associated infections, and up to 41% (seven of 17) in the setting of nosocomial acquisition (Table 2). Of the resistant organisms, 40% (six of 15) were *Enterococcus* species, 27% (four of 15) were *Enterobacter* and 20% (three of 15) were extended-spectrum beta-lactamase-producing *Escherichia coli*. When cases were divided into two time periods according to date of SBP before or after 2008, there was no significant difference in the number of Gram-positive, FQ-resistant or third-generation cephalosporin resistance between these time periods. Therefore, the remaining results were not separated into specific time periods.

Predictors of resistance to third-generation cephalosporins

In the 77 culture-positive patients, the predictors of resistance to third-generation cephalosporins (Table 3) were determined. As expected, the MELD score and the serum creatinine level were highly correlated variables. The likelihood ratio test was used to compare the association of each variable with cephalosporin resistance. Both associations were similar (P=0.07). MELD score was entered into the multivariate model over serum creatinine to provide a combined estimation of both liver and hepatic function. On multivariate analysis (Table 4), nosocomial acquisition of infection was the only predictor of resistance to third-generation cephalosporin antibiotics, with an OR of 4.0 (95% CI 1.04 to 15.2). The use of FQ prophylaxis trended toward predicting resistance to FQ antibiotics (in patients on FQ prophylaxis, 92% of the SBP cases were resistant to FQ antibiotics whereas in patients not on FQ prophylaxis, 62% of SBP cases were resistant; P=0.08); however, FQ use did not contribute to third-generation cephalosporin resistance (P=0.6).

Clinical impact of infection with third-generation cephalosporin-resistant organisms

30-day mortality: Of the 192 patients, eight received a liver transplant within 30 days of presenting with SBP and were, therefore, excluded from the mortality analysis. In the remaining 184 patients, 30-day mortality was 50 of 184 (27%). Cause of death was multisystem organ failure in 62% (31 of 50), sepsis in 30% (15 of 50), variceal hemorrhage in 4% (two of 50); one case developed mesenteric ischemia and a second case developed a small bowel obstruction. In a univariate analysis, serum sodium, MELD score, bilirubin, creatinine and the peripheral leukocyte count were all strongly predictive of mortality. In a model in which the MELD score was entered over bilirubin and creatinine, MELD was the only independent predictor of mortality in the multivariate analysis including all 184 patients (OR 1.12 [1.06 to 1.19]; P=0.001). The peripheral leukocyte count trended toward significance (OR 1.04 [0.99 to 1.09]; P=0.10). There was no significant difference in 30-day mortality between the culture-positive and the culture-negative cases (P=0.24).

TABLE 1
Baseline demographics (n=192)

Variable*	All patients (n=192)	Resistant to third-generation cephalosporins (n=15)	Culture negative OR not resistant to third-generation cephalosporins (n=177)
Age, years	54 (48 to 63)	55 (49 to 63)	54 (47 to 63)
Male sex	126 (66)	10 (67)	116 (65.5)
Etiology of cirrhosis			
Alcohol	75 (39)	5 (33)	70 (40)
Hepatitis C	70 (36.5)	4 (27)	66 (37)
Nonalcoholic fatty liver disease/cryptogenic	25 (13)	2 (13)	23 (13)
Other	22 (11.5)	4 (27)	18 (10)
Sodium, mmol/L (n=189)	133 (129.5 to 136)	134 (129 to 136)	133 (130 to 137)
Peripheral blood leukocytes, ×10^9/L (n=190)	10 (5.7 to 14.9)	5.8 (4.7 to 12)	10.2 (6.1 to 15.0)
International normalized ratio (n=191)	1.6 (1.4 to 1.9)	1.7 (1.4 to 2.1)	1.6 (1.4 to 1.9)
Bilirubin, μmol/L (n=191)	73 (37 to 153)	73 (53 to 146)	73 (36 to 154)
Albumin, g/L (n=184)	27 (23 to 31)	29 (26 to 37)	26 (23 to 31)
Creatinine at diagnosis, μmol/L (n=191)	110 (76 to 175)	142 (130 to 222)	106 (75 to 170)
Model for End-stage Liver Disease score (n=191)	20 (16 to 26)	24 (22 to 30)	20 (15 to 26)
Ascites leukocyte count, ×10^6/L	1795 (804.5 to 4775)	4700 (1790 to 13,600)	1678 (800 to 4413)
Ascites neutrophil count, ×10^6/L	1342.5 (471 to 4191)	4193 (1488 to 13,056)	1141 (463 to 3514)
Any antibiotic use within 30 days	54 (28)	5 (33)	49 (28)
Broad-spectrum antibiotic use within 30 days (with or without fluoroquinolone prophylaxis)	22 (11.5)	3 (20)	19 (11)
Fluoroquinolone prophylaxis	30 (16)	3 (20)	27 (15)
Hepatocellular carcinoma	21 (11)	2 (13)	19 (11)
Variceal bleed at presentation	18 (9)	0 (0)	18 (10)
Diabetes mellitus	31 (16)	1 (7)	30 (17)
Proton pump inhibitor use (n=189)	93 (49)	7 (47)	86 (49)
Culture positive	77 (40)	15 (100)	62 (35)
Gram-positive, n/n (%)	44/77 (57)	7/15 (47)	37/62 (60)
Gram-negative, n/n (%)	33/77 (43)	8/15 (53)	25/62 (40)
Infection acquisition			
Community	72 (37.5)	2 (13)	70 (39.5)
Health care associated	72 (37.5)	6 (40)	66 (37)
Nosocomial	48 (25)	7 (47)	41 (23)

*Data presented as median (interquartile range) or n (%) unless otherwise indicated. *Information available for all 192 patients, unless otherwise indicated*

TABLE 2
Patterns of antibiotic resistance in culture-positive spontaneous bacterial peritonitis

Microorganism	Community acquired (n=25)	Health care associated (n=35)	Nosocomial (n=17)	Total (n=77)
Third-generation cephalosporin-resistant organisms (n=15)				
	2/25 (8%)	6/35 (17%)	7/17 (41%)	–
Viridans group Streptococci	1	0	0	1
Enterococcus	0	2	3	5
Vancomycin-resistant enterococcus	0	0	1	1
Enterobacter	0	2	2	4
ESBL Escherichia coli	0	2	1	3
Bacteroides	1	0	0	1
Third-generation cephalosporin-sensitive organisms (n=62)				
	23/25 (92%)	29/35 (83%)	10/17 (59%)	–
Streptococcus	15	14	6	35
Staphylococcus aureus	1	0	1	2
Escherichia coli	3	12	2	17
Klebsiella	4	2	1	7
Pseudomonas	0	1	0	1

ESBL Extended-spectrum beta-lactamase

To test the impact of third-generation cephalosporin resistance, the mortality analysis was performed again in the culture-positive patients. Of the subset of 77 culture-positive patients, four were excluded from the mortality analysis because they received a transplant within the 30-day follow-up period. Thirty-day mortality in the remaining 73 patients was 33% (24 of 73). Nine of the 13 (69%) patients with cephalosporin resistance died by 30 days versus 25% (15 of 60) of the culture-positive patients without cephalosporin resistance (unadjusted P=0.002 [χ^2 analysis]). Univariate and multivariate regression modelling is shown in Tables 5 and 6. In multivariate analysis, resistance to third-generation cephalosporins (OR 5.3 [1.3 to 22]; P=0.02) and the MELD score (OR 1.14 [1.04 to 1.24]; P=0.005) were independently predictive of 30-day mortality. Cause of death in these 24 patients was multisystem organ failure in 14 and sepsis in 10.

TABLE 3
Univariate analysis: Predictors of resistance to third-generation cephalosporins in culture-positive spontaneous bacterial peritonitis (n=77)

Variable	OR (95% CI)	P
Age	1.0 (0.96 to 1.05)	0.90
Male sex	1.0 (0.3 to 3.4)	0.90
Diabetes mellitus	0.2 (0.03 to 1.8)	0.16
Proton pump inhibitor	0.6 (0.2 to 1.8)	0.40
Peripheral blood leukocytes, ×10^9/L	1.0 (0.9 to 1.1)	1
Model for End-stage Liver Disease	1.08 (0.997 to 1.16)	0.06
Creatinine at diagnosis, μmol/L	1.005 (1.000 to 1.011)	0.05
Ascites leukocyte count	1.0 (1.0 to 1.0)	0.70
Ascites neutrophil count	1.0 (1.0 to 1.0)	0.60
Mode of infection acquisition		
Community	1	–
Health care	2.4 (0.4 to 12.9)	0.32
Nosocomial	8.1 (1.4 to 45.8)	0.02
Nosocomial	4.6 (1.3 to 15.4)	0.015
Any antibiotic exposure within 30 days	2.1 (0.6 to 7.2)	0.25
Fluoroquinolone prophylaxis	1.5 (0.4 to 6.3)	0.60
Exposure to broad-spectrum antibiotics ± fluoroquinolone within 30 days	4.9 (0.9 to 27)	0.07

TABLE 4
Multivariate analysis: Predictors of resistance to third-generation cephalosporins in culture-positive spontaneous bacterial peritonitis (n=77)

Variable	OR (95% CI)	P
Nosocomial infection	4.0 (1.04 to 15.2)	0.04
Exposure to broad-spectrum antibiotics ± fluoroquinolone within 30 days	2.2 (0.3 to 15.7)	0.40
Model for End-stage Liver Disease	1.08 (0.99 to 1.17)	0.09

Renal outcomes: Renal outcomes were evaluable in 187 of 192 (97%) patients. Excluding the four patients on chronic hemodialysis and the one patient without creatinine data, the number of patients with renal insufficiency (creatinine >132 μmol/L at anytime from diagnosis to and including day 7 postdiagnosis) was determined. Of these, 83 of 187 (44%) met the threshold for diagnosis of renal insufficiency during the first seven days. A creatinine level >132 μmol/L within the first seven days postdiagnosis was strongly associated with death within 30 days (51% [40 of 79] versus 10% [10 of 101]; P=0.001).

When the culture-positive patients were considered, excluding the two patients on chronic hemodialysis, renal outcomes were evaluable in 75 of 77 (97%). Forty-one per cent (31 of 75) had a creatinine level >132 μmol/L at anytime from diagnosis to and including day 7 postdiagnosis. Of the evaluable culture-positive patients with third-generation cephalosporin resistance, 62% (eight of 13) developed renal insufficiency. Of the evaluable culture-positive patients without cephalosporin resistance, 37% (23 of 62) developed renal insufficiency. This difference trended toward significance on χ^2 analysis (P=0.10). Again, in this subgroup of culture-positive patients, a creatinine level >132 μmol/L within the first seven days postdiagnosis was strongly associated with death within 30 days (59% [17 of 29] versus 17% [seven of 42]; P=0.001).

DISCUSSION

The present retrospective review of patients with SBP adds third-generation cephalosporin resistance and outcome data from a Canadian tertiary care centre to the predominantly European data. It also provides a summary of the SBP-specific third-generation cephalosporin resistance data in the literature (Table 7) and identifies for the clinician three clinically relevant predictors of resistance to antibiotic therapy.

TABLE 5
Univariate analysis: Predictors of 30-day mortality in culture-positive spontaneous bacterial peritonitis (n=73)*

Variable	OR (95% CI)	P
Age	1.02 (0.98 to 1.06)	0.50
Male sex	0.7 (0.3 to 2.1)	0.60
Sodium, mmol/L	0.98 (0.89 to 1.1)	0.70
Peripheral blood leukocytes, ×10^9/L	1.05 (0.99 to 1.12)	0.08
Albumin, g/L	0.99 (0.91 to 1.08)	0.80
Model for End-stage Liver Disease	1.16 (1.07 to 1.27)	0.001
Creatinine at diagnosis, μmol/L	1.009 (1.003 to 1.015)	0.005
Infection acquisition		
Community acquired	1	–
Health care associated	0.4 (0.1 to 1.2)	0.10
Nosocomial	1.1 (0.3 to 3.9)	0.90
Nosocomial	1.8 (0.6 to 5.7)	0.30
Variceal bleed at presentation	1.0 (0.6 to 5.7)	1.0
Resistance to third-generation cephalosporin antibiotics	6.8 (1.8 to 25)	0.004

*Excluded four culture-positive patients transplanted within 30 days. Thirty-day mortality rate = 24/73 (33%)

TABLE 6
Multivariate analysis: Predictors of 30-day mortality in culture-positive spontaneous bacterial peritonitis (n=73)*

Variable	OR (95% CI)	P
Peripheral blood leukocytes, ×10^9/L	1.03 (0.96 to 1.11)	0.40
Model for End-stage Liver Disease	1.14 (1.04 to 1.24)	0.005
Resistance to third-generation cephalosporin antibiotics	5.3 (1.3 to 22)	0.02

Nineteen per cent of our culture-positive SBP infections were resistant to third-generation cephalosporin antibiotics. This is consistent with the published literature, in which resistance rates between 11% and 45% have been reported (2,6-8, 16-18) (Table 7). With such significant rates of resistance, and the implications for increased morbidity and mortality occurring as a result of inappropriate antibiotic therapy (2,9), predictors of resistance to empirical antibiotic therapy should be considered when determining initial antibiotic therapy in SBP (19-22). Using both our local data and our review of the literature (Table 7), three important predictors of third-generation cephalosporin resistance are identified. Nosocomial acquisition of infection is the most consistent of these predictors (2,6,7), attributed, in part, to more frequent antibiotic exposure as well as exposure to colonized/ infected personnel and the use of indwelling medical devices (urinary and intravascular catheters) in the nosocomial setting (5,23). The recent use of cephalosporin antibiotics has also been recognized as an important predictor (6,7). This variable was tested but was not predictive of resistance in our series, possibly because we limited our antibiotic exposure data collection to within the past 30 days (as opposed to 90 days). This was done in an attempt to enhance the accuracy of the data collected in a retrospective setting. Despite the lack of significance in our series, consistent with published series (6,7) and consistent with infectious disease first principles, this variable should be considered to be a clinically relevant predictor. Importantly, unlike exposure to third-generation cephalosporins, FQ prophylaxis has not impacted the rates of third-generation cephalosporin-resistant SBP infections in our series or others (5). The third relevant predictor is recent colonization or infection with third-generation cephalosporin resistant organisms. Although the latter point was not tested in our group of patients, infection with resistant bacteria in the past three months has been recognized as an independent predictor of third-generation cephalosporin resistance when considered in a series involving multiple types of bacterial infections in cirrhosis and is consistent with infectious disease first principles (2).

TABLE 7
Summary of recent studies (in which the majority of patients with spontaneous bacterial peritonitis [SBP] were recruited within the past 10 years)

	First author (reference), country; years data collected								
	Angeloni (25), Italy; 2004–2007	Ariza (6), Spain; 2001–2009	Cheong (7), Korea; 2000–2009	Present study, Canada; 2003–2011	Fernandez (2), Spain; 2005–2007	Heo (17), Korea; 2005–2006	Novovic (8), Denmark; 2000–2006	Umgelter (16), Germany; 2002–2006	Tandon (18), United States; 2009–2010
Prevalence of third-generation cephalosporin resistance reported	✓	✓	✓ (only for Gram-negative SBP)	✓	✓	✓ (only for Gram-negative SBP)	✓	✓	✓
Overall, n/n (%)	4/9 (44)	53/246 (22)	28/172 (16)	15/77 (19)		6/54 (11)	80/187 (43)	14/42 (33)	5/11 (45)
Community acquired, %		7	10	8	2		33		17
Health care acquired, %		21		17	5				
Nosocomial acquired, %		41	41	41	22		60		80
Independent predictors of third-generation cephalosporin resistance reported (culture-positive infections)	✗	✓	✓ (only for Gram-negative SBP)	✓	✗ (not tested for SBP infection alone)	✗	✗	✗	✗ (not tested for SBP infection alone)
Nosocomial infection		✓	✓	✓					
Cephalosporin use within the past three months		✓	✓	✗					
Other		Ascites neutrophils diabetes UGI bleed	Acute renal failure						

UGI Upper gastrointestinal

In addition to being common, infection with third-generation cephalosporin-resistant organisms has a significant impact on clinical outcomes. In the culture-positive SBP cases in our series, infection with organisms resistant to empirical therapy increased the odds of death by a factor of 5.3. Importantly, this was independent of the MELD score. Sixty-nine per cent of the patients infected with third-generation cephalosporin-resistant organisms died within 30 days. Moreover, patients infected with third-generation cephalosporin-resistant organisms trended to having higher rates of renal insufficiency in the first seven days of SBP diagnosis. These data are supported by the existing literature (2,7,9).

Therefore, based on evaluation of our local data and our review of the existing literature, we plan to modify our local empirical therapy of patients presenting with SBP. As per recommendations from Fernandez et al (2,24), we support the use of carbapenem antibiotics as first-line therapy in patients presenting with nosocomial SBP. Based on infectious disease first principles and literature review, we propose to extend this broad-spectrum coverage to patients who have had exposure to cephalosporin antibiotics in the past 90 days and to patients who are known to be colonized or have had infections with organisms resistant to third-generation cephalosporins in the past 90 days. As with all infections, once antibiotic susceptibilities are available, antibiotic coverage should be narrowed.

The limitations of the current study should be acknowledged. First, it was retrospective in nature and, therefore, although all attempts were made to identify SBP cases, it is probable that some cases were missed. Second, although it can also be regarded as a strength, the sample size of the current study was decreased by the exclusion of cases not receiving antibiotic therapy or in high-risk cases (3,4), intravenous albumin therapy. Third, conclusions were drawn from the small number of culture-positive cases that were resistant to third-generation cephalosporin antibiotics (15 of 77). Despite the small number of cases, our recommendations for local changes in empirical antibiotic therapy are consistent with other studies in the area, particularly with regard to the importance of nosocomial acquisition of infection as a predictor of resistance to third-generation cephalosporin antibiotics. Because rates of resistance are known to vary with centre-dependent antibiotic use patterns and antibiotic stewardship

guidelines, it is probable that some centres, particularly smaller ones, may not have rates of antibiotic resistance as high. Ideally, individual centres should collaborate with experts in microbiology and infections to confirm the generalizability of our findings to their own sites.

CONCLUSION

Third-generation cephalosporin-resistant SBP is a common problem, occurring in one of every five culture-positive SBP cases at our centre and up to 45% in published series. In addition to being common, resistance to third-generation cephalosporins is an independent predictor of mortality in patients with SBP. In an attempt to reduce the mortality associated with third-generation cephalosporin resistance, we plan to modify our local empirical SBP therapy algorithm. Subgroups at high risk for third-generation cephalosporin resistance (nosocomial infections, exposure to cephalosporin antibiotics within 90 days, infection/colonization with cephalosporin-resistant organisms within 90 days) will be given broader empirical antibiotic regimens. The impact of these recommendations on clinical outcomes will require prospective evaluation. Although the identified risk predictors may serve as a guide for many hospitals, ideally, individual sites should evaluate these in the context of their site-specific microbiological SBP profiles and resistance patterns.

KEY MESSAGES

- One in five SBP patients treated at our Canadian tertiary care hospital site are resistant to third-generation cephalosporin antibiotics.
- Third-generation cephalosporin-resistant SBP is an independent predictor of 30-day mortality.
- In an attempt to reduce mortality associated with resistance we suggest that high-risk subgroups receive broader empirical antibiotic coverage. These high-risk subgroups include SBP patients with nosocomial infection; colonization/infection with third-generation cephalosporin-resistant organisms within the past 90 days; and the use of cephalosporin antibiotics within the past 90 days.

REFERENCES

1. Tandon P, Garcia-Tsao G. Bacterial infections, sepsis, and multiorgan failure in cirrhosis. Semin Liver Dis 2008;28:26-42.
2. Fernandez J, Acevedo J, Castro M, et al. Prevalence and risk factors of infections by multiresistant bacteria in cirrhosis: A prospective study. Hepatology 2012;55:1551-61.
3. EASL clinical practice guidelines on the management of ascites, spontaneous bacterial peritonitis, and hepatorenal syndrome in cirrhosis. J Hepatol 2010;53:397-417.
4. Runyon BA. Management of adult patients with ascites due to cirrhosis: An update. Hepatology 2009;49:2087-107.
5. Fernandez J, Navasa M, Gomez J, et al. Bacterial infections in cirrhosis: Epidemiological changes with invasive procedures and norfloxacin prophylaxis. Hepatology 2002;35:140-8.
6. Ariza X, Castellote J, Lora-Tamayo J, et al. Risk factors for resistance to ceftriaxone and its impact on mortality in community, healthcare and nosocomial spontaneous bacterial peritonitis. J Hepatol 2012;56:825-32.
7. Cheong HS, Kang CI, Lee JA, et al. Clinical significance and outcome of nosocomial acquisition of spontaneous bacterial peritonitis in patients with liver cirrhosis. Clin Infect Dis 2009;48:1230-6.
8. Novovic S, Semb S, Olsen H, Moser C, Knudsen JD, Homann C. First-line treatment with cephalosporins in spontaneous bacterial peritonitis provides poor antibiotic coverage. Scand J Gastroenterol 2012;47:212-6.
9. Kumar A, Ellis P, Arabi Y, et al. Initiation of inappropriate antimicrobial therapy results in a fivefold reduction of survival in human septic shock. Chest 2009;136:1237-48.
10. Baquero F. Antibiotic resistance in Spain: What can be done? Task Force of the General Direction for Health Planning of the Spanish Ministry of Health. Clin Infect Dis 1996;23:819-23.
11. Turner PJ. Extended-spectrum beta-lactamases. Clin Infect Dis 2005;41(Suppl 4):S273-S5.
12. Levy SB, O'Brien TF. Global antimicrobial resistance alerts and implications. Clin Infect Dis 2005;41(Suppl 4):S219-S20.
13. Levy SB. Antibiotic resistance worldwide – a Spanish task force responds. Clin Infect Dis 1996;23:824-6.
14. European Antimicrobial Resistance Surveillance System, Annual Report <www.ecdc.europa.eu/en/publications/Publications/antimicrobial-resistance-surveillance-europe-2011.pdf> (Accessed April 9, 2012).
15. Tandon P, Garcia-Tsao G. Renal dysfunction is the most important independent predictor of mortality in cirrhotic patients with spontaneous bacterial peritonitis. Clin Gastroenterol Hepatol 2011;9:260-5.
16. Umgelter A, Reindl W, Miedaner M, Schmid RM, Huber W. Failure of current antibiotic first-line regimens and mortality in hospitalized patients with spontaneous bacterial peritonitis. Infection 2009;37:2-8.
17. Heo J, Seo YS, Yim HJ, et al. Clinical features and prognosis of spontaneous bacterial peritonitis in korean patients with liver cirrhosis: A multicenter retrospective study. Gut Liver 2009;3:197-204.
18. Tandon P, Delisle A, Topal JE, Garcia-Tsao G. High prevalence of antibiotic-resistant bacterial infections among patients with cirrhosis at a US liver center. Clin Gastroenterol Hepatol 2012;10:1291-8.
19. Bartlett JG. A call to arms: The imperative for antimicrobial stewardship. Clin Infect Dis 2011;53(Suppl 1):S4-7.
20. Doron S, Davidson LE. Antimicrobial stewardship. Mayo Clin Proc 2011;86:1113-23.
21. French GL. The continuing crisis in antibiotic resistance. Int J Antimicrob Agents 2010;36(Suppl 3):S3-7.
22. Nicolau DP. Current challenges in the management of the infected patient. Curr Opin Infect Dis 2011;24 (Suppl 1):S1-10.
23. Siegel JD, Rhinehart E, Jackson M, Chiarello L. Management of multidrug-resistant organisms in health care settings, 2006. Am J Infect Control 2007;35(10 Suppl 2):S165-S93.
24. Fernandez J, Gustot T. Management of bacterial infections in cirrhosis. J Hepatol 2012;56(Suppl 1):S1-12.
25. Angeloni S, Leboffe C, Parente A, et al. Efficacy of current guidelines for the treatment of spontaneous bacterial peritonitis in the clinical practice. World J Gastroenterol 2008;14:2757-62.

12

Helicobacter pylori infection and markers of gastric cancer risk in Alaska Native persons: A retrospective case-control study

James W Keck MD MPH[1,2], Karen M Miernyk BS[2,3], Lisa R Bulkow MS[2], Janet J Kelly MS MPH[3], Brian J McMahon MD[2,3], Frank Sacco MD[4], Thomas W Hennessy MD MPH[2], Michael G Bruce MD MPH[2]

JW Keck, KM Miernyk, LR Bulkow, et al. *Helicobacter pylori* infection and markers of gastric cancer risk in Alaska Native persons: A retrospective case-control study. Can J Gastroenterol Hepatol 2014;28(6):305-310.

BACKGROUND: Alaska Native persons experience gastric cancer incidence and mortality rates that are three to four times higher than in the general United States population.

OBJECTIVE: To evaluate pepsinogen I, pepsinogen I/II ratio, anti-*Helicobacter pylori* and cytotoxin-associated gene A (CagA) antibody levels, and blood group for their associations with gastric cancer development in Alaska Native people.

METHODS: The present analysis was a retrospective case-control study that matched gastric cancers reported to the Alaska Native Tumor Registry from 1969 to 2008 to three controls on known demographic risk factors for *H pylori* infection, using sera from the Alaska Area Specimen Bank. Conditional logistic regression evaluated associations between serum markers and gastric cancer.

RESULTS: A total of 122 gastric cancer cases were included, with sera predating cancer diagnosis (mean = 13 years) and 346 matched controls. One hundred twelve cases (91.8%) and 285 controls (82.4%) had evidence of previous or ongoing *H pylori* infection as measured by anti-*H pylori* antibody levels. Gastric cancer cases had a 2.63-fold increased odds of having positive anti-*H pylori* antibodies compared with their matched controls (P=0.01). In a multivariate model, non-cardia gastric cancer (n=94) was associated with anti-*H pylori* antibodies (adjusted OR 3.92; P=0.004) and low pepsinogen I level (adjusted OR 6.04; P=0.04). No association between gastric cancer and blood group, anti-CagA antibodies or pepsinogen I/II ratio was found.

CONCLUSION: Alaska Native people with gastric cancer had increased odds of previous *H pylori* infection. Low pepsinogen I level may function as a precancer marker for noncardia cancer.

Key Words: *Alaska Native; cagA+; Gastric cancer; Helicobacter pylori; Pepsinogen I*

L'infection à *Helicobacter pylori* et les marqueurs de risque de cancer gastrique chez des Autochtones de l'Alaska : une étude cas-témoin rétrospective

HISTORIQUE : Les Autochtones de l'Alaska présentent une incidence et un taux de mortalité de cancer gastrique de trois à quatre fois plus élevés que l'ensemble de la population des États-Unis.

OBJECTIF : Évaluer le pepsinogène I, le ratio du pepsinogène I/II, le taux d'anticorps contre l'*Helicobacter pylori* et le gène A associé à la cytotoxine (CagA) ainsi que le groupe sanguin pour déterminer leur association avec l'apparition du cancer gastrique chez les Autochtones de l'Alaska.

MÉTHODOLOGIE : La présente analyse rétrospective cas-témoins appariait les cancers gastriques déclarés dans le registre des tumeurs des Autochtones de l'Alaska entre 1969 et 2008 à trois contrôles sur les facteurs de risque démographiques connus d'infection à *H pylori*, au moyen de sérums prélevés dans l'*Alaska Area Specimen Bank*. Les chercheurs ont utilisé la régression logistique conditionnelle pour évaluer les associations entre les marqueurs sériques et le cancer gastrique.

RÉSULTATS : Au total, 122 cas de cancer gastrique ont été inclus dans l'étude, les sérums ayant été prélevés avant le diagnostic de cancer (moyenne = 13 ans), de même que 346 sujets-témoins appariés. Cent douze cas (91,8 %) et 285 sujets-témoins (82,4 %) présentaient des manifestations d'infection à *H pylori* antérieure ou en cours d'après la mesure des taux d'anticorps anti-*H pylori*. Les cas de cancer gastrique risquaient 2,63 fois plus de présenter des anticorps anti-*H pylori* positifs que les sujets-témoins appariés (P=0,01). Dans un modèle multivarié, le cancer gastrique ne touchant pas le cardia (n=94) s'associait à des anticorps anti-*H pylori* (RC rajusté 3,92; P=0,004) et à un faible taux de pepsinogène I (RC rajusté 6,04; P=0,04). Les chercheurs n'ont relevé aucune association entre le cancer gastrique et le groupe sanguin, les anticorps anti-CagA ou le ratio du pepsinogène I/II.

CONCLUSION : Les Autochtones de l'Alaska atteints d'un cancer gastrique étaient plus susceptibles d'avoir déjà été infectés par l'*H pylori*. Un faible taux de pepsinogène I peut être un marqueur précancéreux de cancer ne touchant pas le cardia.

Gastric cancer incidence and mortality rates in Alaska Native people are high and exceed those of other population groups in the United States (US). From 2005 to 2007, the mean age-adjusted annual gastric cancer incidence rate was 22.4 per 100,000 Alaska Native people compared with 6.8 per 100,000 in the US white population (1). Gastric cancer is the fifth most frequently diagnosed cancer in Alaska Native people and the third leading cause of cancer mortality. The mortality rate for gastric cancer in Alaska Native people (2003 to 2007) was more than three times higher than the overall US rate (12.7 versus 3.3 per 100,000 population) (2).

One reason for elevated gastric cancer incidence in Alaska Native people may be the high prevalence of *Helicobacter pylori* infection, shown in other populations to be a risk factor for the development of gastric cancer (3,4). In a survey of >2000 samples of blood collected in the 1980s, 75% of Alaska Native people were positive for antibodies to *H pylori*, indicating past or current infection. Childhood infection was common because 32% of children <5 and 67% 5 to 9 years of age had serological evidence of infection (5). Alaska Native people had a higher prevalence of infection than individuals in similar age groups from multiple populations across Asia, Africa and Latin America (6).

The high burden of gastric cancer in the Alaska Native population calls for new prevention and/or treatment strategies to reduce morbidity and mortality. Because *H pylori* infection precedes gastric cancer, one possible strategy is to identify individuals with *H pylori* and aggressively treat them to decrease *H pylori* infection and, subsequently, gastric cancer rates. However, the extremely high prevalence of infection, high proportion of isolates demonstrating antimicrobial resistance (7-9) and frequent reinfection (10) make this solution

[1]*Epidemic Intelligence Service, Office of Surveillance, Epidemiology, and Laboratory Services, Centers for Disease Control and Prevention, Atlanta, Georgia;* [2]*Arctic Investigations Program, Centers for Disease Control and Prevention;* [3]*Alaska Native Tribal Health Consortium;* [4]*Department of Surgery, Alaska Native Medical Center, Anchorage, Alaska, USA*

Correspondence: Dr James W Keck, Arctic Investigations Program, Centers for Disease Control and Prevention, 4055 Tudor Centre Drive, Anchorage, Alaska 99508, USA. e-mail jameswkeck@gmail.com

impractical. Therefore, we sought associations between gastric cancer and serological markers that could form the basis of screening efforts to more efficiently identify individuals at higher risk for cancer so they may be targeted for early detection and treatment.

Studies involving other populations have investigated serum markers and H pylori virulence factors for their association with gastric cancer. Researchers have found associations between exposure to H pylori strains expressing the virulence factor cytotoxin-associated gene A (CagA) and gastric cancer (11,12). Low serum pepsinogen I levels and a low pepsinogen I/II ratio, indicative of chronic gastritis (a precursor of gastric cancer) (13), have shown an association with gastric cancer in some studies but not in others (14,15). Finally, some studies have suggested a possible association between blood group A and gastric adenocarcinoma (16,17), although other studies did not demonstrate this association (18,19). No studies have investigated these potential gastric cancer risk markers in Alaska Native people; furthermore, the aforementioned studies examined the association between the markers and patients at the time of their gastric cancer diagnosis. In the present study, our objective was to measure the association between gastric cancer development in Alaska Native people and potential serological cancer markers from samples obtained years before the cancer diagnosis.

METHODS

Study design

A retrospective matched case-control study was designed to investigate the association between gastric cancer and various serological and serum markers. Cases included Alaska Native individuals diagnosed with gastric adenocarcinoma in adulthood (≥18 years of age) residing in Alaska at the time of diagnosis. Alaska Native people belong to a diverse group of populations indigenous to Alaska. Patients with pathology-confirmed gastric cancer, who had at least one serum specimen in the Alaska Area Specimen Bank collected before their gastric cancer diagnosis, were identified from the Alaska Native Tumor Registry from 1969 through 2008. The Alaska Area Specimen Bank is a collection of >300,000 residual biological specimens from 92,000 people participating in various research studies, public health investigations and clinical testing conducted in Alaska since 1963.

Controls were Alaska Native people without known gastric adenocarcinoma (confirmed by review of the Alaska Native Tumor Registry) who resided in Northwest, Southeast, Southwest or Western Alaska, and had at least one serum specimen available from the Alaska Area Specimen Bank during the time period 1969 to 2008. To control for the known demographic risk factors for H pylori infection within the Alaska Native population (5), controls were matched to cases (3:1) according to region of residence in Alaska (southwest, southeast, west, northwest), age group (10-year age groupings), sex and date of serum specimen collection (±10 years). For cases in which multiple serum samples were available, samples collected >10 years before gastric cancer diagnosis were selected because H pylori serological titres have been reported to decline up to 10 years before cancer diagnosis (20). The study protocol received approval from the Centers for Disease Control and Prevention Institutional Review Board and the Alaska Area Institutional Review Board, including a waiver of informed consent because of the use of deidentified, previously collected medical information from the Alaska Native Tumor Registry. Study approval was received from the Bristol Bay Area and the Yukon-Kuskokwim Health Corporations (southwest), Maniilaq Association (northwest), Norton Sound Health Corporation (west) and the SouthEast Alaska Regional Health Consortium (southeast).

Data abstraction

The Alaska Native Tumor Registry (www.anthc.org/chs/epicenter/), established in 1973, was used to obtain information about the gastric cancers. The Alaska Native Tumor Registry is a full member of the National Cancer Institute Surveillance, Epidemiology, and End Results (SEER) program, and provides comprehensive cancer surveillance of approximately 127,000 Alaska Native people residing in Alaska (21). Additional patient data were obtained from death certificates and RPMS, the health information system used by the Alaska Tribal Health System. The national SEER database (22), a collection of 17 regional registries that provide population-based surveillance for approximately 28% of the US population (http://seer.cancer.gov/), was accessed to obtain national gastric cancer data. SEER*Stat version 6.6.2 (National Cancer Institute, USA) was used to calculate frequencies from the national database (excluding cases from the Alaska Native Tumor Registry) for reported gastric cancers that occurred from 1973 to 2007.

Laboratory testing

Commercial kits were used to test samples for anti-H pylori antibodies (Helicobacter pylori IgA/IgG ELISA; Biohit, Finland), anti-CagA antibodies (Helicobacter pylori p120 [CagA] ELISA; ravo Diagnostika, Germany), pepsinogen I (Pepsinogen I ELISA, Biohit), pepsinogen II (Pepsinogen II ELISA, Biohit) and blood grouping (Affirmagen pooled reagent red blood cells; Ortho Clinical Diagnostics, USA). The manufacturer's test procedures and analysis instructions were followed for all tests. The manufacturer's cut-off values were used for normal versus abnormal levels of pepsinogen I (25 µg/L) and the pepsinogen I/II ratio (2.5). An abnormally low value for either indicates advanced corpus atrophy. Also followed was manufacturer guidance to determine anti-H pylori antibody positivity (≥30 enzyme immune units [EIU]) and anti-CagA antibody positivity (>7.5 units; 5 to 7.5 units indeterminate).

Sample size calculation and statistical analysis

Using previously reported estimates for H pylori and CagA seropositivity in Alaska Native people, sample sizes were calculated under a variety of assumptions. To detect an OR ≥2 at a 95% significance level (P<0.05) with 80% power and 1:3 case-control matching, the calculations produced sample sizes of 107 to 163 cases and 321 to 489 controls (data not shown). Descriptive analyses of case, control and gastric cancer characteristics were undertaken, which are reported as frequencies and percentages; z, χ^2 and paired t tests were used to evaluate differences in proportions and their distributions and paired serological data, as appropriate. The analysis excluded pepsinogen values from five grossly hemolyzed serum samples and anti-H pylori antibody enzyme immunoassay values >1500 (but not the positive test result) due to the instability of the test kit in that range (14 samples). To preserve matching, associations between serological markers and gastric cancer development were checked using univariate and multivariate conditional logistic regression. When more than one serum sample per case was available, the earlier-collected sample was used for modelling. Purposeful backward stepwise regression was used for multivariate models and initially included variables with P≤0.2. In addition, subgroup analyses were performed and restricted to: gastric cancers not located in the cardia region of the stomach (noncardia) because of the reported lack of association between H pylori infection and gastric cancers arising from the cardia of the stomach (3,4,23); cases with serum samples collected ≥10 years before gastric cancer diagnosis due to the reported decline of H pylori antibodies leading up to gastric cancer diagnosis (20); gastric cancer cases diagnosed before 50 years of age (approximately the first age quartile in the sample) because of genetic differences in early onset cancers (24,25); and anti-H pylori antibody-positive cases and controls. All reported P values are two-sided; P<0.05 was considered to be statistically significant. Stata version 10 (StataCorp, USA) was used to perform statistical analyses.

RESULTS

Participant characteristics

Of the 206 reported cases of gastric adenocarcinoma with at least one available serum sample over the 40-year study period, permission from the regional tribal health organizations was granted to include 129 (62.6%) of these cases and initially matched to 377 controls. From this group were

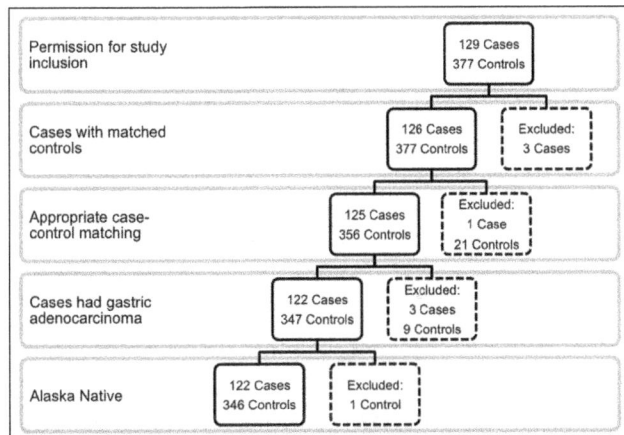

Figure 1) *Reasons for exclusion of seven cases and 31 controls from a matched case-control study of serum markers and gastric cancer in 129 Alaska Native people diagnosed with cancer from 1969 to 2008*

TABLE 1
Demographic and sera characteristics of Alaska Native gastric cancer cases and controls

Characteristic	Case (n=122)	Control (n=346)
Male sex	89 (73.0)	252 (72.8)
Region (Alaska) of residence		
Northwest	28 (23.0)	78 (22.5)
Southeast	8 (6.6)	20 (5.8)
Southwest	59 (48.4)	172 (49.7)
West	27 (22.1)	76 (22.0)
Age at specimen collection*, years	45.2±16.1†	41.2±17.6
Specimen collection time before diagnosis, years*	13.0±7.0	na
Age at gastric cancer diagnosis, years	58.6±15.7	na
25th percentile	47	na
50th percentile	60	na
75th percentile	71	na
Blood group		
A	51 (41.8)	136 (39.3)
AB	8 (6.6)	34 (9.8)
B	12 (9.8)	42 (12.1)
O	51 (41.8)	134 (38.7)
Helicobacter pylori positive‡	112 (91.8)†	285 (82.4)
CagA positive§	116 (95.1)	322 (93.1)
CagA intermediate§		7 (2.0)
H pylori or CagA positive‡§	122 (100.0)	342 (98.8)
Pepsinogen I low¶	5 (4.1)	7 (2.0)
Pepsinogen I/II low**	6 (5.0)	10 (2.9)

*Data presented as n (%) or mean ± SD. *If two specimens collected, earlier specimen collection age used; †P<0.05; ‡Anti-H pylori immunoglobulin (Ig) G/IgA ≥30 enzyme immune units; §Cytotoxin-associated gene A (CagA) IgG: <5 units (negative), 5 to 7.5 units (indeterminate), >7.5 units (positive); ¶Pepsinogen <25 µg/L (one case and four control sample values excluded due to hemolyzed sera); **Pepsinogen I/II ratio <2.5. na Not applicable*

excluded: three cases for lack of matched controls; one case and 21 controls for sex mismatch; three cases with non-adenocarcinoma histologies (two epithelial and one squamous cell) and their nine matched controls; and one control who identified as non-Native. One hundred twenty-two individuals with gastric cancer and 346 matched controls were retained for analysis (Figure 1). Two serum samples were available for 38 (31.1%) cases; the other cases and all of the controls had one sample. Samples obtained from cases predated gastric cancer diagnosis by a mean of 13 years (interquartile range nine to 18 years). Of the gastric cancer group, 73.0% (89 of 122) were male, the group's mean (± SD) age at the time of serum sample collection was 45.2±16.1 years, mean age at time of diagnosis was 58.6±15.7 years and the proportion <50 years of age was 29.5% (36 of 122). The control group was 72.8% (252 of 346) male and had a mean age of 41.2±17.6 years at serum collection. Almost all cases and controls, 92.6% and 92.8%, respectively, identified as Eskimo, and 93.4% and 94.2%, respectively, lived in rural western Alaska communities.

Serum markers and gastric cancer
It was found that 91.8% (112 of 122) of the gastric cancer patients and 82.4% (285 of 346) of the control group had evidence of previous or ongoing H pylori exposure indicated by elevated anti-H pylori antibody levels (Table 1). A greater percentage of cases (95.1% [n=116]) and controls (93.1% [n=322]) had evidence of H pylori exposure as measured by anti-CagA immunoglobulin G (IgG). All of the cases (n=122) and 342 (98.8%) of the controls demonstrated evidence of previous or ongoing H pylori exposure when combining these two serological markers of H pylori infection. Low pepsinogen I level was uncommon, with 4.1% (five of 121) of cases and 2.1% (seven of 342) of controls recording serum pepsinogen I levels <25 µg/L. Equally uncommon was a low pepsinogen I/II ratio: 5.0% (six of 121) of case and 2.9% (10 of 342) of control samples had a calculated ratio <2.5.

Individuals who developed gastric cancer had a 2.59-fold higher odds of positive H pylori serology than their matched controls (P=0.013; [95% CI 1.22 to 5.50]), the only significant univariate association (Table 2). Also calculated were matched ORs using a pepsinogen threshold of 75 µg/L and a pepsinogen I/II ratio of 10; however these analyses did not result in any additional statistically significant associations (data not shown). In the multivariate analysis, which retained variables with P<0.25 (positive H pylori serology and pepsinogen I), only the presence of H pylori antibody was significantly associated with gastric cancer (OR 2.63 [95% CI 1.21 to 5.62]; P=0.01) (Table 2).

Analysis of gastric cancer patient subgroups revealed associations between gastric cancer and H pylori exposure and low pepsinogen I levels, as shown in Table 2. A multivariate model of noncardia gastric

cancer cases (n=94) showed associations with anti-H pylori antibodies (adjusted OR [aOR] 3.92; P=0.004) and low pepsinogen I levels (aOR 6.04; P=0.04). Individuals diagnosed with gastric cancer before 50 years of age (n=36) had a stronger association with anti-H pylori antibodies (aOR 7.96; P=0.047) than cases diagnosed in individuals ≥50 years of age (n=86; aOR 1.88; P=0.14). Gastric cancer patients with serum specimens collected ≥10 years before their cancer diagnosis (n=86) had an association with anti-H pylori antibodies (aOR 3.20; P=0.013), while cases with specimens from <10 years before diagnosis did not (n=36; aOR 0.13; P=0.86). Also investigated were cases and controls positive for anti-H pylori antibodies, which found a nonsignificant association between gastric cancer and antecedent low pepsinogen I level (aOR 4.48; P=0.08). To assess for temporal changes in specimen values and gastric cancer associations, serum specimens collected before and after 1980 were grouped and analyzed. The association of gastric cancer with anti-H pylori and anti-CagA antibodies, pepsinogen I, and the pepsinogen I/II ratio between the two time periods were similar and not significantly different (data not shown). Additionally, the mean values for these serum markers were not statistically different across the two time periods (data not shown).

Paired sera
For 38 of the gastric cancer cases, two separate prediagnosis serum samples were collected a mean of 7.2 years apart (interquartile range four to nine years) (Table 3). Of the measured serum markers, only anti-H pylori antibody levels changed significantly between the earlier and later samples (mean increase = 31.4±90.0 EIU; P=0.04), increasing an average of 5.9 EIU per year. Paired specimen antibody level

TABLE 2
Gastric cancer predictors according to case group

Univariate analysis	All cases (n=122) OR	P	Cases with specimens ≥10 years before diagnosis (n=86) OR	P	Noncardia cases (n=94) OR	P	Helicobacter pylori-positive cases and controls (n=112) OR	P
H pylori positive*	**2.59**	**0.01**	**3.39**	**0.01**	**3.49**	**0.01**	na	na
CagA intermediate and positive†	0.98	0.97	1.32	0.63	0.75	0.56	0.83	0.72
CagA positive†	1.40	0.47	1.95	0.23	1.10	0.84	1.28	0.62
Pepsinogen I <25 µg/L	1.97	0.27	2.50	0.20	3.48	0.11	4.48	0.08
Pepsinogen I/II ratio <2.5	1.72	0.33	2.33	0.19	2.30	0.25	2.22	0.20
Blood group A versus others	1.11	0.62	1.27	0.36	1.15	0.57	1.00	1.00
Multivariate analysis‡								
H pylori positive	**2.63**	**0.01**	**3.32**	**0.01**	**3.92**	**0.004**	na	na
Pepsinogen I, low (<25 µg/L)	2.56	0.15	2.98	0.15	**6.04**	**0.04**	4.48	0.08

*Bolded values indicate statistical significance. *Anti-H pylori immunoglobulin (Ig) G/IgA ≥30 enzyme immune units; †Cytotoxin-associated gene A (CagA) IgG: <5 units (negative), 5 to 7.5 units (indeterminate), >7.5 units (positive); ‡Only variables significant at P<0.2 were retained in the multivariate model. na Not applicable*

TABLE 3
Characteristics of paired sera taken before gastric cancer diagnosis

Characteristic	Specimen Earlier (n=38)	Later (n=38)	Paired, change (Δ) Mean Δ	Mean Δ/year
Anti-Helicobacter pylori antibody*, enzyme immune units	109.6±77.5	141.7±121.7	31.4†	5.9
Anti-cytotoxin-associated gene A antibody, units	29.3±20.6	28.3±19.7	−0.9	−0.4
Pepsinogen I, µg/L	138.6±65.9	140.8±91.2	2.2	0.5
Pepsinogen I/II ratio	8.9±3.9	8.9±5.4	0.01	0.1
Age at serum collection, years	49.3±15.9	56.6±15.3	7.2	
Serum collection before cancer diagnosis, years	12.1±6.5	4.9±5.0	7.2	

*Data presented as mean ± SD unless otherwise indicated. *One sample censored from each case group due to instability of laboratory test at values >1500 enzyme immune units. †P<0.05 for paired t test between earlier and later specimens*

changes varied widely in direction and magnitude, decaying (n=15) or rising (n=23) from −38.1 EIU to 63.5 EIU per year. Anti-H pylori antibody levels and their relation to time before cancer diagnosis from all sera in the cancer group (n=141) were further evaluated and no trend was found (P=0.53).

Gastric cancers
The most frequently occurring histological type of gastric cancer in the sample, as classified by *International Classification of Diseases for Oncology, Third Edition* (ICD-O-3) codes (26), was adenocarcinoma, not otherwise specified (n=81 [66.4%]) followed by signet ring cell (n=19 [15.6%]) and adenocarcinoma, intestinal type (n=8 [6.6%]; Table 4). The distribution of histological cancer types in the sample was not statistically different from the national SEER data (χ^2=9.91; df=12; P=0.62). Most gastric cancers in the study were moderately differentiated (n=35 [28.7%]) or poorly differentiated (n=55 [45.1%]) histologically, which was similar to national data (χ^2=4.24; df=4; P=0.38). The gastric adenocarcinomas occurring in this sample were in a variety of locations in the stomach: 28 (23%) in the cardia; 69 (56.6%) in the body (fundus, greater and lesser curvatures, and antrum); six (4.9%) in the pylorus; four (3.3%) in overlapping regions; and 15 (12.3%) at unspecified locations. This distribution of reported gastric cancer sites was different from national reports (χ^2=59.94; df=8; P<0.001), with a greater proportion of Alaska Native cancers occurring in the greater and lesser curvatures, and fewer occurring in the body and overlapping regions, compared with national data. Summary staging information (27) was available for 101 (82.8%) of the cancers, and 21 (20.8%) of the staged cancers were localized, 44 (43.6%) were regional and 36 (35.6%) were distant, which was similar to the national data (χ^2=4.89; df=3; P=0.18).

DISCUSSION
For the first time, we report an association between the presence of serum anti-H pylori antibodies and the development of gastric cancer in Alaska Native people. This association was larger among people with

noncardia gastric cancer and individuals <50 years of age. The larger OR found in younger individuals likely arises from control H pylori seropositivity increasing with age, which diminishes the association apparent in the older age group. Unlike results reported by most previous studies (11,12), exposure to CagA-positive H pylori strains, as measured by anti-CagA antibody levels, did not appear to increase an individual's risk for gastric cancer in our study population. The near-ubiquitous presence of anti-CagA antibodies (95.1% each of cases and controls), which was significantly higher than reported in other studies (28,29), may have masked any true association between this virulence factor and gastric carcinogenesis. However, other studies have also found no association between infection with CagA-positive H pylori strains and gastric cancer (30), particularly in populations in which H pylori prevalence more closely mirrors that of rural Alaska (31). The high proportion of participants seropositive for CagA is likely due to prevalent H pylori infection and the relative antigenicity of the CagA protein, resulting in persistent CagA antibodies even after clearance of H pylori infection and H pylori IgG antibodies (32).

Few studies have evaluated pepsinogen levels and ratios before gastric cancer diagnosis to determine the predictive or screening value of these markers for gastric cancer. Most studies examined these serum markers in individuals at the time of their gastric cancer diagnosis (14,15,33,34). We found that low pepsinogen I level (<25 µg/L) was significantly associated with the development of noncardia gastric cancer when controlling for H pylori seropositivity. However, only a minority (4.1%) of people who subsequently developed gastric cancer had low pepsinogen levels, suggesting that few cancers would be detected using this marker. Our findings contrast with those of Parsonnet et al (35), who found antecedent low pepsinogen I (<50 µg/L) in 35.2% (45 of 128) of individuals who developed gastric cancer and reported a significant association between low pepsinogen I level and subsequent cancer in individuals with evidence of H pylori infection. A low pepsinogen I/II ratio (<2.5) was not associated with an increased risk for developing gastric cancer in the Alaska Native study population. The disparate frequencies of low pepsinogen I between the present study and other published studies may relate to variations in laboratory methods, particularly duration of sample storage, and is unlikely a reflection of differing gastric cancer pathophysiologies given the similarity of our sample cases to the SEER national sample.

The descriptive pathology of our study sample of Alaska Native gastric cancers was similar to that reported by SEER registries from other US populations. Summary staging information from our study population and from a recent report on cancer in Alaska Natives (36) suggests that gastric cancers in Alaska Native people were diagnosed at a stage similar to those reported in the national SEER database. This finding implies that delayed diagnosis due to access to health care (availability and utilization) is not the main explanation for increased Alaska Native gastric cancer mortality. Histology and histological grade were also similar between the two groups, indicating that Alaska Native people did not experience different or more aggressive tumours than other US populations. The main difference between the two groups was in the recorded sites of the gastric adenocarcinomas, although the differences were mainly in the specific location within the body of the stomach (body, lesser and greater curvatures), which is likely due to variance in surgical reporting and not cancer location. The similarity in descriptive gastric cancer pathologies and stage at diagnosis between the national and study samples suggests that the reason for a higher gastric cancer mortality rate in Alaska Native people is due to elevated cancer incidence in this population.

In the 38 individuals with gastric cancer and available paired serum specimens, we saw a significant increase in anti-H $pylori$ EIU levels from earlier to later specimens, although antibody level changes were heterogeneous, with some individuals experiencing a decline in antibody levels. Our finding counters the report by Tulinius et al (20) describing a decline in H $pylori$ antibody levels approaching cancer diagnosis. The increasing antibody levels apparent in our study may have resulted from the high prevalence of H $pylori$ infection in this population, leading to re-exposure to H $pylori$ and priming of the immune system. Focused exploration of anti-H $pylori$ antibody levels and their temporal relation to gastric cancer diagnosis may further clarify the association.

We aimed to test sera obtained before a diagnosis of gastric cancer. However, because of the retrospective nature of the study, we did not perform endoscopy on individuals to confirm their lack of gastric cancer at the time of serum collection, meaning that we may have included serum samples from individuals (cases) with undiagnosed gastric cancer. However, this scenario is unlikely because 70% of samples predated diagnosis by 10 years and >90% predated diagnosis by at least five years, during which time the likelihood of identifying gastric cancer would have been high. Additionally, our subanalysis was restricted to cases with samples predating diagnosis by at least 10 years had similar findings to the primary analysis (Table 2). Another challenge was the multiple changes made to summary staging and ICD-O-3 code definitions during the 40 years of study data. To correct for this, SEER provides updated coding and staging manuals on a regular basis and recodes data within SEER*Stat to provide uniformity across the multiple years of cancer registry data. Finally, the sample of Alaska Native people with gastric adenocarcinomas may not represent all Alaska Native people because the study population resided primarily in rural areas.

Evidence of H $pylori$ infection was widespread in our study population. Although we demonstrated an association between previous infection and subsequent gastric cancer, the utility of H $pylori$ seropositivity screening to predict gastric cancer in a population with such elevated rates of infection and reinfection is low. While noncardia gastric cancer cases showed an association with previous low pepsinogen I levels, the extremely low sensitivity of this potential screening test for predicting gastric cancer minimizes its clinical utility in this population. Because of the disproportionate burden of gastric cancer in the Alaska Native population, we will continue to examine potential markers of gastric cancer risk and to evaluate potential screening strategies to identify individuals at risk. As a next step,

TABLE 4
Comparison of Alaska Native and nationally reported gastric adenocarcinoma characteristics

	Alaska Native (n=122)	SEER (n=94,251)
Histology*		
Adenocarcinoma, not otherwise specified	81 (66.4)	60,883 (64.6)
Linitis plastica	4 (3.3)	2316 (2.5)
Adenocarcinoma, intestinal type	8 (6.6)	5511 (5.8)
Carcinoma, diffuse type	3 (2.5)	2352 (2.5)
Adenocarcinoma in adenomatous polyp	0 (0.0)	640 (0.7)
Tubular adenocarcinoma	1 (0.8)	477 (0.5)
Carcinoid tumour, malignant	0 (0.0)	2147 (2.3)
Adenocarcinoma with mixed subtypes	0 (0.0)	503 (0.5)
Papillary adenocarcinoma	2 (1.6)	520 (0.6)
Mucinous adenocarcinoma	3 (2.5)	2219 (2.4)
Mucin-producing adenocarcinoma	1 (0.8)	1877 (2.0)
Signet ring cell adenocarcinoma	19 (15.6)	13,744 (14.6)
Other adenocarcinomas	0 (0.0)	1062 (1.1)
Histological grade		
Well differentiated	6 (4.9)	4598 (4.9)
Moderately differentiated	35 (28.7)	20,129 (21.4)
Poorly differentiated	55 (45.1)	46,594 (49.4)
Undifferentiated	2 (1.6)	2514 (2.7)
Unknown	24 (19.7)	20,416 (21.7)
Site†		
Cardia, not otherwise specified	28 (23.0)	22,480 (23.9)
Fundus	7 (5.7)	3966 (4.2)
Body‡	0 (0.0)	7338 (7.8)
Gastric antrum	19 (15.6)	18,368 (19.5)
Pylorus	6 (4.9)	3402 (3.6)
Lesser curvature‡	30 (24.6)	8915 (9.5)
Greater curvature‡	13 (10.7)	4001 (4.2)
Overlapping§	4 (3.3)	8729 (9.3)
Stomach, not otherwise specified	15 (12.3)	17,052 (18.1)
Summary staging¶		
Localized	21 (19.1)	17,835 (23.3)
Regional§	44 (40.0)	23,653 (30.9)
Distant	36 (32.7)	26,432 (34.5)
Unstaged	9 (8.2)	8729 (11.4)

Data presented as n (%). *Histology classification according to International Classification of Diseases for Oncology, Third Edition (ICD-O-3) codes (26). ICD-O-3 cancer types reported that were ≥0.05% of the national total; †Site according to ICD-O-3 topography codes; ‡P<0.001 for z test of proportions between the Alaska Native and national Surveillance Epidemiology and End Results (SEER) groups; §P<0.05 for z test of proportions between the Alaska Native and national SEER groups; ¶Summary staging according to SEER definition (27). Includes only gastric cases diagnosed in 1984 and later because summary staging not available before 1984 in the Alaska Native Tumor Registry

we will characterize H $pylori$ strains circulating in the Alaska Native population to search for genotypes associated with gastric cancer and study how host characteristics predispose individuals to gastric cancer.

ACKNOWLEDGEMENTS: The authors thank Marcella Harker-Jones for her help with blood typing and the Bristol Bay Area Health Corporation, the Yukon-Kuskokwim Health Corporation, the Maniilaq Association, the Norton Sound Health Corporation, and the SouthEast Alaska Regional Health Consortium for their participation in this study.

REFERENCES

1. National Cancer Institute, Surveillance Research Program, Cancer Statistics Branch. Surveillance, Epidemiology, and End Results (SEER) Program SEER*Stat Database: Incidence – SEER 13 Regs Research Data (Katrina/Rita Population Adjustment) – Linked to County Attributes – Total U.S., 1969-2007 Counties, 2010.

2. National Cancer Institute, Surveillance Research Program, Cancer Statistics Branch. Surveillance, Epidemiology, and End Results (SEER) Program SEER*Stat Database: Mortality – All COD, Aggregated With State (Katrina/Rita Population Adjustment), Total U.S. (1990-2007), 2010.

3. Parsonnet J, Friedman GD, Vandersteen DP, et al. *Helicobacter pylori* infection and the risk of gastric carcinoma. N Engl J Med 1991;325:1127-31.

4. Helicobacter and Cancer Collaborative Group. Gastric cancer and *Helicobacter pylori*: A combined analysis of 12 case control studies nested within prospective cohorts. Gut 2001;49:347-53.

5. Parkinson AJ, Gold BD, Bulkow L, et al. High prevalence of *Helicobacter pylori* in the Alaska native population and association with low serum ferritin levels in young adults. Clin Diagn Lab Immunol 2000;7:885-8.

6. Bardhan PK. Epidemiological features of *Helicobacter pylori* infection in developing countries. Clin Infect Dis 1997;25:973-8.

7. Bruce MG, Bruden DL, McMahon BJ, et al. Alaska sentinel surveillance for antimicrobial resistance in *Helicobacter pylori* isolates from Alaska Native persons, 1999-2003. Helicobacter 2006;11:581-8.

8. Carothers JJ, Bruce MG, Hennessy TW, et al. The relationship between previous fluoroquinolone use and levofloxacin resistance in *Helicobacter pylori* infection. Clin Infect Dis 2007;44:e5-8.

9. McMahon BJ, Hennessy TW, Bensler JM, et al. The relationship among previous antimicrobial use, antimicrobial resistance, and treatment outcomes for *Helicobacter pylori* infections. Ann Intern Med 2003;139:463-9.

10. McMahon BJ, Bruce MG, Hennessy TW, et al. Reinfection after successful eradication of *Helicobacter pylori*: A 2-year prospective study in Alaska Natives. Aliment Pharmacol Ther 2006;23:1215-23.

11. Blaser MJ, Perez-Perez GI, Kleanthous H, et al. Infection with *Helicobacter pylori* strains possessing CagA is associated with an increased risk of developing adenocarcinoma of the stomach. Cancer Res 1995;55:2111-5.

12. Parsonnet J, Friedman GD, Orentreich N, Vogelman H. Risk for gastric cancer in people with CagA positive or CagA negative *Helicobacter pylori* infection. Gut 1997;40:297-301.

13. Correa P, Houghton J. Carcinogenesis of *Helicobacter pylori*. Gastroenterology 2007;133:659-72.

14. Kodoi A, Yoshihara M, Sumii K, Haruma K, Kajiyama G. Serum pepsinogen in screening for gastric cancer. J Gastroenterol 1995;30:452-60.

15. Yoshihara M, Hiyama T, Yoshida S, et al. Reduction in gastric cancer mortality by screening based on serum pepsinogen concentration: A case-control study. Scand J Gastroenterol 2007;42:760-4.

16. Aird I, Bentall HH, Roberts JA. A Relationship between cancer of stomach and the ABO blood groups. Br Med J 1953;1:3.

17. You WC, Ma JL, Liu W, et al. Blood type and family cancer history in relation to precancerous gastric lesions. Int J Epidemiol 2000;29:405-7.

18. Pocard M, Panis Y, Valleur P, Sarazin D. No correlation between *H. pylori* and blood groups in gastric cancer. Gastroenterology 1998;114:1.

19. Umlauft F, Keeffe EB, Offner F, et al. *Helicobacter pylori* infection and blood group antigens: Lack of clinical association. Am J Gastroenterol 1996;91:2135-8.

20. Tulinius H, Ogmundsdottir HM, Kristinsson KG, et al. *Helicobacter pylori* antibodies and gastric cancer in Iceland – the decline in IgG antibody level is a risk factor. APMIS 2001;109:835-41.

21. U.S. Census Bureau, Population Division. Table 5. Estimates of the Resident Population by Race Alone or in Combination and Hispanic Origin for the United States and States: July 1, 2009 (SC-EST2009-5), 2010.

22. National Cancer Institute, Surveillance Research Program, Cancer Statistics Branch. Surveillance, Epidemiology, and End Results (SEER) Program SEER*Stat Database. Incidence – SEER 17 Regs Research Data + Hurricane Katrina Impacted Louisiana Cases, Nov 2009 Sub (1973-2007 varying) – Linked to County Attributes – Total U.S. Counties, 1969-2007 2010.

23. Kamangar F, Dawsey SM, Blaser MJ, et al. Opposing risks of gastric cardia and noncardia gastric adenocarcinomas associated with *Helicobacter pylori* seropositivity. J Natl Cancer Inst 2006;98:1445-52.

24. Carvalho R, Milne AN, van Rees BP, et al. Early-onset gastric carcinomas display molecular characteristics distinct from gastric carcinomas occurring at a later age. J Pathol 2004;204:75-83.

25. Milne AN, Sitarz R, Carvalho R, Carneiro F, Offerhaus GJ. Early onset gastric cancer: On the road to unraveling gastric carcinogenesis. Curr Mol Med 2007;7:15-28.

26. Fritz A, Percy C, Jack A, et al. International Classification of Diseases for Oncology, 3rd edn. Geneva: World Health Organization, 2000.

27. Young JL Jr, Roffers SD, Ries LAG, Fritz AG, eds HA. SEER Summary Staging Manual – 2000: Codes and Coding Instructions, Bethesda: National Cancer Institute, NIH, 2001.

28. Ekstrom AM, Held M, Hansson LE, Engstrand L, Nyren O. *Helicobacter pylori* in gastric cancer established by CagA immunoblot as a marker of past infection. Gastroenterology 2001;121:784-91.

29. Wong BC, Lam SK, Ching CK, et al. Seroprevalence of cytotoxin-associated gene A positive *Helicobacter pylori* strains in Changle, an area with very high prevalence of gastric cancer in south China. Aliment Pharmacol Ther 1999;13:1295-302.

30. Yamaoka Y, Kodama T, Kashima K, Graham DY. Antibody against *Helicobacter pylori* CagA and VacA and the risk for gastric cancer. J Clin Pathol 1999;52:215-8.

31. Mitchell HM, Hazell SL, Li YY, Hu PJ. Serological response to specific *Helicobacter pylori* antigens: Antibody against CagA antigen is not predictive of gastric cancer in a developing country. Am J Gastroenterol 1996;91:1785-8.

32. Ye W, Held M, Enroth H, Kraaz W, Engstrand L, Nyrén O. Histology and culture results among subjects with antibodies to CagA but no evidence of *Helicobacter pylori* infection with IgG ELISA. Scand J Gastroenterol. 2005;40:312-8.

33. So JB, Yeoh KG, Moochala S, et al. Serum pepsinogen levels in gastric cancer patients and their relationship with *Helicobacter pylori* infection: A prospective study. Gastric Cancer 2002;5:228-32.

34. Yoshihara M, Sumii K, Haruma K, et al. Correlation of ratio of serum pepsinogen I and II with prevalence of gastric cancer and adenoma in Japanese subjects. Am J Gastroenterol 1998;93:1090-6.

35. Parsonnet J, Samloff IM, Nelson LM, Orentreich N, Vogelman JH, Friedman GD. *Helicobacter pylori*, pepsinogen, and risk for gastric adenocarcinoma. Cancer Epidemiol Biomarkers Prev 1993;2:461-6.

36. Lanier AP, Kelly JJ, Maxwell J, McEvoy T, Homan C. Cancer in Alaska Natives 1969-2003: 35-Year Report. Alaska Native Tribal Health Consortium, 2006.

13

Atypical distribution of inflammation in newly diagnosed ulcerative colitis is not rare

Sang Hyoung Park MD[1], Suk-Kyun Yang MD[1], Soo-Kyung Park MD[1], Jong Wook Kim MD[2], Dong-Hoon Yang MD[1], Kee Wook Jung MD[1], Kyung-Jo Kim MD[1], Byong Duk Ye MD[1], Jeong-Sik Byeon MD[1], Seung-Jae Myung MD[1], Jin-Ho Kim MD[1]

SH Park, S-K Yang, S-K Park, et al. Atypical distribution of inflammation in newly diagnosed ulcerative colitis is not rare. Can J Gastroenterol Hepatol 2014;28(3):125-130.

BACKGROUND: Appendiceal orifice inflammation (AOI) is a common 'skip lesion' in patients with ulcerative colitis (UC). However, other skip lesions are less well known.
OBJECTIVE: To evaluate the atypical distribution of UC lesions, other than AOI, in terms of their frequency, pattern, risk factors and prognostic implications.
METHODS: A retrospective analysis of colonoscopic findings and clinical course of 240 adult UC patients who were initially diagnosed at Asan Medical Center (Seoul, South Korea) was performed.
RESULTS: Of 240 patients, 46 (19.2%) showed an atypical distribution of lesions at initial colonoscopy: eight (3.3%) had rectal sparing (segmental-type UC); and 38 (15.8%) had patchy/segmental skip lesions other than AOI. Skip lesions were detected more frequently in proximal segments of the colon than in distal segments (P=0.001). An atypical distribution was more common in patients with AOI (31.3%) than in those without AOI (10.6%; P<0.001). The clinical course of patients with an atypical distribution was not different from that of patients with a typical distribution in terms of remission, relapse, disease extension, colectomy and mortality. In addition, of the 36 patients with an atypical distribution of lesions at diagnosis who underwent follow-up colonoscopy, 24 (66.7%) demonstrated a typical distribution of lesions.
CONCLUSIONS: Patchy/segmental skip lesions and rectal sparing occur not infrequently in adult patients with newly diagnosed, untreated UC. As such, these features alone should not be considered to be definitive evidence against a diagnosis of UC. There does not appear to be a prognostic implication of an atypical distribution of lesions.

Key Words: Colonoscopy; Diagnosis; Prognosis; Skip lesion; Ulcerative colitis

La répartition atypique de l'inflammation n'est pas rare dans les cas de colite ulcéreuse nouvellement diagnostiquée

HISTORIQUE : L'inflammation de l'orifice appendiculaire (IOA) est une lésion discontinue courante chez les patients atteints de colite ulcéreuse (CU). Cependant, il existe d'autres lésions discontinues, qui sont moins connues.
OBJECTIF : Évaluer la fréquence, l'aspect, les facteurs de risque et les conséquences pronostiques de la répartition atypique des lesions de CU autre que l'IOA.
MÉTHODOLOGIE : Les chercheurs ont procédé à une analyse rétrospective des observations coloscopiques et de l'évolution clinique de 240 patients adultes atteints de CU d'abord diagnostiqués au centre médical Asan de Séoul, en Corée du Sud.
RÉSULTATS : Sur 240 patients, 46 (19,2 %) présentaient une répartition atypique des lésions lors de la coloscopie initiale : chez huit d'entre eux (3,3 %), le rectum était épargné (CU de type segmentaire), tandis que 38 (15,8 %) avaient des lésions discontinues, irrégulières et segmentaires autres qu'une IOA. Les chercheurs ont décelé plus de lésions discontinues dans les segments proximaux que dans les segments distaux du côlon (P=0,001). La répartition atypique était plus courante chez les patients ayant une IOA (31,3 %) que chez ceux sans IOA (10,6 %; P<0,001). L'évolution clinique des patients dont la répartition était atypique ne différait pas de celle des patients qui présentaient une répartition classique sur le plan de la rémission, des récidives, de la dissémination de la maladie, de la colectomie et de la mortalité. De plus, sur les 36 patients dont la répartition des lésions était atypique au diagnostic et qui ont subi une coloscopie de suivi, 24 (66,7 %) ont présenté une répartition classique des lésions.
CONCLUSIONS : Les lésions discontinues irrégulières et segmentaires et l'épargne du rectum ne sont pas rares chez les patients adultes atteints d'une CU non traitée nouvellement diagnostiqués. Ainsi, ces seules caractéristiques ne devraient pas être considérées comme des raisons catégoriques de réfuter un diagnostic de CU. La répartition atypique des lésions ne semble pas avoir d'effets pronostiques.

Ulcerative colitis (UC) is an idiopathic disease characterized by chronic and relapsing inflammation of the colon, and is one of the major conditions belonging to the broad group of inflammatory bowel diseases (IBDs) (1). It is generally accepted that UC always involves the rectum and may progress to involve more proximal portions of the colon in a continuous, nonsegmental fashion (2). However, there are a few exceptions to this general rule. First, endoscopic and histological patchiness and rectal sparing are quite common in treated UC patients (3-5). Second, pediatric, but not adult, patients with new-onset, previously untreated UC often show relative or complete rectal sparing and/or a patchy/segmental involvement of the colon (6-8). Furthermore, absolute or relative rectal sparing is frequently observed (up to 65%) in both pediatric and adult patients with UC associated with primary sclerosing cholangitis (9-12). Finally, up to 75% of patients with distal UC show evidence of periappendiceal inflammation as a 'skip lesion', often referred to as a cecal patch (13,14), appendiceal orifice inflammation (AOI) (15-17) or a periappendiceal red patch (18).

With the increased awareness of these situations and the concomitant advances in endoscopic technologies, studies from Japan identified endoscopic evidence of skip lesions (other than AOI) in newly diagnosed UC patients that manifest as patchy or segmental involvement of the disease in the colon that is discrete from the distal main lesion (19,20). Moreover, 'right-sided' or 'segmental' colitis represent subgroups of UC defined according to extent in Japan (21). However, these lesions sometime lead clinicians to a false diagnosis of other IBDs, such as Crohn disease (CD), because discontinuity of lesions is a characteristic feature in the differential diagnosis of CD and UC (1).

The clinical features and natural course of UC in patients with skip lesions remain unclear. Therefore, we analyzed the endoscopic findings

[1]Department of Gastroenterology, University of Ulsan College of Medicine, Asan Medical Center, Seoul; [2]Division of Gastroenterology, Department of Internal Medicine, Inje University Ilsan Paik Hospital, Ilsanseo-gu, Goyang-si, Gyeonggi-do, Korea
Correspondence: Dr Suk-Kyun Yang, Department of Gastroenterology, University of Ulsan College of Medicine, Asan Medical Center, 88 Olympic-ro 43-gil, Songpa-gu, Seoul 138-736, Korea. e-mail sky@amc.seoul.kr

and pattern of distribution of lesions in patients with newly diagnosed, untreated UC to determine the clinical implications and to evaluate the risk factors associated with this atypical distribution.

METHODS

Patients

Data obtained from the medical and endoscopic records of all patients who were first diagnosed with UC at the Asan Medical Center, a university hospital in Seoul, South Korea, between January 2001 and December 2009 were analyzed retrospectively. UC was definitively diagnosed in those who met all three of the following criteria: a typical history of diarrhea or blood and pus, or both, in the stool for >4 weeks; a typical colonoscopic picture showing diffusely granular, friable or ulcerated mucosa; and characteristic histopathological signs of inflammation on biopsy (22-25). In addition, patients with rectal sparing or skip lesions (either patchy or segmental) were included and considered to have an atypical distribution of UC if their main lesions were typical of UC and their skip lesions had the same characteristics as the main lesions, both endoscopically and histologically. Because AOI is a common feature of UC (found in >50% of patients in some studies [13,16,26]) and requires no further diagnostic workup to exclude CD (as stated in the European consensus [27]), AOI was not considered to be an atypical UC lesion in the present study. Subjects were excluded if they had been prescribed systemic steroids or immunosuppressive agents for any disease at the time of UC diagnosis, or if they did not undergo complete ileocolonoscopy at the time of UC diagnosis. Subjects were also excluded if they had received nonsteroidal anti-inflammatory drugs at the time of UC diagnosis. Thirty-four patients from the authors' previous AOI studies (16,17) were also included in the present study.

Methods

Baseline demographic and clinical features, including sex, age, duration of symptoms, smoking habits, perinuclear antineutrophil cytoplasmic antibody (pANCA) status, extent of disease, endoscopic disease activity and AOI status at the time of UC diagnosis were evaluated. Total colonoscopy, including evaluation of the terminal ileum, was performed in all patients using a video colonoscope (CF-H260AL/CF-240L/CF-230L, Olympus Optical Co, Japan) after bowel preparation using 4 L of polyethylene glycol-electrolyte lavage solution. Photographs were taken of each segment including the terminal ileum, cecum, ascending colon and onward. Colonoscopic photographs were analyzed by one author (SKY) who was blinded to the clinical course of the patients. The extent of disease was classified as proctitis, left-sided colitis or extensive colitis on the basis of the colonoscopic findings. Proctitis was defined as disease involving up to 15 cm from the anal verge; left-sided colitis as disease up to the splenic flexure; and extensive colitis as disease beyond the splenic flexure. The term 'pancolitis' was used to indicate extensive colitis involving the entire colon. In addition, segmental-type UC was defined as UC-like inflammatory lesions (of any extent) in the colon without endoscopic evidence of rectal involvement. AOI and other skip lesions were not considered when classifying the extent of disease. Endoscopic disease activity was classified as mild, moderate or severe according to the endoscopy subscore of the Mayo score (28). Mild disease was characterized as erythema, a decreased vascular pattern and mild friability; moderate disease as marked erythema, an absent vascular pattern, friability and erosions; and severe disease as spontaneous bleeding and/or ulceration.

To investigate changes in the atypical distribution of lesions and the extent of the disease over time, follow-up colonoscopy was performed at one- to three-year intervals, with shorter intervals if clinically indicated. Proximal disease extension was defined as the extension, at any follow-up colonoscopy, of macroscopic inflammation beyond the initially involved segment (ie, from proctitis to left-sided or extensive colitis, or from left-sided colitis to extensive colitis). The subsequent clinical features and follow-up colonoscopic findings were analyzed and compared according to the initial atypical distribution of

lesions. The study protocol was approved by the Institutional Review Board of the Asan Medical Center.

Statistical analysis

Database management and statistical analyses were performed using SPSS version 17.0 (IBM Corporation, USA) for Windows (Microsoft Corporation, USA). When appropriate, results were expressed as proportions or medians and compared using the Mann-Whitney U test. The χ^2 test or Fisher's exact test were used to compare categorical variables. The cumulative rate of disease relapse was calculated using the Kaplan-Meier method, and the values were compared between groups using the log-rank test; $P<0.05$ was considered to be statistically significant.

RESULTS

Baseline characteristics

During the study period, 2200 patients with UC visited the outpatient clinic of the Asan Medical Center. Of these, 267 (12.1%) were initially diagnosed with UC at this institution. Twenty-seven patients were excluded: 10 had received systemic steroids or immunosuppressive agents for diseases other than UC; and 17 did not undergo total colonoscopy at diagnosis. The remaining 240 patients were included in the analysis.

Of the 240 patients, 132 (55.0%) were male and 108 (45.0%) were female, yielding a male-to-female ratio of 1.22:1. The median age at diagnosis was 41 years (range 16 to 79 years) and the median interval from onset of symptoms to diagnosis was 5.3 months (range 0 to 369 months). Of the 240 patients, 44 (18.3%) were current smokers and 87 (36.3%) were pANCA seropositive. At diagnosis, 125 patients (52.1%) had proctitis, 51 (21.3%) had left-sided colitis and 56 (23.3%) had extensive colitis. The remaining eight (3.3%) patients had segmental-type UC. Of the 56 patients with extensive colitis, 39 had pancolitis.

Within the total cohort, 99 (41.3%) patients (54 male and 45 female) were identified as having AOI at diagnosis. If the 39 patients with pancolitis from the total cohort were excluded, AOI was present in 49.3% of patients (99 of 201). Endoscopic disease activity at diagnosis was mild in 101 (42.1%) patients, moderate in 88 (36.7%) and severe in 51 (21.3%).

Atypical distribution of lesions

Of the 240 patients, 46 (19.2%) showed an atypical distribution of lesions at the initial colonoscopy. Eight (3.3%) patients had rectal sparing (segmental-type UC), with no evidence of skip lesions; the distribution of the lesions in these eight patients is summarized in Table 1. The remaining 38 (15.8%) patients had skip lesions other than AOI: 23 (60.5%) had patchy skip lesions (Figure 1A); 13 (34.2%) had segmental skip lesions (Figure 1B); and two (5.3%) had both patchy and segmental skip lesions. Skip lesions were found in 19 (15.2%) of 125 patients with proctitis, nine (17.6%) of 51 with left-sided colitis and 10 (17.9%) of 56 with extensive colitis. Figure 2 shows the location and proportion of lesions in 19 patients with proctitis and skip lesions. Skip lesions were discovered more frequently in the proximal segments of the colon (transverse colon and ascending colon) than at the distal segments (sigmoid colon and descending colon) (P=0.001) (Figure 2).

Table 2 summarizes the baseline characteristics of patients with typical and atypical UC. There were no statistically significant differences between the two groups in terms of demographic findings such as sex distribution, age at diagnosis, duration of symptoms before diagnosis and smoking status. In addition, there were no differences between the two groups regarding clinical features at diagnosis, including pANCA status, disease activity and disease extent. However, AOI was identified in 68 (35.1%) of the 194 patients with typical UC and in 31 (67.4%) of 46 patients with the atypical distribution (P<0.001). If the 39 patients with pancolitis were excluded from the calculations, AOI was present in 68 (43.9%) of the 155 patients with typical UC

TABLE 1
Initial endoscopic findings and follow-up results of eight patients with segmental-type ulcerative colitis

Patient	Age/sex	Cecum	Colon Ascending	Colon Transverse	Colon Descending	Colon Sigmoid	Rectum	Findings on follow-up colonoscopy
1	34/male	+	+					Extensive colitis
2	33/female	+		+				Left-sided colitis*
3	42/male	+				+		Proctitis
4	38/male		+	+				Proctitis
5	50/male			+	+	+		Proctitis*
6	50/male		+					Proctitis*
7	44/female		+	+	+	+		No follow-up
8	71/male			+				No follow-up

Initial proximal lesions remained even after the appearance of rectal involvement, thereby resulting in skip lesions

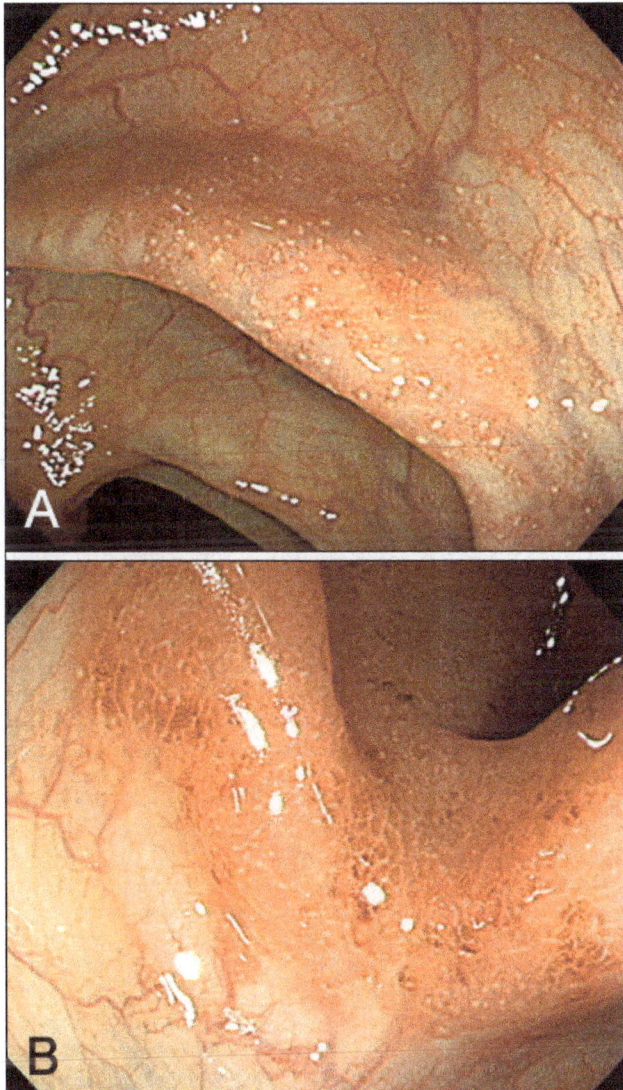

Figure 1) A *Patchy skip lesion in the ascending colon.* **B** *Segmental skip lesion in the transverse colon*

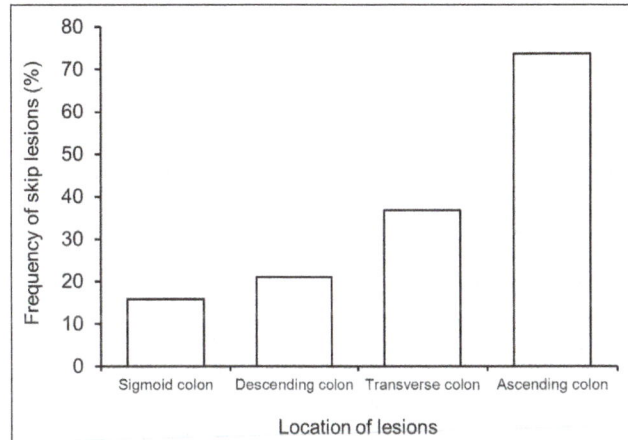

Figure 2) *Location of 'skip lesions' in 19 patients with proctitis and skip lesions. Skip lesions were found more frequently in the proximal segments of the colon (transverse colon and ascending colon) than in the distal segments (sigmoid colon and descending colon) (P=0.001)*

and in 31 (67.4%) of 46 patients with an atypical distribution (P=0.007). Thus, an atypical distribution was more common in patients with AOI (31.3%) than in those without AOI (10.6%; P<0.001).

Clinical course
The clinical courses of UC according to lesion distribution are summarized in Table 3. The median duration of clinical follow-up was 67 months (range one to 139 months) in the 240 patients. There

was no difference in the type of treatment during follow-up, the initial remission rate, the cumulative rate of disease relapse, the rate of colectomy or the mortality rate between the two groups.

Follow-up colonoscopic examinations were performed in 160 (66.7%) of the original cohort of 240 patients (Table 4). The median duration of colonoscopic follow-up was 38 months (range 0.1 to 112 months), with the median number of follow-up colonoscopies being two (range one to seven). There were no differences in baseline characteristics, such as age, sex and endoscopic findings, between patients who were and were not followed-up endoscopically (data not shown). Among the 194 patients with typical UC, 124 (63.9%) underwent follow-up colonoscopy, with proximal extension of the disease detected in 21 (16.9%): from proctitis into left-sided colitis in 12 patients; from proctitis into extensive colitis in four; and from left-sided colitis into extensive colitis in five.

Of the remaining 46 patients with an atypical distribution of lesions (38 with skip lesions, eight with rectal sparing), 36 (78.3%) underwent follow-up colonoscopy, including 30 with skip lesions and six with rectal sparing. Of these 36 patients, 24 (66.7%) showed a typical distribution of lesions on follow-up colonoscopy. Proximal extension of the disease occurred in five (16.7%) of the 30 patients with skip lesions (excluding the six patients with rectal sparing): from proctitis into left-sided colitis in three patients; and from proctitis into extensive colitis in two patients. The proportion of patients with proximal extension was not different between patients with typical distribution and those with skip lesions (P=1.000). In the six patients with rectal sparing, there was evidence of rectal involvement at follow-up, with proctitis being detected in four patients, left-sided colitis in one

TABLE 2
Baseline characteristics of patients with ulcerative colitis according to distribution of lesions

	Distribution		P
	Typical (n=194)	Atypical (n=46)	
Age at diagnosis, years*	41 (17–80)	41 (17–71)	0.217
Sex			1.000
Male	107 (55.2)	25 (54.3)	
Female	87 (44.8)	21 (45.7)	
Smoking			0.880
Never smoker	105 (54.1)	26 (56.5)	
Current smoker	37 (19.1)	7 (15.2)	
Ex-smoker	52 (26.8)	13 (28.3)	
Duration of symptoms before diagnosis, months*	4.0 (0–123)	5.6 (0–369)	0.530
pANCA			0.306
Positive	67 (34.5)	20 (43.5)	
Negative	127 (65.5)	26 (56.5)	
Initial disease extent			0.816
Proctitis	106 (54.6)	19 (41.3)	
Left-sided colitis	42 (21.6)	9 (19.6)	
Extensive colitis	46 (23.7)	10 (21.7)	
Segmental		8 (17.4)	
Initial endoscopic disease activity			0.310
Mild	79 (40.7)	22 (47.8)	
Moderate	70 (36.1)	18 (39.1)	
Severe	45 (23.2)	6 (13.0)	
AOI	68 (35.1)	31 (67.4)	<0.001

*Data presented as n (%). *Data presented as median (range). AOI Appendiceal orifice inflammation; pANCA Perinuclear antineutrophil cytoplasmic antibody*

TABLE 3
Clinical course of patients with ulcerative colitis according to distribution of lesions

	Distribution		P
	Typical (n=194)	Atypical (n=46)	
Duration of clinical follow-up, months*	66 (1–139)	69 (2–138)	0.108
Treatment during follow-up			
5-ASA (topical and/or oral)	194 (100)	46 (100)	
Systemic corticosteroids	68 (35.1)	15 (32.6)	0.864
Azathioprine/ 6-mercaptopurine	10 (5.2)	5 (10.9)	0.173
Infliximab	2 (1.0)	0 (0.0)	1.000
Initial remission rate	193 (99.5)	46 (100.0)	1.000
Cumulative rate of disease relapse, %			0.368
1-year relapse rate	34.8	50.5	
3-year relapse rate	60.2	66.1	
5-year relapse rate	72.6	80.9	
Total proctocolectomy	2 (1.0)	2 (4.3)	0.167
Mortality	3 (1.5)	1 (2.2)	0.576

*Data presented as n (%) unless otherwise indicated. *Data presented as median (range). 5-ASA 5-aminosalicylic acid*

patient and extensive colitis in one patient (Table 1). The median interval from the initial colonoscopy to the identification of rectal involvement was 23.7 months (range 5.8 to 36.6 months) in these six patients. However, initial proximal lesions remained, even after the appearance of rectal involvement, thereby forming skip lesions in three of these six patients. The final diagnosis was not changed to CD in any of the 46 patients who showed an atypical distribution of inflammatory lesions at initial colonoscopy.

DISCUSSION

To our knowledge, the present study was the first to evaluate the frequency and clinical implications of an atypical distribution of inflammatory lesions other than AOI in a large number of adult patients with newly diagnosed UC. The initial colonoscopy showed that 19.2% of patients had rectal sparing (3.3%) or skip lesions other than AOI (15.8%). This atypical distribution is very high if we consider the classical concept that UC always involves the rectum and may progress proximally in a continuous fashion. We hypothesize that this high rate is due to an increased awareness of skip lesions, such as AOI in UC, as well as improved methods used for bowel preparation and advances in endoscopic technology.

Clinical examiners have a tendency to discontinue a colonoscopic evaluation when they reach the margin between the distal inflamed area and the proximal normal mucosa (29). Additionally, total colonoscopy is not recommended for patients with severely active disease for fear of perforating the colon or exacerbating the colitis (30). However, because we previously performed three studies investigating AOI in patients with UC (15-17), we routinely examine the entire colon of UC patients for the presence or absence of periappendiceal skip lesions. Moreover, in our previous prospective study (16), we recognized and briefly discussed the presence of skip lesions other than AOI (16). Since then, we have maintained a consensus among our endoscopists to describe all skip lesions, including AOI, which has led to the frequent discovery of other skip lesions in addition to AOI.

Mutinga et al (31) identified patchy, right-sided colonic inflammation in 12 (3.4%) of 352 patients with UC. This figure is much lower than the findings presented in the present study. Also, in contrast to the present study, Mutinga et al included patients with AOI, and nine patients had only microscopic (but not endoscopic) lesions in the right side of the colon. Therefore, the frequency of macroscopic skip lesions other than AOI in the present study is much higher than that reported by Mutinga et al (31). In contrast, retrospective studies from Japan identified skip lesions other than AOI in 23 (29.9%) of 77 patients with newly diagnosed UC (19) and in 20 (45.5%) of 44 UC patients with AOI (20). Unlike the present study, this Japanese study classified aphthous ulcers at the margin between the distal inflamed area and the proximal normal mucosa as skip lesions, which may account for the higher reported incidence. In addition, if analyzed among the patients with AOI, the frequency of an atypical distribution in the present study would increase to 31.3% (31 of 99), which makes our findings comparable with those of these other Japanese studies.

TABLE 4
Follow-up colonoscopic findings according to distribution of lesions

	Typical distribution (n=194)	Atypical distribution (n=46)	
		Skip lesion (n=38)	Rectal sparing (n=8)
Colonoscopy follow-up	63.9 (124/194)	78.9 (30/38)	75.0 (6/8)
Proximal extension of disease	16.9 (21/124)	16.7 (5/30)	N/A
Change to typical distribution	N/A	70.0 (21/30)	50.0 (3/6)

Data presented as % (n/n). N/A Not applicable

The presence of skip lesions contradicts the conventional concept of UC as a strictly continuous disease. Pathologists may prefer the diagnosis of CD to that of UC when they encounter skip lesions. However, over a median follow-up of 67 months, none of our patients developed any features consistent with CD such as ileal lesions, perianal disease or granuloma. In addition, of the 36 patients with an atypical distribution of lesions at diagnosis who underwent follow-up colonoscopy, 24 (66.7%) showed a typical distribution of lesions, which could be due to the disappearance of skip lesions and/or to the appearance of rectal involvement. As such, we are confident that all of our patients with skip lesions or rectal sparing had UC rather than CD.

The results of the present study have important implications with regard to the diagnosis of IBD. Because our results clearly show that patchy or segmental skip lesions and rectal sparing occur not infrequently in adults with newly diagnosed, untreated UC, these features alone should not be considered definitive evidence against a diagnosis of UC. However, what are the prognostic implications of skip lesions or rectal sparing in UC? Rajwal et al (7) suggested that rectal sparing in pediatric patients with UC indicated a more aggressive disease that is less responsive to medical treatment. However, no study has addressed this issue in the adult population. In our previous study, we found no prognostic implications for the presence of AOI skip lesions on the clinical course of UC (16). Similarly, the present study showed that the presence of an atypical distribution of inflammatory lesions in UC patients had no prognostic implications in terms of rates of remission, relapse, disease extension, colectomy and mortality. Instead, we identified a clear correlation between the presence of an atypical distribution and AOI; however, we cannot offer a logical explanation as to the biological meaning of this relationship.

The present study had several limitations. First, it was retrospective in design. Although there was a consensus among our endoscopists to describe all skip lesions, including AOI, throughout the study period, we cannot exclude the possibility that some minor skip lesions were missed. Therefore, the actual frequency of an atypical distribution of lesions may be higher than reported. Second, we did not evaluate the small bowel using small-bowel follow-through or computed tomography/magnetic resonance enterography to exclude CD. However, we did evaluate the terminal ileum in all patients using colonoscopy; no patients had terminal ileal lesions. Third, we did not perform histopathological analysis in the present study; therefore, some of our patients who were classified as having skip lesions may show histological evidence of continuous lesions. However, the extent of UC is usually classified according to endoscopic appearance rather than histological findings, as set out in the Montreal classification (32) and in the European (30) and American guidelines (33).

CONCLUSION

We showed that an atypical distribution of inflammatory lesions is not a rare finding in patients with newly diagnosed UC. Clinicians and pathologists need to be aware that skip lesions and rectal sparing may occur in untreated patients with UC so as to avoid a misdiagnosis of CD based on the finding of atypical distribution alone can be avoided. Further prospective, large-scale studies are needed to confirm these observations.

FUNDING: This study was supported by a grant of the Korean Health Technology R&D Project, Ministry of Health & Welfare, Republic of Korea (A120176).

DISCLOSURES: Suk-Kyun Yang has received a research grant from Janssen Korea Ltd. None of the other authors have financial disclosures or conflicts of interest to declare.

REFERENCES

1. Podolsky DK. Inflammatory bowel disease. N Engl J Med 2002;347:417-29.
2. Pera A, Bellando P, Caldera D, et al. Colonoscopy in inflammatory bowel disease. Diagnostic accuracy and proposal of an endoscopic score. Gastroenterology 1987;92:181-5.
3. Kim B, Barnett JL, Kleer CG, Appelman HD. Endoscopic and histological patchiness in treated ulcerative colitis. Am J Gastroenterol 1999;94:3258-62.
4. Odze R, Antonioli D, Peppercorn M, Goldman H. Effect of topical 5-aminosalicylic acid (5-ASA) therapy on rectal mucosal biopsy morphology in chronic ulcerative colitis. Am J Surg Pathol 1993;17:869-75.
5. Bernstein CN, Shanahan F, Anton PA, Weinstein WM. Patchiness of mucosal inflammation in treated ulcerative colitis: A prospective study. Gastrointest Endosc 1995;42:232-7.
6. Glickman JN, Bousvaros A, Farraye FA, et al. Pediatric patients with untreated ulcerative colitis may present initially with unusual morphologic findings. Am J Surg Pathol 2004;28:190-7.
7. Rajwal SR, Puntis JW, McClean P, et al. Endoscopic rectal sparing in children with untreated ulcerative colitis. J Pediatr Gastroenterol Nutr 2004;38:66-9.
8. Washington K, Greenson JK, Montgomery E, et al. Histopathology of ulcerative colitis in initial rectal biopsy in children. Am J Surg Pathol 2002;26:1441-9.
9. Faubion WA, Jr., Loftus EV, Sandborn WJ, Freese DK, Perrault J. Pediatric "PSC-IBD": A descriptive report of associated inflammatory bowel disease among pediatric patients with psc. J Pediatr Gastroenterol Nutr 2001;33:296-300.
10. Jorgensen KK, Grzyb K, Lundin KE, et al. Inflammatory bowel disease in patients with primary sclerosing cholangitis: Clinical characterization in liver transplanted and nontransplanted patients. Inflamm Bowel Dis 2012;18:536-45.
11. Loftus EV Jr, Harewood GC, Loftus CG, et al. PSC-IBD: A unique form of inflammatory bowel disease associated with primary sclerosing cholangitis. Gut 2005;54:91-6.
12. Ye BD, Yang SK, Boo SJ, et al. Clinical characteristics of ulcerative colitis associated with primary sclerosing cholangitis in Korea. Inflamm Bowel Dis 2011;17:1901-6.
13. D'Haens G, Geboes K, Peeters M, Baert F, Ectors N, Rutgeerts P. Patchy cecal inflammation associated with distal ulcerative colitis: A prospective endoscopic study. Am J Gastroenterol 1997;92:1275-9.
14. Dendrinos K, Cerda S, Farraye FA. The "cecal patch" in patients with ulcerative colitis. Gastrointest Endosc 2008;68:1006-7.
15. Yang SK, Jung HY, Kang GH, et al. Appendiceal orifice inflammation as a skip lesion in ulcerative colitis: An analysis in relation to medical therapy and disease extent. Gastrointest Endosc 1999;49:743-7.
16. Byeon JS, Yang SK, Myung SJ, et al. Clinical course of distal ulcerative colitis in relation to appendiceal orifice inflammation status. Inflamm Bowel Dis 2005;11:366-71.
17. Park SH, Yang SK, Kim MJ, et al. Long term follow-up of appendiceal and distal right-sided colonic inflammation. Endoscopy 2012;44:95-8.
18. Rubin DT, Rothe JA. The peri-appendiceal red patch in ulcerative colitis: Review of the University of Chicago experience. Dig Dis Sci 2010;55:3495-501.
19. Murano M, Inoue T, Kuramoto T, et al. Endoscopic findings of initial active ulcerative colitis. Stom Intest (Tokyo) 2009;44:1492-504.
20. Tanaka T, Okawa K, Ueda W, et al. Clinical study of ulcerative colitis with skipped lesions at the orifice of the appendix. Stom Intest (Tokyo) 2009;44:1534-40.
21. Hisabe T, Hirai F, Matsui T. Diagnosis of ulcerative colitis. J Jpn Soc Coloproctol 2011;64:807-16.
22. Yang SK, Hong WS, Min YI, et al. Incidence and prevalence of ulcerative colitis in the Songpa-Kangdong District, Seoul, Korea, 1986-1997. J Gastroenterol Hepatol 2000;15:1037-42.
23. Garland CF, Lilienfeld AM, Mendeloff AI, Markowitz JA, Terrell KB, Garland FC. Incidence rates of ulcerative colitis and Crohn's disease in fifteen areas of the United States. Gastroenterology 1981;81:1115-24.

24. Binder V, Both H, Hansen PK, Hendriksen C, Kreiner S, Torp-Pedersen K. Incidence and prevalence of ulcerative colitis and Crohn's disease in the county of Copenhagen, 1962 to 1978. Gastroenterology 1982;83:563-8.

25. Tysk C, Jarnerot G. Ulcerative proctocolitis in Orebro, Sweden: A retrospective epidemiologic study, 1963-1987. Scand J Gastroenterol 1992;27:945-50.

26. Matsumoto T, Nakamura S, Shimizu M, Iida M. Significance of appendiceal involvement in patients with ulcerative colitis. Gastrointest Endosc 2002;55:180-5.

27. Stange EF, Travis SP, Vermeire S, et al. European evidence-based Consensus on the diagnosis and management of ulcerative colitis: Definitions and diagnosis. J Crohns Colitis 2008;2:1-23.

28. Schroeder KW, Tremaine WJ, Ilstrup DM. Coated oral 5-aminosalicylic acid therapy for mildly to moderately active ulcerative colitis. A randomized study. N Engl J Med 1987;317:1625-9.

29. Okawa K, Aoki T, Sano K, Harihara S, Kitano A, Kuroki T. Ulcerative colitis with skip lesions at the mouth of the appendix: A clinical study. Am J Gastroenterol 1998;93:2405-10.

30. Dignass A, Eliakim R, Magro F, et al. Second European evidence-based consensus on the diagnosis and management of ulcerative colitis Part 1: Definitions and diagnosis. J Crohns Colitis 2012;6:965-90.

31. Mutinga ML, Odze RD, Wang HH, Hornick JL, Farraye FA. The clinical significance of right-sided colonic inflammation in patients with left-sided chronic ulcerative colitis. Inflamm Bowel Dis 2004;10:215-9.

32. Silverberg MS, Satsangi J, Ahmad T, et al. Toward an integrated clinical, molecular and serological classification of inflammatory bowel disease: Report of a Working Party of the 2005 Montreal World Congress of Gastroenterology. Can J Gastroenterol 2005;19 Suppl A:5-36.

33. Kornbluth A, Sachar DB. Ulcerative colitis practice guidelines in adults (update): American College of Gastroenterology, Practice Parameters Committee. Am J Gastroenterol 2004;99:1371-85.

14

Patient-reported outcome measures in inflammatory bowel disease

Wael El-Matary MBBCh MD MSc FRCPCH FRCPC

W El-Matary. Patient-reported outcome measures in inflammatory bowel disease. Can J Gastroenterol Hepatol 2014;28(10):536-542.

Patient-reported outcome measures (PROMs) are increasingly used in both research and clinical health settings. With the recent development of United States Food and Drug Administration guidance on PROMs, more attention is being devoted to their role and importance in health care. Several methodological challenges in the development, validation and implementation of PROMs must be resolved to ensure their appropriate utilization and interpretation. The present review discusses recent developments and updates in PROMs, with specific focus on the area of inflammatory bowel disease.

Key Words: HRQoL; IBD; PROMs

Les mesures de résultats déclarés par le patient en cas de maladie inflammatoire de l'intestin

Les mesures de résultats déclarés par le patient (MRDP) sont de plus en plus utilisées dans les milieux de recherche et les milieux cliniques. Depuis les directives récentes de la *Food and Drug Administration* des États-Unis sur le sujet, on s'intéresse davantage au rôle et à l'importance de ces mesures dans les soins. Il faut résoudre plusieurs problèmes méthodologiques liés à l'élaboration, à la validation et à la mise en œuvre des MRDP pour en assurer l'utilisation et l'interprétation adéquates. La présente analyse traite des récents ajouts et mises à jour aux MRDP, particulièrement les maladies inflammatoires de l'intestin.

Patient-reported outcome (PRO) measures (PROMs) are measures of the outcome of treatment and disease management that are reported directly by the patient or the caregiver. They highlight patients' experience with a disease and its treatment, including thoughts, impressions, perceptions and attitudes (1).

These outcomes may include symptoms, health/functional status, health-related quality of life (HRQoL), satisfaction with treatment and outcomes, and perceptions of the humanity of care through short, self-completed questionnaires most commonly used to measure patients' symptoms, functional status or HRQoL before and after an intervention (1-4). PRO instruments can be used in risk management programs because they are tools that measure the benefits and risks of exposure to pharmaceutical products from the patient's perspective. Clinical measures of improvement in some disease states may not necessarily correlate with improvements in a patient's ability to perform daily activities (5).

This category of health outcome measurement was developed following a significant global shift in the philosophy and understanding of health care and how it is measured. It is important to distinguish PROMs from patient-reported experience measures, which focus on aspects of the humanity of care such as being treated with dignity or being kept waiting (6).

Several thousand generic and disease-specific PROMs have emerged. Generic PROMs usually focus on general aspects (eg, mobility, ability to self-care). A single PROM can be comprised of numerous scales and domains (3,4).

Initially, PROMs were meant to be an additional outcome for clinical trials. However, over the years, PROMs have become a target to collect in several health care systems to help with better administration and planning of health services (7).

The first nationwide application of PROMs in clinical care was in the United Kingdom (UK) in 2008 in a voluntary audit of mastectomy and breast reconstruction, followed in April 2009 by a mandatory audit of all providers of hip and knee replacement, groin hernia repair and varicose vein surgery (8). Since April 2009, the National Health Service in the UK became the first health system in the world to advocate routinely collecting PROMs (4).

In 2006, the United States Food and Drug Administration (FDA) published new guidelines recommending PROMs to be used as end points in clinical trials. It was recommended that "the use of PRO instruments is part of a general movement toward the idea that the patient, properly queried, is the best source of information about how he or she feels" (9). These guidelines recommended a systematic cascade or cycle for creating a PRO instrument, which usually entails several important steps including item generation, selection of a method of administration, recall period and response scales (9). Any PRO instrument must be evaluated for validity, reliability and its ability to detect a meaningful change. The guidance also described how sponsors of new drugs or devices can use study results measured by PRO instruments to support claims on labels or the advertising of approved products (9).

A Patient-Centered Outcomes Research Institute (PCORI) has been created in the United States to support research that can produce answers generated through using rigorous, valid, patient-centred methods (10). The PCORI has adopted the following mission statement to guide their work: "help people make informed health care decisions, and improves health care delivery and outcomes, by producing and promoting high-integrity, evidence-based information that comes from research guided by patients, caregivers, and the broader healthcare community" (11).

PATIENTS' VIEWS OR CLINICIANS' VIEWS

Although many physicians are questioning the objectivity of PROMs in clinical practice and how patients may be affected by many other confounders when they complete PROM questionnaires, many other health care workers believe in incorporating patients' feedback and recognize the benefits of PROMs (12,13).

The skepticism of those who are opposed is based on the belief that only physicians can objectively recognize improvement of symptoms and subsequent improvement in quality of life (QoL).

In contrast, those who advocate for routine use of PROMs in health care are appreciative of how patients welcome being involved, and this may have significant health benefits in itself. Patient response rates are invariably better than those of clinicians, which may be

Section of Pediatric Gastroenterology, Department of Pediatrics, and Manitoba Institute of Child Health, Faculty of Medicine, University of Manitoba, Winnipeg, Manitoba. Dr El-Matary is also affiliated with the University of Alexandria, Egypt
Correspondence: Dr Wael El-Matary, Section of Pediatric Gastroenterology, Faculty of Medicine, University of Manitoba, AE 408, Health Sciences Centre, 840 Sherbrook Street, Winnipeg, Manitoba R3A 1S1. e-mail welmatary@hsc.mb.ca.

explained by the fact that a patient has to complete only one questionnaire, whereas a clinician must complete a questionnaire for every patient. Moreover, to a large extent, PROMs avoid observer bias, which is inevitable if physicians are assessing their own practice (3).

Considering patients' views increases public accountability of health services and health care professionals; assists physicians to provide better and more patient-centred care; assesses and compares the quality of providers; and provides data for evaluating different practices (3). Whether these data are confounded by many other factors remain a matter of debate. These confounders include how and where the interview/survey is being conducted, how patients feel about health care providers including their own physicians, patients' socioeconomic status, cultural background and patients' health comorbidities (13).

PROMs IN CLINICAL TRIALS

Outcome selection and reporting in clinical trials can be a challenging task. Heterogeneity and lack of validation of outcomes measured across different studies for the same disorder or therapy could compromise synthesis of high-quality evidence (13). Several items of PROMs can be ill-defined depending on how the survey is designed (structured versus semistructured or nonstructured) (13-15); consequently, reporting the outcome can be difficult. A proposed solution to this problem is the development of core outcome sets (COSs). COSs are an agreed minimum set of outcome domains to be measured and reported in all trials of a particular treatment or condition (ie, standardization of a minimum set of outcomes that can be measured across all the studies for the same disease or treatment) (14). This should significantly reduce outcome reporting bias (15,16). Currently, however, there is no consensus in several disciplines on what these COSs should be.

PROMs IN INFLAMMATORY BOWEL DISEASE

Several questionnaire and survey tools, including HRQoL tools, examining views and feedback of patients with inflammatory bowel disease (IBD) have been developed over the years. Several examples include Inflammatory Bowel Disease Stress Index (IBDSI), Inflammatory Bowel Disease Questionnaire (IBDQ-32), Rating Form of IBD Patient Concerns (RFIPC), Cleveland Global Quality of Life (Faszio Score), Inflammatory Bowel Disease Quality of Life Questionnaire (IBDQOL), Inflammatory Bowel Disease Questionnaire – short form (IBDQ-9), Short Inflammatory Bowel Disease Questionnaire and Work Productivity and Activity Impairment: Crohn's Disease (WPAI: CD) (17-25) (Table 1).

Many of these tools have been used primarily in the research setting and are frequently used as end points for clinical trials in IBD. Several examples include reporting significant improvement of HRQoL in patients with IBD treated with several biologics (26-35). Both generic and disease-specific tools were used in these studies including the EQ-5D (26,30-33).

Nonetheless, until recently, the term 'PROMs' has not been formally used to describe these tools. On the other hand, very few studies have developed their own PROMs based on previous similar tools, patients' feedback and expert opinion.

A recent study by Kappelman et al (36), used the Patient-Reported Outcomes Measurement Information System (PROMIS) initiative of the National Institutes of Health, which was developed to address, investigate and promote implementation of PROMs among patients with chronic disease (37,38). In this study, the investigators performed cross-sectional and longitudinal analyses using an Internet cohort of adults with IBD to evaluate the performance PROMIS measures in relation to validated activity indexes and disease-specific HRQoL (36). They built their own PROMs questionnaire based on previous literature, investigators' experience and patients' feedback. The main domains included were anxiety, depression, fatigue, sleep disturbance, satisfaction with social role and pain interference. They used the Short IBD Questionnaire (24) to measure HRQoL. Disease activity was assessed using the Short Crohn's Disease Activity Index (SCDAI) for Crohn's

TABLE 1
Characteristics of inflammatory bowel disease (IBD)-specific patient-reported outcome measures (PROMs) used in adult patients with IBD

PROMs	Outcome measured	Items, n
Inflammatory Bowel Disease Stress Index (IBDSI) (17)	Overall life satisfaction, worries about health, relationships, sexuality, body image, recreation and psychosomatic symptomatology	8
Inflammatory Bowel Disease Questionnaire (IBDQ)-32 (18)	Quality of life	32
Rating Form of IBD Patient Concerns (RFIPC) (19)	Concerns associated with IBD and treatments	25
Cleveland Global Quality of Life (Faszio Score) (CGQL) (20)	Quality of life after pouch surgery	3
Inflammatory Bowel Disease Quality of Life Questionnaire (IBDQOL) (21)	Quality of life	36
Inflammatory Bowel Disease Questionnaire- short form (IBDQ)-9 (22,23)	Quality of life	9
Short Inflammatory Bowel Disease Questionnaire (SIBDQ) (24)	Quality of life	10
Work Productivity and Activity Impairment: Crohn's Disease (PAI:CD) (25)	Work and activity impairment	6

disease (CD) (39) and the Simple Clinical Colitis Activity Index (SCCAI) for ulcerative colitis and indeterminate colitis (40). More than 10,000 patients with IBD were able to complete PRO testing. In the cross-sectional part of the study, and compared with the general population, IBD patients in this cohort reported more depression, anxiety, fatigue, sleep disturbance and pain interference; they also had less social satisfaction. In each PROMIS domain, there was worse functioning with increased disease activity and worsening Short IBD Questionnaire scores. Longitudinal analyses showed improved PROMIS scores with improved disease activity and worsening PROMIS scores with worsening disease. Based, on these results, the authors concluded that the use of PROMs should advance patient-centred outcomes research in IBD (36).

In a study from Norway (41) that used the term 'PROMs', Jelsness-Jørgensen et al (42) used the Short Form 36 (SF-36), Inflammatory Bowel Disease Questionnaire (N-IBDQ) (43) and the Rating Form of IBD Patient Concerns (RFIPC) (16) instruments as PROMs at baseline and after one year to examine the impact of conventional versus nurse-led follow-up on PROMs of 140 patients with IBD (41). Conventional follow-up was described as regular visits to a clinic that was operated by experienced consultant gastroenterologists. Nurse-led follow-up was performed in the form of three monthly visits to a clinic that was led by an IBD nurse. Periods of hospitalization, surgery and number of relapses were also recorded at baseline and during follow-up. There was no significant difference in any of the study outcomes, except for a shorter interval from the start of a relapse to starting treatment in the nurse-led follow-up group (41).

In a small group of patients with CD, Dur et al (44) examined determinants of health (DH) that are most important to patients and explored which DH(s) were covered by commonly used PROMs for CD (44). They found that social support, self-efficacy, job satisfaction and occupational balance were the most meaningful DHs for patients with CD. While social support and self-efficacy were covered by several PROMs, such as the Inflammatory Bowel Disease – Self Efficacy Scale (IBD-SES), job satisfaction, occupational balance, secondary gain from illness, sense of coherence, vocational gratification and work-life balance are not covered by any of the 18 identified PROMs (44).

PROMs AND INTERNATIONAL CLASSIFICATION OF FUNCTIONING, DISABILITY AND HEALTH IN IBD

The WHO's International Classification of Functioning, Disability and Health (ICF) has been used worldwide for many different goals (45-47). The ICF is a generic classification for functionality and has been used for evaluating functional outcomes in other chronic disorders (eg, stroke) (48). It provides a unified, holistic and standardized language to describe health, disease and disease consequences. It also connects, through several domains, disease-related disability with other factors that may influence heath conditions including social, personal and environmental factors (49,50).

Several investigators have suggested linking measurements of health status in patients with IBD and the ICF (45,51,52). In a recent systematic review by Achleitner et al (45), who were trying to create a link between several IBD-related PROMs and ICF, they defined PROMs as outcome measures in which patients respond to a number of standardized questions asked in a paper-pencil format. The items of the identified PROMs were linked to the ICF. The authors identified 46 studies reporting the use of IBD-specific PROMs. Of note was that these studies did not use the term 'PROMs' for these specific tools; however, these questionnaires were mainly addressing QoL for patients with IBD (16-24). Nearly 70% of the 129 items identified could be linked to specific categories of the ICF (45). However, none of those already existing IBD PROMs contained all items that could be linked to ICF (45). Consequently, there is room to create and validate new PROMs that involve all necessary ICF-based items. This tool can be used for clinical and research purposes.

Peyrin-Biroulet et al (53) performed a literature search investigating disability evaluation in IBD in relation to ICF. Although the several available tools for QoL measurement in IBD capture some aspects of functioning, it was obvious that disability was poorly investigated in the IBD literature. Moreover, compared with other chronic diseases, such as rheumatoid arthritis (RA), the consequences of disability in the management of IBD was underestimated. The authors recommended identifying ICF COSs for IBD that were already implemented in other chronic diseases such as depression and obesity. In addition, and similar to Achleitner et al (45), they also recommended the development of a validated tool including all aspects of limitations of functions in patients with IBD that can be used for both clinical practice and research purposes (46). This tool should be considered to be under the umbrella of PROMs, and should be designed to consider the different personal and environmental factors for individual patients with IBD.

Hence, the international IBD disability index (IBD-DI) was developed as a result of the collaborative work of several investigators (The IPNIC group) (52). The index was developed through several steps including four preparatory studies and is currently being validated (53-55). ICF IBD-DI consists of 19 categories assessed through 28 questions covering the five domains of overall health, body function (seven categories), body structures (two categories), activity participation (five categories) and environmental factors (five categories) (52). The IBD-DI was specifically designed to exclude the use of any questions that examine patients' subjective coping and feelings (53,55). It addresses the extent of disability and limitations in several areas such as sleep, work, social events and exacerbating effects of medication, food, family and health care professionals. Similar to other ICF scores, positive scores were proportional to absence of limitations and good functioning, while negative scores were indicative of greater disability. Scores from each question were combined into domain totals and a final composite score representative of the overall degree of disability ranging from −80 (maximum degree of disability) to 22 (no disability) with '0' as the anticipated point of neutrality. Scores of severe, moderate, mild and minimal disability correlated with the ability to work <50%, 50% to 75%, 76% to 99% and 100% of work hours in the previous week (53,55).

In a validation study, Leong et al (55) measured IBD-DI, IBD-Q and WPA:I in an adult cohort with IBD. They also examined disease-related clinical outcomes, including CDAI, in those with CD (75 patients) and partial Mayo score in patients with ulcerative colitis (41 patients); they also recruited 50 healthy controls. IBD-DI significantly correlated with CDAI, partial Mayo score and IBD-Q. IBD-DI was the only outcome predictive of unemployment status.

PROMs IN OTHER DISCIPLINES

Cancer care

Several PROMs have been used in both clinical care and research involving cancer patients (56-64). In the most widely cited model of PRO measurement, Wilson and Cleary (59) highlighted an interesting, unique perception of PROs in the form of different 'levels' of PROs along a scale with regard to their 'proximal' (symptoms) versus 'distal' (overall QoL) relationship to the disease or treatment involved (59). The model indicated that more distal PROs were subject to greater mediation by personal and environmental factors than were more proximal PROs. The most distal outcome, overall QoL, was affected not only by health status but also by nonmedical factors (eg, bereavement, financial stress, environmental factors). Intermediate levels of PROMs are available as health-related or disease-specific QoL measures, which limit assessment to the impacts of health in general or a particular condition (58,59).

Soreide and Soreide (60) emphasized the increasing importance of PROMs in addition to the classical outcomes for clinical patient-centred decision making in patients with cancer.

Three main approaches to measuring PROMs in patients with cancer have been suggested. One is the generic approach to health status measurement that allows comparison across different health conditions (61). The second approach is the cancer-generic approach, which is more specific to patients with any cancer, regardless of type (62-64). The third is more focused to the specific cancer subtype (65,66).

PROMIS is also developing measures of self-reported health domains specifically targeted to cancer, such as sleep/wake function, sexual function, cognitive function and the psychosocial impacts of the illness experience (ie, stress response and coping, shifts in self-concept, social interactions and spirituality) (67). Future directions include reviewing the current PROMs in oncology to ensure continuing validity (58).

RA

Standardization of disease assessment in RA have been formulated through the Outcome Measures in Rheumatology Clinical Trials (OMERACT) meetings, leading to a 'core set' of eight outcomes as an international standard in RA clinical trials (68,69). Interestingly, these outcomes did not include fatigue, which is an integral part of RA experienced by almost all patients (70,71). Nicklin et al (72) developed draft PROMs not only to measure fatigue in patients with RA but also to develop the wording for it in a way that patients can understand and express. Fatigue descriptors included 'exhausted', 'tired', 'drained', 'lethargic', etc. Nonetheless, this set of PROMs has not yet been fully evaluated for validity or reliability (72). This study highlighted the importance of collaboration with patients to develop PROMs.

In their systematic review to appraise PROMs that focussed on RA of the foot, Walmsley et al (73) identified 11 PROMs that were utilized in this context; however, only one was disease specific. Examples of nondisease-specific PROMs would include the Foot Function Index (74), The Manchester Foot Pain and Disability Questionnaire (75), The Podiatry Health Questionnaire (76), The Bristol Foot Score (77), The Foot Health Status Questionnaire (78) and The Rowan Foot Pain Assessment Questionnaire (79). The disease-specific PROM was The Juvenile Arthritis Foot Disability Index (80). The review concluded that there was a need to develop an RA-disease and foot-specific PROM with a greater emphasis on cognitive pretesting methods and patient preference-based qualities (73).

Asthma

A recent inquiry from the UK identified several concerns regarding outcome measures in patients with allergy (81). Worth et al (82) are currently conducting a systematic review to identify validated generic and disease-specific PROMs for asthma and related allergic conditions in adults and children. Blanco-Aparicio et al (83) preformed a prospective cohort study that included 108 adult patients with asthma. Patients were asked to complete a survey to determine the ability of brief specific HRQoL questionnaires to predict emergency department visits and hospitalizations in patients with asthma. They used the AQ20, which is a specific questionnaire validated for patients with asthma (84). They also used chronic obstructive pulmonary disease-specific questionnaires in another group of patients with chronic obstructive pulmonary disease (85,86). The AQ20 predicted exacerbations in asthma during the first year of follow-up but not during the second year (83).

The Living with Asthma Questionnaire is a validated asthma-specific QoL instrument for assessing patients' own subjective experiences of asthma. The scale has 68 items and covers 11 domains of asthma experience. They were developed from extensive interactions with patients with asthma (87).

Diabetes

A diabetes QoL (DQoL) instrument has been developed and validated in patients (both adolescents and adults) with type 1 diabetes (88). The DQoL is a multiple-choice assessment tool with four primary scales that includes 46 core items. These scales are satisfaction, impact, diabetes worry, social/vocational worry. This tool does not identify specific types of treatment or self-monitoring. Consequently, it can be used for patients using different methods of diabetes management (88). However, it has been recently identified that currently there are no PROMs that are strongly associated with variations in therapeutic strategies of diabetes (89). Moreover, PROMs are poorly utilized in diabetes care (89).

Surgery

Several generic and disease-specific PROMs have been used in patients who have undergone surgeries. Generic PROMs include EQ-5D and EQ-VAS (90-93). Examples of surgery-specific PROMs include Aberdeen Varicose Vein Questionnaire (AVVQ), Oxford Hip Score (OHS) and Oxford Knee Score (OKS) (93-96).

PEDIATRIC CARE

Children are not small adults. Interviewing children and adolescents requires knowledge of their specific cognitive, linguistic, social, cultural and developmental characteristics to better understand their perspective (97,98). Developing the knowledge in advance of key words the children use, for example, by asking parents, will allow the interviewer to quickly connect with the child. Parental interviews should provide information about the child's history as well as clarify each parent's view of the child. Questions asked to children should be simple and precise (98). Careful attention should be devoted to the use of age-appropriate language throughout the interview (99). These issues must be taken into consideration when health care providers plan and develop pediatric-specific PROMs and assess HRQoL. Several validated tools have been developed for several pediatric diseases.

In the area of pediatric IBD, generic and disease-specific instruments have been developed, validated and utilized in many settings. Generic tools include the Pediatric Quality of Life Inventory (PedsQL), which examined HRQoL in children with IBD and compared them with healthy peers and with children with other chronic diseases (100-103). Disease-specific tools include the IMPACT questionnaire, which measures six domains including bowel-related symptoms, systematic symptoms, functionality including social interaction, body image, emotional aspects and treatment-related concerns (104,105).

Other disease-specific instruments include the TNO-AZL Children's Quality of Life questionnaire (TACQOL), which includes seven domains (106), and IMPACT II (NL), which includes six domains (107).

A recent systematic review recently examined the available literature that investigated psychosocial functioning and HRQoL in children and young adults with IBD and identified 12 studies that included >5000 children and young adults (790 with IBD, <18 years of age) and fulfilled its inclusion criteria (108). Several studies examined HRQoL (106,107,109,110) but only one study was a prospective longitudinal study using IMPACT III instrument (110). Overall, and despite concerns about design and methodological flaws in several of those studies, HRQoL appeared to be lower in children and young adults with IBD (108).

In an attempt to develop a self-efficacy scale for children with IBD (111), a recent pediatric study followed the FDA cycle for developing PROMs (9). The investigators initially conducted a survey in the form of semistructured questionnaire to obtain the input of patients attending a pediatric gastroenterology clinic. Self-efficacy themes related to disease management were reviewed and followed by arranging a consensus panel of gastroenterologists and psychologists to review the initially constructed items. These specific items were then reviewed and adjusted by a panel of participants for content and understandability using cognitive interview methods. This eventually resulted in four domains that include a three-item self-efficacy scale (112). Validation studies are needed before this scale can be widely used (112).

PROMs have been developing with promising results in other areas of pediatrics and child care including children with mental health problems, eye problems and obesity (113-115).

FINAL REMARKS

In a recent Canadian survey (116), 52% of Canadians believed that the current health system needs fundamental changes and 10% believed that the system needs to be completely rebuilt. These challenges are not unique to Canada but occur across the world (117).

Many Canadian health care leaders were interviewed seeking their views on the challenges that the system is currently facing, especially with regard to quality improvement (118). The results of these interviews highlighted the need for engaging physicians and patients in quality agenda. One of the themes identified in this survey was the need to commit to measurement and reporting on performance and quality outcomes. Quality measurements and indicators are crucial for health care improvement. PROMs can add unique aspects of quality and performance measurement. Moreover, they can inform health care providers on issues related inequities in health status. National surveys, such as the Canadian Community Health Survey, can be utilized to provide meaningful PROMs.

Under the Excellent Care for All Act, The Ontario government has legalized the performance of yearly surveys for patients' satisfaction. The results of these surveys should be used to guide health care providers in improving the quality of care. However, there is a need for development, validation and implementation of quality indicators that can be linked to improved outcomes (119).

On the other hand, several health care providers are debating whether patient-satisfaction scores are linked to improvement in overall outcomes (120). A recent study showed that increased patient satisfaction was associated with health care-related costs and higher overall mortality (121). The authors speculated that the cause of their conclusion may be related to the fact that there is currently an increasing utilization of discretionary care (medical management for which there is no proven benefit) with higher chances of overtreatment and iatrogenic harm, an explanation that has been addressed previously (121,122).

Several questions related to PROMs and their use, including those for IBD, still require answers as to the best way to define patient satisfaction, how to develop them and whether FDA guidelines must be followed in development, how to objectively measure it and whether the improvement is truly beneficial (120). Although developing the IBD-DI is an important step, it remains unclear whether it will help in answering these questions, and how practical its routine use in clinical and research setting will be.

ACKNOWLEDGEMENT: Dr El-Matary is funded by a grant from the Manitoba Institute of Child Health and Winnipeg Children's Hospital Foundation.

REFERENCES

1. Smith S, Cano S, Lamping D, et al. Patient-reported outcome measures (PROMs) for routine use in treatment centres: Recommendations based on a review of the scientific evidence. London: Health Services Research Unit, London School of Hygiene and Tropical Medicine, 2005.

2. Bradley C. Feedback on the FDA's February 2006 draft guidance on patient reported outcome (PRO) measures from a developer of PRO measures. Health Qual Life Outcomes 2006;4:78.

3. Black N, Jenkinson C. Measuring patients' experiences and outcomes. BMJ 2009;339:b2495.

4. Medical Research Council (MRC). Patient Reported Outcome Measures (PROMs): Identifying UK research priorities. London: MRC, 2009

5. Breitscheidel L, Stamenitis S. Using patient-reported outcome assessments in clinical practice and their importance in risk management. J Med Econ 2009;12:180-1.

6. Black N. Patient reported outcome measures could help transform healthcare. BMJ 2013;346:f167.

7. Greenhalgh J. The application of PROs in clinical practice: What are they, do they work and why? Qual Life Res 2009;18:115-23.

8. Jeevan R, Cromwell D, Browne J, et al. Fourth Annual National Mastectomy and Breast Reconstruction Audit 2011. London: The NHS Information Centre, 2011.

9. Food and Drug Administration. Guidance for industry: Patient reported outcome measures: Use in medical product development to support labelling claims. Draft Guidance. Health Qual Life Outcomes 2006;4:79.

10. Washington AE, Lipstein SH. The patient-centered outcomes research institute promoting better information, decisions, and health. N Engl J Med 2011;365:e31.

11. Gabriel SE, Normand SL. Getting the methods right – the foundation of patient-centered outcomes research. N Engl J Med 2012;367:787-90.

12. Ousey K, Cook L. Understanding patient reported outcome measures (PROMs). Br J Community Nurs 2011;16:80-2.

13. Bredart A, Marrel A, Abetz-Wbb L, et al. Interviewing to develop patient-reported outcome (PRO) measures for clinical research: Eliciting patients' experience. Health Qual Life Outcomes 2014;12:15.

14. Williamson PR, Altman DG, Blazeby JM, et al. Developing core outcome sets for clinical trials: Issues to consider. Trials 2012;13:132.

15. Macefield RC, Jacobs M, Korfage IJ, et al. Developing core outcomes sets: Methods for identifying and including patient-reported outcomes (PROs). Trials 2014;15:49.

16. Bren L. The importance of patient-reported outcomes. Its all about the patients. FDA Consumer Magazine, November/December. Food and Drug Adminstration. <http://permanent.access.gpo.gov/lps1609/www.fda.gov/fdac/features/2006/606_patients.html> (Accessed April 5, 2014).

17. Joachin G, Milne B. Inflammatory bowel disease: Effects on lifestyle. J Adv Nurs 1987;12:483-7.

18. Guyatt G, Mitchell A, Irvine EJ, et al. A new measure of health status for clinical trials in inflammatory bowel disease. Gastroenterology 1989;96:804-10.

19. Drossman DA, Leserman J, Li ZM, Mitchell CM, Zagami EA, Patrick DL. The rating form of IBD patient concerns: A new measure of health status. Psychosom Med 1991;53:701-12.

20. Fazio VW, O'Riordain MG, Lavery IC, et al. Long-term functional outcome and quality of life after stapled restorative proctocolectomy. Ann Surg 1999;230:575-84.

21. Love JR, Irvine EJ, Fedorak RN. Quality of life in inflammatory bowel disease. J Clin Gastroenterol 1992;14:15-9.

22. Alcalá MJ, Casellas F, Prieto L, Malagelada JR. Development of a short questionnaire for quality of life specific for inflammatory bowel disease. Gastroenterology 2001;120(Suppl 1):A450.

23. Alcalá MJ, Casellas F, Fontanet G, Prieto L, Malagelada JR. Shortened questionnaire on quality of life for inflammatory bowel disease. Inflamm Bowel Dis 2004;10:383-91.

24. Irvine EJ, Zhou Q, Thompson AK. CCRPT Investigators. The Short Inflammatory Bowel Disease Questionnaire: A quality of life instrument for community physicians managing inflammatory bowel disease. Canadian Crohn's Relapse Prevention Trial. Am J Gastroenterol 1996;91:1571-8.

25. Reilly MC, Zbrozek AS, Dukes EM. The validity and reproducibility of a work productivity and activity impairment instrument. Pharmacoeconomics 1993;4:353-65.

26. Probert CS, Hearing SD, Schreiber S, et al. Infliximab in moderately severe glucocorticoid resistant ulcerative colitis: A randomised controlled trial. Gut 2003;52:998-1002.

27. Lichtenstein GR, Bala M, Han C, et al. Infliximab improves quality of life in patients with Crohn's disease. Inflamm Bowel Dis 2002;8:237-43.

28. Feagan BG, Yan S, Bala M, Bao W, Lichtenstein GR. The effects of infliximab maintenance therapy on health-related quality of life. Am J Gastroenterol 2003;98:2232-8.

29. Sands BE, Blank MA, Patel K, et al. Long-term treatment of rectovaginal fistulas in Crohn's disease: Response to infliximab in the ACCENT II Study. Clin Gastroenterol Hepatol 2004;2:912-20.

30. Loftus EV, Feagan BG, Colombel JF, et al. Effects of adalimumab maintenance therapy on health-related quality of life of patients with Crohn's disease: Patient-reported outcomes of the CHARM trial. Am J Gastroenterol 2008;103:3132-41.

31. Colombel JF, Sandborn WJ, Rutgeerts P, et al. Comparison of two adalimumab treatment schedule strategies for moderate-to-severe Crohn's disease: Results from the CHARM trial. Am J Gastroenterol 2009;104:1170-9.

32. Lichtiger S, Binion DG, Wolf DC, et al. The CHOICE trial: Adalimumab demonstrates safety, fistula healing, improved quality of life and increased work productivity in patients with Crohn's disease who failed prior infliximab therapy. Aliment Pharmacol Ther 2010;32:1228-39.

33. Panaccione R, Loftus EV Jr, Binion D, et al. Efficacy and safety of adalimumab in Canadian patients with moderate to severe Crohn's disease: Results of the Adalimumab in Canadian Subjects with Moderate to Severe Crohn's Disease (ACCESS) trial. Can J Gastroenterol 2011;25:419-25.

34. Watanabe M, Hibi T, Lomax KG, et al. Adalimumab for the induction and maintenance of clinical remission in Japanese patients with Crohn's disease. J Crohns Colitis 2012;6:160-73.

35. Feagan BG, Coteur G, Tan S, et al. Clinically meaningful improvement in health-related quality of life in a randomized controlled trial of certolizumab pegol maintenance therapy for Crohn's disease. Am J Gastroenterol 2009;104:1976-83.

36. Kappelman M, Long MD, Martin C, et al. Evaluation of patient-reported outcome measurement information system in a large cohort of patients with inflammatory bowel diseases. Clin Gastroenterol Hepatol 2014;12:1315-23.

37. Adler D. Developing the Patient-Reported Outcomes Measurement Information System (PROMIS). Med Care 2007;45(Suppl 1):S1–S2.

38. Cella D, Yount S, Rothrock N, et al. The Patient-Reported Outcomes Measurement Information System (PROMIS): Progress of an NIH roadmap cooperative group during its first two years. Med Care 2007;45:S3-S11.

39. Thia K, Faubion WA Jr, Loftus EV Jr, et al. Short CDAI: Development and validation of a shortened and simplified Crohn's disease activity index. Inflamm Bowel Dis 2011;17:105-11.

40. Jowett SL, Seal CJ, Phillips E, et al. Defining relapse of ulcerative colitis using a symptom-based activity index. Scand J Gastroenterol 2003;38:164-71.

41. Jelsness-Jørgensen L, Bernklev T, Henrikson M, et al. Is patient reported outcome (PRO) affected by different follow-up regimens in inflammatory bowel disease (IBD)? A one year prospective, longitudinal comparison of nurse-led versus conventional follow-up. J Crohn's Colitis 2012;6:887-94

42. Ware JE, Sherbourne CD. The MOS 36-ltem short-form health survey (SF-36): I. Conceptual framework and item selection. Med Care 1992;30:473-83.

43. Irvine EJ, Feagan B, Rochon J, et al. Quality of life: A valid and reliable measure of therapeutic efficacy in the treatment of inflammatory bowel disease. Canadian Crohn's Relapse Prevention Study Group. Gastroenterology 1994;106:287-96.

44. Dur M, Sadlonova M, Haider S, et al. Health determining concepts important to people with Crohn's disease and their coverage by patient-reported outcomes of health and wellbeing. J Crohns Colitis 2014;8:45-55.

45. Achleitner U, Coenen M, Colombel JF, et al. Identification of areas of functioning and disability addressed in inflammatory bowel disease-specific patient reported outcome measures. J Crohns Colitis 2012;6:507-17.

46. World Health Organization (WHO). International Classification of Functioning, Disability and Health (ICF). Geneva: World Health Organization, 2001.

47. Cieza A, Stucki G. Content comparison of health-related quality of life (HRQOL) instruments based on the international classification of functioning, disability and health (ICF). Qual Life Res 2005;14:1225-37.

48. Geyh S, Cieza A, Kollerits B, Grimby G, Stucki G. Content comparison of health-related quality of life measures used in stroke based on the International Classification of Functioning, Disability and Health (ICF): A systematic review. Qual Life Res 2007;16:833-51.

49. Nordenfelt L. Action theory, disability and ICF. Disabil Rehabil 2003;25:1075-9.

50. Martins AI, Quieros A, Crequeira M, Rocha N, Teixeira M. The International Classification of Functioning, Disability and Health as a conceptual model for the evaluation of environmental factors. Procedia Computer Science 2012;14:293-300.

51. Peyrin-Biroulet L, Cieza A, Sandborn WJ, et al. Disability in inflammatory bowel diseases: Developing ICF core sets for patients with inflammatory bowel diseases based on the International Classification of Functioning, Disability, and Health. Inflamm Bowel Dis 2010;16:15-22.

52. Reichel C, Streit J, Wunsch S. Linking Crohn's disease health status measurements with International Classification of Functioning, Disability and Health and vocational rehabilitation outcomes. J Rehabil Med 2010;42:74-80.

53. Peyrin-Biroulet L, Cieza A, Sandborn WJ, et al. Development of the first disability index for inflammatory bowel disease based on the international classification of functioning, disability and health. Gut 2012;61:241-7.

54. Williet N, Sandborn WJ, Peyrin-Biroulet L. Patient-reported outcomes as primary end points in clinical trials of inflammatory bowel disease. Clin Gastroenterol Hepatol 2014;12:1246-56.

55. Leong RW, Huang T, Ko Y, et al. Prospective validation study of the International Classification of Functioning, Disability and Health score in Crohn's disease and ulcerative colitis. J Crohns Colitis March 21, 2014 (Epub ahead of print).

56. Pearce NJ, Sanson-Fisher R, Campbell HS. Measuring quality of life in cancer survivors: A methodological review of existing scales. Psychooncology 2008;17:629-40.

57. Edwards B, Ung L. Quality of life instruments for caregivers of patients with cancer: A review of their psychometric properties. Cancer Nurs 2002;25:342-9.

58. Luckett T, King MT. Choosing patient-reported outcome measures for cancer clinical research – practical principles and an algorithm to assist non-specialist researchers. Eur J Cancer 2010;46:3149-57.

59. Wilson IB, Cleary PD. Linking clinical variables with health-related quality of life. A conceptual model of patient outcomes. JAMA 1995;273:59-65.

60. Soreide K, Soreide KH. Using patient-reported outcome measures for improved decision-making in patients with gastrointestinal cancer – the last clinical frontier in surgical oncology? Front Oncol 2013;3:157.

61. Cella D, Rosenbloom SK, Beaumont JL, et al. Development and validation of 11 symptom indexes to evaluate response to chemotherapy for advanced cancer. J Natl Compr Canc Netw 2011;9:268-78.

62. Blazeby JM, Fayers P, Conroy T, Sezer O, Ramage J, Rees M. Validation of the European Organization for Research and Treatment of Cancer QLQ- LMC21 questionnaire for assessment of patient-reported outcomes during treatment of colorectal liver metastases. Br J Surg 2009;96:291-8.

63. Bottomley A, Flechtner H, Efficace F, et al. Health related quality of life outcomes in cancer clinical trials. Eur J Cancer 2005;41:1697-709.

64. Sloan JA, Berk L, Roscoe J, et al. Integrating patient-reported out-comes into cancer symptom management clinical trials supported by the National Cancer Institute-sponsored clinical trials networks. J Clin Oncol 2007;25:5070-7.

65. Byrne C, Griffin A, Blazeby J, Conroy T, Efficace F. Health-related quality of life as a valid outcome in the treatment of advanced colorectal cancer. Eur J Surg Oncol 2007;33(Suppl 2):S95-S104.

66. Pusic AL, Cemal Y, Albornoz C, et al. Quality of life among breast cancer patients with lymphedema: A systematic review of patient-reported outcome instruments and outcomes. J Cancer Surviv 2013;7:83-92.

67. Garcia D, Cella D, Caluser SB, et al. Standardizing patient-reported outcomes assessment in cancer clinical trials: A patient-reported outcomes measurement information system Initiative. J Clin Oncol 25:5106-12.

68. Felson DT, Anderson JJ, Boers M, et al. The American College of Rheumatology preliminary core set of disease activity measures for rheumatoid arthritis clinical trials. Arthritis Rheum 1993;36:729-40.

69. Boers M, Brooks P, Strand CV, Tugwell P. The OMERACT filter for outcome measures in rheumatology. J Rheumatol 1998;25:198-9.

70. Milton HV, Hewlett S, Kirwan JR. Fatigue in rheumatoid arthritis. Rheumatology (Oxford) 2002;(41 Suppl):73. (Abst)

71. Wolfe F, Hawley DJ, Wilson K. The prevalence and meaning of fatigue in rheumatic disease. J Rheumatol 1996;23:1407-17.

72. Nicklin J, Cramp F, Kirwan J, Urban M, Hewlett S. Collaboration with patients in the design of patient-reported outcome measures: Capturing the experience of fatigue in rheumatoid arthritis. Arthritis Care Res 2010;62:1552-8.

73. Walmsley S, Williams AE, Ravey M, Graham A. The rheumatoid foot: A systematic literature review of patient-reported outcome measures. J Foot Ankle Res 2010;3:12.

74. Budiman-Mak E, Conrad KJ, Roach KE. The Foot Function Index: A measure of foot pain and disability. J Clin Epidemiol 1991;44:561-70.

75. Garrow AP, Papageorgiou AC, Silman AJ, Thomas E, Jayson MI, Macfarlane GJ. Development and validation of a questionnaire to assess disabling foot pain. Pain 2000,85:107-13.

76. Macran S, Kind P, Collingwood J, Hull R, McDonald I, Parkinson L. Evaluating podiatry services: Testing a treatment specific measure of health status. Quality Life Res 2003;12:177-88.

77. Barnett S, Campbell R, Harvey I. The Bristol Foot Score: Developing a patient-based foot-health measure. J Am Podiatr Med Assoc 2005,95:264-72.

78. Bennett PJ, Patterson C, Wearing S, Baglioni T. Development and validation of a questionnaire designed to measure foot-health status. J Am Podiatr Med Assoc 1998,88:419-28.

79. Rowan K. The development and validation of a multi-dimensional measure of chronic foot pain: The Rowan Foot Pain Assessment Questionnaire (ROFPAQ). Foot Ankle Int 2001;22:795-809.

80. Andre M, Hagelberg S, Stenstrom CH. The juvenile arthritis foot disability index: Development and evaluation of measurement properties. J Rheumatol 2004;31:2488-93.

81. House of Lords Science and Technology Committee. Allergy, 6th Report of Session 2006-2007. London: The Stationery Office, 2007.

82. Worth A, Hammersley VS, Nurmatov U, Sheikh A. Systematic literature review and evaluation of patient reported outcome measures (PROMs) for asthma and related allergic diseases. Prim Care Respir J 2012;21:455.

83. Blanco-Aparicio M, Vázquez I, Pita-Fernández S, Pértega-Diaz S, Verea-Hernando H. Utility of brief questionnaires of health-related quality of life (Airways Questionnaire 20 and Clinical COPD Questionnaire) to predict exacerbations in patients with asthma and COPD. Health Qual Life Outcomes 2013;11:85.

84. Quirk FH, Jones PW. Repeatability of two new short airways questionnaires. Thorax 1994;49:1075.

85. Van der Molen T, Willemse BW, Schokker S, Ten Hacken NH, Postma DS, Juniper EF. Development, validity and responsiveness of the clinical COPD questionnaire. Health Qual Life Outcomes 2003;1:13.

86. Jones PW, Quirk FH, Baveystock CM, Littlejohns P. A self-complete measure of health status for chronic airflow limitation: The St. George's Respiratory Questionnaire. Am Rev Respir Dis 1992;145:1321-7.

87. Hyland ME. The Living with Asthma Questionnaire. Respir Med 1991;(85 Suppl B):13-16.

88. Reliability and validity of a diabetes quality-of-life measure for the diabetes control and complications trial (DCCT). The DCCT Research Group. Diabetes Care 1988;11:725-32.

89. Brazil F, Pontarolo R, Correr CJ. Patient Reported Outcomes Measures (PROMs) in diabetes: Why are they still rarely used in clinical routine? Diabetes Res Clin Pract 2012;97:e4-e5.

90. Brooks R, EuroQol Group. EuroQol: The current state of play. Health Policy 1996;37:53-72.

91. Cheung K, Oemar M, Oppe M, Rabin R. EQ-5D User Guide: Basic Information on how to use the EQ-5D. Version 2.0. Rotterdam: EuroQoL Group; 2009.

92. The EuroQol group. Euroqol - a new facility for the measurement of health-related quality of life. Health Policy 1990;16:199-208.

93. Garratt AM, Macdonald LM, Ruta DA, Russell IT, Buckingham JK, Krukowski ZH. Towards measurement of outcome for patients with varicose veins. Qual Health Care 1993;2:5-10.

94. Dawson J, Fitzpatrick R, Carr A, Murray D. Questionnaire on the perceptions of patients about total hip replacement. J Bone Joint Surg Br 1996;78:185-90.

95. Dawson J, Fitzpatrick R, Murray D, Carr A. Questionnaire on the perceptions of patients about total knee replacement. J Bone Joint Surg Br 1998;80-B:63-9.

96. Baker PN, Petheram T, Jameson TT, et al Comparison of patient-reported outcome measures following total and unicondylar knee replacement. J Bone Joint Surg Br 2012;94-B:919-27

97. Eiser C, Twamley S. Talking to children about health and illness. In: Murray M, Chamberlain K, eds. Qualitative Health Psychology: Theories and Methods. London: Sage, 1999:133-45.

98. Collins D. Pretesting survey instruments: An overview of cognitive methods. Qual Life Res 2003;12:229-38.

99. Kirk S. Methodological and ethical issues in conducting qualitative research with children and young people: A literature review. Int J Nurs Stud 2007;44:250-60.

100. Varni JW, Seid M, Kurtin PS. Reliability and validity of the pediatric quality of life inventory version 4.0 generic core scales in healthy and patient populations. Med Care 2001;39:800-12.

101. Kunz JH, Hommel KA, Greenley RN. Health-related quality of life of youth with inflammatory bowel disease: A comparison with published data using the PedsQL 4.0 generic core scale. Inflamm Bowel Dis 2010;16:939-46.

102. Drotar D, Schwartz L, Palermo TM, Burant C. Factor structure of the child health questionnaire-parent form in pediatric populations. J Pediatr Psychol 2006;31:127-38.

103. Marcus SB, Strople JA, Neighbors K, et al. Fatigue and health-related quality of life in pediatric inflammatory bowel disease. Clin Gastroenterol Hepatol 2009;7:554-61.

104. Griffiths AM, Nicholas D, Smith C, et al. Development of a quality-of life index for pediatric inflammatory bowel disease: Dealing with differences related to age and IBD type. J Pediatr Gastroenterol Nutr 1999;28:S46-52.

105. Otley A, Smith C, Nicholas D, et al. The IMPACT questionnaire: A valid measure of health-related quality of life in pediatric inflammatory bowel disease. J Pediatr Gastroenterol Nutr 2002;35:557-63.

106. Loonen HJ, Grootenhuis MA, Last BF, Koopman HM, Derkx HH. Quality of life in paediatric inflammatory bowel disease measured by a generic and a disease specific questionnaire. Acta Paediatr 2002;91:348-54.

107. Loonen HJ, Grootenhuis MA, Last BF, de Haan RJ, Bouquet J, Derkx BH. Measuring quality of life in children with inflammatory bowel disease: The impact-II (NL). Qual Life Res 2002;11:47-56.

108. Ross SC, Strachan J, Russell RK, Wilson SL. Psychosocial functioning and health-related quality of life in pediatric inflammatory bowel disease. J Pediatr Gastroenterol Nutr 2011;53:480-8.

109. De Boer M, Grootenhuis M, Derkx B, et al. Health-related quality of life and psychosocial functioning of adolescents with inflammatory bowel disease. Inflamm Bowel Dis 2005;11:400-6.

110. Otley AR, Griffiths AM, Hale S, et al. Health-related quality of life in the first year after a diagnosis of pediatric inflammatory bowel disease. Inflamm Bowel Dis 2006;12:684-91

111. Izaguirre MR, Keefer L. Development of a self-efficacy scale for adolescents and young adults with inflammatory bowel disease. J Pediatr Gastroenterol Nutr2014;59:29-32.

112. Ebach DR. PROs and CONcepts. J Pediatr Gastroenterol Nutr 2014;59:4-5.

113. Wolpert M, Ford T, Trustman E. Patient-reported outcomes in child and adolescent mental health services (CAMHS): Use of idiographic and standardized measures. J Ment Health 2012;21:165-73.

114. Tadic V, Hogan A, Septi N, et al. Patient-reported outcome measures (PROMs) in paediatric ophthalmology: A systematic review. Br J Ophthalmol 2013;97:1369-81.

115. Riazi A, Shakoor S, Dundas I, Eiser C, McKenzie S. Health-related quality of life in a clinical sample of obese children and adolescents. Health Qual Life Outcomes 2010;8:134.

116. Bierman A. The PROMise of quality improvement in healthcare: Will Canada choose the right road. Healthc Pap 2011;11:55-60.

117. Schoen C, Osborn R, Doty MM, Bishop M, Peugh J, Murukutla N. Towards higher performance health systems: Adults. Health care experiences in seven countries. Health Affairs 2007;27:w717-34.

118. Sullivan D, Ashbury FD, Pun J, Pitts B, Stipich N, Neeson J. Responsibilities for Canada's healthcare quality agenda: Interviews with Canadian leaders. Healthc Pap 2011;11:10-21.

119. Detsky J, Shaul RZ. Incentives to increase patient satisfaction: Are we doing harm than good? CMAJ 2013;185:13-4.

120. Manary MP, Boulding W, Staelin R, et al. The patient experience and health outcomes. N Engl J Med 2013;368:201-3.

121. Fenton JJ, Jerant AF, Bertakis KD, et al. The cost of satisfaction. Arch Intern Med 2012;172:405-11.

122. Fisher ES, Welch HG. Avoiding the unintended consequences of growth in medical care. JAMA 1999;281:446-53.

15

Surveillance patterns after curative-intent colorectal cancer surgery in Ontario

Jensen Tan MD MSc FRCSC[1], Jennifer Muir MD[1], Natalie Coburn MD MPH FRCSC FACS[1,2],
Simron Singh MD MPH FRCPC[2], David Hodgson MD MPH FRCPC[3,4], Refik Saskin MSc[3], Alex Kiss PhD[3,5],
Lawrence Paszat MD MSc FRCPC[2,3], Abraham El-Sedfy MD MSc[2,6], Eva Grunfeld MD DPhil FCFP[3,7],
Craig Earle MD MSc FRCPC[2,3], Calvin Law MD MPH FRCSC[1,2,3,5]

J Tan, J Muir, N Coburn, et al. Surveillance patterns after curative-intent colorectal cancer surgery in Ontario. Can J Gastroenterol Hepatol 2014;28(8):427-433.

BACKGROUND: Postoperative surveillance following curative-intent resection of colorectal cancer (CRC) is variably performed due to existing guideline differences and to the limited data supporting different strategies.

OBJECTIVES: To examine population-based rates of surveillance imaging and endoscopy in patients in Ontario following curative-intent resection of CRC with no evidence of recurrence, as well as patient or disease factors that may predispose certain groups to more frequent versus less frequent surveillance; to provide insight to the care patients receive in the presence of conflicting guidelines, in efforts to help improve care of CRC survivors by identifying any potential underuse or overuse of particular surveillance modalities, or inequalities in access to surveillance.

METHOD: A retrospective cohort study was conducted using data from the Ontario Cancer Registry and several linked databases. Ontario patients undergoing curative-intent CRC resection from 2003 to 2007 were identified, excluding patients with probable disease relapse. In the five-year period following surgery, the number of imaging and endoscopic examinations was determined.

RESULTS: There were 4960 patients included in the study. Over the five-year postoperative period, the highest proportion of patients who underwent postoperative surveillance received the following number of tests for each modality examined: one to three abdominopelvic computed tomography (CT) scans (n=2073 [41.8%]); one to three abdominal ultrasounds (n=2443 [49.3%]); no chest CTs, one to three chest x-rays (n=2385 [48.1%]); and two endoscopies (n=1845 [37.2%]). Odds of not receiving any abdominopelvic imaging (CT or abdominal ultrasound) were higher in those who did not receive adjuvant chemotherapy (OR 6.99 [95% CI 5.26 to 9.35]) or those living in certain geographical areas, but were independent of age, sex and income. Nearly all patients (n=4473 [90.2%]) underwent ≥1 endoscopy at some point during the follow-up period.

CONCLUSION: In contrast to findings from similar studies in other jurisdictions, most Ontario CRC survivors receive postoperative surveillance with imaging and endoscopy, and care is equitable across sociodemographic groups, although unexplained geographical variation in practice exists and warrants further investigation.

Key Words: *Colorectal adenocarcinoma; Curative-intent surgery; Postoperative imaging; Surgery; Surveillance*

Les profils de surveillance après des opérations de cancers colorectaux à visée curative en Ontario

HISTORIQUE : La surveillance postopératoire après une résection de cancer colorectal (CCR) à visée curative est variable, en raison de différences dans les lignes directrices et de données limitées en appui à diverses stratégies.

OBJECTIFS : Examiner les taux de surveillance en population de l'imagerie et de l'endoscopie chez des patients de l'Ontario après une résection de CCR à visée curative sans preuve de récurrence, de même que les facteurs liés aux patients ou à la maladie susceptibles de prédisposer certains groupes à une surveillance plus fréquente. Donner un aperçu des soins reçus en présence de directives contradictoires. Ce faisant, chercher à améliorer les soins aux survivants du CCR en déterminant toute sous-utilisation ou surutilisation potentielle de certaines modalités de surveillance toute d'inégalité d'accès à la surveillance.

MÉTHODOLOGIE : Les chercheurs ont mené une étude de cohorte rétrospective au moyen des données du Registre des cas de cancer de l'Ontario et de plusieurs bases de données qui y sont liées. Ils ont repéré les patients de l'Ontario qui avaient subi une résection de CCR à visée curative entre 2003 à 2007, à l'exception des récurrences éventuelles. Dans les cinq ans suivant l'opération, ils ont répertorié le nombre d'examens d'imagerie et d'endoscopie.

RÉSULTATS : Un total de 4 960 patients ont participé à l'étude. Pendant la période postopératoire de cinq ans, la plus forte proportion de patients qui s'étaient soumis à une surveillance postopératoire a subi le nombre suivant de tests par modalité examinée : de une à trois tomodensitométries abdomino-pelviennes (n=2 073 [41,8 %]); de une à trois échographies abdominales (n=2 443 [49,3 %]); aucune tomodensitométrie du thorax, de une à trois radiographies pulmonaires (n=2 385 [48,1 %]) et deux endoscopies (n=1 845 [37,2 %]). Le risque de ne pas subir d'imagerie abdomino-pelvienne (par tomodensitométrie ou échographie abdominale) était plus élevé chez les patients qui ne recevaient pas de chimiothérapie adjuvante (RR 6,99 [95 % IC 5,26 à 9,35]) ou qui vivaient dans certaines régions géographiques, mais ne dépendaient pas de l'âge, du sexe ou du revenu. Presque tous les patients (n=4 473 [90,2 %]) ont subi au moins une endoscopie pendant la période de suivi.

CONCLUSION : Contrairement aux observations découlant d'études similaires menées dans d'autres territoires, la plupart des survivants du CCR de l'Ontario ont reçu une surveillance postopératoire par imagerie et endoscopie, et les soins sont équitables entre les divers groupes sociodémographiques. Cependant, il existe des variations géographiques inexpliquées en pratique, qui justifient un examen plus approfondi.

In Canada, colorectal cancer (CRC) is the third most common cancer in men and women (13.8% and 11.6%, respectively), but is the second most common cause of cancer death in men and third most common cause of cancer death in women (12.7% and 11.6%, respectively) (1). The Canadian Cancer Society estimated that 23,900 Canadians were diagnosed with CRC in 2013 and 9200 died from the disease (1).

[1]*Department of General Surgery, University of Toronto;* [2]*Odette Cancer Centre, Sunnybrook Health Sciences Centre;* [3]*Institute for Clinical and Evaluative Sciences;* [4]*University Health Network;* [5]*Sunnybrook Research Institute, Sunnybrook Health Sciences Centre, Toronto, Ontario;* [6]*Department of Surgery, Saint Barnabas Medical Center, Livingston, New Jersey, USA;* [7]*Department of Family and Community Medicine, University of Toronto, Toronto, Ontario*
Correspondence: Dr Calvin Law, Sunnybrook Health Sciences Centre, Suite T2-025, 2075 Bayview Avenue, Toronto, Ontario M4N 3M5.
e-mail calvin.law@sunnybrook.ca

TABLE 1
Variation in surveillance guidelines for patients after a curative-intent colorectal cancer resection

Guideline, year (reference)	Abdominopelvic imaging	Chest imaging	Endoscopy
ASCO, 2005 (16)	CT abdo/pelvis every 12 months for 3 years in high-risk patients*	CT chest every 12 months for 3 years in high-risk patients*	Colonoscopy at 3 years after resection for colon cancer survivors; sigmoidoscopy every 6 months for 5 years for rectal cancer survivors
ASCO, 2013 (20)	CT abdo/pelvis every 12 months for 3 years in high-risk patients	CT chest every 12 months for 3 years in high-risk patients	Colonoscopy 1 year after resection; if normal, repeat at 5 years. If not performed before diagnosis, colonoscopy should be performed after completion of adjuvant chemotherapy (before 1 year)
CCO, 2003 (19)	May undergo liver imaging at time of clinical assessment†	May have chest imaging at time of clinical assessment*	Colonoscopy before or within 6 months of resection; if normal, repeat at 3 to 5 years; if tubular or villous adenoma >1 cm, repeat at 1 year
CCO, 2012 (17)	CT abdo/pelvis every 12 months for 3 years. OR liver U/S every 6 to 12 months for 3 years then every 12 months for 2 years	CT chest every 12 months for 3 years. OR chest x-ray every 6 to 12 months for 3 years then every 12 months for 2 years	Colonoscopy 1 year after resection; if normal, repeat at 5 years
NCCN, 2003 (18)	CT abdo/pelvis if symptoms develop	CT chest if symptoms develop	Colonoscopy at 1 year after resection

*Did not define high risk; †Called for clinical assessment every six months for three years, then every 12 months for five years for high-risk (stage IIb-III) patients, and every 12 months for low-risk (stage I-IIa) patients. abdo Abdominal; ASCO American Society of Clinical Oncology; CCO Cancer Care Ontario; CT Computed tomography; NCCN National Comprehensive Cancer Network; U/S Ultrasound

Specifically in Ontario, it was estimated that were 8700 new cases of CRC in 2013 and that 3350 died from the disease, representing some of the highest rates in the world (1,2). While annual age-adjusted incidence has remained relatively stable (59 to 65 cases per 100,000 Canadians) since 1985, a decrease in age-adjusted CRC mortality from 33 deaths per 100,000 Canadians in 1985 to 24 in 2007 may reflect improvements in screening, diagnosis, treatment and surveillance of CRC patients (1). Nevertheless, approximately 30% to 50% of patients receiving curative-intent treatment experience a recurrence (3), and 90% of these recurrences occur in the first five years after treatment (4). More intensive follow-up of curatively treated cancers may improve survival if there are additional treatment options available (5); however, this surveillance may be costly and may pose problems such as increased exposure to radiation and increased patient distress (6).

Several studies have investigated the means and effectiveness of surveillance following primary CRC resection (7-13); a 2008 Cochrane review examining many of these studies (14) has concluded that there has been a significant improvement in five-year survival with more-intensive versus less-intensive follow-up strategies. Substantial variation among the follow-up strategies used in the included studies precluded any determination of optimal method and frequency of follow-up. Furthermore, recent conference proceedings from Mant et al (15) comparing four different surveillance strategies following curative resection of CRC revealed that performing a computed tomography (CT) scan and obtaining a carcinoembryonic antigen level within the first one to two years after surgery was equivalent to more intensive follow-up strategies. Their results suggest that a single evaluation at 12 to 18 months identifies a majority of patients who would benefit from subsequent surgical intervention, which would likely be more cost effective (15). Given the variation in surveillance regimens noted in the literature, it is not surprising that guidelines regarding CRC surveillance also vary considerably in their recommendations (16-19), although the American Society of Clinical Oncology (ASCO) recently adopted guidelines similar to Cancer Care Ontario (CCO), with addition of several qualifying statements (20) (Table 1).

Accordingly, we sought to examine population-based rates of surveillance imaging and endoscopy in patients in Ontario, as well as patient or disease factors that may predispose certain groups to more frequent versus less frequent surveillance. We limited our population of interest to individuals who underwent curative-intent resection for CRC and who remained free of recurrence for at least five years of follow-up after operation. The present study provides insight to the care patients receive in the presence of conflicting guidelines, and may

help to improve care of CRC survivors by identifying any potential underuse or overuse of particular surveillance modalities or inequalities in access to surveillance.

METHODS

A retrospective cohort study was performed at the Institute for Clinical and Evaluative Sciences (ICES, Toronto, Ontario). Source information included the Ontario Cancer Registry (OCR) and the following linked administrative databases: the Canadian Institutes of Health Information Discharge Abstract Database (CIHI-DAD), the Ontario Health Insurance Plan (OHIP), the ICES physician database, and the Registered Persons database. Research Ethics Board approval for the present study was obtained from the Sunnybrook Health Sciences Centre and the University of Toronto, Toronto, Ontario.

Patient selection criteria

Patients 18 to 80 years of age, with an *International Classification of Diseases, Ninth Revision* (ICD-9) diagnosis of colon or rectal cancer and an ICD-0-2 histology code of adenocarcinoma were identified from the OCR from January 1, 2003 through December 31, 2007. Patients with a diagnosis of any other neoplasm at any time based on OCR records were excluded to remove the confounding effect of receiving imaging or follow-up care for tumours other than CRC. Patients who underwent a CRC resection were identified by searching for linked OHIP billings and CIHI-DAD procedures, starting from 14 days before the diagnosis date to ensure inclusion of patients who did not have a preoperative diagnosis of CRC (eg, those who presented emergently with an obstruction or perforation). Either one OHIP claim or one CIHI code for CRC resection was considered to be sufficient for classifying a patient as having undergone surgery. Patients who did not undergo a colorectal resection or who underwent a CRC resection >120 days after diagnosis were excluded because the population of interest was limited to those who underwent a potentially curative CRC resection, and resections performed >120 days from diagnosis were not likely for curative intent.

Once the cohort of patients who underwent curative-intent resection had been identified, additional series of exclusion criteria were applied to eliminate patients who likely developed a recurrence. These patients were excluded to avoid contamination of results with tests performed for diagnosis or treatment planning rather than surveillance. Thus, patients experiencing the following within the entire five-year follow-up period after primary CRC resection were excluded: death; a diagnosis of advanced (secondary) disease, based on CIHI diagnosis codes for hospital admissions; evidence of early relapse of

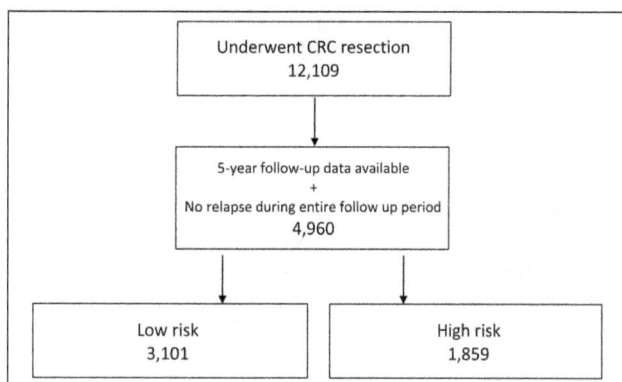

Figure 1) *Patient selection. CRC Colorectal cancer*

disease via lung or liver procedures (resection, destruction, or biopsy); a palliative care consult, determined by OHIP fee codes; the first claim for chemotherapy >120 days following primary resection; and the number of days between first and last chemotherapy claim exceeding 270 days, between days 0 and 395 after CRC resection. The fifth exclusion is based on data from the Cancer Quality Council of Ontario indicating that approximately 85% of patients will initiate a course of adjuvant chemotherapy within four months of primary CRC resection (21). Initiation of chemotherapy later than this suggests treatment of early disease relapse. The final exclusion was applied because the usual duration of a course of adjuvant chemotherapy is 180 days. Allowing time for breaks in treatment due to side effects or delays, or duration of chemotherapy >270 days, likely represents ongoing treatment for metastatic disease or relapse.

Finally, patients were excluded if they lacked five years of follow-up data, residence within one of the 14 health regions in Ontario referred to as Local Health Integration Network (LHIN) of residence, or income information. Patients residing in the southeast LHIN were also excluded due to the alternative funding plan used by this LHIN, which affects the completeness of OHIP billings.

Patient follow-up
The follow-up period was defined as commencing on the date of primary surgery and patients were followed for five full years thereafter. Modalities of follow-up care that were measured included: abdominopelvic imaging, defined as CT of the abdomen/pelvis (CT A/P) or abdominal ultrasound (AUS); chest imaging, defined as chest x-ray (CXR) or CT of the chest; and endoscopy, defined as flexible sigmoidoscopy or colonoscopy.

Patient-related variables
Demographic variables collected included sex, age at diagnosis of CRC, LHIN of residence, mean neighbourhood income and rural versus urban residence. Mean neighbourhood income quintiles were derived from the Registered Persons database, postal codes and census tract information (census year 2001). Rural status was based on the Statistics Canada definition, namely, residence in a community population <10,000 based on the 2001 census.

Receipt of chemotherapy was used as a proxy for stage to classify relapse risk because stage information was not available in the OCR for the time period of the present study. Patients were labelled as high risk for recurrence if they received chemotherapy in their immediate postoperative period (within four months of operation); otherwise, they were considered to be low risk for recurrence.

Statistical analysis
Descriptive statistics were performed on variables of interest with categorical variables summarized using counts and percentages. For patients with complete five-year follow-up data with no evidence of recurrence, descriptive tables were generated by counts of each type of surveillance modality for the follow-up period, stratifying the cohorts

according to low-risk and high-risk patients. To explore factors associ-

TABLE 2
Multivariable logistic regression analysis for patients receiving neither abdominopelvic computed tomography scan nor abdominal ultrasound during the five-year follow-up period

	OR (95% CI)	P
Age, years		
<50	Reference	
50–64	0.97 (0.68–1.39)	0.88
65–74	1.07 (0.75–1.52)	0.73
>75	1.21 (0.83–1.74)	0.32
Sex		
Male	Reference	
Female	0.85 (0.71–1.02)	0.08
Risk category		
High	Reference	
Low	**6.99 (5.26–9.35)**	**<0.01**
Rural		
No	Reference	
Yes	1.00 (0.77–1.31)	0.99
Income quintile		
1 (low)	Reference	
2	1.08 (0.81–1.43)	0.62
3	0.94 (0.70–1.26)	0.67
4	1.07 (0.80–1.44)	0.63
5 (high)	1.07 (0.80–1.43)	0.64
Local Health Integration Network		
1	Reference	
2	1.03 (0.70–1.52)	0.86
3	1.32 (0.78–2.21)	0.30
4	1.11 (0.75–1.63)	0.60
5	**1.90 (1.26–2.86)**	**<0.01**
6	1.06 (0.74–1.52)	0.76
7	1.03 (0.66–1.60)	0.90
8	1.43 (0.93–2.18)	0.10
9	1.14 (0.68–1.92)	0.62
10	0.41 (0.16–1.07)	0.07
11	**2.03 (1.38–2.98)**	**<0.01**
12	**0.61 (0.37–0.99)**	**0.05**
13	1.20 (0.75–1.92)	0.44

Bolded values indicate statistical significance

ated with receiving no abdominal imaging (CT or ultrasound) in the entire follow-up period, univariate and multivariable logistic regression analyses were performed with the outcome of zero abdominal imaging modalities versus one or more. The predictor variables of interest were patient age category, sex, LHIN of residence, rural status, income quintile and risk category of the primary tumour. The estimates from the models were presented as ORs and their associated 95% CIs. All tests were two-sided; $P<0.05$ was considered to be statistically significant. All analyses were performed using SAS version 9.1.3 for Unix (SAS Institute, USA).

RESULTS
In total, 12,109 patients who underwent curative CRC resection for colorectal adenocarcinoma, with no other primary malignancy, were identified from the OCR from January 1, 2003 through December 31, 2007 (Figure 1). These patients underwent a CRC resection from 14 days before to 120 days after the OCR diagnosis date and were disease free at the beginning of the follow-up period. After application of exclusion criteria, of these 12,109 patients, 4960 (41%) had complete

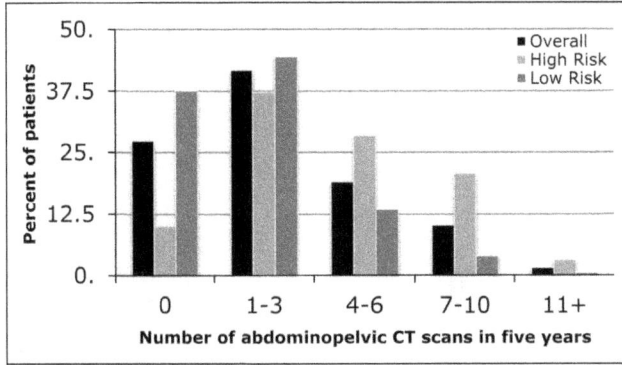

Figure 2) *The number of abdominopelvic computed tomography (CT) scans received in the five-year follow-up period, stratified according to high and low risk for recurrence*

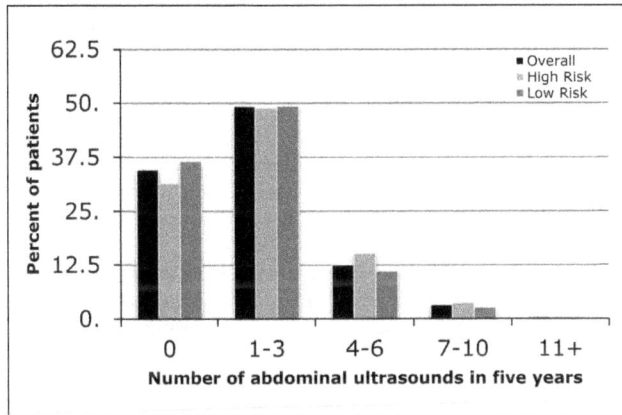

Figure 3) *The number of abdominal ultrasounds received in the five-year follow-up period, stratified according to high and low risk for recurrence*

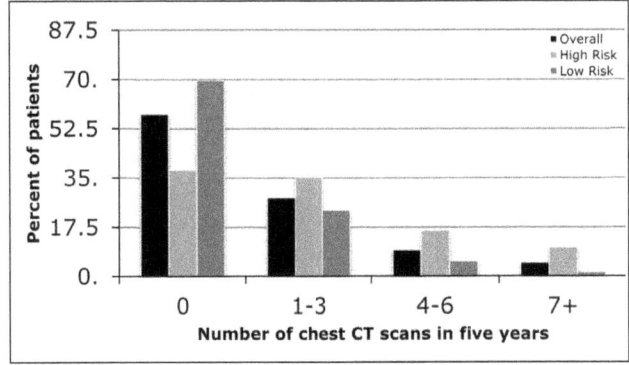

Figure 4) *The number of chest computed tomography (CT) scans received in the five-year follow-up period, stratified according to high and low risk for recurrence*

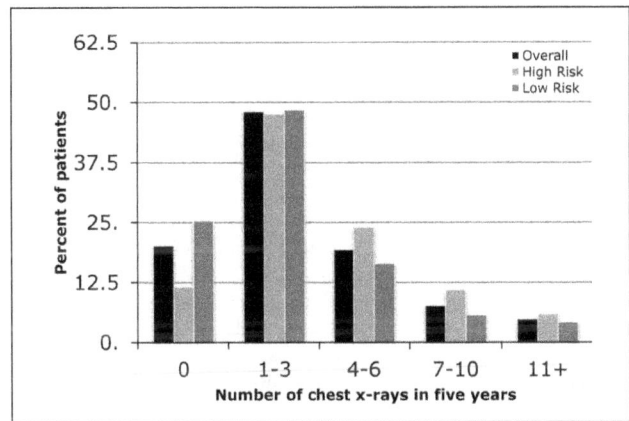

Figure 5) *The number of chest x-rays received in the five-year follow-up period, stratified according to high- and low-risk for recurrence*

five-year data to examine frequencies of follow-up modalities, no out-migration and no disease recurrence or death between years 1 and 5 after resection. In total, 3101 (62.5%) patients were considered to be low risk and 1859 (37.5%) high risk. Overall patient characteristics are summarized in Table 2.

Abdominopelvic imaging
Over the five-year follow-up period, 1354 (27.3%) patients did not undergo any CT A/P (Figure 2). The largest proportion of patients (n=2073 [41.8%]) underwent between one and three CT A/P in the follow-up period, with progressively smaller numbers of patients undergoing four to six, seven to 10 and ≥11 scans, respectively. This analysis was repeated by stratifying the cohort according to low- and high-risk primary tumours. While 1166 (37.6%) low-risk patients did not receive any CT A/P in the entire follow-up period, only 188 (10.1%) high-risk patients did not receive a single CT A/P.

Frequency of abdominal ultrasound (AUS) was also examined throughout the follow-up period. Overall, 1177 (34.6%) did not receive any AUS, while almost one-half (2443 [49.3%]) underwent one to three AUS (Figure 3). Results were similar when stratified according to high- and low-risk patients.

To understand the proportion of patients that did not undergo any abdominopelvic imaging whatsoever, the subgroup of patients who did not receive any CT A/P was analyzed for the frequency of AUS performed. Of the 1354 patients who did not receive CT A/P during the follow-up period, 592 (43.7%) also did not receive AUS (11.9% of cohort). This group was comprised primarily of patients at low risk for recurrence (538 [91.9%]). No differences in the proportion of patients with no abdominopelvic imaging were noted according to age, sex, income or rural residence (Table 2). However, compared with the referent LHIN (LHIN 1), there was a significant variation in the proportion

of patients without abdominopelvic imaging depending on LHIN (Table 2). The strongest association was observed for patients with low-risk primary cancers to have increased odds of not receiving any abdominal imaging (OR 6.99 [95% CI 5.26 to 9.35]).

Chest imaging
The majority of patients did not receive any CT scans of the chest (2863 [57.7%]) (Figure 4). High-risk patients were slightly more likely to receive CT chest in each frequency category. The number of CXRs patients received during the five-year follow-up period was also examined (Figure 5). Patients most frequently underwent one to three CXRs in each of the overall (2385 [48.1%]), high-risk (885 [47.6%]) and low-risk (1500 [48.4%]) categories.

Endoscopy
Most patients (4473 [90.2%]) underwent endoscopy at some point during the follow-up period, with the highest proportion of patients undergoing two endoscopies in each of the overall (1845 [37.2%]), low-risk (1133 [36.5%]) and high-risk (712 [38.3%]) groups (Figure 6).

Univariate and multivariate analysis was performed to test for associations of surveillance endoscopies with age, sex, LHIN of residence, income and risk category. As income quintile increased, there was a trend toward more patients undergoing ≥4 endoscopies and fewer patients undergoing zero endoscopies (Figure 7).

DISCUSSION
In the present population-based cohort study, the actual imaging and endoscopic surveillance received by Ontario patients post curative-intent CRC resection was examined. For both imaging studies and endoscopy, patients were noted to have undergone a variable number

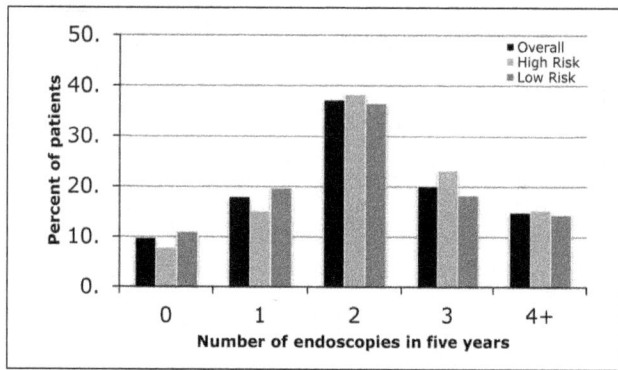

Figure 6) *The number of endoscopies received in the five-year follow-up period, stratified according to high and low risk for recurrence*

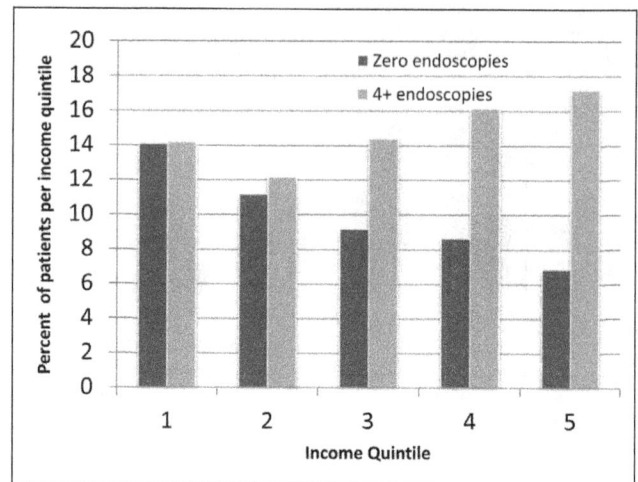

Figure 7) *Comparison of percentage of patients undergoing zero versus four or more endoscopies, stratified according to income quintile*

of tests during their five-year follow-up period. This is not unexpected given the heterogeneity of guidelines at the time of our study, but it is interesting to note the wide variation that existed in the number of tests. For example, while some patients did not receive a single CT A/P or AUS during their follow-up, some patients received ≥11. While those receiving many scans may have undergone imaging for reasons other than CRC surveillance, it is also possible that different patients and physicians have different attitudes regarding the benefits and necessity of imaging surveillance after curative-intent CRC resection. This would be consistent with the finding that, among the subgroup of patients who received no abdominopelvic surveillance imaging, most had low-risk primary tumours. Both patients and physicians may believe there to be a lesser need for surveillance imaging in patients judged to have a lower risk for recurrence.

Variations among LHINs in the ORs for receiving no abdominopelvic surveillance imaging during the five-year follow-up period is concerning for potential health care inequity. However, such variations are not unexpected given that Cooper et al (22) previously demonstrated similar geographical variations in surveillance patterns in the United States. However, our results must be interpreted cautiously given that other potential confounders, such as patient preference, number of medical comorbidities or patient distance from nearest imaging facility, were not taken into account.

Income quintile was not an independent predictor for receiving no abdominopelvic surveillance imaging in the present study. This is in contrast to findings by Elston Lafata et al (23) in the United States showing that lower income patients had a decreased chance of receiving surveillance metastatic disease testing in the form of CT, ultrasound, magnetic resonance imaging, CXR or serum transaminases. While no other Ontario study has examined patient income as a predictor for CRC imaging surveillance, Booth et al (24) did demonstrate decreased overall and cancer-specific survivals for lower-income Ontario patients. However, Grunfeld et al (25) noted small differences (<2%) between income quintiles when examined as a predictor of imaging surveillance for breast cancer patients. It is possible that surveillance imaging patterns are not influenced by income in Ontario because of our universal health care system, and that Booth et al's results were, thus, not related to surveillance imaging practices.

However, the income equality noted in our study for surveillance imaging did not persist when surveillance endoscopy was considered. On the contrary, more affluent Ontarians are more likely to receive four or more endoscopies and less likely to receive zero endoscopies compared with less affluent individuals. The lack of association between income and imaging surveillance in Ontario, but the presence of this association for endoscopic surveillance may be a result of endoscopy being a relatively scarce resource compared with imaging modalities such as CT scans and ultrasounds. Further study involving individual level data and actual household income may be useful in further defining the relationship between receipt of surveillance

endoscopy and socioeconomic status. It is not until these potential explanatory mechanisms are elucidated that further intervention, such as knowledge translation initiatives or deployment of resources, can be used to address socioeconomic status as a potential barrier to receiving surveillance endoscopy.

The finding that most patients receive at least one endoscopic evaluation postoperatively is consistent with both the 2003 CCO guideline, which called for colonoscopy before or within six months of surgery, and the 2009 NCCN guideline, which recommended colonoscopy at three years following resection (26). However, the American Society of Clinical Oncology guideline, while suggesting colonoscopy at one year for colon cancer survivors, also suggested sigmoidoscopy every six months for rectal cancer patients. The latter should lead to rectal cancer survivors undergoing approximately 10 endoscopic evaluations over the course of their five-year follow-up, which clearly very few patients achieved (16). The subset of patients receiving no endoscopy postoperatively may reflect individuals too unwell to undergo the procedure itself (or any treatment that would be indicated should a recurrence be noted), those who preferred to forego the examination, or perhaps those who, in accordance with the CCO guideline, only received preoperative endoscopy.

With respect to chest imaging, it is important to note that CCO's recommendations at the time of the present study did not address CT scanning and did not define a recommended frequency for CXR (19). As such, it is not surprising that relatively few Ontario patients received surveillance chest CT. More patients received CXR, but this result could be confounded because CXR are common tests ordered for a wide range of indications, not just CRC surveillance.

Other studies have also examined adherence to CRC surveillance guidelines, with mixed results. A study involving 409 French patients (27) showed poor adherence to French guidelines at the time, with 65% of patients undergoing fewer than the recommended number of AUS, 52% undergoing fewer than the recommended number of CXR and 20% undergoing fewer than the recommended number of colonoscopies. In the United States, a study focusing on patients >65 years of age demonstrated that 60% of patients received less than the recommended amount of postoperative surveillance (28). In contrast, a smaller single-centre Norwegian study demonstrated a 62% compliance rate with Norwegian surveillance recommendations, including 85% undergoing liver ultrasound and 55% undergoing colonoscopy within one year (29). The latter study was aimed primarily at determining patient compliance because all patients were ordered testing in accordance with guidelines by their treating physician. Relative to these observations in other nations, it would appear that Ontario physicians' and patients' adherence to guidelines regarding colonoscopy is quite good. It is difficult to make generalized statements about compliance with imaging in the current study because guidelines at the time were nonspecific.

It is interesting to compare the results of the present study with those of a survey conducted by Earle et al (30) in 2003 to measure Canadian physicians' surveillance strategies following curative-intent CRC resection. Surgeons, medical oncologists and radiation oncologists all specializing in CRC were presented with a hypothetical patient – a 50-year-old man, otherwise healthy, with stage III disease after a curative CRC resection – and asked to provide their recommendations for follow-up. Of the 160 physicians who completed the survey, <10% recommended body surveillance by abdominal CT in any follow-up year, and only approximately one-third recommended AUS imaging in any follow-up year. In contrast, approximately 90% of physicians recommended bowel surveillance with colonoscopy in follow-up year 1. Opinions regarding chest imaging were not solicited in the survey. Clearly, with almost 90% of patients in the current study receiving at least one abdominopelvic CT or ultrasound within five years of follow-up, patients are receiving more body surveillance than the study by Earle et al (30) would predict. This could be a result of changing practice because the survey was conducted in 2003, differences in practice between Ontario and other Canadian provinces, or contamination of our study data with imaging obtained for an alternate indication. The high proportion of physicians recommending surveillance endoscopy in the study by Earle et al is consistent with our findings that most Ontario patients receive at least one postoperative endoscopy.

Limitations to the present study were primarily related to the use of administrative data. Although such population-level data generate a large sample size, the data at the individual level are lost. For example, unlike the Surveillance, Epidemiology, and End Results database from the National Cancer Institute, our administrative data do not identify patient race or ethnicity, which would allow us to evaluate other social elements that may affect postoperative CRC surveillance patterns in addition to income level. Also in the present study, lack of information on the indications for CT, AUS, CXR and endoscopic evaluations may have allowed confounding of surveillance data to occur if these tests were ordered for indications other than CRC surveillance. Furthermore, an additional limitation to the present study arises from

the application of strict exclusion criteria, which reduced our sample size for analysis from 12,109 to 4960 patients to eliminate bias caused by additional testing around the time of detection of disease relapse. However, it is still possible that a small number of patients with disease relapse were included in the sample, which could skew results toward higher use of all surveillance modalities. An additional limitation of our study involved trying to determine the number of patients that received a colonoscopy within one year of resection, as recommended by most guidelines. In the use of administrative data, it is extremely problematic to develop rules to define and determine adherence to guidelines. For example, a one-year follow-up colonoscopy can be performed anywhere between 10 and 14 months after resection, but this represents an arbitrary range. If a specific cutoff was used at 12 months postresection, many one-year follow-up colonoscopies may be systematically excluded. However, we are able to measure whether any surveillance was performed during the five-year follow-up period, which will reflect issues of follow-up and access to care. Therefore, we reported the number of colonoscopies over the five-year follow-up period. Given these limitations, the present study provides a seminal overview of current surveillance patterns in the province of Ontario and these observations should be further studied and confirmed with individual-level data in a variety of settings throughout the province, including both academic and nonacademic centres, as well as urban and rural centres. Further study is recommended in determining the current knowledge guidelines of physicians who provide CRC follow-up, as well as access to resources in the area where they practice.

ACKNOWLEDGEMENTS: This study was conducted with the support of the Ontario Institute for Cancer Research and Cancer Care Ontario through funding provided by the Government of Ontario. This study was supported by the Institute for Clinical Evaluative Sciences (ICES), which is funded by an annual grant from the Ontario Ministry of Health and Long-Term Care (MOHLTC). The opinions, results and conclusions reported in this paper are those of the authors and are independent from the funding sources. No endorsement by ICES or the Ontario MOHLTC is intended or should be inferred. Dr Coburn (Career Scientist Award) and Dr Law (Hanna Family Research Chair in Surgical Oncology) held support grants.

REFERENCES

1. Canadian Cancer Society's Steering Committee on Cancer Statistics. Canadian cancer statistics 2013. Toronto: Canadian Cancer Society, 2013.
2. Ferlay J, Shin HR, Bray F, Forman D, Mathers C, Parkin DM. Estimates of worldwide burden of cancer in 2008: GLOBOCAN 2008. Int J Cancer 2011;127:2893-917.
3. Tjandra JJ, Chan MK. Follow-up after curative resection of colorectal cancer: A meta-analysis. Dis Colon Rectum 2007;50:1783-99.
4. Pfister DG, Benson AB III, Somerfield MR. Clinical practice. Surveillance strategies after curative treatment of colorectal cancer. N Engl J Med 2004;350:2375-82.
5. Furman MJ, Lambert LA, Sullivan ME, Whalen GF. Rational follow-up after curative cancer resection. J Clin Oncol 2013;31.1.1130-3.
6. Virgo KS, Wade TP, Longo WE, Coplin MA, Vernava AM, Johnson FE. Surveillance after curative colon cancer resection: Practice patterns of surgical subspecialists. Ann Surg Oncol 1995;2:472-82.
7. Castells A, Bessa X, Daniels M, et al. Value of postoperative surveillance after radical surgery for colorectal cancer: Results of a cohort study. Dis Colon Rectum 1998;4:714-23; discussion 23-4.
8. Kjeldsen BJ, Kronborg O, Fenger C, Jorgensen OD. A prospective randomized study of follow-up after radical surgery for colorectal cancer. Br J Surg 1997;84:666-9.
9. Makela JT, Laitinen SO, Kairaluoma MI. Five-year follow-up after radical surgery for colorectal cancer. Results of a prospective randomized trial. Arch Surg 1995;130:1062-7.
10. Ohlsson B, Breland U, Ekberg H, Graffner H, Tranberg KG. Follow-up after curative surgery for colorectal carcinoma. Randomized comparison with no follow-up. Dis Colon Rectum 1995;38:619-26.
11. Pietra N, Sarli L, Costi R, Ouchemi C, Grattarola M, Peracchia A. Role of follow-up in management of local recurrences of colorectal cancer: A prospective, randomized study. Dis Colon Rectum 1998;41:1127-33.
12. Rodriguez-Moranta F, Salo J, Arcusa A, et al. Postoperative surveillance in patients with colorectal cancer who have undergone curative resection: A prospective, multicenter, randomized, controlled trial. J Clin Oncol 2006;24:386-93.
13. Schoemaker D, Black R, Giles L, Toouli J. Yearly colonoscopy, liver CT, and chest radiography do not influence 5-year survival of colorectal cancer patients. Gastroenterology 1998;114:7-14.
14. Jeffery M, Hickey BE, Hider PN. Follow-up strategies for patients treated for non-metastatic colorectal cancer. Cochrane Database Syst Rev 2007(1):CD002200.
15. Mant D, Perera R, Gray A, et al. Effect of 3-5 years of scheduled CEA and CT follow-up to detect recurrence of colorectal cancer: FACS randomized controlled trial. 2013 ASCO Annual Meeting. J Clin Oncol 2013 (Suppl): A3500.
16. Desch CE, Benson AB III, Somerfield MR, et al. Colorectal cancer surveillance: 2005 update of an American Society of Clinical Oncology practice guideline. J Clin Oncol 2005;23:8512-9.
17. Earle C, Annis R, Sussman J, Haynes AE, Vafaei A. Follow up care, surveillance protocol, and secondary prevention measures for survivors of colorectal cancer. Toronto: Cancer Care Ontario. Program in Evidence based Care Evidence Based Series, 2012;26(2).

18. Engstrom PF, Benson AB III, Saltz L. Colon cancer. Clinical practice guidelines in oncology. J Natl Compr Canc Netw 2003;1:40-53.

19. Figueredo A, Rumble RB, Maroun J, et al. Follow-up of patients with curatively resected colorectal cancer: A practice guideline. BMC Cancer 2003;3:26.

20. Meyerhardt JA, Mangu PB, Flynn PJ, et al. Follow-up care, surveillance protocol, and secondary prevention measures for survivors of colorectal cancer: American Society of Clinical Oncology clinical practice guideline endorsement. J Clin Oncol 2013;31:4465-70.

21. Cancer Care Ontario, Informatics Centre of Excellence. Wait time between Diagnosis and Adjuvant Chemotherapy. Cancer Quality Council of Ontario, 2013.

22. Cooper GS, Yuan Z, Chak A, Rimm AA. Geographic and patient variation among Medicare beneficiaries in the use of follow-up testing after surgery for nonmetastatic colorectal carcinoma. Cancer 1999;85:2124-31.

23. Elston Lafata J, Johnson CC, Ben-Menachem T, Morlock RJ. Sociodemographic differences in the receipt of colorectal cancer surveillance care following treatment with curative intent. Med Care 2001;39:361-72.

24. Booth CM, Li G, Zhang-Salomons J, Mackillop WJ. The impact of socioeconomic status on stage of cancer at diagnosis and survival: A population-based study in Ontario, Canada. Cancer 2010;116:4160-7.

25. Grunfeld E, Hodgson DC, Del Giudice ME, Moineddin R. Population-based longitudinal study of follow-up care for breast cancer survivors. J Oncol Pract 2010;6:174-81.

26. Engstrom PF, Arnoletti JP, Benson AB III, et al. NCCN Clinical Practice Guidelines in Oncology: Colon cancer. J Natl Compr Canc Netw 2009;7:778-831.

27. Boulin M, Lejeune C, Le Teuff G, et al. Patterns of surveillance practices after curative surgery for colorectal cancer in a French population. Dis Colon Rectum 2005;48:1890-9.

28. Cooper GS, Kou TD, Reynolds HL Jr. Receipt of guideline-recommended follow-up in older colorectal cancer survivors: A population-based analysis. Cancer 2008;113:2029-37.

29. Korner H, Soreide K, Stokkeland PJ, Soreide JA. Systematic follow-up after curative surgery for colorectal cancer in Norway: A population-based audit of effectiveness, costs, and compliance. J Gastrointest Surg 2005;9:320-8.

30. Earle CC, Grunfeld E, Coyle D, Cripps MC, Stern HS. Cancer physicians' attitudes toward colorectal cancer follow-up. Ann Oncol 2003;14:400-5.

16

Inflammatory bowel disease nurses in Canada: An examination of Canadian gastroenterology nurses and their role in inflammatory bowel disease care

Jennifer G Stretton NP MN BScN[1], Barbara K Currie NP MN BNRN[2], Usha K Chauhan NP MN BScN[3]

JG Stretton, BK Currie, UK Chauhan. Inflammatory bowel disease nurses in Canada: An examination of Canadian gastroenterology nurses and their role in inflammatory bowel disease care. Can J Gastroenterol Hepatol 2014;28(2):89-93.

BACKGROUND/OBJECTIVE: Inflammatory bowel disease (IBD) is a chronic relapsing illness primarily including Crohn disease and ulcerative colitis. The disease course often fluctuates over time, and requires maintenance therapy and acute interventions to target disease flares. IBD management requires a multidisciplinary approach, with care from physicians, nurses, dieticians, social workers and psychologists. Because nurses play a pivotal role in managing chronic disease, the aim of the present study was to assess and determine how many nurses work primarily with IBD patients in Canada.

METHODS: A 29-question survey was developed using an Internet-based survey tool (www.surveymonkey.com) to investigate nursing demographics, IBD nursing roles and nursing services provided across Canada. Distribution included the Canadian Society of Gastroenterology Nurses and Associates, the Canadian Association of Gastroenterology, Progress (AbbVie Corporation, USA) and BioAdvance (Janssen Inc, USA) coordinators (via e-mail), and online availability for 15 weeks.

RESULTS: Of 275 survey respondents, 98.2% were female nurses, with 68.7% employed in full-time positions. Among them, 42.5% were between 51 and 60 years of age, and 32.4% were between 41 and 50 years of age. In addition, 53.8% were diploma-prepared registered nurses, 35.3% were Baccalaureate-prepared nurses and 4.4% were Masters-prepared nurses. Almost one-half (44% [n=121]) were employed in Ontario, followed by 19.6% (n=54) in Alberta and 9.1% (n=25) in British Columbia. All provinces were represented with the exception of Nunavut and the Northwest Territories. Forty-three per cent (n=119) of nurses identified as working in endoscopy units. Of the 90% who responded as working with IBD patients, only 30% (n=79) had a primary role in IBD care. Among these 79 nurses with a primary role in IBD care, 79.7% worked with the adult population, 10.1% with the pediatric population, and 10.1% worked with both adult and pediatric patients. Their major service was an outpatient setting (67.1%).

CONCLUSIONS: Survey results showed that only a small percentage of Canadian gastroenterology nurses provide clinical IBD care. Many have multiple roles and responsibilities, and provide a variety of services. The exact depth of care and service is unclear and further study is needed.

Key Words: *Inflammatory bowel disease; Nursing; Nursing roles*

Les infirmières en maladies inflammatoires de l'intestin au Canada : un examen des infirmières canadiennes en gastroentérologie et leur rôle dans les soins des maladies inflammatoires de l'intestin

HISTORIQUE ET OBJECTIF : Les maladies inflammatoires de l'intestin (MII), des maladies chroniques récidivantes, incluent surtout la maladie de Crohn et la colite ulcéreuse. Elles fluctuent souvent au fil du temps et exigent un traitement d'entretien et des interventions aiguës pour cibler les exacerbations. Il faut adopter une démarche multidisciplinaire pour prendre en charge les MII, qui incluent les soins de médecins, d'infirmières, de diététistes, de travailleurs sociaux et de psychologues. Puisque les infirmières jouent un rôle essentiel dans la prise en charge des maladies chroniques, la présente étude visait à évaluer et à déterminer le nombre d'infirmières qui travaillent surtout avec des patients atteints d'une MII au Canada.

MÉTHODOLOGIE : Un sondage de 29 questions a été élaboré au moyen d'un outil virtuel de création de sondages (www.surveymonkey.com), afin d'explorer la démographie des soins infirmiers, les rôles des infirmières à l'égard des MII et les services de soins infirmiers prodigués au Canada. Ce sondage, qui est demeuré en ligne 15 semaines, a été distribué à la Société canadienne des infirmières et infirmiers en gastroentérologie et travailleurs associés, à l'Association canadienne de gastroentérologie et aux coordonnateurs de Progress (AbbVie Corporation, États-Unis) et BioAdvance (Janssen Inc, États-Unis) (par courriel).

RÉSULTATS : Sur les 275 répondants au sondage, 98,2 % étaient des infirmières (et non des infirmiers), et 68,7 % avaient un emploi à temps plein. De ce nombre, 42,5 % avaient de 51 à 60 ans, et 32,4 %, de 41 à 50 ans. De plus, 53,8 % possédaient un diplôme en soins infirmiers, 35,3 %, un baccalauréat en soins infirmiers et 4,4%, une maîtrise en soins infirmiers. Près de la moitié (44 % [n=121]) occupait un emploi en Ontario, suivie de 19,6 % (n=54) en Alberta et de 9,1 % (n=25) en Colombie-Britannique. Toutes les provinces étaient représentées, à l'exception du Nunavut et des Territoires du Nord-Ouest. Quarante-trois pour cent des infirmières (n=119) ont précisé travailler dans une unité d'endoscopie. Des 90 % qui ont affirmé travailler avec des patients atteints d'une MII, seulement 30 % (n=79) jouaient un rôle primaire en soins des MII. Chez les 79 infirmières ayant un rôle primaire en soins des MII, 79,7 % travaillaient auprès de la population adulte, 10,1 % auprès de la population d'âge pédiatrique et 10,1 % auprès des patients adultes et d'âge pédiatrique. Elles travaillaient surtout en consultations externes (67,1 %).

CONCLUSIONS : Les résultats du sondage ont démontré que seul un petit pourcentage d'infirmières canadiennes en gastroentérologie donne des soins cliniques des MII. Bon nombre ont des rôles et responsabilités multiples et offrent des services variés. On n'a pu établir clairement l'ampleur exacte de leurs soins et de leurs services. D'autres études s'imposent.

Managing patients living with inflammatory bowel disease (IBD) requires a multidisciplinary approach using the expertise of physicians, nurses, dieticians, social workers and psychologists.

The literature has reported the emergence of the 'nurse specialist' in IBD and the significant contribution nurses play in the management of IBD (1). Not only do nurses provide patients with education, counselling and support, but with the evolving roles of advanced practice nurses (APNs), investigating, diagnosing, prescribing and/or monitoring therapy is also within their scopes of practice.

IBD is a chronic disease and includes both Crohn disease (CD) and ulcerative colitis (UC). IBD is a chronic relapsing condition that can negatively impact quality of life and contribute significant cost to the

[1]*Division of Gastroenterology, St Joseph's Healthcare Hamilton, Hamilton, Ontario;* [2]*Division of Gastroenterology, QEII Health Sciences Centre, Halifax, Nova Scotia;* [3]*Division of Gastroenterology, Hamilton Health Sciences, Hamilton, Ontario*
Correspondence and reprints: Jennifer G Stretton, Division of Gastroenterology, St Joseph's Healthcare Hamilton, 50 Charlton Avenue East, Room H429, Hamilton, Ontario L8N 4A6. e-mail jstretto@stjoes.ca

health care system (2). Disease activity often fluctuates over time and, therefore, requires maintenance therapy and acute interventions to target disease flares. The medical model of care is often reactive (3). Currently there is no preventive treatment for IBD and comprehensive management is required. Disease management aims to maximize time in remission, alleviate or reduce symptoms, resolve complications and improve quality of life.

The Canadian Nurses Association emphasizes the patients' central role in the management of their illness (4). Patient education surrounding the disease process and medications helps patients achieve the best possible quality of life with their chronic conditions. Registered nurses (RNs) and nurse practitioners (NPs) play an integral role in chronic disease management.

Nursing is a self-regulated profession, and through provincial and territorial legislation, nursing regulatory bodies are accountable for the protection of the public (5). In Canada, there are three nursing roles – registered practical nurse/licensed practical nurse (RPN/LPN), RN and APN. APNs include both NPs and clinical nurse specialists. An RPN/LPN obtains a two-year diploma in practical nursing through a community college, whereas an RN completes a four-year Bachelor's degree in nursing. Both RPN/LPNs and RNs write a certification examination. In practice, an RPN/LPN manages stable patients and is able to assist with health education and medication management. An RN manages both acute and chronic patients, can perform physical examinations, provides patient education and is able to monitor medical therapy. The clinical nurse specialist is a registered nurse who holds a Master's or Doctoral degree in nursing. They have advanced knowledge and clinical expertise in a nursing specialty (6). The NP has additional experience/training with a Masters in nursing degree and can autonomously diagnose, order and interpret diagnostic tests; prescribe pharmaceuticals; and perform procedures within their legislated scope of practice.

Nightingale et al (7) studied the effects of IBD nurse specialists on outcomes in patients with IBD. Patients were provided with educational materials on lifestyle, health promotion, medications and diagnostic tests. Patients also had telephone access to the specialist nurse. IBD nurses provided improved patient education, satisfaction and disease management. Patient satisfaction improved with access to information on IBD. The study reported a 38% decrease in hospital visits and a 19% decrease in the length of hospital stays. The authors concluded that IBD nurse specialists were valuable and cost-effective members of the team.

In 2010, Hernandez-Sampelayo et al (8) reviewed the scientific evidence regarding the quality of care in IBD patients in relation to nurses. The review highlighted the importance of having IBD specialist nurses and indicated that patients with access to this service were reported to experience beneficial outcomes. The authors identified methodological limitations of the studies reviewed and suggested further research – specifically in nursing interventions and patient outcomes.

In 2011, The Royal College of Nursing in the United Kingdom (UK) published findings from its national IBD nursing audit (9). The goals of the audit were to: evaluate the IBD nursing services and identify areas for improvement; provide national evidence of IBD nurse numbers, activity and effectiveness; and provide feedback to nurses demonstrating the impact of IBD nursing service. This audit provided national data supporting the important contribution IBD nurses make to patients living with IBD in the UK.

Furthermore, in May 2011, 240 IBD nurses from across the UK were invited to complete an online survey related to their professional background, service and daily activity. The results identified several important factors regarding the IBD nursing profile, service profile and activity, namely, job specifics, nursing education, nonmedical prescribing, managerial responsibilities, clinical responsibilities, workplace environment, nursing educational activities and patient education materials.

The survey revealed that the number of IBD nurses across the UK is increasing. The majority of IBD nurses also had other gastroenterology (GI)-related roles and only a percentage of their patient load was committed to IBD patients. Many similarities within their roles were identified such as emergency telephone contact and advice, patient information, counselling, monitoring and administration of IBD therapy. Much of the IBD nurse specialist activity was centred in acute hospital settings, and they were often the link between primary and secondary care.

As reported in previous research (7,8), the management of IBD is a complex process and nursing plays an invaluable and necessary role in the treatment and care of individuals with IBD. The UK audit emphasized several important points that are critical for the successful treatment of IBD – namely, the number of nurses, activities and services in which they participate. Unlike the valuable information that was obtained in the UK, Canadian nursing support, roles in IBD care and management is poorly understood and documented. Canada has among the highest reported prevalence and incidence of IBD in the world. As highlighted in the Crohn's and Colitis Foundation of Canada report *The Impact of Inflammatory Bowel Disease in Canada 2012* (10), there are approximately 233,000 Canadians living with IBD (129,000 with CD and 104,000 with UC). The report also suggested that >10,200 new cases of IBD are diagnosed every year. Given the staggering numbers of people living with IBD, one hopes that there are sufficient numbers of nurses specialized in this field to consistently provide ongoing care and disease-management support. Unfortunately, this may not be the case.

Recognizing the documentation of the valuable work performed in the UK, it was decided that the role of the nurse specialist in IBD should be evaluated in Canada. The authors developed a Canadian IBD Nurses Survey with the purpose of conducting a geographical assessment of GI nurses working with IBD patients in Canada. The goals were to gain an understanding of the community of nurses impacting the care of IBD patients and garner an appreciation of the demographics of IBD nurses including age, sex, years of experience, educational preparation, employment setting and scope of practice. With the results of this survey, the authors would determine whether there was interest among those surveyed in establishing a Canadian IBD Nurses Interest Group.

METHODS

The Canadian Inflammatory Bowel Disease Nurse's Survey was developed by the authors and was targeted at GI nurses (RPN/LPNs, RNs and APNs) who had a role in caring for patients with IBD. The 29-question survey was developed using an Internet-based survey tool (www.surveymonkey.com), to assess nursing demographics, the role of the IBD nurse and nursing services provided across Canada.

In October 2012, the survey was distributed through Survey Monkey to GI nurses across the country. In collaboration with the Canadian Society of Gastroenterology Nurses and Associates (CSGNA) and the Canadian Association of Gastroenterology (CAG), the survey was circulated to their memberships via e-mail. The survey was e-mailed to 395 CSGNA members and 439 CAG clinical members. The authors believed it was important to include the large number of nurses in the community that work with IBD patients. The survey was also distributed to nurses working within the 'Progress' (AbbVie Corporation, USA [n=47]) and 'BioAdvance' (Janssen Inc, USA [n=75]) patient support programs. The Progress and BioAdvance programs offer support and care to patients receiving biologic therapy. The authors invited known IBD nurse specialists from across the country to assist in disseminating the survey to GI nurses. The authors also connected with nursing colleagues from past nursing conferences, nursing advisory board meetings and research investigator meetings.

The survey was administered online and remained open for an extended period of time to ensure and encourage participation, particularly from those in the patient-support programs. It concluded at the end of January 2013.

The study cohort was characterized using standard descriptive statistics. χ^2 tests were used to determine the association between job titles and the categorical variables. For continuous variables, ANOVA was used to test for differences among the nursing groups. Statistical analysis was performed using SAS statistical software version 9.1 (SAS Institute Inc, USA). All tests were two-tailed and P<0.05 was considered to be statistically significant.

RESULTS

Demographics

The survey generated feedback from 275 nurses. Of those surveyed, with the exception of Nunavut and the Northwest Territories, 44% (n=121) of nurses were employed in Ontario, followed by 19.6% (n=54) in Alberta and 9.1% (n=25) in British Columbia (Figure 1).

Of the 275 respondents, 98.2% were female; among them, 68.7% were employed in full-time positions and the remainder in part-time positions. Of the part-time nurses surveyed, 19.8% worked <35 h per week and, of these, 8.3% worked <20 h per week. Two per cent of nurses were working 'casual' hours or <10 h per week. Of the nurses surveyed, 53.8% were diploma-prepared RNs, 35.3% were Baccalaureate-prepared nurses and 4.4% were Masters-prepared nurses.

Overall, 5.8% of nurses surveyed were between 21 and 30 years of age; 13.1% were between 31 and 40; 32.4% were between 41 and 50; 42.5% were between 51 and 60; and 6.2% were between 61 and 70. Slightly more than 63% of the nurses surveyed had >25 years of nursing experience.

Nursing role and geographical variation

Of the 275 GI nurses surveyed, 90% reported that they worked with IBD patients; however, only 79 (28.7%) indicated that their primary nursing role was in IBD care (Figure 1). The proportion of primary nursing role in IBD care showed significant variation across the provinces (from 20% to 100%; P=0.0045). The job titles of nurses also showed a significant variation among the provinces (P<0.0001) (Table 1).

IBD nursing services

A total of 118 nurses were identified as working in endoscopy units. Although this group is essential to nursing care for those with IBD, their roles are well defined and understood within the nursing community; therefore, their responses were removed from this analysis. Of the 79 respondents with a clinical focus in IBD nursing care, results showed that 31.6% worked in inpatient care whereas 67.1% provided outpatient services (Table 2).

Further analysis of nurses who worked primarily in IBD care showed that 79.7% worked with the adult population, 10.1% worked with the pediatric population and 10.1% worked with both adult and pediatric patients with IBD.

Staff RNs and nurse clinicians represented 39% of the IBD nurses identified (Table 2). Of these, 45% provided inpatient care and 90% provided outpatient care. In the outpatient setting, RNs/nurse clinicians provided the largest overall service to IBD patients – most of which was within the telephone advice, rapid access and transition services.

IBD research nurses/coordinators represented 16.5% of respondents. The majority of research coordinators worked predominantly in

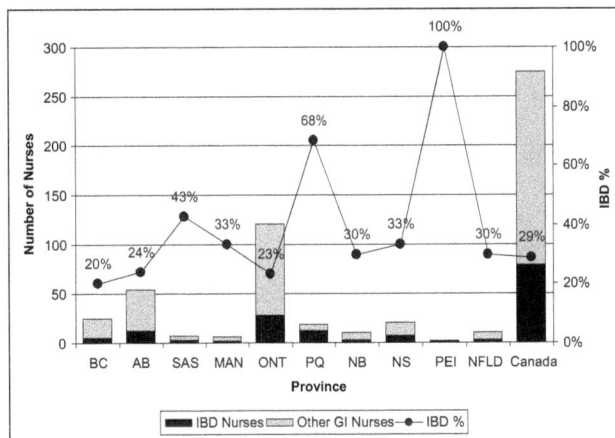

Figure 1) *Geographical distribution of the respondents and their role in inflammatory bowel disease (IBD). AB Alberta; BC British Columbia; GI Gastroenterology; MAN Manitoba; NB New Brunswick; NFLD Newfoundland and Labrador; NS Nova Scotia; ONT Ontario; PEI Prince Edward Island; PQ Quebec; SAS Saskatchewan*

outpatient settings (76.9%, Table 2). In addition to providing clinical care, research nurses are responsible for coordinating clinical research, ensuring participant safety, confirming accuracy of data collection, recording, ongoing maintenance of informed consent and guaranteeing the overall integrity of protocol implementation (11).

The 'other' respondents (13.9%) reported having various titles such as Clinic coordinator, Nurse manager, Endoscopy nurse, Research assistant, Director of clinic services, Nurse endoscopist, Nurse-performed flexible sigmoidoscopy coordinator, Research nurse, Field case manager, Clinical leader and Case manager/coordinator. Almost three-quarters (72.7%) of this group provided biologic services followed by telephone advice (36.4%), rapid access clinic (18.2%) and transition services (27.3%).

All services, including inpatient, outpatient, telephone advice line, rapid access clinics, transition and biologic, are offered within the nursing population but to varying degrees. In assessing the average nursing time devoted to individual services (Table 3), findings showed that most IBD nurses devoted their clinical time to the outpatient setting (39.3%), whereas inpatient care represented only 8.6% of their duties. Nurse clinicians devoted almost one-half of their time (43.9%) to providing telephone advice whereas the remainder of the group devoted just <15%.

DISCUSSION

The overall response rate for the present survey exceeded the authors' expectations by reaching 275 GI nurses across Canada. Results indicated that almost one-half of the nurses were >50 years of age, with 63.6% having >20 years of nursing experience. The majority of respondents (92.7%) worked with IBD patients, yet only 28.7% described IBD as their primary role. The majority of IBD nurses worked

TABLE 1
Job titles of gastroenterology nurses according to province

Job title	Canada (n=275)	BC (n=25)	AB (n=54)	SAS (n=7)	MAN (n=6)	ONT (n=121)	PQ (n=19)	NB (n=10)	NS (n=21)	PEI (n=2)	NFLD (n=10)
Advanced practice nurse	12 (4.4)	2 (8.0)	1 (1.9)	0 (0.0)	0 (0.0)	7 (5.8)	1 (5.3)	0 (0.0)	1 (4.8)	0 (0.0)	0 (0.0)
Nurse clinician	24 (8.7)	4 (16.0)	5 (9.3)	1 (14.3)	0 (0.0)	4 (3.3)	10 (52.6)	0 (0.0)	0 (0.0)	0 (0.0)	0 (0.0)
Staff nurse	145 (52.7)	18 (72.0)	29 (53.7)	5 (71.4)	2 (33.3)	67 (55.4)	2 (10.5)	3 (30.0)	11 (52.4)	1 (50.0)	7 (70.0)
Research coordinator	15 (5.5)	0 (0.0)	2 (3.7)	0 (0.0)	2 (33.3)	8 (6.6)	2 (10.5)	0 (0.0)	1 (4.8)	0 (0.0)	0 (0.0)
LPN/RPN	5 (1.8)	0 (0.0)	4 (7.4)	0 (0.0)	0 (0.0)	0 (0.0)	0 (0.0)	0 (0.0)	1 (4.8)	0 (0.0)	0 (0.0)
BioAdvance*/Progress† coordinator	32 (11.6)	1 (4.0)	6 (11.1)	1 (14.3)	0 (0.0)	17 (14.0)	2 (10.5)	1 (10.0)	3 (14.3)	1 (50.0)	0 (0.0)
Other	42 (15.3)	0 (0.0)	7 (13.0)	0 (0.0)	2 (33.3)	18 (14.9)	2 (10.5)	6 (60.0)	4 (19.0)	0 (0.0)	3 (30.0)

*Data presented as n (%). *Janssen Inc, USA; †AbbVie Corporation, USA. AB Alberta; BC British Columbia; LPN Licenced practical nurse; MAN Manitoba; NB New Brunswick; NFLD Newfoundland and Labrador; NS Nova Scotia; ONT Ontario; PEI Prince Edward Island; PQ Quebec; RPN Registered practical nurse; SAS Saskatchewan*

TABLE 2
Nursing services provided by those who indicated inflammatory bowel disease care was their primary nursing role

Nursing service	Overall (n=79)	Advanced practice nurse (n=5)	Nurse clinician (n=13)	Staff nurse (n=18)	Research coordinator (n=13)	BioAdvance*/ Progress† coordinator (n=19)	Other (n=11)
Inpatient care	25 (31.6)	2 (40.0)	8 (61.5)	6 (33.3)	4 (30.8)	0 (0.0)	5 (45.5)
Outpatient care	53 (67.1)	5 (100.0)	13 (100.0)	15 (83.3)	10 (76.9)	4 (21.1)	6 (54.5)
Telephone advice line	31 (39.2)	4 (80.0)	13 (100.0)	4 (22.2)	2 (15.4)	4 (21.1)	4 (36.4)
Rapid access clinic	19 (24.1)	4 (80.0)	6 (46.2)	3 (16.7)	2 (15.4)	2 (10.5)	2 (18.2)
Transitional care service	19 (24.1)	4 (80.0)	5 (38.5)	4 (22.2)	1 (7.7)	2 (10.5)	3 (27.3)
Management of biological service	44 (55.7)	2 (40.0)	4 (30.8)	8 (44.4)	3 (23.1)	19 (100.0)	8 (72.7)

Data presented as n (%). *Janssen Inc, USA; †AbbVie Corporation, USA

TABLE 3
Average time devoted to services

Nursing service	Overall (n=79)	Advanced practice nurse (n=5)	Nurse clinician (n=13)	Staff nurse (n=18)	Research coordinator (n=13)	BioAdvance*/ Progress† coordinator (n=19)	Other (n=11)	P‡
Inpatient care	8.6	10.0	3.5	15.9	10.4	0.0	15.0	0.1624
Outpatient care	39.3	58.0	41.5	54.6	63.9	12.8	21.4	0.0001
Telephone advice line	15.7	14.0	43.9	11.2	3.2	10.6	12.3	<0.0001
Rapid access clinic	4.3	10.0	12.7	2.1	2.1	1.1	2.7	0.1244
Transitional care service	3.6	4.0	5.0	5.1	0.8	3.1	3.2	0.8766
Management of biological service	30.1	4.0	5.0	21.2	4.2	71.9	45.5	<0.0001

Data presented as % unless otherwise indicated. *Janssen Inc, USA; †AbbVie Corporation, USA; ‡ANOVA test

with adults in the outpatient setting but services including inpatient care, telephone advice line, rapid access clinics, transition and biologic were offered. The exact depth of care and service provided is unclear and requires further investigation. There was variation among job titles in those surveyed. Variability existed even among similar roles such as in research nurse/research coordinator. The survey results also revealed that many respondents have multiple roles and responsibilities including managerial, nurse endoscopist, reimbursement specialist, infusion clinic coordinator, endoscopy nurse and enterostomal therapist. Along with GI nursing, some nurses also worked outside of GI in cardiology, internal medicine, oncology, dermatology and nephrology. They also treated patients with gastrointestinal illnesses other than IBD including hepatology, colorectal cancer screening and management, celiac disease and gastroesophagel reflux disease.

IBD is a chronic condition and resources are needed for high-quality management. The Crohn's and Colitis Foundation of Canada report identified several challenges facing the IBD community (10). Social awareness of IBD, access to IBD specialists and timely access for consultation, diagnosis, treatment and therapy were discussed in the 2012 *Impact of Inflammatory Bowel Disease in Canada* report (10). The report found that both new and long-standing IBD patients endure long wait times for consultation, investigations and therapy. In addition, there exists a decline in the number of gastroenterologists in Canada with a greater number of specialists approaching retirement. This concern also impacts nursing in Canada, with current pressures on the nursing workforce that include increased workloads, shortage in full-time nursing positions and, as the present study shows, an aging nursing population close to retirement. These data support the concern that the average age of nurses in Canada is increasing and it is critical to consider a succession plan.

Historically, nurses have been an important part of the multidisciplinary approach to IBD management. Nurses have been shown to provide consistent, high-quality care, improve continuity in patient care and act as the liaison between specialists, primary care providers and those within the multidisciplinary team. Nurses are relied on to provide patient education, counselling, and physical and emotional support.

A challenge for IBD nurses in Canada is to provide evidence supporting the relevance of their role in caring for IBD patients. The degree to which nurses impact IBD-specific patient outcomes requires further exploration. Nurses are in a unique position to measure hospital admission rates, emergency department visits, surgical rates, complication rates, medication compliance and patient quality of life. Although this is important for patient care, it will also contribute to the validation of nursing roles in IBD management and for estimates of health human resource requirements.

With the existing challenges facing IBD patients and their health care providers, the concept of 'nurse-led' IBD clinics needs to be explored and documented in greater detail. IBD nurse specialists, in collaboration with their IBD physician counterpart, could reduce wait times for consultation, diagnosis and initiation of therapy. Unlike in the UK, services such as telephone helplines, outpatient clinics, biologic and immunosuppression services, rapid access clinic and transitional care services are not widely available throughout Canada. With ongoing growth and expansion of the nurse specialist role in IBD in Canada, further development of these services could be possible. With additional investment in IBD nursing resources, the potential for shorter wait times, reductions in emergency department visits, decreased length of inpatient stay, increased patient quality of life and decreased complication rates may also be achievable. This approach has been implemented and is effective in many other disease states such as diabetes and hypertension (10). Although the aim of many nursing initiatives is to improve patient outcomes, there is limited quality research on the extent of nursing's influence on IBD health outcomes.

The survey also provided each respondent with an opportunity to provide comments regarding the questionnaire and their professional needs. Many nurses suggested that additional support and mentoring is needed for novice IBD nurses in Canada. Further development and expansion of IBD nursing roles was addressed, along with the need for learning opportunities and networking with other nurses. There was interest expressed in developing a national IBD Nurses Interest Group as a forum to address these needs.

The present survey provided insight into the numbers of Canadian nurses impacting the care of IBD patients, and the demographics of

IBD nurses including age, sex, years of nursing experience, educational preparation, employment setting and scope of practice. As a result of this exercise, several additional questions have been identified. Further exploration into specific nursing services in Canada, educational preparation, scope of nursing practice, nursing responsibilities and the educational needs of IBD nurses in Canada is still required.

Limitations to the present study were identified. The response rate was not calculated because distribution numbers were unclear. The survey was distributed through several organizations. The authors reached out to nurses through gastroenterologists and members of the CAG, CSGNA, BioAdvance and Progress. The authors relied on these individuals to distribute the survey to nurses who may not have been part of the initial distribution group. There is a possibility that relevant nurses were missed and did not receive the survey. In addition, the survey used was not validated. It was presented in English and was not available in French for Quebec colleagues. There appeared to be confusion regarding job title description in some of the surveys submitted. Definitions of 'Nurse clinician' and 'Staff nurse' (endoscopy, ward, outpatient clinic, community physician offices) may have been helpful for respondents. Definitions regarding services, such as 'transition' and 'biologic', may have been helpful to those who may not be familiar with these programs.

ACKNOWLEDGEMENTS: The authors thank Dr Jiming Fang, biostatistical consultant in Toronto, Ontario, who provided statistical assistance and suggestions for this study.

REFERENCES

1. Marin L, Torrejon A, Oltra L, et al. Nursing resources and responsibilities according to hospital organizational model for management of inflammatory bowel disease in Spain. J Crohns Colitis 2011;5:211-7.
2. Randell RL, Long MD, Martin CF, et al. Patient perception of chronic illness care in a large inflammatory bowel disease cohort. Inflamm Bowel Dis 2013;19:1428-33.
3. Sack C, Phan VA, Grafton R, et al. A chronic care model significantly decreases costs and healthcare utilisation in patients with inflammatory bowel disease. J Crohns Colitis 2012;6:302-10.
4. Canadian Nurses Association. Effectiveness of Registered Nurses and Nurse Practitioners in Supporting Chronic Disease Self-Management March 2012. Ottawa: Canadian Nurses Association.
5. College of Nurses of Ontario. Practice Standard: Professional Standards, Revised June 2009. Toronto: College of Nurses of Ontario.
6. Hamric AB, Spross JA The Clinical Nurse Specialist in Theory and Practice. Philadelphia: Saunders, 1989: 466.
7. Nightingale AJ, Middleton W, Middleton SJ, Hunter JO. Evaluation of the effectiveness of a specialist nurse in the management of inflammatory bowel disease (IBD). Eur J Gastroenterol Hepatol 2000;12:967-73.
8. Hernandez-Sampelayo P, Seoane M, Oltra L, et al. Contribution of nurses to the quality of care in management of inflammatory bowel disease: A synthesis of the evidence. J Crohns Colitis 2010;4:611-22.
9. Mason I, Holbrook K, Kemp K, Garrick V, Johns K, Kane M. Inflammatory bowel disease nursing: Results of an audit exploring the roles, responsibilities and activity of nurses with specialist/advanced roles. London: Royal College of Nursing.
10. Crohn's and Colitis Foundation of Canada. Impact of Inflammatory Bowel Disease in Canada 2012. Toronto: Crohn's and Colitis Foundation of Canada.
11. Hastings C. Clinical Research Nursing. <http://clinicalcenter.nih.gov/nursing/crn/crn_2010.html> (2010) (Accessed August 15, 2013).

17

Timing of rebleeding in high-risk peptic ulcer bleeding after successful hemostasis: A systematic review

Sara El Ouali MD[1], Alan N Barkun MD MSc[1,2], Myriam Martel BSc[1], Davide Maggio MD[1]

S El Ouali, AN Barkun, M Martel, D Maggio. Timing of rebleeding in high-risk peptic ulcer bleeding after successful hemostasis: A systematic review. Can J Gastroenterol Hepatol 2014;28(10):543-548.

BACKGROUND: Peptic ulcer rebleeding (PUR) usually occurs within three days following endoscopic hemostasis. However, recent data have increasingly suggested delayed rebleeding.
OBJECTIVE: To better characterize the timing of PUR (Forrest Ia to IIb) following initially successful endoscopic hemostasis.
METHODS: An exhaustive literature search (1989 to 2013), with cross-referencing, was performed to identify pertinent randomized controlled trial (RCT) arms. Patients receiving high-dose proton pump inhibitor (PPI) infusion following successful modern-day endoscopic hemostasis were included. A sensitivity analysis included any patients receiving PPI doses >40 mg daily. The main outcome measure was 30-day rebleeding, while weighted mean averages at t = three, seven, 14 and 28 to 30 days are also reported.
RESULTS: Of 756 citations, six RCTs were included (561 patients; 58.5% to 89.5% male; 55.3 to 67.5 years of age). Among patients receiving high-dose PPI (five RCTs [393 patients]), 11.5% (95% CI 8.4% to 14.7%) experienced rebleeding, 55.6% (95% CI 41.1% to 70.1%) rebled within three days, 20% (95% CI 8.3% to 31.7%) between four and seven days, 17.8% (95% CI 6.6% to 28.9%) at eight to 14 days, and 6.7% (95% CI 0% to 14%) at 15 to 28 to 30 days. Using the relaxed lower PPI dosing threshold, similar respective rates were 14.4% (95% CI 11.5% to 17.3%) overall, with interval rates of 39.5% (95% CI 28.9% to 50.15%), 34.6% (95% CI 24.2% to 44.9%), 19.7% (95% CI 11% to 28.4%) and 6.2% (95% CI 0.95% to 11.5%). Qualitative review of patient characteristics, limited by small sample size, possible bias and study heterogeneity, suggested increased patient comorbidity and postendoscopic use of lower PPI dosing may predict delayed rebleeding.
CONCLUSION: In patients with high-risk PUR undergoing successful endoscopic hemostasis, most rebled within three days, with many experiencing later rebleeding. Additional research is needed to better predict such an outcome.

Key Words: Endoscopic therapy; High-risk stigmata; Peptic ulcer bleeding; Rebleeding; Timing

Le moment de la reprise du saignement d'un ulcère gastroduodénal à haut risque après une hémostase réussie : une analyse systématique

HISTORIQUE : La reprise du saignement d'un ulcère gastroduodénal (RSUG) se produit généralement dans les trois jours suivant l'hémostase endoscopique. Cependant, des données récentes indiquent de plus en plus une reprise tardive du saignement.
OBJECTIF : Mieux caractériser le moment de la RSUG (Forrest Ia à IIb) après une hémostase endoscopique d'abord réussie.
MÉTHODOLOGIE : Les chercheurs ont procédé à une analyse bibliographique complète (de 1989 à 2013) avec référencement pour extraire les essais aléatoires et contrôlés pertinents (EAC). Étaient inclus les patients qui recevaient une infusion d'un inhibiteur de la pompe à protons (IPP) à forte dose après une hémostase endoscopique moderne réussie. L'analyse de sensibilité incluait tous les patients ayant reçu une dose quotidienne d'IPP supérieure à 40 mg. La principale mesure d'issue était une reprise du saignement dans les 30 jours, tandis que les moyennes pondérées à t=trois, sept, 14 et 28 à 30 jours étaient également précisées.
RÉSULTATS : Six EAC faisaient partie des 756 articles (561 patients; 58,5 % à 89,5 % d'hommes; 55,3 à 67,5 ans). Chez les patients qui avaient reçu un IPP à forte dose (cinq EAC [393 patients]), 11,5 % (95 % IC 8,4 % à 14,7 %) ont subi une reprise des saignements, 55,6 % (95 % IC 41,1 % à 70,1 %) se sont remis à saigner dans les trois jours, 20 % (95 % IC 8,3 % à 31,7 %) au bout de quatre à sept jours, 17,8 % (95 % IC 6,6 % à 28,9 %) au bout de huit à 14 jours, et 6,7 % (95 % IC 0 % à 14 %) au bout de 15 à entre 28 et 30 jours. Selon un seuil posologique rabaissé d'IPP, les taux similaires respectifs étaient de 14,4 % (95 % IC 11,5 % à 17,3 %) dans l'ensemble, selon des taux d'intervalle de 39,5 % (95 % IC 28,9 % à 50,15 %), 34,6 % (95 % IC 24,2 % à 44,9 %), 19,7 % (95 % IC 11 % à 28,4 %) et 6,2 % (95 % IC 0,95 % à 11,5 %). Une analyse qualitative des caractéristiques des patients, limitée par la petite taille de l'échantillon, les biais possibles et l'hétérogénéité des études, a laissé supposer qu'une comorbidité accrue des patients et une utilisation postendoscopique de posologies d'IPP plus faibles peuvent être prédictives d'une reprise tardive du saignement.
CONCLUSION : La plupart des patients très vulnérables à une RSUG qui subissent une hémostase endoscopique réussie se remettent à saigner dans les trois jours, et bon nombre présentent une reprise tardive du saignement. D'autres recherches s'imposent pour mieux prédire un tel résultat.

Acute upper gastrointestinal bleeding accounts for >400,000 hospitalizations per year in the United States, with the majority of cases being nonvariceal in origin. Peptic ulcer bleeding accounts for most cases of nonvariceal upper gastrointestinal bleeding and is a major cause of morbidity and mortality (1,2). Recent advances in endoscopic hemostatic techniques and the use of high-dose intravenous (IV) proton pump inhibitors (PPIs) have been shown to improve outcomes in peptic ulcer bleeding (3). However, approximately 11% to 16% of patients with ulcers with high-risk stigmata (Forrest Ia to IIb) rebled after initial endoscopic hemostasis, with most rebleeding reported to occur in the first 72 h (4-6).

The finding that most rebleeding occurs within the first three days is supported by several studies in which endoscopic follow-up of Forrest Ia to IIb ulcers showed healing with a clean base by day 3 to 4 (7-11); however, most of these older studies excluded patients with comorbidities, or patients on anticoagulants or nonsteroidal anti-inflammatory drugs (NSAIDs), which is not reflective of a contemporary patient population (7,9,11). In addition to these landmark studies, most of the current data on peptic ulcer rebleeding are derived from trials using endoscopic hemostatic techniques or pharmacological therapies that are not consistent with current recommendations, with use of epinephrine injection alone, low PPI doses or

Divisions of ¹Gastroenterology and ²Clinical Epidemiology, McGill University, Montreal, Quebec
Correspondence: Dr Alan N Barkun, Division of Gastroenterology, The McGill University Health Centre, Montreal General Hospital site, 1650 Cedar Avenue, Room D7-346, Montreal, Quebec H3G 1A4. e-mail alan.barkun@muhc.mcgill.ca

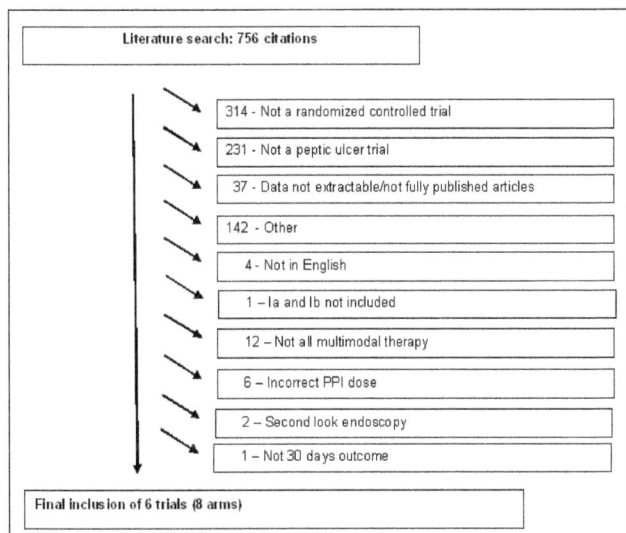

Figure 1) *STROBE (STrengthening the Reporting of OBservational studies in Epidemiology) diagram. PPI Proton pump inhibitor*

no PPI pharmacotherapy. In fact, more recent data from randomized trials suggest higher rates of rebleeding after three days (12-18).

The timing of rebleeding in the era of high-dose PPI and modern-day endoscopic therapy thus remains unclear. In the context of increasing health care costs and pressure to discharge patients sooner, with many centres not tightly adhering to guidelines (19,20), it is particularly important to clarify the timing of rebleeding.

The aim of the present systematic review was, accordingly, to examine the timing of peptic ulcer rebleeding in patients who exhibited high-risk stigmata having received recommended contemporary endoscopic and pharmacological therapies.

METHODS
Search strategy
A comprehensive computerized medical literature search was performed using the MEDLINE, EMBASE, Cochrane library and ISI Web of Knowledge databases from 1989 to September 2013. A highly sensitive search strategy was used to identify randomized controlled trials with a combination of controlled vocabulary and text words related to "upper gastrointestinal bleeding", "endoscopic therapy" and "PPIs". In addition, recursive searches and cross-referencing were performed; manual searches of articles identified after the initial search were also conducted.

Study selection
All human, adult studies published in French or English were considered. All randomized controlled trials were included if the study population fulfilled the following criteria: patients with peptic ulcer bleeding exhibiting high-risk stigmata (Forrest Ia to IIb); patients in whom successful initial hemostasis was achieved using contemporary endoscopic hemostatic methods (excluding epinephrine monotherapy), followed by PPIs at a dose >40 mg once daily. In addition, recorded outcomes needed to include rebleeding at different time points, up to 30 days. Any treatment arms of any of the studies not fulfilling these criteria were excluded, as were patients who underwent second-look endoscopy.

Validity assessment and data abstraction
Two reviewers independently identified and examined the relevant studies. A third independent reviewer resolved disagreements on specific studies. The quality of each study was assessed using modified Jadad criteria, in which an additional point was attributed for the description of allocation concealment, a priori sample size estimation, description and number of drop-outs, adequate description of the population selection and characteristics, for a total of 10 points from

the initial five-point score (21). The Cochrane risk-of-bias tool (22) was also used.

Assessment of heterogeneity
Comparative qualitative analyses evaluated the homogeneity of study characteristics, such as patient populations, interventions and outcomes across studies, guiding possible sensitivity analyses.

Statistical heterogeneity was not sought because no inferential calculations were performed as part of the present analysis.

Principal outcome, data synthesis and analysis
Among all trials selected, only the arms satisfying the aforementioned criteria were considered.

Only descriptive data were generated from the present analysis, including patient characteristics and the main outcome of time to rebleeding.

Rebleeding at different time points – three days, seven days, 14 days, and 28 to 30 days – was examined. Weighted averages of rebleeding rates among all included studies were calculated for each time point; 95% CIs were also reported. Additional data pertaining to different patient characteristics and previously recognized predictors of rebleeding were extracted and analyzed. The primary analysis included the assessment of study arms having administered only high-dose IV PPI (80 mg bolus followed by 8 mg/h for three days); a planned sensitivity analysis examined studies including any dose of PPI >40 mg daily.

All statistical analyses were performed using SAS version 9.2 (SAS Institute Inc, USA).

RESULTS
Study identification
A total of 756 citations were initially identified; reasons for excluding studies are listed in Figure 1. Randomized controlled trials were excluded if epinephrine monotherapy was used in part of the patient population, such as in the study by Sung et al (15). Overall, eight arms from six full-text randomized controlled trials (13,16,18,23-25) were included, yielding a total of 561 patients.

High-dose PPI (80 mg IV bolus followed by 8 mg/h for 72 h) was used in five study arms (13,16,18,23,24), which comprised the primary analysis, yielding a total of 393 patients. The sensitivity analysis included any studies using PPI doses >40 mg (total of the above eight arms).

Study characteristics
Characteristics of the included studies are shown in Table 1 and summarized below.

Study populations: All patients exhibited bleeding gastric or duodenal ulcers demonstrating high-risk stigmata. Most studies used the Forrest classification and included Forrest type Ia to IIb ulcers (Ia: spurting; Ib: oozing; IIa: visible vessel; and IIb: adherent clot). One study classified ulcers according to stigmata of recent hemorrhage (16), either major or minor in type, as described in the study by Yang et al (10). The patients ranged in age from 55.3 to 67.5 years, with 58.5% to 89.5% being male. Active bleeding (Forrest Ia and Ib) occurred in 14.3% patients (18) to up to 53.3% (24). The presence of ≥1 comorbidities ranged from 24.5% of patients (13) to 100% of patients in the study by Cheng et al (16). Hemodynamic instability or shock was recorded in four of six studies. It ranged from 13.3% (24) to up to 46.8% of patients in the study by Chiu et al (25). The proportion of patients categorized according to American Society of Anesthesiologists (ASA) scores varied (Table 1). The use of NSAIDs was recorded in almost all studies and ranged from 18% (13) to up to 57.9% (18). Mean (± SD) ulcer size ranged from to 0.9±0.5 cm (25) to 1.4±1.2 cm (18).

Outcome definition
The definition of rebleeding was similar among all studies. Rebleeding was defined clinically according to different parameters, including the presence of melena, hematemesis or fresh blood in the nasogastric

TABLE 1
Study characteristics

Characteristic	Chen et al (23), 2012	Chiu et al (25), 2003 (low-dose PPI)*	Lau et al (24), 2000	Cheng et al (16), 2005	Cheng et al (16), 2005 (low-dose PPI)	Zargar et al (13), 2006	Choi et al (18), 2009	Choi et al (18), 2009 (low-dose PPI)
				Author (reference), year				
Forrest classification	Ia to IIa	Ia to IIb	Ia to IIa	SRH, Major	SRH, Major	Ia to IIa	Ia to IIb	Ia to IIb
Study period	January 2008 to August 2010	August 1999 to January 2001	May 1998 to July 1999	January 2001 to April 2003	January 2001 to April 2003	January 2001 to August 2003	May 2004 to April 2008	May 2004 to April 2008
n in arm	100	100	120	52	53	102	19	21
ASA score (1 to 5)	1 or 2: 65% 3: 26% 4: 8%	1: 43% 2: 37% 3: 15% 4: 1%	1 or 2: 58.3% 3: 26.7% 4: 15%	2: 7% 3: 26% 4: 19% 5: 1%	2: 4% 3: 29% 4: 19% 5: 0%	N/A	N/A	N/A
Hemodynamic Instability, %	28.00	46.80	13.30	N/A	N/A	27.50	N/A	N/A
Comorbid illness, %	N/A	69.10	25	100	100	24.5	42.1	47.60
Active bleeding, %	42.00	49	53.3	N/A	N/A	36.3	31.6	14.3
Ulcer size, cm, mean ± SD	1.09±0.54	0.9±0.5	1.2±1.1	1.2±0.8	1.2±1	1.2±0.8	1.4±1.2	1.4±0.8
Duodenal ulcer, %	47.00	57.00	54.20	36.50	37.70	82.40	57.90	38.10
Gastric ulcer, %	53.00	43.00	44.00	53.80	54.70	17.60	42.10	61.90
Endoscopic treatment	Epinephrine injection + heater probe	Epinephrine injection + heater probe	Epinephrine injection + heater probe	Epinephrine injection + heater probe	Epinephrine injection + heater probe	Epinephrine injection + heater probe	Epinephrine injection + APC or hemoclips	Epinephrine injection + APC or hemoclips
Pharmacological treatment	Pantoprazole 80 mg IV bolus then 8 mg/h × 72 h	Omeprazole 40 mg IV BID × 3 days	Omeprazole 80 mg IV bolus then 8 mg/h × 72 h	Omeprazole 80 mg IV bolus then 200 mg/day × 72 h	Omeprazole 80 mg IV bolus then 80 mg/day × 72 h	Pantoprazole 80 mg IV bolus then 8 mg/h × 72 h	Pantoprazole 80 mg IV bolus then 8 mg/h × 72 h	Pantoprazole 40 mg IV bolus then 4 mg/h × 72 h
NSAID use, %	39	6.4[†]	32.5	25	22.60	18	57.90	57.10
Age, years, mean ± SD	65.5 (15)	67.5 (12.6)	64 (17.2)	62.5 (12.5)	65.8 (13.8)	55.3 (9.2)	61 (16.5)	57.4 (14.5)
Sex, male/female, %/%	79/21	66/34	66.7/33.3	69.2/30.8	58.5/41.5	68.6/31.4	89.5/10.5	85.7/14.3
Modified Jadad score	9	6	8	6	6	10	6	6

*No second-look endoscopy arm; †Only acetylsalicylic acid use reported. APC Argon plasma coagulation; ASA American Association of Anesthesiologists; BID Twice per day; IV Intravenous; N/A Not applicable; NSAID Nonsteroidal anti-inflammatory drug; PPI Proton pump inhibitor; SRH Stigmata of recent hemorrhage

tube, a change in vital signs (systolic blood pressure <90 mmHg, heart rate >100 beats/min to 110 beats/min), drop in hemoglobin level, or sudden increase in transfusion requirements. Following clinical suspicion, rebleeding was then confirmed on endoscopy.

Performance of endoscopy and adjuvant therapy
Initial endoscopy was performed within 24 h of admission in all studies. In five of the six trials, endoscopic therapy involved epinephrine injection combined with thermocoagulation. In the study by Choi et al (18), epinephrine was used in addition to argon plasma coagulation and/or application of hemoclips.

Different PPI regimens were used among the studies with lower PPI dosing. One arm of the trial by Choi et al (18) used pantoprazole 40 mg IV bolus followed by 4 mg/h for 72 h (18). One arm of the study by Cheng et al (25) used omeprazole 80 mg IV bolus followed by 80 mg infusion per day for three days, and Chiu et al (16) used omeprazole 40 mg IV twice daily for three days (25).

One-half of the trials used pantoprazole (13,18,23), while the other one-half used omeprazole (16,24,25).

Study quality
The quality of studies on the modified Jadad score varied from 6 to 10 points (Table 1), with a mean of 7.5±1.8. The Cochrane risk-of-bias tool revealed overall low bias with a potential of bias for Choi et al (18) and Chen et al (23), in which the treatment allocation was not blinded (Figure 2).

Primary analysis: rebleeding in patients receiving high-dose PPIs
Among the 393 patients receiving high-dose PPI, 45 rebled within the first 30 days, corresponding an overall rate of rebleeding of 11.5%

(95% CI 8.4% to14.7%). The rebleeding rate, broken down according to time following initial endoscopic hemostasis, is shown in Figure 3, with 55.6% rebleeding occurring within the first three days.

Sensitivity analysis: rebleeding in patients receiving PPI doses >40 mg once daily
When including all patients receiving PPI at a dose >40 mg once daily, 81 of 561 patients rebled at 30 days, corresponding to an overall rebleeding rate of 14.4% (95% CI 11.5% to 17.3%). In this broader patient population, among those who rebled, 39.5% (95% CI 28.9% to 50.15%) did so within three days.

Of note, in the study by Cheng at al (16), rebleeding rates showed a different trend. In the high-dose PPI arm, the overall rebleeding rate was 40.4% at 30 days. Among the patients who rebled, 38.1% did so by day 3, 14.3% between days 4 and 7, 38.1% between seven and 14 days, and 9.5% between day 14 and 28 to 30. An exploratory a posteriori sensitivity analysis was subsequently performed. When excluding this study, the rebleeding rate among studies using high-dose PPI at day 3 was 70.8%, 25% between days 4 and 7, and 4.2% between day 15 and 28 to 30. Among studies using all PPI doses, rebleeding was 48.6%, 48.6% and 2.7% at day 3, between days 4 to 7, and between day 14 and 28 to 30, respectively.

DISCUSSION
The timing of rebleeding after endoscopic hemostasis in peptic ulcer bleeding remains unclear in the era of high-dose PPI and contemporary endoscopic therapy. Most of the current data regarding the timing of peptic ulcer rebleeding are obtained from studies using endoscopic hemostatic techniques and pharmacological therapies that are not

Figure 2) *Risk of bias summary*

Figure 3) *Rebleeding rates at different time points in patients receiving high-dose proton pump inhibitors (95% CIs represented by vertical lines)*

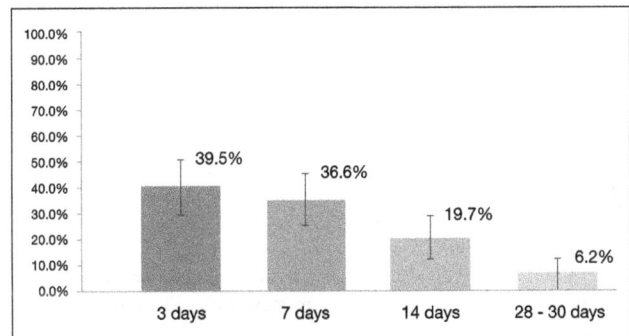

Figure 4) *Rebleeding rates at different time points in patients receiving lower doses of proton pump inhibitors*

consistent with current recommendations, with no PPI pharmacotherapy or low PPI doses, as well as epinephrine injection alone.

The finding that most rebleeding occurs within the first three days is also supported by several landmark studies in which endoscopic follow-up of ulcers showed healing with a clean base by day 3 to 4; however, most of these older studies excluded patients on NSAIDs or anticoagulants, and patients with any comorbidities, which is not reflective of a contemporary patient population (7,9,11).

The aim of the present systematic review was, thus, to better examine the timing of peptic ulcer rebleeding in patients exhibiting high-risk stigmata who received recommended contemporary endoscopic and pharmacological therapies.

Our primary analysis evaluated studies using high-dose PPI infusion. Among patients who rebled, 55.6% did so within three days. This is higher than what has been reported in the literature, with rebleeding rates of up to 95% in the first three days (7,8,11,26).

When analyzing rebleeding rates among the included studies, the study by Cheng et al (16) appears to stand out, demonstrating different trends in rebleeding with an overall high rate of rebleeding of 40.4%. Furthermore, among patients who rebled, only 38.1% did so by day 3. When excluding this outlier study, 70.8% of patients rebled by day 3, which is more consistent with rates reported in the literature.

We closely examined the study by Cheng et al (16) to better understand the difference in rebleeding trends reported in this trial. In this study, patients had to have at least one comorbidity to be included. In other words, 100% of their patients had at least one other coexisting illness, which is higher than all other included studies that enrolled

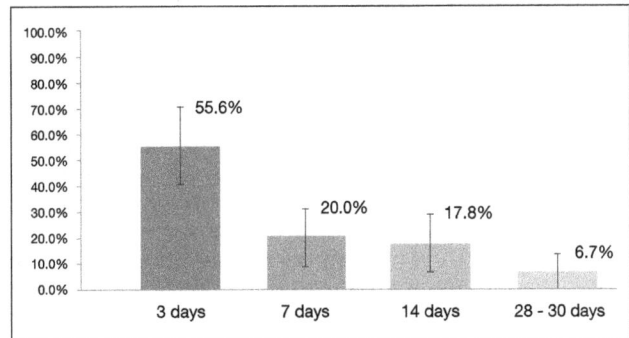

patient populations without comorbidities in proportions of up to 75%. Furthermore, in the study by Cheng et al (16), up to 48.1% had ≥2 comorbidities. Although they did not report the rates of hemodynamic instability or shock, 48% of their patients had an ASA score ≥3, demonstrating a sicker patient profile than all other included studies. When including all studies using PPI doses >40 mg daily, only 39.5% of patients who rebled did so within the first 72 h, with the remainder rebleeding mostly between days 4 and 7. When excluding the 'outlier' study by Cheng et al (16), the trend toward increased delayed rebleeding persisted, with 51.3% of patients rebleeding after the three-day period, including 48.6% bleeding by day 7.

To determine why most patients rebled after the three-day period in the lower-dose PPI analysis, we performed an explorative qualitative review, comparing patient characteristics among the included studies. Unfortunately, no patient-level data were available. However, on qualitatively reviewing the data, several factors appeared to be possibly associated with delayed rebleeding.

First, higher rates of delayed rebleeding were found when including studies using PPIs at lower doses, which suggests that PPI dosing may not only affect rebleeding rates, as it is already established, but may also impact the timing of rebleeding. Interestingly, a recently published RCT demonstrated decreased rates of delayed peptic ulcer rebleeding among high-risk patients receiving a prolonged 11-day course of twice daily PPI dosing (27).

In addition to lower PPI doses, the presence of coexisting illness may also impact the timing of rebleeding. Among the included studies, trials enrolling patients with higher rates of comorbidities appear to demonstrate delayed rebleeding. Cheng et al (16), as described above, included all patients with at least one comorbidity and had higher rates of delayed rebleeding. Another included study, by Chiu et al (25), had patients with high rates of comorbidities (up to 69.1%). Rebleeding was also delayed in this trial, with most patients rebleeding between days 4 and 7. Choi et al (18) included up to 47.6% of patients with comorbidities (up to 42.1% in the high-dose PPI arm). In these arms, the only patient who rebled did so on day 6 – after the 72 h period.

The presence of comorbidities as a factor leading to increased rebleeding and mortality has been demonstrated in the literature (3,28-30); however, its association with delayed rebleeding had not yet been shown. In the present systematic review, no data could be extracted regarding the different types of comorbidities because most studies reported these without further categorization according to system. Cheng et al (16) identified the presence of hypoalbuminemia (albumin <30 g/L) as well as having ≥2 comorbidities as associated with a higher trend of rebleeding between days 4 and 14 in univariable analysis. End-stage renal disease (ESRD) was also associated, but with more delayed rebleeding. Only ESRD was significantly increased among patients who rebled between days 15 to 28 in multivariable analysis.

Patients with renal disease and ESRD are not only at increased risk for upper gastrointestinal bleeding (31), but also appear to have worse outcomes related to peptic ulcer bleeding. Patients with ESRD exhibit higher rates of rebleeding (up to 40.6% in study by Cheung et al [32]), as well as increased delayed rebleeding (beyond seven days) (16,33). ESRD has also been associated with increased long-term peptic ulcer rebleeding (34).

Patients with ESRD may be at higher risk for peptic ulcer rebleeding due to multiple factors, mainly bleeding diathesis. This is believed to be due to platelet dysfunction in the context of uremia, as well as impaired platelet-vessel wall interaction (35). Dialysis may also contribute to increased bleeding through exposure to heparin as well as through continuous platelet activation, due to interaction of blood with artificial surfaces (35,36).

In addition, ESRD is associated with lower albumin levels and poor nutrition, thereby possibly leading to slower ulcer healing and, perhaps, a greater risk of rebleeding (33). The impact of gastric acid secretion remains unclear because it has been shown to be increased in some studies, and decreased or normal in others (33,37).

Hemodynamic instability and higher ASA scores have also been shown in the literature to be associated with higher rates of rebleeding and overall poorer prognosis (3,38-40).

Interestingly, in the present analysis, studies demonstrating higher rates of delayed rebleeding had higher rates of unstable patients as well as a higher number of patients with an ASA score >3 (16,25). However, hemodynamic instability and ASA score were not systematically recorded in all included studies.

CONCLUSION

The results of the present systematic review appear to demonstrate higher rates of delayed rebleeding when including studies using modern-day endoscopic hemostatic technique as well as intravenous PPI. A qualitative review of patient characteristics from studies exhibiting delayed rebleeding suggests that possible associations may include increased patient comorbidity and use of lower doses of PPI following endoscopic hemostasis, as well as increased hemodynamic instability and higher ASA scores. However, such associations are limited by lack of patient-level data and the limited number of studies available. In addition, there existed significant clinical heterogeneity. Timing of rebleeding among patients receiving modern-day therapy and determinants of delayed rebleeding should be further explored in future research, as this could greatly impact on the outcomes of patients with peptic ulcer bleeding (and perhaps other etiologies) by adapting care to patients at increased risk for delayed rebleeding, through the use of second-look endoscopy, or better adapted follow-up oral PPI dosing.

DISCLOSURES: Dr Alan Barkun is a consultant for Olympus and Takeda Canada; is a speaker for Takeda Canada and AstraZeneca; is on the advisory board for Pendopharm Canada; and received research funding from Boston Scientific and Cook. Dr Sara El Ouali, Ms Myriam Martel and Dr Davide Maggio have no financial disclosures or conflicts of interest to declare.

FUNDING: None.

AUTHOR'S CONTRIBUTIONS: Conception and design: Sara El Ouali, Alan N Barkun, Myriam Martel and Davide Maggio; analysis and interpretation of data: Sara El Ouali, Alan N Barkun, Myriam Martel and Davide Maggio. Drafting of the manuscript: Sara El Ouali, Alan N Barkun, Myriam Martel and Davide Maggio. Critical revision of the article for important intellectual content: Sara El Ouali, Alan N Barkun, Myriam Martel and Davide Maggio. Final approval of the article: Sara El Ouali, Alan N Barkun, Myriam Martel and Davide Maggio.

REFERENCES

1. Garcia-Iglesias P, Villoria A, Suarez D, et al. Meta-analysis: Predictors of rebleeding after endoscopic treatment for bleeding peptic ulcer. Aliment Pharmacol Ther 2011;34:888-900.
2. Gralnek IM, Barkun AN, Bardou M. Management of acute bleeding from a peptic ulcer. N Engl J Med 2008;359:928-37.
3. Barkun AN, Bardou M, Kuipers EJ, et al. International consensus recommendations on the management of patients with nonvariceal upper gastrointestinal bleeding. Ann Intern Med 2010;152:101-13.
4. Barkun A, Sabbah S, Enns R, et al. The Canadian Registry on Nonvariceal Upper Gastrointestinal Bleeding and Endoscopy (RUGBE): Endoscopic hemostasis and proton pump inhibition are associated with improved outcomes in a real-life setting. Am J Gastroenterol 2004;99:1238-46.
5. Peura DA, Lanza FL, Gostout CJ, Foutch PG. The American College of Gastroenterology Bleeding Registry: Preliminary findings. Am J Gastroenterol 1997;92:924-8.
6. Vreeburg EM, Snel P, de Bruijne JW, Bartelsman JF, Rauws EA, Tytgat GN. Acute upper gastrointestinal bleeding in the Amsterdam area: Incidence, diagnosis, and clinical outcome. Am J Gastroenterol 1997;92:236-43.
7. Hsu PI, Lai KH, Lin XZ, et al. When to discharge patients with bleeding peptic ulcers: A prospective study of residual risk of rebleeding. Gastrointest Endosc 1996;44:382-7.
8. Hsu PI, Lin XZ, Chan SH, et al. Bleeding peptic ulcer – risk factors for rebleeding and sequential changes in endoscopic findings. Gut 1994;35:746-9.
9. Lau JY, Chung SC, Leung JW, Lo KK, Yung MY, Li AK. The evolution of stigmata of hemorrhage in bleeding peptic ulcers: A sequential endoscopic study. Endoscopy 1998;30:513-8.
10. Yang CC, Shin JS, Lin XZ, Hsu PI, Chen KW, Lin CY. The natural history (fading time) of stigmata of recent hemorrhage in peptic ulcer disease. Gastrointest Endosc 1994;40:562-6.
11. Lin HJ, Perng CL, Lee FY, Lee CH, Lee SD. Clinical courses and predictors for rebleeding in patients with peptic ulcers and non-bleeding visible vessels: A prospective study. Gut 1994;35:1389-93.
12. Laine L, Jensen DM. Management of patients with ulcer bleeding. Am J Gastroenterol 2012;107:345-60.
13. Zargar SA, Javid G, Khan BA, et al. Pantoprazole infusion as adjuvant therapy to endoscopic treatment in patients with peptic ulcer bleeding: Prospective randomized controlled trial. J Gastroenterol Hepatol 2006;21:716-21.
14. Jensen DM, Pace SC, Soffer E, Comer GM, Study G. Continuous infusion of pantoprazole versus ranitidine for prevention of ulcer rebleeding: A U.S. multicenter randomized, double-blind study. Am J Gastroenterol 2006;101:1991-9.
15. Sung JJ, Barkun A, Kuipers EJ, et al. Intravenous esomeprazole for prevention of recurrent peptic ulcer bleeding: A randomized trial. Ann Intern Med 2009;150:455-64.
16. Cheng HC, Kao AW, Chuang CH, Sheu BS. The efficacy of high- and low-dose intravenous omeprazole in preventing rebleeding for patients with bleeding peptic ulcers and comorbid illnesses. Dig Dis Sci 2005;50:1194-201.
17. Chiu PW, Lam CY, Lee SW, et al. Effect of scheduled second therapeutic endoscopy on peptic ulcer rebleeding: A prospective randomised trial. Gut 2003;52:1403-7.
18. Choi KD, Kim N, Jang IJ, et al. Optimal dose of intravenous pantoprazole in patients with peptic ulcer bleeding requiring endoscopic hemostasis in Korea. J Gastroenterol Hepatol 2009;24:1617-24.

19. Barkun AN, Bhat M, Armstrong D, et al. Effectiveness of disseminating consensus management recommendations for ulcer bleeding: A cluster randomized trial. CMAJ 2013 19;185:E156-66.

20. Hayes SM, Murray S, Dupuis M, Dawes M, Hawes IA, Barkun AN. Barriers to the implementation of practice guidelines in managing patients with nonvariceal upper gastrointestinal bleeding: A qualitative approach. Can J Gastroenterol 2010;24:289-96.

21. Jadad AR, Moore RA, Carroll D, et al. Assessing the quality of reports of randomized clinical trials: Is blinding necessary? Control Clin Trials 1996;17:1-12.

22. Higgins JP, Green S, Cochrane Collaboration. Cochrane handbook for systematic reviews of interventions. Chichester: Hoboken: Wiley-Blackwell, 2008.

23. Chen CC, Lee JY, Fang YJ, et al. Randomised clinical trial: High-dose vs. standard-dose proton pump inhibitors for the prevention of recurrent haemorrhage after combined endoscopic haemostasis of bleeding peptic ulcers. Aliment Pharmacol Ther 2012;35:894-903.

24. Lau JY, Sung JJ, Lee KK, et al. Effect of intravenous omeprazole on recurrent bleeding after endoscopic treatment of bleeding peptic ulcers. N Engl J Med 2000;343:310-6.

25. Chiu PW, Lam CY, Lee SW, et al. Effect of scheduled second therapeutic endoscopy on peptic ulcer rebleeding: A prospective randomised trial. Gut 2003;52:1403-7.

26. Laine L, Jensen DM. Management of patients with ulcer bleeding. Am J Gastroenterol 2012;107:345-60.

27. Cheng HC, Wu CT, Chang WL, Cheng WC, Chen WY, Sheu BS. Double oral esomeprazole after a 3-day intravenous esomeprazole infusion reduces recurrent peptic ulcer bleeding in high-risk patients: A randomised controlled study. Gut March 21, 2014 (Epub ahead of print).

28. Cappell MS, Nadler SC. Increased mortality of acute upper gastrointestinal bleeding in patients with chronic obstructive pulmonary disease. A case controlled, multiyear study of 53 consecutive patients. Dig Dis Sci 1995;40:256-62.

29. Lin HJ, Wang K, Perng CL, Lee FY, Lee CH, Lee SD. Natural history of bleeding peptic ulcers with a tightly adherent blood clot: A prospective observation. Gastrointest Endosc 1996;43:470-3.

30. Cheng HC, Chuang SA, Kao YH, Kao AW, Chuang CH, Sheu BS. Increased risk of rebleeding of peptic ulcer bleeding in patients with comorbid illness receiving omeprazole infusion. Hepatogastroenterology 2003;50:2270-3.

31. Wasse H, Gillen DL, Ball AM, et al. Risk factors for upper gastrointestinal bleeding among end-stage renal disease patients. Kidney Int 2003;64:1455-61.

32. Cheung J, Yu A, LaBossiere J, Zhu Q, Fedorak RN. Peptic ulcer bleeding outcomes adversely affected by end-stage renal disease. Gastrointest Endosc 2010;71:44-9.

33. Tseng GY, Fang CT, Lin HJ, et al. Efficacy of an intravenous proton pump inhibitor after endoscopic therapy with epinephrine injection for peptic ulcer bleeding in patients with uraemia: A case-control study. Aliment Pharmacol Ther 2009;30:406-13.

34. Wu CY, Wu MS, Kuo KN, Wang CB, Chen YJ, Lin JT. Long-term peptic ulcer rebleeding risk estimation in patients undergoing haemodialysis: A 10-year nationwide cohort study. Gut 2011;60:1038-42.

35. Boccardo P, Remuzzi G, Galbusera M. Platelet dysfunction in renal failure. Semin Thromb Hemost 2004;30:579-89.

36. Kaw D, Malhotra D. Platelet dysfunction and end-stage renal disease. Semin Dial 2006;19:317-22.

37. Ponticelli C, Passerini P. Gastrointestinal complications in renal transplant recipients. Transpl Int 2005;18:643-50.

38. Garcia-Iglesias P, Villoria A, Suarez D, et al. Meta-analysis: Predictors of rebleeding after endoscopic treatment for bleeding peptic ulcer. Aliment Pharmacol Ther 2011;34:888-900.

39. Chiu PW, Joeng HK, Choi CL, Kwong KH, Ng EK, Lam SH. Predictors of peptic ulcer rebleeding after scheduled second endoscopy: Clinical or endoscopic factors? Endoscopy 2006;38:726-9.

40. Corley DA, Stefan AM, Wolf M, Cook EF, Lee TH. Early indicators of prognosis in upper gastrointestinal hemorrhage. Am J Gastroenterol 1998;93:336-40.

18

Single-dose infliximab in hepatitis C genotype 1 treatment-naive patients with high serum levels of tumour necrosis factor-alpha does not influence the efficacy of pegylated interferon alpha-2b/ribavirin therapy

Curtis Cooper MD[1], Stephen Shafran MD[2], Susan Greenbloom MD[3], Robert Enns MD[4], John Farley MD[5], Nir Hilzenrat MD[6], Kurt Williams MD[7], Magdy Elkashab MD[8], Nabil Abadir MD[9], Manuela Neuman PhD[10]

C Cooper, S Shafran, S Greenbloom, et al. Single-dose infliximab in hepatitis C genotype 1 treatment-naive patients with high serum levels of tumour necrosis factor-alpha does not influence the efficacy of pegylated interferon alpha-2b/ribavirin therapy. Can J Gastroenterol Hepatol 2014;28(1):35-40.

BACKGROUND: Serum tumour necrosis factor-alpha (TNF-α) levels correlate negatively with hepatitis C virus (HCV) antiviral response.
OBJECTIVES: To test the hypothesis that a single infliximab induction dose would positively influence on-treatment virological response and sustained virological response (SVR).
METHODS: The present study was a phase IIIB, randomized, prospective, open-label pilot trial conducted at eight Canadian sites. Treatment-naive HCV genotype 1-infected patients 18 to 65 years of age with high serum TNF-α values (>300 pg/mL) were randomly assigned to receive a single pretreatment induction infliximab infusion (5 mg/kg) seven days before antiviral therapy (arm A) or no pretreatment (arm B). All patients received pegylated interferon α2b (1.5 µg/kg/week) plus weight-based ribavirin (800 mg/day to 1400 mg/day) for up to 48 weeks.
RESULTS: Eighty-five patients (arm A [n=41], arm B [n=44]; 70% male) received pegylated interferon α2b. The mean age (48.1 years), race (81% white) and METAVIR fibrosis stage (F0–2 = 79%, F3–4 = 21%) were similar between groups. Infliximab was well tolerated without attributable severe adverse events; 56.5% completed the study (arm A [n=21], arm B [n=27]). Most discontinuations were due to virological failure at weeks 12 (n=20 [23.5%]) and 24 (n=7 [8.2%]) and did not differ according to group. Numerically lower proportions of infliximab recipients achieved rapid virological response (19.5% versus 36.4%), complete early virological response (43.9% versus 59.1%) and SVR (34.1% versus 52.3%). However, between-group differences did not reach statistical significance. No differences in adverse event profile or laboratory measures were noted.
CONCLUSION: A single infliximab dose before pegylated-interferon α2b and ribavirin therapy did not result in greater viral decline during the first 12 weeks of HCV therapy or improved SVR.

Key Words: HCV; Infliximab; Interferon; TNF-alpha; Viral kinetics

Une seule dose d'infliximab chez des patients atteints d'hépatite C de génotype 1 naïfs au traitement présentant des taux sériques élevés de facteur de nécrose tumorale alpha n'influe pas sur l'efficacité d'une thérapie à l'interféron pégylé alpha 2b et à la ribavirine

HISTORIQUE : Les taux sériques de facteur de nécrose tumorale alpha (TNF-α) ont une corrélation négative avec la réponse antivirale au virus de l'hépatite C (VHC).
OBJECTIFS : Vérifier l'hypothèse selon laquelle une seule dose d'induction à l'infliximab aurait une influence positive sur la réponse virologique pendant le traitement et sur la réponse virologique soutenue (RVS).
MÉTHODOLOGIE : Le présent essai pilote ouvert aléatoire et prospectif de phase IIIB a été mené dans huit établissements canadiens. Les chercheurs ont réparti au hasard des patients de 18 à 65 ans infectés par le VHC de génotype 1 naïfs au traitement dont les valeurs de TNF-α étaient élevées (plus de 300 pg/mL) entre une seule infusion d'induction d'infliximab (5 mg/kg) sept jours avant l'antivirothérapie (volet A) et aucun traitement préalable (volet B). Tous les patients ont reçu de l'interféron pégylé α2b (1,5 µg/kg/ semaine) associé à de la ribavirine administrée selon le poids (800 mg/jour à 1 400 mg/jour) pendant un maximum de 48 semaines.
RÉSULTATS : Quatre-vingt-cinq patients (volet A [n=41], volet B [n=44]; 70 % d'hommes) ont reçu de l'interféron pégylé α2b. L'âge moyen (48,1 ans), la race (81% de blancs) et le stade de fibrose selon la classification Métavir (F0–2 = 79 %, F3–4 = 21 %) étaient similaires entre les groupes. L'infliximab était bien toléré et ne s'associait à aucuns événements indésirables graves; 56,5 % ont terminé l'étude (volet A [n=21], volet B [n=27]). La plupart des abandons étaient attribuables à un échec virologique lors des semaines 12 (n=20 [23,5 %]) et 24 (n=7 [8,2 %]), ce qui ne différait pas entre les groupes. Moins de patients ayant reçu de l'infliximab ont obtenu une réponse virologique rapide (19,5 % par rapport à 36,4 %), une réponse virologique précoce complète (43,9 % par rapport à 59,1 %) et une RVS (34,1 % par rapport à 52,3 %). Cependant, les différences entre les groupes n'atteignaient pas de signification statistique. Les chercheurs n'ont remarqué aucunes différences sur le plan du profil d'effets indésirables ou des mesures de laboratoire.
CONCLUSION : Une seule dose d'infliximab administrée avant une thérapie à l'interféron pégylé α2b et à la ribavirine ne suscite pas de diminution de la charge virale ou d'amélioration de la RVS pendant les 12 premières d'une thérapie contre le VHC.

Viral and host factors involved in determining the natural course of hepatitis C virus (HCV) disease are only partially defined. It is known that an effective host response against HCV infection requires a coordinated effort involving both nonspecific and HCV antigen-specific immune responses. Nonspecific immune responses include those of the interferon system, a family of related proteins that act against many phases of the viral life cycle; complement, which can serve to disrupt the viral envelope and lead to enhanced opsonization of viruses by phagocytic cells; and natural killer cells, which lyse infected cells. Activation of Kupffer cells, which are the resident

[1]University of Ottawa, Ottawa Hospital Research Institute, Ottawa, Ontario; [2]University of Alberta, Edmonton, Alberta; [3]Toronto Digestive Disease Associates, Toronto, Ontario; [4]St Paul's Hospital, University of British Columbia; [5]Private Practice, Vancouver, British Columbia; [6]Jewish General Hospital and McGill University, Montreal, Quebec; [7]Royal University Hospital, Saskatoon, Saskatchewan; [8]Private practice, Toronto, Ontario; [9]Merck Canada Inc, Kirkland, Quebec; [10]University of Toronto, Toronto, Ontario

Correspondence: Dr Curtis Cooper, University of Ottawa, The Ottawa Hospital Division of infectious Diseases, G12-501 Smyth Road, Ottawa, Ontario K1H 8L6. e-mail ccooper@toh.on.ca

macrophages within the liver, produce cytokines (eg, tumour necrosis factor-alpha [TNF-α]) that have important effects on viral replication and transcription (1,2).

Cytokines are signalling proteins transiently produced after cellular activation (2). Cytokines play a key role in the cell-to-cell communication necessary for the regulation of immunity and inflammation within the liver (2-4). Interferon alpha (IFN-α), which is a key component of current standard of care for HCV antiviral treatment, is an endogenous cytokine that stimulates T lymphocyte antiviral response by signalling the immune system to prevent activated T cell death during infection. Evaluation of the cytokine network may provide important insights into the mechanism of viral persistence in chronic HCV infection. In patients with chronic HCV infection, measurement of serum proinflammatory cytokine levels may also be useful for the selection of patients with higher probability of virological response with HCV antiviral therapy (5-9). Furthermore, modulation of the cytokine network may be beneficial as a therapeutic intervention (10).

Infliximab is a chimeric immunoglobulin G16 monoclonal antibody that neutralizes the biological activity of TNF-α by high-affinity binding of soluble and transmembrane forms of TNF-α and inhibition of TNF-α binding with its receptors (11). Given the potential influence of high TNF-α levels on the pathogenesis of HCV infection (12), we evaluated the safety and efficacy of a single, low-dose infliximab induction therapy injection on virological response and sustained virological response (SVR) in HCV-infected study participants receiving pegylated IFN-α2b and ribavirin-based antiviral treatment.

METHODS

The present phase IIIB, randomized, prospective, open-label pilot trial was conducted at eight Canadian sites. Treatment-naive HCV genotype 1-infected patients 18 to 65 years of age with high serum TNF-α levels (>300 pg/mL) were included. Clinical evidence of liver decompensation and cirrhosis on biopsy were exclusionary. The degree of fibrosis was assessed using METAVIR score. Other exclusion criteria included HCV infection acquired within the preceding 12 months, pregnancy or breastfeeding, hepatitis B virus or HIV coinfection, alcohol consumption >350 g per week, injection drug use within six months of screening, active and severe psychiatric illness, and weight <40 kg or >125 kg. Previous exposure to TNF-α inhibitors, interferon or ribavirin was exclusionary. Chronic systemic steroid use, antiviral agents and herbal remedies specific for the liver were prohibited. Tuberculosis screening was conducted by inquiring about exposure and previous infection history, chest x-ray and tuberculin skin testing. Active tuberculosis or a tuberculin skin reaction >5 mm precluded eligibility.

Participants were randomly assigned to receive either a single pretreatment induction infusion of infliximab (5 mg/kg) seven days before antiviral therapy or no pretreatment. All patients received pegylated IFN-α2b (1.5 μg/kg/wk) plus weight-based ribavirin (800 mg/day to 1400 mg/day) for up to 48 weeks.

HCV RNA levels were assessed before infliximab dosing, on day 0 of HCV antiviral therapy, and at weeks 2, 4, 6, 8, 12, 24, 48 and 72. HCV-RNA results were given in IU/mL (1 IU/mL × 2.7 copies/IU = copies/mL). HCV was quantified using polymerase chain reaction for HCV RNA. Initially, the Amplicor HCV Monitor test (Roche Diagnostics, Canada) was used. The test is specifically designed for assessing viral load with the low linear sensitivity 6×10^2 and lower limit of detection (ie, 50 IU/mL). The procedure is based on five major steps required by the specimen preparation, reverse transcription of target RNA to generate complementary DNA, polymerase chain reaction amplification of target complementary DNA using HCV-specific complementary primers, hybridization of the amplified DNA to oligonucleotide probes specific to the target and detection of the probe bind amplifier. The lower limit of detection is 15 IU/mL. For the final 30 patients enrolled in the study, the newly automated, sensitive method CobasAmpliprep-Amplicor/Taqman HCV test (Roche

Diagnostics, Canada) was used. The equivalence of the methods were validated. To ascertain the validity of the conclusions, the HCV RNA of the SVRs that have been judged by Amplicor HCV Monitor has been retested using the Taqman HCV test.

TNF-α levels (pg/mL) were quantitatively determined in serum using ELISA at the same time points. Cytoscreen immunoassay kits (Biosource International, InVitrogen, USA) were used, with a sensitivity and specificity of 96% and 92%, respectively. Standards and reference reagents, available from the National Institute for Biological Standards and Controls (Herts, United Kingdom), were used. These methods are standardized in one of the author's (MN) laboratory according to the procedures described (5-7).

Clinical and laboratory safety measures where determined at each visit. The Short-Form 36 quality of life questionnaire was completed by the patient at the screening visit, at treatment weeks 12 and 48, and at week 72 before any study visit procedures.

As a primary outcome, the SVR 24 weeks before completion of therapy was compared between randomized treatment arms. The rapid virological response (RVR) at week 4 and complete early virological responses (EVR) at week 12 were assessed as secondary outcomes. Safety was also evaluated as a secondary outcome. The originally planned target of 96 participants provided 80% power to identify a clinically relevant increase in SVR from 48% to 75% assuming a 15% drop-out rate. However, enrollment was interrupted at 89 participants due to slow accrual. Efficacy analysis was conducted on a modified intent-to-treat population, defined as all participants receiving at least one dose of study medication. Descriptive statistics were performed for all study variables. Between-group differences were tested for statistical significance using Fisher's exact test. Viral outcome measures were assessed using univariable and multivariable logistic regression.

All sites obtained local research ethics approval before initiation of the present study. All participants provided informed consent.

RESULTS

Eighty-five of 89 randomized patients (70% male) received pegylated IFN-α2b and ribavirin and were included in the modified intent-to-treat analysis (Figure 1). Forty-three received infliximab and 46 did not. Mean age (48.1 years), race (81% white) and METAVIR liver fibrosis stage (F0–2 = 79%, F3–4 = 21%) were similar between randomized groups (Table 1). Interferon dose per kg and ribavirin dose per kg were similar according to group (data not shown).

Forty-eight participants (56.5%) completed the study (21 infliximab recipients and 27 controls). Over the course of the study, 37 (43.5%) discontinued prematurely (20 infliximab recipients and 17 controls). Treatment arms did not differ statistically in terms of mean treatment duration (infliximab recipients = 3.81 months versus controls = 3.49 months; P=0.29). The majority of discontinuations were due to virological failure at week 12 (n=20 [23.5%]) and week 24 (n=7 [8.2%]) and did not differ statistically according to group.

No change in HCV RNA was observed in the week following infliximab dosing (data not shown). Following the initiation of HCV antiviral therapy, the slope of HCV RNA decay was similar between groups (Figure 2). A positive correlation between TNF-α and HCV RNA decline was identified that was similar between randomized groups (data not shown). Numerically lower proportions of patients achieved week 4 RVR (19.5% versus 36.4%), week 12 complete EVR (43.9% versus 59.1%) and SVR 24 weeks after completion of therapy (34.1% versus 52.3%) in infliximab recipients compared with the control arm. However, between-group differences did not reach statistical significance in any of these outcome measures based either on an observed case analysis or a dropout-equals-failure analysis. Although potentially limited by sample size, mean HCV RNA levels did not differ statistically at any time point over the course of the study. The mean time to undetectable HCV RNA was 109 days (95% CI 88 to 130 days) in infliximab recipients and 83 days (95% CI 64 to 101 days) in the control group (P=0.22) (Figure 2).

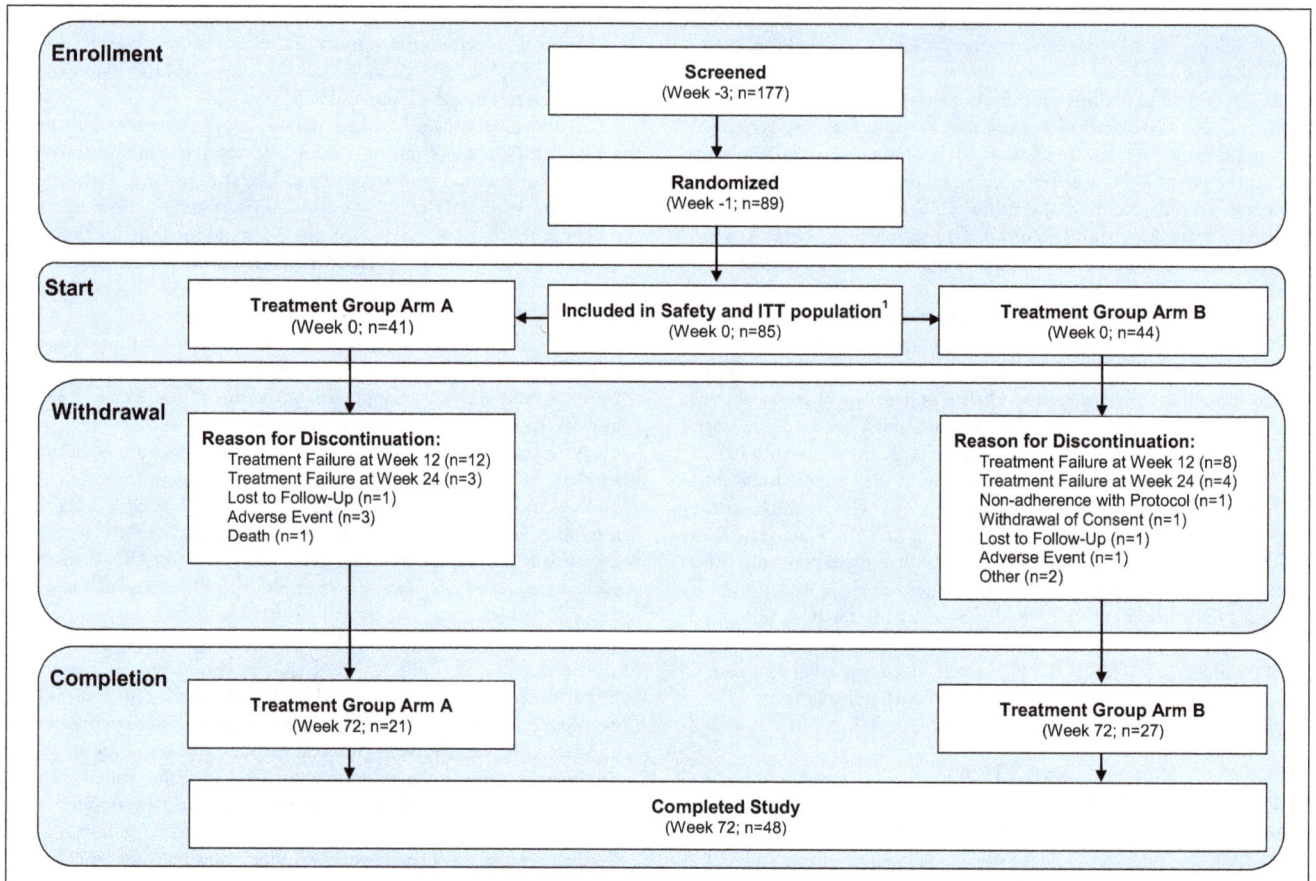

Figure 1) *Participant flow diagram. Intent-to-treat (ITT) population defined as all randomized subjects who received at least one dose of study medication (n=85 [89%]; 70% male). Four subjects did not receive any study medication. One patient reported two reasons for discontinuation including adverse event and treatment failure at week 24 in arm B. One patient completed the initial 17 visits but did not return at visit 18 (week 72); this patient was not considered as discontinued*

TABLE 1
Patient demographics according to treatment group – ITT

	Arm A (n=41)	Arm B (n=44)	Total (n=85)	P
Age, years				
Mean (median)	47.9 (49.4)	48.3 (50.3)	48.1 (49.8)	0.433[*]
Sex				
Male	30 (73.2)	31 (70.5)	61 (71.8)	0.781[†]
Female	11 (26.8)	13 (29.5)	24 (28.2)	
Race				
Caucasian	32 (78.0)	37 (84.1)	69 (81.2)	0.239[†]
Asian	5 (12.2)	3 (6.8)	8 (9.4)	
Hispanic	1 (2.4)	0 (0.0)	1 (1.2)	
Black	0 (0.0)	3 (6.8)	3 (3.5)	
Native Indian	1 (2.4)	1 (2.3)	2 (2.4)	
Other[‡]	2 (4.9)	0 (0.0)	2 (2.4)	
Fibrosis score – historical liver biopsy (METAVIR System)				
F0	0 (0.0)	1 (2.3)	1 (1.2)	0.688[§]
F1	15 (36.6)	18 (40.9)	33 (38.8)	
F2	17 (41.5)	16 (36.4)	33 (38.8)	
F3	9 (22.0)	8 (18.2)	17 (20.0)	
F4	0 (0.0)	1 (2.3)	1 (1.2)	

*Data presented as n (%) unless otherwise indicated. Percentages are based on the total number of patients with available data in each group (Arm A Infliximab recipients; Arm B Control arm) at each visit. *Assessed with the independent samples t test for continuous variables; †Assessed using the Fisher's exact test for categorical variables; ‡Other includes a multiracial (n=1) and Métis (n=1) participant; §Assessed using the Pearson χ^2 test. ITT Intent to treat*

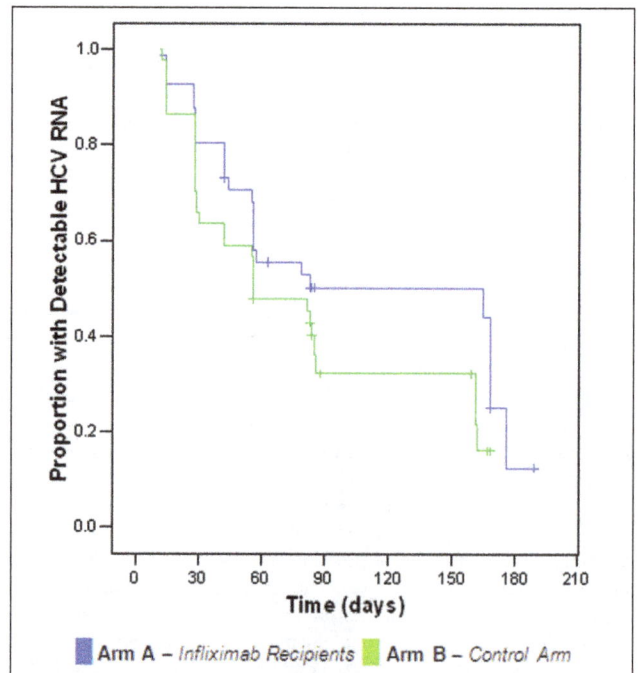

Figure 2) *Time to undetectable hepatitis C virus (HCV) RNA levels – intention to treat. Following the initiation of HCV antiviral therapy, the slope of HCV RNA decay was similar between groups. The mean time to undetectable HCV RNA was 109 days (95% CI 88 to 130 days) in infliximab recipients and 83 days (95% CI 64 to 101 days) in the control group (P=0.22)*

TABLE 2
Rapid virological response according to fibrosis score – intent to treat

| | Arm A (n=41) | | Arm B (n=44) | | Total (n=85) | | |
Fibrosis score	Yes	No	Yes	No	Yes	No	P*
F0	0 (0.0)	0 (0.0)	0 (0.0)	1 (100.0)	0 (0.0)	1 (100.0)	NC
F1	5 (33.3)	10 (66.7)	6 (33.3)	12 (66.7)	11 (33.3)	22 (66.7)	>0.999
F2	2 (11.8)	15 (88.2)	8 (50.0)	8 (50.0)	10 (30.3)	23 (69.7)	0.026†
F3	1 (11.1)	8 (88.9)	2 (25.0)	6 (75.0)	3 (17.6)	14 (82.4)	0.576
F4	0 (0.0)	0 (0.0)	0 (0.0)	1 (100.0)	0 (0.0)	1 (100.0)	NC

*Data presented n (%) unless otherwise indicated. Percentages are based on the total number of patients with available data in each group at each visit. *Assessed with the Fisher's Exact test; †Statistically significant result. Arm A Infliximab recipients; Arm B Control arm; NC Not calculable*

TABLE 3
Complete early virological response according to fibrosis score – intent to treat

| | Arm A (n=41) | | Arm B (n=44) | | Total (n=85) | | |
Fibrosis score	Yes	No	Yes	No	Yes	No	P*
F0	0 (0.0)	0 (0.0)	0 (0.0)	1 (100.0)	0 (0.0)	1 (100.0)	NC
F1	6 (42.9)	8 (57.1)	13 (76.5)	4 (23.5)	19 (61.3)	12 (38.7)	0.075
F2	10 (62.5)	6 (37.5)	10 (71.4)	4 (28.6)	20 (66.7)	10 (33.3)	0.709
F3	2 (25.0)	6 (75.0)	3 (37.5)	5 (62.5)	5 (31.3)	11 (68.8)	>0.999
F4	0 (0.0)	0 (0.0)	0 (0.0)	1 (100.0)	0 (0.0)	1 (100.0)	NC

*Data presented as n (%) unless otherwise indicated. Percentages are based on the total number of patients with available data in each group at each visit. *Assessed using Fisher's exact test. Arm A Infliximab recipients; Arm B Control arm; NC Not calculable*

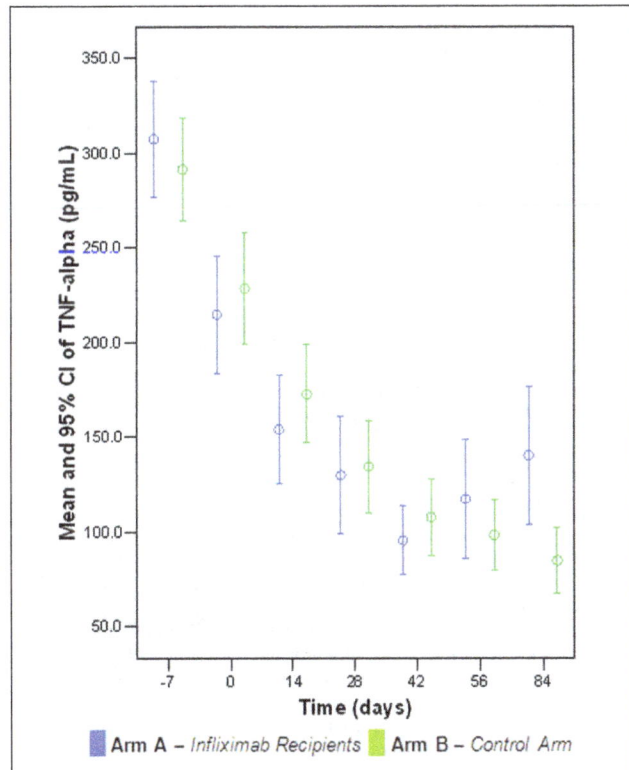

Figure 3) *Tumour necrosis factor-alpha (TNF-α) levels at each visit according to treatment group. The baseline levels of TNF-α were similar between study arms. A rapid decline in serum TNF-α level was noted one week following dosing of infliximab and preceeding the initial dosing of pegylated interferon α-2b and ribavirin. This rapid decline continued following the dosing of pegylated interferon α-2b and ribavirin, and positively correlated with hepatitis C virus RNA decline over the initial four weeks of dosing. However, the slope of decline was similar in both groups, irrespective of infliximab dosing*

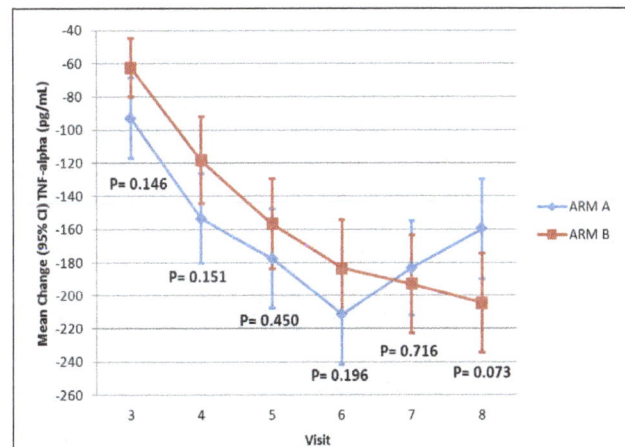

Figure 4) *Changes in tumour necrosis factor-alpha (TNF-α) levels between day 0 (visit 3) and week 12 (visit 8). Between-group P value, assessed using independent samples t test, revealed no statistical differences in the decline of unadjusted mean change of serum TNF-α in the two arms between day 0 (visit 3) and week 12 (visit 8) of pegylated interferon and ribavirin therapy. A numerical difference in the value of serum TNF-α level was observed until week 6 (visit 6), suggesting a larger reduction in inflammation in treatment arm A (infliximab recipients) compared with arm B (control arm). The effect dissipated over time*

RVR and EVR were assessed as a function of fibrosis (Tables 2 and 3). As would be expected, RVR and EVR diminished with advancing fibrosis. No consistent difference was observed between randomized groups.

Figure 3 illustrates the kinetics of serum TNF-α during the entire study. The baseline levels of TNF-α were similar between study arms. Figure 4 illustrates the decline of serum TNF-α levels in the two arms between day 0 (visit 3) and week 12 (visit 8). There were no statistical differences between the two arms. However, until week 6 (visit 6) there was a numerical difference in the value of serum TNF-α, suggesting a larger reduction in inflammation in treatment arm A compared with arm B. The effect dissipated over time.

In general, laboratory parameters, vital signs and physical examination were stable, and similar between study arms and most visits. Specifically, the slope of aspartate and alanine aminotransferase level decline was similar according to group (data not shown). No differences between infliximab recipients and control participants in quality of life scores were identified over the course of treatment (data not shown). Infliximab was well tolerated without attributable severe adverse events. Over the course of the 72-week study, a total of 1147 treatment-emergent adverse events were reported in 100% of participants. Of these, 21 serious adverse events (SAE) in 12 (14.1%) participants were identified. Possible or probable relationship to the study drug was assigned in eight of 10 SAEs in infliximab-recipients and seven of 11 in the control arm. One participant discontinued therapy due to a SAE (lobar pneumonia) in the infliximab-recipient group. This SAE was determined to be likely related to study drug. One death due to arteriosclerosis coronary artery disease occurred in the infliximab arm, which was judged to be not likely related to the study drug.

DISCUSSION

The use of a single dose of TNF-α inhibitor was demonstrated to be safe and well tolerated in HCV-infected study participants, corroborating the current body of evidence (13). However, there was no evidence of any beneficial effect on HCV RNA decline, SVR or alanine aminotransferase response. This is consistent with other studies that have assessed the influence of TNF-α inhibition on liver enzymes and viremia (14). In contrast to our results, a pilot study evaluating the influence of TNF-α inhibition on HCV treatment outcome demonstrated both improved tolerability of interferon-based treatment and improved on-treatment virological response (15). Of note, SVR rates did not differ significantly between etanercept (42%) and placebo (32%) recipients. Potential explanations for the differences between our study results and those of Zein (15) include the use of multiple doses of TNF-α inhibitor while on antiviral therapy, the use of a different TNF-α inhibitor (ie, etanercept) and a small sample size, increasing the risk of a type II statistical error. In our study, there was no evidence of improved pegylated IFN and ribavirin tolerance in the weeks immediately following dosing and no evidence of more rapid virological decline within the first four weeks of HCV antiviral therapy; a period in which we would have expected a maximal effect of infliximab, if present. Furthermore, no difference in on-treatment liver enzyme level decline was identified.

A rapid decline in serum TNF-α level was noted one week following dosing of infliximab and proceeding the initial dosing of pegylated IFN α-2b and ribavirin (Figure 3). This rapid decline continued following the dosing of pegylated IFN α-2b and ribavirin and positively correlated with HCV RNA decline over the initial four weeks of dosing. However, the slope of decline was similar in both groups, irrespective of infliximab dosing. Serum TNF-α levels >300 pg/mL at screening were required for inclusion. We noted that at the time of infliximab dosing, levels were lower than this cut-point, which is likely indicative of a regression to the mean phenomenon. This may have served to diminish the impact of infliximab. We do not believe that this change in TNF-α level from screening to infliximab dosing was due to altered alcohol consumption because excess alcohol use was an exclusionary for participation in the present study. A subanalysis of those with serum TNF-α levels >300 pg/mL, both at screening and at the time of infliximab dosing, did not reveal any evidence that this was the case (data not shown). The observation that the slope of serum TNF-α decline was similar with pegylated IFN α-2b and ribavirin dosing, irrespective of infliximab administration, indicated that these HCV antiviral medications and/or their influence on HCV infection have a far more potent influence on serum TNF-α levels than infliximab in the context of chronic HCV infection.

The strengths of the present study include the randomized allocation of treatment and frequent clinical and laboratory monitoring of participants. However, several limitations are acknowledged. First, the study lasted longer than expected and was interrupted before the calculated sample size was achieved. Also, the assay used to quantify HCV RNA was changed midway through the conduct of the study. Although not ideal, we do not believe that this had a major influence on our findings because only 15 of 89 (17%) of participants underwent HCV RNA evaluations using both assays. Furthermore, the initial 12 weeks of HCV RNA testing was conducted using either one or the other assay but not both. As well, it is unlikely that the primary outcome (SVR) would be misclassified given the minimal

difference in lower limit of detection between assays (ie, 50 IU/mL versus 15 IU/mL) because HCV RNA levels would have fully rebounded to baseline levels by week 24 post-therapy in unsuccessful HCV antiviral recipients. Interleukin (IL) 28B status was unavailable for our analysis because the present study was conducted before the identification of this as a key predictor of HCV antiviral outcome (16). Although it is likely that IL28B distribution was balanced between treatment arms in the present randomized study, it would have been valuable to evaluate the influence of infliximab as a function of IL28B genotype.

CONCLUSION

Infliximab can be safely administered to patients infected with HCV. This is clinically relevant because HCV infection is occasionally identified in those with concurrent disorders requiring TNF-α inhibitor therapy (13,14,17). Our study demonstrates that manipulation of endogenous TNF-α levels with a single dose of infliximab treatment proceeding combination pegylated IFNα-2b and ribavirin therapy does not result in greater viral decline during the first 12 weeks of therapy or improved SVR rates, and should not be considered as an adjunctive treatment for HCV.

ACKNOWLEDGEMENTS: The authors thank the participants, research associates and monitors who contributed to this study and JSS for statistical analysis. Special thanks to J-F Pouliot, P Egli, E Levesque and Schering-Plough-Merck PEGADE team that enabled the study. Schering-Plough-Merck provided the investigational drugs and funded this work. Dr Neuman greatly appreciates the assistance of D Murphy and J Chamberland, *Institute Nationale de Santé Publique du Québec*, for contributing their assistance in validating the TaqMan® HCV Test methodology.

REFERENCES

1. Koziel MJ, Dudley D, Afdhal N, et al. Hepatitis C virus (HCV)-specific cytotoxic T lymphocytes recognize epitopes in the core and envelope proteins of HCV. J Virol 1993;67:7522-32.
2. Jacobson Brown PM, Neuman MG. Immunopathogenesis of hepatitis C viral infection: Th1/Th2 responses and the role of cytokines. Clin Biochem 2001;34:167-71.
3. Koziel MJ. Cytokines in viral hepatitis. Semin Liver Dis 1999;19:157-69.
4. Tilg H, Wilmer A, Vogel W, et al. Serum levels of cytokines in chronic liver diseases. Gastroenterology 1992;103:264-74.
5. Neuman MG, Benhamou JP, Martinot M, et al. Predictors of sustained response to alpha interferon therapy in chronic hepatitis C. Clin Biochem 1999;32:537-45.
6. Neuman MG, Benhamou JP, Bourliere M, et al. Serum tumour necrosis factor-alpha and transforming growth factor-beta levels in chronic hepatitis C patients are immunomodulated by therapy. Cytokine 2002;17:108-17.
7. Neuman MG, Benhamou JP, Malkiewicz IM, et al. Cytokines as predictors for sustained response and as markers for immunomodulation in patients with chronic hepatitis C. Clin Biochem 2001;34:173-82.
8. Fukuda R, Ishimura N, Ishihara S, et al. Intrahepatic expression of pro-inflammatory cytokine mRNAs and interferon efficacy in chronic hepatitis C. Liver 1996;16:390-9.
9. Larrea E, Garcia N, Qian C, Civeira MP, Prieto J. Tumor necrosis factor alpha gene expression and the response to interferon in chronic hepatitis C. Hepatology 1996;23:210-7.
10. Neuman MG, Benhamou JP, Malkiewicz IM, et al. Kinetics of serum cytokines reflect changes in the severity of chronic hepatitis C presenting minimal fibrosis. J Viral Hepat 2002;9:134-40.
11. Nahar IK, Shojania K, Marra CA, Alamgir AH, Anis AH. Infliximab treatment of rheumatoid arthritis and Crohn's disease. Ann Pharmacother 2003;37:1256-65.
12. Gonzalez-Amaro R, Garcia-Monzon C, Garcia-Buey L, et al. Induction of tumor necrosis factor alpha production by human hepatocytes in chronic viral hepatitis. J Exp Med 1994;179:841-8.

13. Brunasso AM, Puntoni M, Gulia A, Massone C. Safety of anti-tumour necrosis factor agents in patients with chronic hepatitis C infection: A systematic review. Rheumatology (Oxford) 2011;50:1700-11.

14. Peterson JR, Hsu FC, Simkin PA, Wener MH. Effect of tumour necrosis factor alpha antagonists on serum transaminases and viraemia in patients with rheumatoid arthritis and chronic hepatitis C infection. Ann Rheum Dis 2003;62:1078-82.

15. Zein NN. Etanercept as an adjuvant to interferon and ribavirin in treatment-naive patients with chronic hepatitis C virus infection: A phase 2 randomized, double-blind, placebo-controlled study. J Hepatol 2005;42:315-22.

16. Ge D, Fellay J, Thompson AJ, et al. Genetic variation in IL28B predicts hepatitis C treatment-induced viral clearance. Nature 2009;461:399-401.

17. Li S, Kaur PP, Chan V, Berney S. Use of tumor necrosis factor-alpha (TNF-alpha) antagonists infliximab, etanercept, and adalimumab in patients with concurrent rheumatoid arthritis and hepatitis B or hepatitis C: A retrospective record review of 11 patients. Clin Rheumatol 2009;28:787-91.

19

Hepatitis C drugs: The end of the pegylated interferon era and the emergence of all-oral, interferon-free antiviral regimens: A concise review

Alan Hoi Lun Yau MD, Eric M Yoshida MD MHSc FRCPC

AHL Yau, EM Yoshida. Hepatitis C drugs: The end of the pegylated interferon era and the emergence of all-oral, interferon-free antiviral regimens: A concise review. Can J Gastroenterol Hepatol 2014;28(8):445-451.

Between 2001 and 2011, the standard of care for chronic hepatitis C virus (HCV) infection was a combination of pegylated interferon (PEG-IFN) and ribavirin (RBV). In May 2011, boceprevir and telaprevir, two first-generation NS3/4A protease inhibitors, were approved in combination with PEG-IFN and RBV for 24 to 48 weeks in hepatitis C virus genotype 1 infections. In December 2013, simeprevir, a second-generation NS3/4A protease inhibitor, was approved for use with PEG-IFN and RBV for 12 weeks in genotype 1, while sofosbuvir, a NS5B nucleotide polymerase inhibitor, was approved for use with PEG-IFN and RBV for 12 weeks in genotypes 1 and 4, as well as with RBV alone for 12 weeks in genotype 2 and for 24 weeks in genotype 3. Sofosbuvir combined with simeprevir or an NS5A replication complex inhibitor (ledipasvir or daclatasvir) with or without RBV for 12 weeks in genotype 1 resulted in a sustained virological response >90%, irrespective of previous treatment history or presence of cirrhosis. Similarly impressive sustained virological response rates have been shown with ABT-450/r (ritonavir-boosted NS3/4A protease inhibitor)-based regimens in combination with other direct-acting antiviral agent(s) with or without RBV for 12 weeks in genotype 1. The optimal all-oral interferon-free antiviral regimen likely entails a combination of an NS5B nucleotide polymerase inhibitor with either a second-generation NS3/4A protease inhibitor or an NS5A replication complex inhibitor with or without RBV. Further research is needed to determine the role of resistance testing, clarify the optimal follow-up duration post-treatment, and evaluate the antiviral efficacy and safety in difficult-to-cure patient populations.

Key Words: *All-oral; Hepatitis C; Interferon-free; Simeprevir; Sofosbuvir*

Les médicaments contre l'hépatite C : la fin de l'ère de l'interféron pégylé et l'émergence d'une posologie antivirale entièrement orale et sans interféron : une analyse concise

Entre 2001 et 2011, la norme des soins de l'infection par le virus de l'hépatite C (VHC) chronique était une polythérapie d'interféron pégylé (IFN-PEG) et de ribavirine (RBV). En mai 2011, le bocéprévir et le télaprévir, deux inhibiteurs de la protéase NS3/4A de première génération, ont été approuvés en combinaison avec l'IFN-PEG et la RBV pour un traitement de 24 à 48 semaines contre l'infection par le VHC de génotype 1. En décembre 2013, le siméprévir, un inhibiteur de la protéase NS3/4A de seconde génération, a été approuvé en combinaison avec l'IFN-PEG et la RBV pour un traitement de 12 semaines contre le génotype 1, tandis que le sofosbuvir, un inhibiteur nucléotidique de la polymérase NS5B, a été approuvé en combinaison avec l'IFN-PEG et la RBV pour un traitement de 12 semaines contre les génotypes 1 et 4, ainsi qu'avec la RBV seule pour un traitement de 12 semaines contre le génotype 2 et de 24 semaines contre le génotype 3. Le sofosbuvir en combinaison avec le siméprévir ou un inhibiteur du complexe de réplication NS5A (lédipasvir ou daclatasvir), accompagné ou non de RBV et administré pendant 12 semaines pour traiter le génotype 1, a suscité une réponse virologique soutenue de plus de 90 %, quels que soient les antécédents thérapeutiques et en présence ou en l'absence de cirrhose. De même, les posologies à base d'ABT-450/r (inhibiteur de la protéase NS3/4A rehaussé de ritonavir), combinées à d'autres antiviraux à action directe avec ou sans RBV pour un traitement de 12 semaines contre le génotype 1, entraînent un taux de réponse virologique soutenu impressionnant. La posologie antivirale entièrement orale et sans interféron optimale se compose probablement d'un inhibiteur nucléotidique de la polymérase NS5B combiné à un inhibiteur de la protéase NS3/4A de seconde génération ou à un inhibiteur du complexe de réplication NS5A, accompagné ou non de RBV. Il faudra mener d'autres recherches pour déterminer le rôle des tests de résistance, établir la durée de suivi optimale après le traitement et évaluer l'efficacité et l'innocuité antivirale au sein des populations de patients difficiles à soigner.

Chronic hepatitis C virus (HCV) infection has been estimated to affect 2% to 3% (170 million individuals) of the population worldwide (1) and 0.8% (275,000 individuals) of Canadians (2). In Canada, HCV-related morbidity and mortality increased by 15% to 18% annually between 1994 and 2004 (3). In response to the increasing medical and economic burden of HCV on the Canadian health care system, the landscape of HCV antiviral therapy has changed rapidly in the past three years (Table 1) (4). Between 2001 and 2011, the standard of care for chronic HCV infection was a combination of pegylated interferon (PEG-IFN) and ribavirin (RBV), with a sustained virological response (SVR) of up to 40% to 50% in genotype 1 (G1) and up to 70% to 80% in genotypes 2 and 3 (G2/3) (5,6). However, PEG-IFN is contraindicated in decompensated cirrhosis (7) and is associated with constitutional, neuropsychiatric, autoimmune and hematological side effects (8), whereas RBV is contraindicated in renal failure (9) and is associated with cough, rash, hemolysis and teratogenesis (8). Hence, many patients are ineligible for or intolerant to PEG-IFN and RBV therapy.

DIRECT-ACTING ANTIVIRAL AGENTS IN COMBINATION WITH PEG-IFN AND RBV: WHAT IS CURRENTLY AVAILABLE

The limited efficacy and tolerability of PEG-IFN and RBV have prompted the development of many direct-acting antiviral agents (DAAs) that target specific proteins involved in HCV replication (Table 2) (10). In May 2011, boceprevir (BOC) and telaprevir (TVR), two first-generation NS3/4A protease inhibitors, were approved for use in HCV G1, but must be used in combination with PEG-IFN and RBV to prevent the rapid emergence of resistance-associated variants (11-13). Although BOC and TVR have significantly improved the SVR to 60% to 75% in G1 treatment-naive patients (11-13), the SVR remained suboptimal (30% to 40%) in difficult-to-cure populations such as patients with cirrhosis (14), G1a (15), and previous null responders to PEG-IFN and RBV (defined as failure to achieve at least a 2 log reduction in HCV RNA at week 12 of therapy) (16,17). Moreover, protease inhibitors are associated with additional side effects including

Department of Medicine, Division of Gastroenterology, University of British Columbia, Vancouver, British Columbia
Correspondence: Dr Eric Yoshida, Vancouver General Hospital, Division of Gastroenterology, 5153-2775 Laurel Street, Vancouver,
British Columbia V5Z 1M9. e-mail eric.yoshida@vch.ca

TABLE 1
Currently approved hepatitis C treatment regimens

Year	Treatment regimen	Genotype	SVR, %	Study (reference)
2001	PEG-IFN + RBV × 48 weeks	1 or 4	42–46	Manns et al (5), Fried et al (6)
2001	PEG-IFN + RBV × 24 weeks	2 or 3	76–82	Manns et al (5), Fried et al (6)
2011	PEG-IFN + RBV + BOC × 24–48 weeks	1	56–75	SPRINT-1 (11), SPRINT-2 (12)
2011	PEG-IFN + RBV + TVR × 24–48 weeks	1	69–75	ADVANCE (13)
2013	PEG-IFN + RBV + SMV × 12 weeks*	1	80–81	QUEST-1 (19), QUEST-2 (20), PILLAR (21)
2013	PEG-IFN + RBV + SOF × 12 weeks	1	89–91	NCT01188772 (25), ATOMIC (26), NEUTRINO (27)
2013	PEG-IFN + RBV + SOF × 12 weeks	4	96	NEUTRINO (27)
2013	RBV + SOF × 12 weeks	2	92–100	FISSION (27), POSITRON (35), VALENCE (36)
2013	RBV + SOF × 24 weeks	3	92–94	VALENCE (36)

Followed by pegylated interferon (PEG-IFN) + ribavirin (RBV) for 12 weeks in treatment-naive or previous relapsers and 36 weeks in previous partial or null responders. Sofosbuvir (SOF) + RBV is recommended in hepatocellular carcinoma patients awaiting liver transplantation for up to 48 weeks or until transplant. BOC Boceprevir; SMV Simeprevir; SVR Sustained virological response in treatment-naive patients; TVR Telaprevir

TABLE 2
General characteristics of direct-acting antiviral agents

Direct-acting antiviral agents	Antiviral efficacy	Resistance barrier	Genotypic coverage	Side effects	Drug interactions
NS3/4A protease inhibitor (first generation)	++	+	Genotype 1	+++	+++
NS3/4A protease inhibitor (second generation)	+++	++	Multiple genotypes	+	++
NS5A replication complex inhibitor	+++	++	Multiple genotypes	+	++
NS5B nucleotide polymerase inhibitor	+++	+++	All genotypes	+	+
NS5B non-nucleoside polymerase inhibitor	++	+	Genotype 1	++	++

+ Minimal; ++ Intermediate; +++ Significant; NS Nonstructural protein

anemia and dysgeusia for BOC and anemia, and rash and anorectal symptoms for TVR (18). Finally, the use of triple therapy is associated with a heavy pill burden, complex dosing schedule and numerous drug interactions, even though the treatment duration could be shortened from 48 weeks to 24 to 28 weeks through response-guided therapy.

Following the approval of BOC and TVR, second-generation NS3/4A protease inhibitors, such as simeprevir (SMV), were being developed. In December 2013, SMV was approved for use with PEG-IFN and RBV for 12 weeks in G1. The approval was based on data from the QUEST-1 (19), QUEST-2 (20) and PILLAR (21) clinical trials in which SMV in combination with PEG-IFN and RBV for 12 weeks followed by PEG-IFN and RBV alone for an additional 12 to 36 weeks produced an SVR of 80% to 81% in G1 treatment-naive patients. A similar SVR (79%) was shown with the same treatment regimen in G1 previous relapsers to PEG-IFN and RBV in the PROMISE study (22). This was further confirmed in the ASPIRE study, in which 12 weeks of SMV given with 48 weeks of PEG-IFN and RBV resulted in an SVR of 77% in previous relapsers; however, a lower SVR of 65% and 53% was found in previous partial and null responders, respectively (23). In all of these studies (19-23), the SVR in G1a was significantly lower (58% if Q80K positive, 75% if Q80K negative) than in G1b (>80%) due to the presence of the Q80K polymorphism, which is commonly found in 30% to 47% of G1a infections and significantly decreases susceptibility to SMV (24). This has strong clinical implications in North America, where G1a is the most prevalent HCV subgenotype and where Q80K polymorphism testing is recommended in G1a patients before treatment with SMV.

Because first- and second-generation protease inhibitors may develop cross-resistance, other classes of DAA, such as nucleotide NS5B polymerase inhibitors, which include sofosbuvir (SOF), were being developed. In December 2013, SOF was approved for use with PEG-IFN and RBV for 12 weeks in G1 and G4 infections. The approval was based on data from the NCT01188772 (25), ATOMIC (26) and NEUTRINO (27) clinical trials in which SOF in combination with PEG-IFN and RBV for 12 weeks produced an SVR of 89% to 91% in G1 treatment-naive patients. The NEUTRINO study also reported an SVR of 96% in G4 treatment-naive patients who received PEG-IFN, RBV and SOF for 12 weeks. G1a was present in 69% to

77% among these studies and cirrhosis was identified as a negative predictor of SVR (80% with cirrhosis, 92% without cirrhosis) in the NEUTRINO study. G2 and G3 treatment-naive patients also appear to benefit from the same treatment regimen, with an SVR of 92% to 96% in the NCT01188772 (25) and PROTON (28) studies. A similar SVR (83% to 96%) was demonstrated with this regimen in G2 and G3 treatment-experienced patients, in whom compensated cirrhosis was present in 50% of enrolled patients in the LONESTAR-2 study (29).

The addition of a DAA to the backbone of PEG-IFN and RBV has clearly improved the likelihood of achieving an SVR; however, SOF appears to be superior to BOC, TVR and SMV in enhancing antiviral efficacy. The first-generation protease inhibitors BOC and TVR are associated with significant adverse effects, which are in addition to those of PEG-IFN and RBV. The commercial availability of SMV and SOF offers patients a shortened treatment course and a lack of adverse effects experienced with BOC and TVR. The continued use of PEG-IFN and RBV in these new antiviral combinations, however, remains problematic because patients with decompensated cirrhosis and significant medical and/or psychiatric comorbidities are excluded from treatment. Moreover, the need for intensive monitoring of patients on PEG-IFN- and RBV-containing regimens imposes a heavy clinical burden on nursing care in chronic HCV.

DAAs WITHOUT PEG-IFN: EARLY CLINICAL TRIALS AND WHAT IS CURRENTLY AVAILABLE

The limited safety and tolerability of interferon (IFN)-based regimens (Table 3) have led to the development of IFN-free regimens that have been shown to have a superior impact on health-related quality of life and cost effectiveness (30-32). In 2010, Gane et al (33) published the first proof-of-concept study (INFORM-1) that demonstrated that potent viral suppression could be achieved with IFN-free DAA combination therapy whereby danoprevir (NS3/4A protease inhibitor) and mericitabine (NS5B nucleotide polymerase inhibitor) in combination for two weeks produced a 4.9 IU/mL and 5.1 $\log_{10}$ IU/mL decrease in HCV RNA in G1 treatment-naive and previous null responder patients, respectively. In 2012, Lok et al (34) published the first curative-intent study that showed that an SVR could be achieved with an IFN-free regimen whereby asunaprevir (NS3/4A protease

TABLE 3
Common adverse events of simeprevir (SMV)- and sofosbuvir (SOF)-based regimens

Treatment regimen	Adverse events
PEG-IFN + RBV + SMV	Anemia, fatigue, headache, hyperbilirubinemia, influenza-like illness, neutropenia, photosensitivity, pruritus, rash
PEG-IFN + RBV + SOF	Anemia, fatigue, headache, influenza-like illness, insomnia, nausea, neutropenia, rash, thrombocytopenia
RBV + SOF	Anemia, diarrhea, fatigue, headache, insomnia, nausea, pruritus, rash

PEG-IFN Pegylated interferon; RBV Ribavirin

inhibitor) and daclatasvir (NS5A complication complex inhibitor) given for 24 weeks to G1 previous null responders produced an SVR of 36%, which was interesting given the presence of G1a HCV subgenotype in 82% and non-CC IL28B genotype in 91%.

Subsequent clinical trials involving IFN-free regimens have shown more promising efficacy (Table 4). In December 2013, SOF was approved for use with RBV for 12 weeks in G2 and for 24 weeks in G3 based on results from the following studies. In G2 treatment-naive patients, SOF and RBV for 12 weeks produced an SVR of 92% to 97% in noncirrhotics and 94 to 100% in cirrhotics in the FISSION (27), POSITRON (35) and VALENCE (36) clinical trials. In G2 treatment-experienced patients, SOF and RBV for 12 weeks resulted in a SVR of 91% to 96% in noncirrhotics and 60% to 88% in cirrhotics in FUSION (35) and VALENCE (36). In G3 treatment-naive patients, SOF and RBV for 12 weeks produced a SVR of 68% in noncirrhotics and 21% to 56% in cirrhotics in FISSION (27) and POSITRON (35); however, extending the duration of SOF and RBV to 24 weeks improved the SVR to 94% in noncirrhotics and 92% in cirrhotics in VALENCE (36). In G3 treatment-experienced patients, SOF and RBV for 12 to 16 weeks resulted in an SVR of 37% to 63% in noncirrhotics and 19% to 61% in cirrhotics in FUSION (35). Extending the duration of SOF and RBV to 24 weeks improved the SVR to 87% in noncirrhotics but the SVR remained suboptimal (60%) in cirrhotics in VALENCE (36). However, the SVR did improve to 83% in G3 treatment-experienced cirrhotics when PEG-IFN was added to SOF and RBV for 12 weeks in LONESTAR-2 (29). In summary, an excellent SVR was demonstrated with SOF and RBV for 12 weeks in G2 and for 24 weeks in G3 irrespective of previous treatment history or presence of cirrhosis, with the exception of G3 treatment-experienced cirrhotics who required the addition of PEG-IFN to SOF and RBV for 12 weeks.

The use of SOF and RBV for 24 weeks could also be considered in G1 patients who are ineligible for PEG-IFN, although the efficacy appears to be more limited (Table 4). In G1 treatment-naive patients, SOF and RBV for 12 weeks produced an SVR of 84% in noncirrhotics in ELECTRON (37), but only 56% in a patient population consisting of 4% to 8% cirrhotics in QUANTUM (38). Extending the duration of SOF and RBV to 24 weeks in QUANTUM did not improve the SVR which remained suboptimal at 52% (38). However, combination DAA with SMV and SOF with or without RBV for 12 weeks produced a SVR of 67% to 100% in G1 treatment-naive cirrhotics in COSMOS (39-41). In G1 previous null responders, SOF and RBV for 12 weeks resulted in a disappointing SVR of 10% in noncirrhotics in ELECTRON (37). However, combination DAAs with SMV and SOF with or without RBV for 12 weeks in G1 previous null responders produced an impressive SVR of 93% to 96% in noncirrhotics and 80% to 100% in cirrhotics in COSMOS (39-41). In summary, a modest SVR was demonstrated with SOF and RBV for 12 weeks in G1 treatment-naive noncirrhotics, whereas a combination os DAAs with SMV and SOF with or without RBV for 12 weeks was required for G1 treatment-naive cirrhotics and G1 prior null responders with or without cirrhosis. It appears that the addition of RBV may not be needed to achieve a SVR when two potent DAAs are used in combination, as shown in COSMOS (39-41); however, RBV appears to be necessary when a single DAA is used as shown in ELECTRON (37), in which SOF with and without RBV for 12 weeks produced an SVR of 100% and 60%, respectively, in G2/3 treatment-naive noncirrhotics. It has been postulated that RBV may accelerate viral clearance and, thereby, suppress the emergence of DAA resistance (42).

DAAs WITHOUT PEG-IFN: RECENT CLINICAL TRIALS AND WHAT MAY BE AVAILABLE IN THE FUTURE

Following the success of SMV and SOF in COSMOS (39), several other SOF-based regimens in combination with another DAA have also shown impressive results (Table 4). In G1 treatment-naive noncirrhotic patients, SVR with ledipasvir (LDV) (NS5A replication complex inhibitor) and SOF with or without RBV for eight weeks was 93% to 100% in ION-3 (43) and LONESTAR (44); daclatasvir (DCV) (NS5A replication complex inhibitor) and SOF with or without RBV for 12 weeks was 95% to 100% in AI444040 (45); and GS-9669 (NS5B non-nucleoside polymerase inhibitor) and SOF with RBV for 12 weeks was 92% in ELECTRON (46). In G1 treatment-naive patients in whom cirrhosis was present in 16%, LDV and SOF with or without RBV for 12 weeks resulted in a SVR of 97% to 99% in ION-1 (47). In G1 previous null-responders to PEG-IFN and RBV, an SVR of 100% was produced with GS-9669, SOF, and SOF for 12 weeks in noncirrhotic patients and with LDV, SOF, and RBV for 12 weeks in noncirrhotics and cirrhotics in ELECTRON (46). In G1 patients with previous virological failure to protease inhibitor-based regimens (ie, BOC or TVR), DCV and SOF with or without RBV for 24 weeks produced a SVR of 95 to 100% in noncirrhotics in AI444040 (45), whereas LDV and SOF with or without RBV for 12 weeks resulted in a SVR of 94% to 100% in a patient population consisting of cirrhosis in 20% in ION-2 (48) and in 55% in LONESTAR (44). Importantly, these findings demonstrated that failing the protease inhibitor class of DAAs does not preclude treatment success with another class. Finally, the AI444040 (45) study showed that DCV and SOF with or without RBV for 24 weeks produced a SVR of 92% in G2 and 89% in G3 treatment-naive noncirrhotic patients. In summary, an impressive SVR >90% was demonstrated in G1 with SOF in combination with LDV or DCV or GS-9669 with or without RBV for 12 weeks irrespective of treatment history or the presence of cirrhosis. Furthermore, the majority of patients in these studies had unfavourable characteristics including G1a HCV subgenotype and non-CC IL-28B genotype, which strongly suggest that their relevance in IFN-free regimens is minor.

Aside from SOF, another NS5B nucleotide polymerase inhibitor, mericitabine (MCB), was also evaluated in clinical trials although results were less encouraging. In G1 treatment-naive noncirrhotic patients, MCB in combination with ritonavir-boosted danoprevir (NS3/4A protease inhibitor) and RBV for 24 weeks produced a SVR of only 41% which was significantly lower in G1a at 26% compared with G1b (71%) in INFORM-SVR (49). In G1b treatment-experienced noncirrhotics, the same treatment regimen resulted in a SVR of 39% in previous partial responders and 55% in previous null responders in MATTERHORN (50). Based on these disappointing results, MCB is unlikely to be selected as an optimal candidate in DAA combination therapy.

High rates of SVR have also been shown without using NS5B nucleotide polymerase inhibitors as backbone in ABT-450/r (ritonavir-boosted NS3/4A protease inhibitor) -based regimens (Table 4). In G1 treatment-naive noncirrhotic patients, ABT-450/r in combination with ombitasvir (ABT-267) (NS5A replication complex inhibitor) for 12 weeks produced a SVR of 95% in G1b in PEARL-I (51) but only 60% in M12-998 (52) in which G1a was present in 80% of enrolled patients. The decrease in SVR in G1a was also observed in previous clinical trials with protease inhibitor-based regimens. However, the SVR improved to 100% with the addition of RBV in M12-998 (52) and to

TABLE 4
Sustained virological response (SVR) of sofosbuvir (SOF)- and ABT-450/r-based regimens

Genotype (%)	Treatment history	Cirrhosis status	Antiviral regimen	SVR, %	n	Study (reference)
G1a (88)	TN	NC	SOF + RBV x 12 weeks	84	25	ELECTRON (37)
G1a (80)	TN	NC	SOF + LDV ± RBV × 8 weeks	93–94	431	ION-3 (43)
G1a (88)	TN	NC	SOF + LDV ± RBV × 8 weeks	95–100	41	LONESTAR (44)
G1a (82)	TN	NC	SOF + DCV ± RBV × 12 weeks	95–100	82	AI444040 (45)
G1a (84)	TN	NC	SOF + GS-9669 + RBV × 12 weeks	92	25	ELECTRON (46)
G1b (100)	TN	NC	ABT-450/r + ABT-267 × 12 weeks	95	42	PEARL-I (51)
G1a (80)	TN	NC	ABT-450/r + ABT-267 × 12 weeks	60	10	M12-998 (52)
G1a (73)	TN	NC	ABT-450/r + ABT-072 + RBV × 12 weeks	91	11	PILOT (55)
G1a (80)	TN	NC	ABT-450/r + ABT-267 + RBV × 12 weeks	100	10	M12-998 (52)
G1a (85)	TN	NC	ABT-450/r + ABT-333 + RBV × 12 weeks	93–95	33	CO-PILOT (56)
G1a (66)	TN	NC	ABT-450/r + ABT-267 + ABT-333 × 12 weeks	89	79	AVIATOR (53)
G1a (100)	TN	NC	ABT-450/r + ABT-267 + ABT-333 × 12 weeks	90	205	PEARL-IV (54)
G1a (60)	TN	C (6%)	SOF + RBV × 12–24 weeks	52–56	50	QUANTUM (38)
G1a (68)	TN	C (16%)	SOF + LDV ± RBV × 12 weeks	97–99	431	ION-1 (47)
G1a (81)	TN	C	SOF + SMV ± RBV × 12 weeks	67–100	9	COSMOS (39-41)
G1a (67)	TN	C	ABT-450/r + ABT-267 + ABT-333 + RBV × 12 weeks	94	86	TURQUOISE-II (58)
G1a (90)	TE	NC	SOF + RBV × 12 weeks	10	10	ELECTRON (37)
G1a (89)	TE	NC	SOF + LDV + RBV × 12 weeks	100	9	ELECTRON (46)
G1a (81)	TE	NC	SOF + DCV ± RBV × 24 weeks	95–100	41	AI444040 (45)
G1a (90)	TE	NC	SOF + GS-9669 + RBV × 12 weeks	100	10	ELECTRON (46)
G1a (76)	TE	NC	SOF + SMV ± RBV × 12 weeks	93–96	41	COSMOS (39-41)
G1b (100)	TE	NC	ABT-450/r + ABT-267 × 12 weeks	90	40	PEARL-I (51)
G1a (94)	TE	NC	ABT-450/r + ABT-333 + RBV × 12 weeks	47	17	CO-PILOT (56)
G1a (62)	TE	NC	ABT-450/r + ABT-267 + ABT-333 + RBV × 12 weeks	93	45	AVIATOR (53)
G1a (58)	TE	NC	ABT-450/r + ABT-267 + ABT-333 + RBV × 12 weeks	96	297	SAPPHIRE-II (57)
G1a (79)	TE	C (20%)	SOF + LDV ± RBV × 12 weeks	94–96	220	ION-2 (48)
G1a (85)	TE	C (55%)	SOF + LDV ± RBV × 12 weeks	95–100	40	LONESTAR (44)
G1a (78)	TE	C	SOF + LDV ± RBV × 12 weeks	100	9	ELECTRON (46)
G1a (81)	TE	C	SOF + SMV ± RBV × 12 weeks	80–100	9	COSMOS (39-41)
G1a (67)	TE	C	ABT-450/r + ABT-267 + ABT-333 + RBV × 12 weeks	87–97	122	TURQUOISE-II (58)
G2	TN	NC	SOF + RBV ×12 weeks	92	92	POSITRON (35)
G2	TN	NC	SOF + RBV × 12 weeks	97	30	VALENCE (36)
G2	TN	NC	SOF + DCV ± RBV × 24 weeks	92	26	AI444040 (45)
G2	TN	NC	ABT-450/r + ABT-267 + RBV × 12 weeks	80	10	M12-998 (52)
G2	TN	C (20%)	SOF + RBV × 12 weeks	97	70	FISSION (27)
G2	TN	C	SOF + RBV × 12 weeks	94	17	POSITRON (35)
G2	TN	C	SOF + RBV × 12 weeks	100	2	VALENCE (36)
G2	TE	NC	SOF + RBV × 12 weeks	91	33	VALENCE (36)
G2	TE	NC	SOF + RBV × 12 weeks	96	26	FUSION (35)
G2	TE	C	SOF + RBV × 12 weeks	60	10	FUSION (35)
G2	TE	C	SOF + RBV × 12 weeks	88	8	VALENCE (36)
G3	TN	NC	SOF + RBV × 12 weeks	68	84	POSITRON (35)
G3	TN	NC	SOF + RBV × 24 weeks	94	92	VALENCE (36)
G3	TN	NC	SOF + DCV ± RBV × 24 weeks	89	18	AI444040 (45)
G3	TN	NC	ABT-450/r + ABT-267 + RBV × 12 weeks	50	10	M12-998 (52)
G3	TN	C (20%)	SOF + RBV × 12 weeks	56	183	FISSION (27)
G3	TN	C	SOF + RBV × 12 weeks	21	14	POSITRON (35)
G3	TN	C	SOF + RBV × 24 weeks	92	13	VALENCE (36)
G3	TE	NC	SOF + RBV × 12 weeks	37	38	FUSION (35)
G3	TE	NC	SOF + RBV × 16 weeks	63	40	FUSION (35)
G3	TE	NC	SOF + RBV × 24 weeks	87	100	VALENCE (36)
G3	TE	C	SOF + RBV × 12 weeks	19	26	FUSION (35)
G3	TE	C	SOF + RBV × 16 weeks	61	23	FUSION (35)
G3	TE	C	SOF + RBV × 24 weeks	60	45	VALENCE (36)

ABT-267 Ombitasvir; ABT-333 Dasabuvir; C Cirrhotic; DCV Daclatasvir; G Genotype; LDV Ledipasvir; NC Noncirrhotic; r Ritonavir; RBV Ribavirin; SMV Simeprevir; TE Treatment experienced; TN Treatment naive

89% to 90% with the addition of dasabuvir (ABT-333) (NS5B non-nucleoside polymerase inhibitor) in AVIATOR (53), in which G1a was present in 61% to 68%, and in PEARL-IV (54), in which G1a was present in 100%. Similarly, ABT-450/r and RBV in combination with ABT-072 (NS5B non-nucleoside polymerase inhibitor) for 12 weeks produced a SVR of 91% in PILOT (55) in which G1a was present in 73%, whereas ABT-450/r and RBV in combination with dasabuvir for 12 weeks produced a SVR of 93% to 95% in CO-PILOT (56) in which G1a was present in 79% to 90%. Importantly, one patient experienced a late relapse at 36 weeks post-treatment in PILOT (55), raising the concern that longer follow-up beyond 24 weeks may be needed with IFN-free regimens. In G1 treatment-experienced noncirrhotic patients, ABT-450/r and ombitasvir given for 12 weeks resulted in an SVR of 90% in G1b in PEARL-I (51), whereas ABT-450/r, dasabuvir and RBV given for 12 weeks produced a relatively disappointing SVR of 47% in CO-PILOT (56), in which G1a was present in 94% of study patients. However, when ombitasvir was added as a third DAA, the SVR improved significantly to 93% in AVIATOR (53), in which G1a was present in 62% and to 96% in SAPPHIRE-II (57), in which G1a was present in 58%. In G1 treatment-naive and experienced cirrhotic patients (Child-Pugh class A), ABT-450/r, ombitasvir, dasabuvir and RBV given for 12 weeks produced an SVR of 94% and 87% to 97%, respectively, in TURQUOISE-II (58). Finally, the M12-998 study (52) showed that 12 weeks of ABT-450, ombitasvir and RBV produced an SVR of 80% in G2 but only 50% in G3 treatment-naive noncirrhotic patients. In summary, an SVR >90% was demonstrated in G1b noncirrhotics regardless of treatment history with ABT-450/r and ombitasvir for 12 weeks; in G1a treatment-naive noncirrhotics with ABT-450/r combined with either another DAA and RBV or two other DAAs for 12 weeks; and in G1a treatment-experienced noncirrhotics and G1 cirrhotics irrespective of treatment history with ABT-450/r, ombitasvir, dasabuvir and RBV for 12 weeks. Treatment was well tolerated in all of these clinical trials.

Other treatment regimens that included three DAAs (NS3/4A protease inhibitor, NS5A replication complex inhibitor and NS5B non-nucleoside polymerase inhibitor) also appeared to improve SVR. Asunaprevir (NS3/4A protease inhibitor) in combination with DCV (NS5A replication complex inhibitor) for 24 weeks in G1 previous null responder noncirrhotic patients produced an SVR of 65% to 100% in G1b (59-61) but only 36% in a patient population in which G1a was present in 82% (34). The SVR remained suboptimal (23%) with the addition of RBV (61). However, ASV, DCV and BMS-791325 (NS5B non-nucleoside polymerase inhibitor) given for 12 to 24 weeks in G1 treatment-naive noncirrhotic patients resulted in a SVR of 89% to 94% in NCT01455090 (62), in which G1a was present in 72% to 75% of patients. On the other hand, unexpectedly disappointing results have been recently published involving G1 treatment-naive noncirrhotics whereby vedroprevir (VDV) (NS3/4A protease inhibitor), LDV (NS5A replication complex inhibitor), tegobuvir (NS5B non-nucleoside polymerase inhibitor) and RBV for

12 to 24 weeks produced a surprisingly low SVR of only 54 to 63% in the QUAD trial (63) in which G1a was present in 67% to 76% of patients. Finally, MK-5172 (NS3/4A protease inhibitor), MK-8472 (NS5A replication complex inhibitor), and RBV for 12 weeks resulted in a remarkable SVR of 96% to 100% in C-WORTHY trial (64) in which G1a was present in 70% to 76% of patients.

CONCLUSION

As the present brief review indicates, there are many DAAs that have been through clinical trials, both currently and in the recent past, that seek to provide an efficacious, IFN-free treatment for the long-term clearance of HCV. Clearly not all of these agents will survive to licensure and the marketplace. It is commonly accepted that the ideal DAA combination should include such primary characteristics as potent antiviral efficacy, high genetic barrier to resistance, broad genotypic coverage, minimal side effects and favourable safety profile, whereas secondary characteristics should include low pill burden, short treatment duration, no dietary restriction, few drug interactions and affordable drug cost (10). The optimal antiviral regimen likely entails combination of an NS5B nucleotide polymerase inhibitor with either a second-generation NS3/4A protease inhibitor or a NS5A replication complex inhibitor. The role of RBV requires further clarification but appears to be unnecessary when two DAAs with potent antiviral efficacy and high genetic barrier to resistance are used. Although it is too early to declare that PEG-IFN is 'dead', clearly in the near future, its role in HCV treatment will continue to diminish. Despite the recent advances in DAA drug development, many questions remain unanswered. Whether resistance testing is warranted before treatment initiation or in virological failure to IFN-free regimens remains to be elucidated. It is also unclear whether prolonged follow-up beyond 24 weeks post-treatment is necessary with IFN-free regimens. Finally, more data from future research are needed in HCV G4, G5 and G6, and in difficult-to-cure patient populations, which include decompensated cirrhosis, renal failure, HIV coinfection, solid organ transplantation, and pre- and post-liver transplantation. The most important question of whether long-term HCV clearance will also result in clinical improvement in patients with early decompensated cirrhosis, as has been the situation in hepatitis B, remains unknown and awaits further experience with IFN-free DAAs.

DISCLOSURES: Dr Yau does not have any competing interests. Dr Yoshida has been an investigator in hepatitis C clinical trials sponsored by Hoffmann LaRoche, Merck Inc, Vertex Inc, Gilead Sciences Inc, Pfizer Inc, Norvartis Inc, Boehringer Ingelheim Inc, Janssen Inc and AbbVie Inc. He has participated in Advisory Board meetings of Hoffmann LaRoche Canada, Vertex Canada and Boehringer Ingelheim Canada. He has received honoraria for CME lectures provided by Vertex Canada, Gilead Canada and Merck Canada.

REFERENCES

1. World Health Organization (WHO). Viral Hepatitis – Resolutions from the 63rd World Health Assembly, 2010.
2. Remis R. Modeling the incidence and prevalence of hepatitis C infection and its sequelae in Canada, 2007 final report. Public Health Agency of Canada. 2007.
3. Myers RP, Liu MF, Shaheen AAM. The burden of hepatitis C virus infection is growing: A Canadian population-based study of hospitalizations from 1994 to 2004. Can J Gastroenterol 2008;22:381-7.
4. Dungum M, O'Shea R. Hepatitis C virus: Here comes all-oral treatment. Cleve Clin J Med 2014;81:159-72.
5. Manns MP, McHutchison JG, Gordon SC, et al. Peginterferon alfa-2b plus ribavirin compared with interferon alfa-2b plus ribavirin for initial treatment of chronic hepatitis C: A randomized trial. Lancet 2001;358:958-65.
6. Fried MW, Shiffman ML, Reddy R, et al. Peginterferon alfa-2a plus ribavirin for chronic hepatitis C virus infection. N Engl J Med 2002;347:975-82.
7. Hézode C, Fontaine H, Dorival C, et al. Triple therapy in treatment-experienced patients with HCV-cirrhosis in a multicenter cohort of the French Early Access Programme (ANRS CO20-CUPIC) – NCT01514890. J Hepatol 2013;59:434-41.
8. Ward RP, Kugelmas M. Using pegylated interferon and ribavirin to treat patients with chronic hepatitis C. Am Fam Physician 2005;72:655-62.
9. Bruchfeld A, Lindahl K, Stahle L, et al. Interferon and ribavirin treatment in patients with hepatitis C-associated renal disease and renal insufficiency. Nephrol Dial Transplant 2003;18:1573-80.
10. Schinazi R, Halfon P, Marcellin P, Asselah T. HCV direct-acting antiviral agents: The best interferon-free combinations. Liver Int 2014;34(S1):69-78.

11. Kwo PY, Lawitz EJ, McCone J, et al. Efficacy of boceprevir, an NS3 protease inhibitor, in combination with peginterferon alfa-2b and ribavirin in treatment-naïve patients with genotype 1 hepatitis C infection (SPRINT-1): An open-label, randomized, multicenter phase 2 trial. Lancet 2010;376:705-16.

12. Poordad F, McCone J, Bacon BR, et al. Boceprevir for untreated chronic HCV genotype 1 infection. N Engl J Med 2011;364:1195-206.

13. Jacobson IM, McHutchison JG, Dusheiko G, et al. Telaprevir for previously untreated chronic hepatitis C virus infection. N Engl J Med 2011;364:2405-16.

14. Lange CM, Zeuzem S. Perspectives and challenges of interferon-free therapy for chronic hepatitis C. J Hepatol 2013;58:583-92.

15. Stedman CA. Current prospects for interferon-free treatment of hepatitis C in 2012. J Gastroenterol Hepatol 2013;28:38-45.

16. Bacon BR, Gordon SC, Lawitz E, et al. Boceprevir for previously treated chronic HCV genotype 1 infection. N Engl J Med 2011;364:1207-17.

17. Zeuzem S, Andreone P, Pol S, et al. Telaprevir for retreatment of HCV infection. N Engl J Med 2011;364:2417-28.

18. González-Moreno J, Payeras-Cifre A. Hepatitis C virus infection: Looking for interferon free regimens. Scientific World Journal 2013;2013(825375):1-11.

19. Jacobson IM, Dore GJ, Foster GR, et al. Simeprevir (TMC435) with peginterferon/ribavirin for chronic HCV genotype-1 infection in treatment-naïve patients: Results from QUEST-1, a phase III trial. J Hepatol 2013;58:S567-577. Abst 1425.

20. Manns M, Marcellin P, Poordad FPF, et al. Simeprevir (TMC435) with peginterferon/ribavirin for treatment of chronic HCV genotype-1 infection in treatment-naïve patients: Results from QUEST-2, a phase III trial. J Hepatol 2013;58(S567-S577): Abst 1413.

21. Fried MW, Buti M, Dore GJ, et al. Once-daily simeprevir (TMC435) with pegylated interferon and ribavirin in treatment-naïve genotype 1 hepatitis C: The randomized PILLAR study. Hepatology 2013;58:1918-29.

22. Lawitz E, Zeuzem S, Gane E, et al. Simeprevir (TMC435) with pegylated interferon-α-2a/ribavirin for treatment of chronic HCV genotype 1 infection in patients who relapsed after previous interferon-based therapy: Efficacy and safety in patient sub-populations in the PROMISE phase III trial. 64th Annual Meeting of the American Association for the Study of Liver Diseases, Washington DC, November 1 to 5, 2013.

23. Zeuzem S, Berg T, Gane E, et al. Simeprevir increases rate of sustained virologic response among treatment-experienced patients with HCV genotype-1 infection: A phase IIb trial. Gastroenterology 2014;146:430-41.

24. Bae A, Sun SC, Qi X, et al. Susceptibility of treatment-naïve hepatitis C virus (HCV) clinical isolates to HCV protease inhibitors. Antimicrob Agents Chemother 2010;54:5288-97.

25. Lawitz E, Lalezari JP, Hassanein T, et al. Sofosbuvir in combination with peginterferon alfa-2a and ribavirin for non-cirrhotic, treatment-naïve patients with genotypes 1, 2, and 3 hepatitis C infection: A randomized, double-blind, phase 2 trial. Lancet Infect Dis 2013;13:401-8.

26. Kowdley KV, Lawitz E, Crespo I, et al. Sofosbuvir with pegylated interferon alfa-2a and ribavirin for treatment-naïve patients with hepatitis C genotype-1 infection (ATOMIC): An open-label, randomized, multicentre phase 2 trial. Lancet 2013;381:2100-7.

27. Lawitz E, Mangia A, Wyles D, et al. Sofosbuvir for previously untreated chronic hepatitis C infection. N Engl J Med 2013;368:1878-87.

28. Lalezari J, Lawitz E, Rodriguez-Torres M, et al. Once daily PSI-7977 plus PegIFN/RBV in a phase 2b trial: Rapid virologic suppression in treatment-naive patients with HCV GT2/GT3. J Hepatol 2011;54(S25-S44):Abst 61.

29. Lawitz E, Poordad F, Brainard DM, et al. Sofosbuvir in combination with PegIFN and ribavirin for 12 weeks provides high SVR rates in HCV-infected genotype 2 or 3 treatment-experienced patients with and without compensated cirrhosis: Results from the LONESTAR-2 study. 64th Annual Meeting of the American Association for the Study of Liver Diseases, Washington DC, November 1 to 5, 2013.

30. Younossi ZM, Stepanova M, Henry L, et al. Minimal impact of sofosbuvir and ribavirin on health related quality of life in chronic hepatitis C (CH-C). J Hepatol 2014;60:741-7.

31. Younossi ZM, Stepanova M, Henry L, et al. Effects of sofosbuvir-based treatment, with and without interferon, on outcome and productivity of patients with chronic hepatitis C. Clin Gastroenterol Hepatol 2013;S1542-3565(13)01838-7.

32. Younossi ZM, Singer ME, Mir HM, et al. Impact of interferon free regimens on clinical and cost outcomes for chronic hepatitis C genotype 1 patients. J Hepatol 2014;60:530-7.

33. Gane EJ, Roberts SK, Stedman CA, et al. Oral combination therapy with a nucleoside polymerase inhibitor (RG7128) and danoprevir for chronic hepatitis C genotype 1 infection (INFORM-1): A randomized, double-blind, placebo-controlled, dose-escalation trial. Lancet 2010;376:1467-75.

34. Lok AS, Gardiner AF, Lawitz E, et al. Preliminary study of two antiviral agents for hepatitis C genotype 1. N Engl J Med 2012;366:216-24.

35. Jacobson IM, Gordon SC, Kowdley KV, et al. Sofosbuvir for hepatitis C genotype 2 or 3 in patients without treatment options. N Engl J Med 2013;368:1867-77.

36. Zeuzem S, Dusheiko GM, Salupere R, et al. Sofosbuvir + ribavirin for 12 or 24 weeks for patients with HCV genotype 2 or 3: The VALENCE trial. 64th Annual Meeting of the American Association for the Study of Liver Diseases, Washington DC, November 1 to 5, 2013.

37. Gane EJ, Stedman CA, Hyland RH, et al. Nucleotide polymerase inhibitor sofosbuvir plus ribavirin for hepatitis C. N Engl J Med 2013;368:34-44.

38. Lalezari JP, Nelson DR, Hyland RH, et al. Once-daily sofosbuvir plus ribavirin given for 12 or 24 weeks in treatment-naive patients with HCV infection: The QUANTUM study. J Hepatol 2013;58:S229-407.

39. Jacobson IM, Ghalib RH, Rodriguez-Torres M, et al. SVR results of a once-daily regimen of simeprevir (TMV435) plus sofosbuvir (GS-7977) with or without ribavirin in cirrhotic and non-cirrhotic HCV genotype 1 treatment-naïve and prior null responder patients: The COSMOS study. 64th Annual Meeting of the American Association for the Study of Liver Diseases, Washington DC, November 1 to 5, 2013. Abst LB-3.

40. Sulkowski M, Jacobson IM, Ghalib R, et al. Once-daily simeprevir (TMC435) plus sofosbuvir (GS-7977) with or without ribavirin in HCV genotype 1 prior null responders with metavir F0-2: COSMOS study subgroup analysis. J Hepatol 2014;60:S4. A7 (Abst).

41. Lawitz E, Ghalib R, Rodriguez-Torres M, et al. Simeprevir plus sofosbuvir with/without ribavirin in HCV genotype 1 prior null-responder/treatment-naïve patients (COSMOS study). Primary endpoint (SVR12) results in patients with metavir F3-4 (Cohort 2). J Hepatol 2014;60(1):S524:A165 (Abst).

42. Sharma P, Lok AS. Interferon-free treatment regimens for hepatitis C: Are we there yet? Gastroenterology 2011,141.1963-7.

43. Kowdley KV, Gordon SC, Reddy KR, et al. Ledipasvir and sofosbuvir for 8 or 12 weeks for chronic HCV without cirrhosis. N Engl J Med 2014;370:1879-88.

44. Lawitz E, Poordad FF, Pang PS, et al. Sofosbuvir and ledipasvir fixed-dose combination with and without ribavirin in treatment-naïve and previously treated patients with genotype 1 hepatitis C virus infection (LONESTAR): An open-label, randomized, phase 2 trial. Lancet 2014;383:515-23.

45. Sulkowski MS, Gardiner DF, Rodriguez-Torres M, et al. Daclatasvir plus sofosbuvir for previously treated or untreated chronic HCV infection. N Engl J Med 2014;370:211-21.

46. Gane EJ, Stedman CA, Hyland RH, et al. Efficacy of nucleotide polymerase inhibitor sofosbuvir plus the NS5A inhibitor ledipasvir or the NS5B non-nucleoside inhibitor GS-9669 against HCV genotype 1 infection. Gastroenteroloy 2014;146:736-43.

47. Afdhal N, Zeuzem S, Kwo P, et al. Ledipasvir and sofosbuvir for untreated HCV genotype 1 infection. N Engl J Med 2014;370:1889-98.

48. Afdhal N, Reddy R, Nelson DR, et al. Ledipasvir and sofosbuvir for previously treated HCV genotype 1 infection. N Engl J Med 2014;370:1483-93.

49. Gane EJ, Pockros P, Zeuzem S, et al. Interferon-free treatment with a combination of mericitabine and danoprevir with or without ribavirin in treatment-naïve HCV genotype 1-infected patients. J Hepatol 2012;56:S555-6.

50. Feld JJ, Jacobson IM, Jensen DM, et al. Up to 100% SVR4 rates with ritonavir-boosted danoprevir (DNVr), mericitabine (MCB) and ribavirin (R) +/- peginterferon alfa-2a (40KD) (P) in HCV genotype 1-infected partial and null responders: results from the MATTERHORN study. Hepatology 2012;56(S4):231A-232A.

51. Lawitz E, Hezode C, Varunok P, et al. Interferon- and ribavirin-free regimen of ABT-450/r + ABT-267 in HCV genotype 1b-infected treatment-naïve patients and prior null responders (Abstr 75). 64th Annual Meeting of the American Association for the Study of Liver Diseases, Washington, DC, November 1 to 5, 2013. (Abst)

52. Lawitz E, Sullivan G, Rodriguez-Torres M, et al. A 12-week trial of interferon-free regimens containing ABT-450/r and ABT-267 +/- ribavirin (RBV) in treatment-naïve patients with HCV genotypes 1-3. Hepatol Int 2013;7(S1):S358-9.

53. Kowdley KV, Lawitz E, Poordad F, et al. Phase 2b trial of interferon-free therapy for hepatitis C virus genotype 1. N Engl J Med 2014;370:222-32.

54. Ferenci P, Bernstein D, Lalezari J, et al. ABT-450/r-ombitasvir and dasabuvir with or without ribavirin for HCV. N Engl J Med 2014;370:1983-92.

55. Lawitz E, Poordad F, Kowdley KV, et al. A phase 2a trial of 12-week interferon-free therapy with two direct-acting antivirals (ABT-450/r, ABT-072) and ribavirin in IL28B C/C patients with chronic hepatitis C genotype 1. J Hepatol 2013;59:18-23.

56. Poordad F, Lawitz E, Kowdley KV, et al. Exploratory study of oral combination antiviral therapy for hepatitis C. N Engl J Med 2013;368:45-53.

57. Zeuzem S, Jacobson IM, Baykal T, et al. Retreatment of HCV with ABT-450/r-ombitasvir and dasabuvir with ribavirin. N Engl J Med 2014;370:1604-14.

58. Poordad F, Hezode C, Trinh R, et al. ABT-450/r-ombitasvir and dasabuvir with ribavirin for hepatitis C with cirrhosis. N Engl J Med 2014;370:1973-82.

59. Chayama K, Takahashi S, Toyota J, et al. Dual therapy with the nonstructural protein 5A inhibitor, daclatasvir, and the nonstructural protein 3 protease inhibitor, asunaprevir, in hepatitis C virus genotype 1b-infected null responders. Hepatology 2012;55:742-8.

60. Suzuki Y, Ikeda K, Suzuki F, et al. Dual oral therapy with daclatasvir and asunaprevir for patients with HCV genotype 1b infection and limited treatment options. J Hepatol 2013;58:655-62.

61. Lok AS, Gardiner DF, Hezode C, et al. Randomized trial of daclatasvir and asunaprevir with or without PegIFN/RBV for hepatitis C virus genotype 1 null responders. J Hepatol 2014;60:490-9.

62. Everson GT, Sims KD, Rodriguez-Torres M, et al. Efficacy of an interferon- and ribavirin-free regimen of daclatasvir, asunaprevir, and BMS-791325 in treatment-naïve patients with HCV genotype 1 infection. Gastroenterology 2014;146:420-9.

63. Wyles DL, Rodriguez-Torres M, Lawitz E, et al. All-oral combination of ledipasvir, vedroprevir, tegobuvir, and ribavirin in treatment-naïve patients with genotype 1 HCV infection. Hepatology 2014 (Epub ahead of print).

64. Lawitz E, Vierling J, Murillo A, et al. High efficacy and safety of the all-oral combination regimen, MK-5172/MK-8742 +/- RBV for 12 weeks in HCV genotype 1 infected patients: The C-WORTHY study. 64th Annual Meeting of the American Association for the Study of Liver Diseases, Washington, DC, November 1 to 5, 2013.

20

Initial management of noncirrhotic splanchnic vein thrombosis: When is anticoagulation enough?

Pranavi Ravichandran MD[1], Kris P Croome MD MS[1,2], Michael J Kovacs MD FRCPC[3],
Alejandro Lazo-Langner MD MSc[3,4], Roberto Hernandez-Alejandro MD[1,2]

P Ravichandran, KP Croome, MJ Kovacs, A Lazo-Langner, R Hernandez-Alejandro. Initial management of noncirrhotic splanchnic vein thrombosis: When is anticoagulation enough? Can J Gastroenterol Hepatol 2014;28(4):207-211.

BACKGROUND: The optimal initial treatment of splanchnic vein thrombosis is uncertain. Anticoagulant therapy has been shown to be associated with vessel recanalization and decreased recurrence. Furthermore, information regarding potential predictors of chronic complications is not well understood.

METHODS: A retrospective cohort study involving consecutive patients diagnosed with first-episode noncirrhotic splanchnic vein thrombosis referred to the thrombosis clinic of the authors' institution between 2008 and 2011 was conducted. Demographic and clinical information was collected. The response to initial anticoagulant therapy was evaluated by determining radiographic recanalization of vessels and clinical resolution (defined as the absence of ongoing splanchnic vein thrombosis symptoms or complications requiring treatment beyond anticoagulant therapy.)

RESULTS: Twenty-two patients were included. Anticoagulant therapy alone resulted in vessel recanalization in 41% of patients and 68% achieved clinical resolution. Two patients experienced bleeding events. Factors associated with a lack of clinical resolution included signs of portal hypertension/liver failure on presentation, complete vessel occlusion at diagnosis, presence of a myeloproliferative disorder or JAK2[V617F] tyrosine kinase mutation and the absence of a local/transient predisposing factor.

CONCLUSIONS: Anticoagulant therapy appeared to be an effective initial treatment in patients with splanchnic vein thrombosis. Clinical factors may help to identify patients who are at risk for developing complications thus requiring closer monitoring. These findings were limited by the small sample size and need to be explored in larger prospective studies.

Key Words: Anticoagulation; Portal hypertension; Splanchnic vein thrombosis; Therapy

La prise en charge initiale de la thrombose veineuse splanchnique non cirrhotique : quand l'anticoagulation suffit-elle?

HISTORIQUE : On ne connaît pas le traitement initial optimal de la thrombose veineuse splanchnique. L'anticoagulothérapie s'associe à une recanalisation des vaisseaux et à une diminution des récurrences. De plus, on comprend mal les données sur les prédicteurs potentiels des complications chroniques.

MÉTHODOLOGIE : Les auteurs ont mené une étude rétrospective de cohorte auprès de patients consécutifs ayant un diagnostic de premier épisode de thrombose veineuse splanchnique aiguillés vers la clinique de thrombose de leur établissement entre 2008 et 2011. Ils ont colligé des renseignements démographiques et cliniques. Ils ont évalué la réponse à l'anticoagulothérapie initiale en déterminant la recanalisation radiographique des vaisseaux et leur résolution clinique (définie comme l'absence de symptômes continus de thrombose veineuse splanchnique ou de complications exigeant un traitement en plus de l'anticoagulothérapie).

RÉSULTATS : Vingt-deux patients ont participé à l'étude. L'anticoagulothérapie seule a assuré la recanalisation des artères chez 41 % des patients, dont 68 % ont profité d'une résolution clinique. Deux patients ont souffert d'hémorragies. Les facteurs associés à l'absence de résolution clinique incluaient les signes d'hypertension portale ou d'insuffisance hépatique à la présentation, une occlusion complète des vaisseaux au diagnostic, la présence d'un trouble myéloprolifératif ou de la mutation de la tyrosine kinase JAK2[V617F] et l'absence de facteur prédisposant local ou transitoire.

CONCLUSIONS : L'anticoagulothérapie semblait efficace comme traitement initial de la thrombose veineuse splanchnique. Des facteurs cliniques peuvent contribuer à dépister les patients vulnérables aux complications et qui ont donc besoin d'une surveillance plus attentive. Ces observations étaient limitées par la petite taille de l'échantillon et devront être évaluées dans le cadre d'études prospectives plus vastes.

Splanchnic vein thrombosis unrelated to primary liver disease is a rare and poorly understood clinical phenomenon; information pertaining to its optimal management is limited (1-4). Anticoagulant therapy in patients with splanchnic vein thrombosis has been shown to be effective in recanalizing thrombosed vessels and alleviating symptoms (2). For chronic splanchnic vein thrombosis with ongoing risk factors, prolonged or indefinite anticoagulant therapy has been credited with decreasing recurrence rates and preventing symptom progression (4,5).

When medical management is not effective, progressive or recurrent splanchnic vein thrombosis can cause mesenteric ischemia or portal hypertension requiring surgical or endoscopic management. Given its reported safety and efficacy, most clinicians begin management with anticoagulant therapy alone, resorting to more invasive interventions following an ineffective trial of medical management (2-4,6). In the present study, we aimed to describe our experience with the treatment of splanchnic vein thrombosis and to identify potential predictors of the need for additional interventions beyond anticoagulant therapy.

METHODS

A retrospective cohort study including consecutive adult patients with a newly diagnosed first episode of noncirrhotic splanchnic vein thrombosis referred to the Thrombosis Clinic at the London Health Sciences Centre in London, Ontario, between January 2008 and August 2011 was conducted. Information regarding demographic and clinical

[1]*Department of Surgery, Division of General Surgery, University of Western Ontario;* [2]*Multi-Organ Transplant Program, London Health Sciences Centre;*
[3]*Department of Medicine, Division of Hematology;* [4]*Department of Epidemiology and Biostatistics, University of Western Ontario, London, Ontario*
Correspondence: Dr Alejandro Lazo-Langner, Division of Hematology, Department of Medicine, University of Western Ontario,
800 Commissioners Road East, Room E6-216A, London, Ontario N6A 5W9. e-mail alejandro.lazolangner@lhsc.on.ca

TABLE 1
Splanchnic vein involvement and degree of occlusion at maximally occlusive site (n=22)

Vessel(s) involved	Complete	Partial	Not specified	Total, n (%)
Isolated splanchnic vein thrombosis				
Portal vein	2	2	2	6 (27.3)
SMV		5	1	6 (27.3)
Multivessel disease				
Portal vein + SMV + SV	2		3	5 (22.7)
Portal vein + SV	1			1 (4.5)
Portal vein + SMV	1			1 (4.5)
Portal vein + SMV + DVT	1			1 (4.5)
Portal vein + DVT	1			1 (4.5)
Portal vein + BCS	1			1 (4.5)

BCS Budd-Chiari syndrome with hepatic vein thrombosis; DVT Left deep vein thrombosis; SMV Superior mesenteric vein; SV Splenic vein

TABLE 2
Risk factors for splanchnic vein thrombosis (n=22)

Factor	n (%)
Local/transient etiology	11 (50)
Malignancy*	5 (22.7)
Recent abdominal surgery*	7 (31.8)
Idiopathic small bowel obstructions	1 (4.5)
Diverticulitis	1 (4.5)
Chronic pancreatitis with recent stenting	1 (4.5)
Systemic thrombophilia	8 (36.4)
Myeloproliferative disorder/JAK2V617F tyrosine kinase mutation†	6 (27.3)
Prothrombin gene G20210A variant	2 (9.1)
Factor V Leiden	4 (18.2)
Multiple thrombophilia	4 (18.2)
Unknown	3 (13.6)

In three patients, abdominal surgery was due to malignancy; †In one patient, myeloproliferative disorder was biopsy proven but JAK2 negative

variables, predisposing factors and thrombophilia was collected. The index date was the date an objectively confirmed diagnosis of portal, splenic and/or superior mesenteric veins was made. Thrombophilia screening was performed in all patients and included prothrombin gene G20210A variant, Factor V Leiden, protein C deficiency, protein S deficiency, antithrombin deficiency, anticardiolipin antibodies, lupus anticoagulant and paroxysmal nocturnal hemoglobinuria. The duration of anticoagulation therapy was also recorded. Patients were classified as having a myeloproliferative disorder if they carried the JAK2V617F tyrosine kinase mutation (7) or if they met current diagnostic criteria for overt myeloproliferative disorder in the absence of the JAK2V617F mutation (8).

The response to initial anticoagulant therapy was assessed by determining radiographic recanalization of vessels on follow-up imaging and clinical resolution. The latter was defined as the absence of ongoing splanchnic vein thrombosis symptoms or complications requiring treatment beyond anticoagulant therapy. Also assessed were the occurrence of major bleeding events according to the definition from the International Society on Thrombosis and Haemostasis (9) as well as clinically relevant nonmajor bleeding. Groups were compared using the Mann-Whitney or Fisher's exact tests, as appropriate; P<0.05 was considered to be statistically significant.

RESULTS

Patient characteristics
Between January 2008 and August 2011, 22 patients (nine female; mean age 51 years [range 29 to 67 years]) who received anticoagulant therapy and did not demonstrate primary cirrhotic disease were referred to the authors' clinic and included in the study. Table 1 summarizes the distribution of vessels involved. Comorbid conditions included history of deep vein thrombosis or pulmonary embolism (n=5), hypertension (n=4), type 2 diabetes (n=1), obesity (n=1), inflammatory bowel disease (n=2), recent or ongoing nonhepatic malignancy (n=5), and recent abdominal surgery (n=6). A local or transient risk factor for splanchnic vein thrombosis formation was identified in 50% of the patients. Among the remaining patients, eight had thrombophilic disorders identified (Table 2). Myeloproliferative disorders were identified in six patients (27.3%). No underlying risk factors for splanchnic vein thrombosis were identified in three patients.

Four patients were diagnosed incidentally on staging computed tomography scans for colorectal cancer or lymphoma. Another patient was initially imaged due to recurrent, transiently elevated liver enzyme levels. All symptomatic patients were diagnosed with splanchnic vein thrombosis within 24 h to three weeks from the onset of symptoms.

The most common presenting symptom was abdominal pain (54.5%). Other presenting complaints included abdominal distension and decreased bowel movements, marked hepatosplenomegaly secondary to myelofibrosis and fever in a patient with a history of recurrent diverticulitis. Of note, one patient presented with upper and lower gastrointestinal bleeding and an acute surgical abdomen secondary to intestinal ischemia. Four patients had documented signs of portal hypertension or hepatic dysfunction at the time of diagnosis of splanchnic vein thrombosis. These included nonbleeding gastroesophageal varices (n=2), hepatosplenomegaly (n=3), ascites (n=2) and jaundice (n=2). Screening endoscopy was not routinely offered to all patients included in the present review, and information pertaining to the presence or absence of gastroesophageal varices was only available for these four patients.

All patients included in the study received anticoagulant therapy promptly after diagnosis. Treatment consisted of unfractionated heparin or low molecular weight heparin followed by oral vitamin K antagonists. Patients who recurred were switched to long-term treatment with low molecular weight heparin at the discretion of the treating physician who also determined the duration of anticoagulant therapy. All of the 11 patients with only clear local or transient risk factors completed a short course of anticoagulant therapy (six months in 10 patients and three months in a patient whose course was stopped early in anticipation of an unrelated surgical procedure). All remaining patients were prescribed indefinite anticoagulation.

No patients underwent thrombolytic therapy. In one patient who was diagnosed with mesenteric vein thrombosis intraoperatively, visible thrombi were manually removed during laparotomy and anticoagulant therapy was started postoperatively. The mean follow-up period for all patients was 22 months.

Treatment outcomes and predictors
Follow-up imaging was available for 21 patients because one patient died during follow-up from concurrent metastatic colorectal cancer. Vessel recanalization was documented in nine patients (41%) and clinical resolution was achieved in 15 (68%). Of the 11 patients who received short-course anticoagulation for splanchnic vein thrombosis associated with only local or transient risk factors, eight (73%) obtained vessel recanalization and 10 (91%) resolved clinically. The local/transient risk factor group had an increased association with recanalization (P=0.008) and tended to achieve clinical resolution more frequently (P=0.063) than individuals with identified thrombophilias or unknown etiologies. The clinical complications and subsequent interventions made in patients who did not achieve clinical resolution are descibed in Table 3.

TABLE 3
Complications and subsequent interventions in patients failing to achieve clinical resolution

Patient	Thrombosed vessels	Clinical complications	Interventions
1	Portal vein	Deceased (ongoing malignancy)	
2	Portal vein	Development of new nonbleeding varices	Beta-blockers
3	Portal vein	Persistence of nonbleeding varices	Beta-blockers
	Superior mesenteric vein	Massive splenomegaly + compressive gastric	Splenectomy
	Splenic vein	outlet obstruction	
4	Portal vein	Transient rethrombosis and abdominal pain	
	Splenic vein		
5	Portal vein	Portocaval shunt occlusion	Urgent liver transplant
	Hepatic veins (Budd-Chiari syndrome)	Liver failure	
	Portocaval shunt		
6	Portal vein	Enlargement of nonbleeding varices	Discontinuation of anticoagulant therapy
	Deep vein thrombosis (leg)		Beta-blockers
		Rethrombosis (deep vein thrombosis)	Resume anticoagulant therapy
			Splenectomy
			Devascularization of gastroesophageal junction
		Variceal hemorrhage	Discontinuation of anticoagulant therapy
			Variceal band ligation
		Rethrombosis: Portal vein	Restart indefinite anticoagulant therapy
		New thrombosis: Inferior vena cava and left renal vein	
7	Mesenteric veins (diagnosed intraoperatively)	Acute ischemic gut at initial presentation	Manual thrombectomy
			Small bowel resection

Factors associated with a lack of clinical resolution (and subsequent need for further interventions) included signs of portal hypertension/liver failure on presentation (P=0.005), complete vessel occlusion at diagnosis (P=0.029), presence of a myeloproliferative disorder or $JAK2^{V617F}$ tyrosine kinase mutation (P=0.004) and the absence of a local/transient predisposing factor (P=0.034). There did not appear to be any statistically significant association between outcome and age, sex or clinical presentation. Of the four patients with incidental diagnoses in the context of active or treated malignancy, three attained persistent radiographic recanalization and one died from concurrent metastatic colonic malignancy.

There was one event each of major and clinically relevant nonmajor bleeding. One patient experienced recurrent lower gastrointestinal bleeding that ceased on completion of a six-month course of anticoagulant therapy, and variceal hemorrhage occurred in one patient who subsequently underwent endoscopic variceal band ligation followed by resumption of prolonged anticoagulant therapy for recurrent splanchnic vein thrombosis.

DISCUSSION

In the present study, we report our experience with the treatment of patients with noncirrhotic splanchnic vein thrombosis using anticoagulant therapy. We found that approximately one-half of the patients achieved recanalization of the involved vessels, particularly among patients with a transient or local risk factor. Other studies have also reported partial or complete recanalization in 33% to 90% of cases with anticoagulant therapy alone (1,2,4,10). However, in addition to vessel recanalization, the presence of clinical resolution (and avoidance of additional therapies) is also a clinically relevant parameter that has not been frequently studied. In fact, studies investigating lower-extremity deep vein thrombosis have not demonstrated that radiographic resolution alone is associated with improved rates of symptom-free survival or recurrence (11). In this regard, we found that clinical resolution occurred more frequently in patients with transient/local risk factors, in those with partial vein occlusions, in those without signs of portal hypertension or liver failure, and in those without the $JAK2^{V617F}$ mutation. This information may help to identify patients at higher risk for developing chronic complications and, thus, requiring closer monitoring. There did not appear to be any

statistically significant association between outcome and age, sex or clinical presentation in the current study.

In patients with ongoing prothrombotic disorders, prolonged anticoagulant therapy has been found to decrease the rate of recurrent thrombotic complications by >60% (4,5). While there are no trial data available to identify specific patient groups in which prolonged anticoagulant therapy is necessary to prevent splanchnic vein thrombosis complications, some authors suggest prescribing long-term anticoagulant therapy for all patients with thrombophilic disorders and any patient who presents with mesenteric vein thrombosis due to the risk of recurrent bowel ischemia (1,3,5).

However, the use of anticoagulant therapy has been associated with an increased risk for bleeding, particularly in the presence of additional risk factors. Therefore, the risk of using anticoagulant therapy should be carefully considered in each patient. Based on a retrospective cohort study involving 136 patients, Condat et al (5) reported no significant association between anticoagulant therapy and the risk or severity of variceal bleeding in splanchnic vein thrombosis patients. They published a risk-benefit ratio that favoured the use of anticoagulant therapy to prevent thrombus progression, thereby preventing further increases in portal pressure (5). In contrast, some authors have advised against the use of long-term anticoagulant therapy in light of significant variceal hemorrhage rates; however, these recommendations were based on study populations that included patients with cirrhotic splanchnic vein thrombosis (12). The natural history of variceal bleeding in primary splanchnic vein thrombosis patients appears to differ from that of cirrhotic patients, with decreased severity when matched for similar variceal characteristics, decreased frequency of bleeds and overall better outcomes (3,6). This may be due to an intact coagulation pathway in the context of normal liver function (3). Even in cirrhotic patients, however, anticoagulation may be beneficial. In a recent randomized trial involving 70 advanced cirrhotic patients, Villa et al (13) demonstrated that prophylactic low molecular weight heparin was both safe and effective in preventing the development of portal vein thrombosis. They cited improved survival in the anticoagulation group, less hepatic decompensation and no bleeding complications.

In cirrhotic and noncirrhotic patients, variceal size, endoscopic features and a history of previous bleeds can help to predict future bleeding risk and may guide the decision to proceed with endoscopic treatment before anticoagulant therapy or to institute a thorough endoscopic screening protocol. It may be advisable to screen all patients with portal venous thrombosis endoscopically (14). Alternatively, one could restrict endoscopic assessment to patients with ultrasonographic features suggestive of esophageal varices (15). While some have proposed that the presence of nonbleeding varices may be an indication to hold or shorten anticoagulation courses (12), this does not optimally minimize morbidity and mortality due to the poor outcomes of progressive splanchnic vein thrombosis. Recanalization is the best treatment for varices formed secondary to splanchnic thrombosis and, as such, withholding anticoagulation should probably be discouraged in the absence of high bleeding risk (16). Beta blockade remains an effective means of preventing variceal bleeding in general (3), although variceal band ligation may be preferable in the setting of portal vein thrombosis (14) and is effective 90% of the time in hemorrhage prevention (16). A dual approach of endoscopic and medical management has led to more pronounced variceal regression (14). Therefore, a pragmatic approach may involve prophylactic endoscopic variceal band ligation with concurrent anticoagulant therapy (3). In the setting of variceal hemorrhage, endoscopic eradication significantly reduces the risk of recurrent bleeding in these patients, allowing for ongoing anticoagulation for treatment of their underlying thrombotic pathology (3).

Taking the previous information into consideration, it is our practice to consider anticoagulation for all patients with newly diagnosed splanchnic vein thrombosis if there is no contraindication, particularly esophageal varices with endoscopic high-risk bleeding features. For patients with events associated with transient risk factors, we consider three to six months of anticoagulation. For patients without associated risk factors and in the presence of high-risk thrombophilias (eg, combined defects, antiphospholipid antibodies, myeloproliferative neoplasms), we consider indefinite anticoagulation. However, periodic reassessments are performed to re-evaluate bleeding risk and thrombus resolution. In patients without evidence of improvement during follow-up (eg, thrombus persistence with development of collaterals and/or cavernomatous transformation), we consider discontinuation of anticoagulants due to futility.

Given the efficacy and safety of anticoagulant therapy and the overall low mortality rate associated with splanchnic vein thrombosis, the general consensus is to reserve invasive procedures such as transjugular intrahepatic portosystemic shunt procedures for cases in which anticoagulant therapy and endoscopy are ineffective (2,3,6,10). Additionally, several surgical techniques have been used in this patient population, including splanchnic-intrahepatic portal bypass, splenectomy and devascularization of the gastroesophageal junction, which has reportedly been more effective in spontaneous splanchnic vein thrombosis than in cirrhotic patients (3). Given the heterogeneity of splanchnic vein thrombosis, its complications and its predisposing factors, the choice of interventions is difficult to standardize and is best informed by patient factors.

In addition to splanchnic vein thrombosis itself, concomitant diseases – particularly cancer and myeloproliferative disorders – are an important cause of morbidity and mortality in these patients (3,4,6). The relatively recent description of the association between splanchnic vein thrombosis and the presence of the $JAK2^{V617F}$ tyrosine kinase mutation found in myeloproliferative disorders should prompt its investigation in all patients because these disorders require further hematological work-up (7,17,18). In addition, some authors suggest screening for thrombophilic disorders in splanchnic vein thrombosis patients regardless of apparent local etiology because both local and thrombophilic factors are believed to interact in the pathogenesis of splanchnic vein thrombosis (4,19). It is our practice to investigate patients with idiopathic noncirrhotic splanchnic vein thrombosis for thrombophilia, although the clinical value of this practice is yet to be determined. Finally, the role of screening for other potential prothrombotic conditions, such as paroxysmal nocturnal hemoglobinuria, is at

present unclear, particularly given its rarity, although patients with this condition have been reported to frequently develop splanchnic vein thrombosis (20).

The limitations of the present study were those inherent in its single-centre retrospective design, as well as the observational approach required to analyze a rare, heterogenous and potentially life-threatening condition. Another limitation was that six of our patients had the diagnosis made incidentally on computed tomography scan. The significance of an incidental finding of splanchnic vein thrombosis is not certain. Finally, other limitations include the small study population and nonstandardized treatment and screening algorithms. In the absence of randomized controlled trials, observational studies may help to inform treatment practices; however, our findings should certainly be regarded as hypothesis generating.

CONCLUSION

Based on our experience and that of others, the use of initial anticoagulant therapy appears to be a reasonable option in the initial management of patients with splanchnic vein thrombosis in the absence of contraindications to anticoagulation. The presence of certain clinical factors may help to identify patients at higher risk for developing chronic complications and need for further therapy, thus requiring closer monitoring. These findings need to be further explored in larger prospective studies to provide robust clinical recommendations.

DISCLOSURES: Presented in poster format at the Canadian Surgery Forum, Calgary Alberta, in September 2012 and at the American Society of Hematology Annual Meeting, Atlanta, Georgia, USA, in December 2012.

REFERENCES

1. Amitrano L, Guardascione MA, Scaglione M, et al. Prognostic factors in noncirrhotic patients with splanchnic vein thromboses. Am J Gastroenterol 2007;102:2464-70.
2. Condat B, Pessione F, Denninger MH, et al. Recent portal or mesenteric vein thrombosis: Increased recognition and frequent recanalization on anticoagulant therapy. Hepatology 2000;32:465-70.
3. Webster GJM, Burroughs AK, Riordan SM. Review article: Portal vein thrombosis – new insights into aetiology and management. Aliment Pharmacol Ther 2005;21:1-9.
4. Turnes J, Garcia-Pagan JC, Gonzalez M, et al. Portal hypertension-related complications after acute portal vein thrombosis: Impact of early anticoagulation. Clin Gastroenerol Hepatol 2008;6:1412-7.
5. Condat B, Pessione F, Hillaire S, et al. Current outcome of portal vein thrombosis in adults: Risk and benefit of anticoagulant therapy. Gastroenterology 2001;120:490-7.
6. Janssen HLA, Wijngoud A, Haagsma EB, et al. Extrahepatic portal vein thrombosis: Aetiology and determinants of survival. Gut 2001;49:720-4.
7. Orr DW, Patel RK, Lea NC, et al. The prevalence of the activating JAK2 tyrosine kinase mutation in chronic porto-splenomesenteric venous thrombosis. Alimen Pharmacol Ther 2010;31:1330-6.
8. Tefferi A, Vardiman JW. Classification and diagnosis of myeloproliferative neoplasms: The 2008 World Health Organization criteria and point-of-care diagnostic algorithms. Leukemia 2008;22:14-22.
9. Schulman S, Kearon C; Subcommittee on Control of Anticoagulation of the Scientific and Standardization Committee of the International Society on Thrombosis and Haemostasis. Definition of major bleeding in clinical investigations of antihemostatic medicinal products in non-surgical patients. J Thromb Haemost 2005;3:692-4.
10. Plessier A, Darwish-Murad S, Hernandez-Guerra M, et al. Acute portal vein thrombosis unrelated to cirrhosis: A prospective multi-centre follow-up study. Hepatology 2010;51:210-8.
11. Rodger MA, Kahn SR, Wells PS, et al. Identifying unprovoked thromboembolism patients at low risk for recurrence who can discontinue anticoagulation therapy. CMAJ 2008;179:417-26.
12. Thatipelli MR, McBane RD, Hodge DO, et al. Survival and recurrence in patients with splanchnic vein thrombosis. Clin Gastroenterol Hepatol 2010;8:200-5.

13. Villa E, Camma C, Marietta M, et al. Enoxaparin prevents portal vein thrombosis and liver decompensation in patients with advanced cirrhosis. Gastroenterology 2012;143:1253-60.

14. Sogaard KK, Astrup LB, Vilstrup H, et al. Portal vein thrombosis; risk factors, clinical presentation and treatment. BMC Gastroenterol 2007;7:34.

15. Brintintan A, Chira RI, Mircea PA. Non-invasive ultrasound-based diagnosis and staging of esophageal varices in liver cirrhosis. A systematic review of the literature published in the third millennium. Med Ultrason 2013;15:116-24.

16. Spahr L, Boehlen F, de Moerloose P, et al. Anticoagulants in portal vein thrombosis: Don't be so shy! Blood 2009;113:5031-2.

17. Regina S, Herault O, D'Alteroche L, et al. JAK2 V617F is specifically associated with idiopathic splanchnic vein thrombosis. J Thromb Haemost 2007;5:859-61.

18. De Stefano V, Rossi E, Za T, et al. JAK2 V617F mutational frequency in essential thrombocythemia associated with splanchnic or cerebral vein thrombosis. Am J Hematol 2011;86:526-8.

19. Denninger MH, Chait Y, Casadevall N, et al. Cause of portal or hepatic venous thrombosis in adults: The role of multiple concurrent factors. Hepatology 2000;31:587-91.

20. Lee JW, Jang JH, Kim HS, et al. Clinical signs and symptoms associated with increased risk of thrombosis in patients with paroxysmal nocturnal hemoglobinuria from a Korean registry. Int J Hematol 2013;97:749-57.

21

Outcomes of pediatric laparoscopic fundoplication: A critical review of the literature

Kathryn Martin MD, Catherine Deshaies MD CM, Sherif Emil MD CM

K Martin, C Deshaies, S Emil. Outcomes of pediatric laparoscopic fundoplication: A critical review of the literature. Can J Gastroenterol Hepatol 2014;28(2):97-102.

BACKGROUND/OBJECTIVE: Laparoscopic fundoplication for gastroesophageal reflux disease (GERD) is one of the most common procedures performed in children. A critical literature review was performed to evaluate the level and quality of evidence supporting the efficacy of this procedure.

METHODS: Systematic reviews of the EMBASE, PubMed and CENTRAL databases were conducted to retrieve all articles published over a 15-year period (1996 to 2010) reporting medium- to long-term outcomes (minimum six months follow-up) of laparoscopic fundoplication for the treatment of pediatric GERD. Articles were critically appraised using the Newcastle-Ottawa quality assessment scale and the Cochrane risk of bias assessment tool. Extracted outcomes included GERD recurrence, need for reoperation, postoperative morbidity and mortality.

RESULTS: A total of 5302 articles were retrieved. Thirty-six studies met inclusion and exclusion criteria, including five prospective (level 2b), four retrospective comparative (level 3b) and 27 case series (level 4). No studies compared laparoscopic fundoplication with medical treatment. Thirty-six per cent of studies did not describe the symptoms used to suspect GERD; 11% did not disclose the diagnostic modalities used; and 41% did not report the findings of diagnostic modalities. Only 17% of studies provided a definition of recurrence, and only 14% attempted to control for confounding variables. The follow-up intervals were inconsistently reported, ranging between two months and nine years. Significant heterogeneity among studies limited the ability to pool outcomes. Mean (± SD) recurrence rates varied between 0% and 48±19.6% of patients. Reoperation was required in 0.69±0.95% to 17.7±8.4% of patients. Mortality ranged between 0% and 24±16.7%.

CONCLUSION: The level and quality of the evidence supporting laparoscopic fundoplication are extremely poor. Higher-quality data are required before the procedure can be considered to be an effective intervention in the treatment of pediatric GERD.

Key Words: *Fundoplication; Gastroesophageal reflux disease; Laparoscopic; Pediatric*

Les résultats de la fundoplication laparoscopique en pédiatrie : une analyse bibliographique critique

HISTORIQUE ET OBJECTIF : La fundoplication laparoscopique pour traiter le reflux gastro-œsophagien pathologique (RGOP) est l'une des interventions les plus effectuées chez les enfants. Les chercheurs ont procédé à une analyse bibliographique critique pour évaluer la qualité et la catégorie des preuves en corroborant l'efficacité.

MÉTHODOLOGIE : Les chercheurs ont procédé à l'analyse systématique des bases de données EMBASE, PubMedet CENTRAL pour en extraire tous les articles publiés sur une période de 15 ans (1996 à 2010) rendant compte des résultats à moyen et long terme (minimum de six mois de suivi) de la fundoplication laparoscopique pour traiter le RGOP en pédiatrie. Ils ont effectué l'évaluation critique des articles au moyen de l'échelle d'évaluation de la qualité de Newcastle-Ottawa et de l'outil d'évaluation du risque de biais de Cochrane. Les résultats obtenus incluaient la récurrence du RGOP, le besoin de réopérer, la morbidité postopératoire et la mortalité.

RÉSULTATS : Au total, les chercheurs ont extrait 5 302 articles. Trente-six études respectaient les critères d'inclusion et d'exclusion, soit cinq études prospectives (catégorie 2b), quatre études comparatives prospectives (catégorie 3b) et 27 séries de cas (catégorie 4). Aucune étude ne comparait la fundoplication laparoscopique avec le traitement médical. Trente-six pour cent des études ne décrivaient pas les symptômes retenus pour présumer un RGOP, 11 % ne révélaient pas les modalités diagnostiques utilisées et 41 % ne précisaient pas les résultats des modalités diagnostiques. Seulement 17 % des études incluaient une définition de la récurrence et seulement 14 % cherchaient à contrôler les variables confusionnelles. Les intervalles de suivi, qui n'étaient pas transmis de façon uniforme, variaient entre deux mois et neuf ans. En raison de l'hétérogénéité importante des études, la possibilité de regrouper les résultats était limitée. Le taux de récurrence moyen (± ÉT) variait entre 0 % et 48±19,6 % des patients. Il a fallu réopérer de 0,69±0,95 % à 17,7±8,4 % des patients. Le taux de mortalité se situait entre 0 % et 24±16,7 %.

CONCLUSION : La qualité et la catégorie des preuves en appui à la fundoplication laparoscopique sont extrêmement faibles. Il faudra des données de meilleure qualité avant que l'intervention puisse être considérée comme efficace pour traiter le RGOP en pédiatrie.

The treatment of gastroesophageal reflux disease (GERD) in infants and children presents an ongoing challenge to physicians and surgeons. A step-up approach is recommended beginning with conservative therapies and progressing to acid suppression if symptoms persist (1,2). Laparoscopic fundoplication (LF) is considered when medical treatments have failed (1,2). However, the definition of failure is largely subjective and clinician dependent. Currently, there are no studies comparing medical therapies with LF for the treatment of pediatric GERD. While complications of LF are well documented, the indications are often vague and objective documentation of refractory reflux is often missing (2-4). Despite this, LF remains one of the most common operations performed by pediatric surgeons in the United States.

Published reviews of LF have simply analyzed the data from individual studies without assessment of their quality (5-7). Position papers and treatment guidelines have been formulated by national and international surgical organizations based on the same data, typically without comment on the level of the evidence (6,8). To fill this gap, we conducted a critical review of all articles published from 1996 to 2010 that reported the medium- to long-term outcomes of LF. Our primary goal was to assess the quality of the literature. Our secondary goal was to evaluate reported outcomes.

METHODS

Systematic searches of the EMBASE, PubMed and CENTRAL databases from 1996 to 2010 were conducted in conjunction with

Division of Pediatric General and Thoracic Surgery, The Montreal Children's Hospital; McGill University Health Centre, Montreal, Quebec
Correspondence: Dr Sherif Emil, Division of Pediatric General and Thoracic Surgery, Montreal Children's Hospital, 2300 Tupper Street, Room C-818, Montreal, Quebec H3H 1P3.e-mail sherif.emil@mcgill.ca

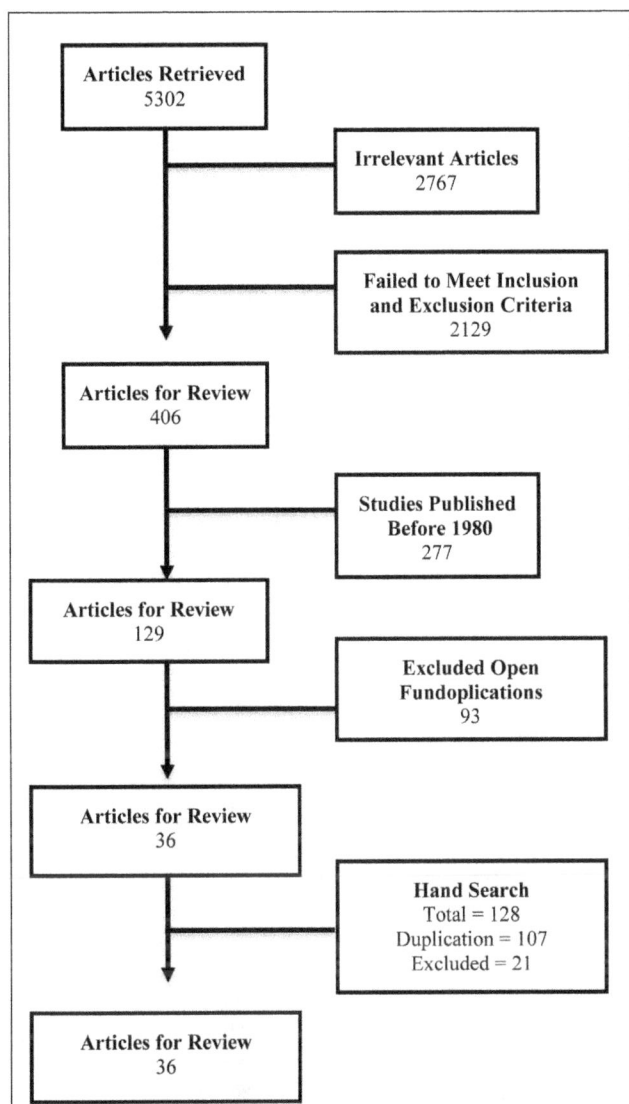

Figure 1) *Article selection*

librarians at the Montreal Children's Hospital, McGill University Health Centre (Montreal, Quebec). All studies reporting the medium- to long-term outcomes of LF in the treatment of pediatric GERD were retrieved. No language limitations were placed. Separate search strategies were formulated for each database using database-specific subject terms, syntax and free-text forms. Queries included a combination of exploded and nonexploded subject headings including the following: "gastroesophageal reflux disease", "GERD", "fundoplication", "anti-reflux surgery" and "pediatrics". Review articles, case series involving <20 patients, editorials and letters were excluded. Articles reporting <50% follow-up at six months were also excluded.

A single investigator reviewed all retrieved citations' titles and abstracts to eliminate those that clearly did not meet inclusion and exclusion criteria. Two independent reviewers reviewed the remaining articles in their entirety for final selection based on the standardized eligibility criteria. Any disagreements in the selection process were resolved through discussion between reviewers. The references of the selected articles were manually searched to identify any additional relevant articles.

The articles were reviewed in detail for quality assessment and data extraction. Data were then pooled and discrepancies dealt with through re-review until consensus was reached. Article quality was determined by study design, a standardized quality assessment form based on the Newcastle-Ottawa quality assessment scale and the

Cochrane risk-of-bias assessment tool. Data were extracted using a standardized data extraction form. Extracted data included baseline demographics, diagnostic criteria, study intervention, follow-up details and outcomes, including postoperative mortality, GERD recurrence and need for reoperation.

Quality assessments are reported qualitatively with special attention devoted to study design, confounders, biases and length of follow-up reporting. Outcomes are reported as proportions with 95% CIs. Pooled estimates are presented where appropriate, based on χ^2 testing for heterogeneity.

RESULTS

The literature search retrieved a total of 5302 articles, 36 of which met inclusion and exclusion criteria (Figure 1). A summary of the selected articles is presented in Table 1.

Quality assessment

The retrieved studies all constituted low-level evidence: five prospective comparative studies (level 2b) (9-13), four retrospective comparative studies (level 3b) (14-17) and 27 case series (level 4) (18-44). Three of the prospective studies compared LF in neurologically impaired versus neurologically intact patients. There were no randomized controlled trials of LF versus medical therapy. All nonrandomized comparative studies compared LF with open fundoplication or minor technical modifications in the laparoscopic technique; none compared LF with medical therapy. There were three before-and-after studies (11-13). However, none of these studies clearly described the treatments, if any, that patients received before LF. Thus, the preoperative disease status was largely unknown, making the outcomes difficult to interpret (11-13).

Table 2 outlines the quality features of the selected articles. Only five studies attempted to control for confounders in their analysis. The factors controlled for varied among studies and included age, sex, comorbidities, respiratory status and surgical technique. The percentage of neurological impairment was reported in 78% of studies; however, the majority did not control for this factor in their analysis. Similarly, the rates of esophageal atresia were reported in 22% of studies, none of which controlled for its presence during analysis. No studies controlled for the confounding effects of the learning curve associated with LF.

Bias was present throughout, with only two studies clearly attempting to reduce bias (10,33). The first was a prospective study involving a cohort of institutionalized patients (10). To reduce detection bias, this study used universal pH testing at 12 months postoperatively to detect recurrence and had no patients lost to follow-up. However, the authors did not describe how patients were assigned to LF, raising the possibility of a significant selection bias (10). The second study (33) was a case series that used clear selection criteria for LF, routine pH testing at 12 months to detect recurrence and had no loss to follow-up.

The remaining studies were prone to selection, detection, reporting and attrition bias. With regard to selection bias, the studies failed to adequately describe why patients were selected for LF over other surgical or medical treatments. They also failed to describe the background population from which the reported samples were derived. Detection bias was prevalent due to the lack of a definition of recurrence, which was only present in 17% of studies, as well as the reliance on patient- and caregiver-reported symptoms to trigger further investigations. Only two studies used a standardized follow-up interview with blinded assessors (12,13). Reporting bias was prevalent because studies failed to indicate which outcomes were being investigated a priori. Furthermore, studies failed to report the absence of many common complications, making it unclear whether these did not occur, were not investigated or were omitted. Finally, attrition bias was a common problem because patients were lost to follow-up over time, particularly in studies reporting extended follow-up periods. All studies failed to indicate the features of participants lost to follow-up compared with those remaining in the sample. Follow-up protocols were rarely reported.

TABLE 1
Summary of articles

Author (reference), year	n	Study design	Population	Fundoplication technique
Esposito et al (9), 2001	36	Prospective cohort	<1 year of age	Nissen; Toupet
Cheung et al (10), 2006	20	Prospective cohort	Neurologically impaired	Nissen
Capito et al (11), 2008	127	Prospective cohort	Mixed	Nissen-Rossetti
Engelmann et al (12), 2010	40	Prospective cohort	Mixed	Thal
Engelmann et al (13), 2010	26	Prospective cohort	Mixed	Thal
Somme et al (14), 2002	53	Retrospective cohort	<1 year of age	Nissen
Diaz et al (15), 2005	456	Retrospective cohort	Mixed	Nissen
Barsness et al (16), 2007	26	Retrospective cohort	<1 year of age	Nissen
Curtis et al (17), 2010	384	Retrospective cohort	Mixed	Nissen
Longis et al (18), 1996	30	Case series	Mixed	Nissen-Rossetti; Toupet
Thompson et al (19), 1996	25	Case series	<1 year of age	Nissen
Rothenberg et al (20), 1997	56	Case series	Respiratory disease	Nissen; Nissen-Rossetti
Tovar et al (21), 1998	27	Case series	Mixed	Nissen
Hopkins and Stringel (22), 1999	25	Case series	Mixed	Nissen
Dick and Potts (23), 1999	50	Case series	Mixed	Modified Nissen
Esposito et al (24), 2000	289	Case series	Mixed	Nissen-Rossetti; Toupet
Schleef et al (25), 2000	30	Case series	Mixed	Thal
Liu et al (26), 2001	117	Case series	Mixed	Nissen-Rossetti
Allal et al (27), 2001	142	Case series	Mixed	Nissen; Toupet
Mattioli et al (28), 2002	70	Case series	Mixed	Nissen-Rossetti
Van der Zee et al (29), 2002	149	Case series	Mixed	Nissen; Thal
Pimpalwar et al (30), 2002	54	Case series	Neurologically impaired	Nissen
Mattioli et al (31), 2002	288	Case series	Mixed	Nissen; Toupet; Thal
Esposito et al (32), 2003	80	Case series	Neurologically impaired	Nissen; Thal
Mattioli et al (33), 2004	48	Case series	Neurologically normal	Nissen-Rossetti
Kwiecien et al (34), 2004	132	Case series	Mixed	Toupet
Lima et al (35), 2004	47	Case series	Neurologically impaired	Nissen; Toupet; Dor
Kawahara et al (36), 2004	56	Case series	Neurologically impaired	Nissen; Thal
Okuyama et al (37), 2004	42	Case series	Neurologically impaired	Nissen
Liu et al (38), 2006	368	Case series	Mixed	Nissen-Rossetti
Esposito et al (39), 2006	238	Case series	Neurologically normal	Nissen; Toupet; Thal
Boesch and Acton (40), 2007	25	Case series	Respiratory disease	Nissen
Tannuri et al (41), 2008	151	Case series	Mixed	Nissen
Perger et al (42), 2008	44	Case series	Mixed	Nissen
Mathei et al (43), 2008	106	Case series	Mixed	Nissen
Shariff et al (44), 2008	79	Case series	<1 year of age	Nissen

Outcomes

Mortality was reported by 58% of the studies. All mortalities were attributed to progression of the patients' underlying cardiac, neurological or respiratory disorders. Figure 2 illustrates the reported mortality rates with 95% CIs. The mean (± SD) pooled mortality rate in neurologically impaired children was found to be 17.9±4.9% (χ^2 for heterogeneity P=0.549).

Recurrence rates following LF were reported by 83% of studies. However, only six studies used an explicit definition of recurrence. The reported recurrence rates ranged between 0% and 48±19.6% (Figure 3). Significant heterogeneity existed among the studies, preventing pooling of data (χ^2 for heterogeneity P<0.001).

The need for reoperation following LF was reported in 50% of the studies. A consistent definition of indications for reoperation was absent. Some studies reported the percentage of re-do fundoplications due to recurrent GERD, while others included reoperation for wrap stenosis, pyloroplasty and recurrent hiatal hernia. The rate of reoperation was reported to be between 0.69±0.95% and 17.7±8.4% (Figure 4). Studies reporting neurologically impaired and neurologically normal populations were sufficiently homogenous to allow pooling (χ^2 for heterogeneity P=0.16 and P=0.528, respectively). The pooled estimate for reoperation in neurologically impaired patients was 15.4±4.2%. The pooled estimate for reoperation in neurologically

TABLE 2
Summary of quality features

Quality feature	Percentage of studies
Description of % of population with neurological impairment	78
Description of % of population with history of esophageal atresia	22
Description of patient symptoms	64
Description of diagnostic tests	89
Results of diagnostic tests	52
Description of surgical techniques	75
Median and range of follow-up provided	33
Relevant outcomes reported (recurrence, reoperation or death)	100
Clear definition of recurrence given	17
Details regarding complications	92
Attempts to control for confounders	14
Attempts to reduce bias	6

normal patients was 7.0±3.3%. The neurologically impaired group underwent significantly more reoperations than the neurologically normal group (χ^2 P=0.003).

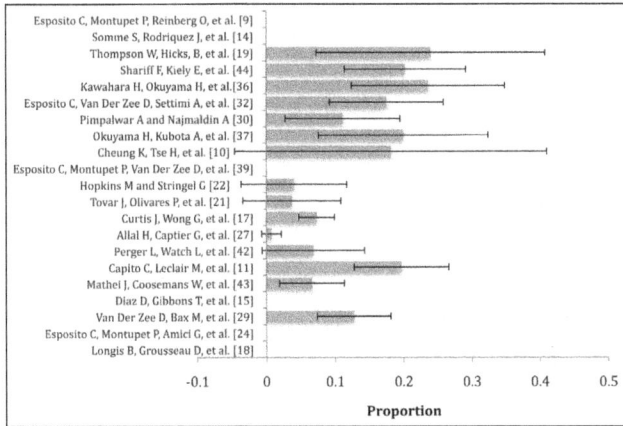

Figure 2) *Mortality rates. Bars represent 95% CIs*

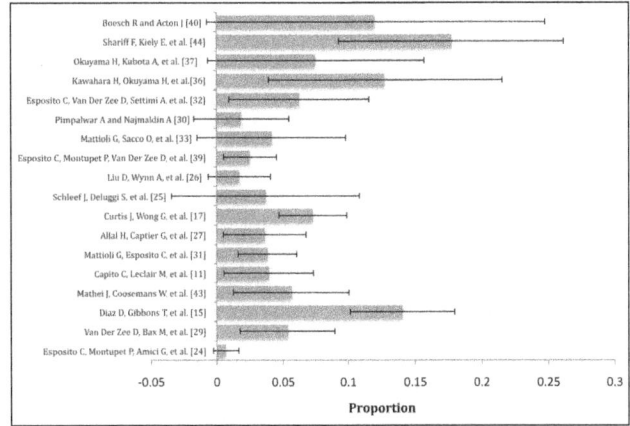

Figure 4) *Reoperation rates. Bars represent 95% CIs*

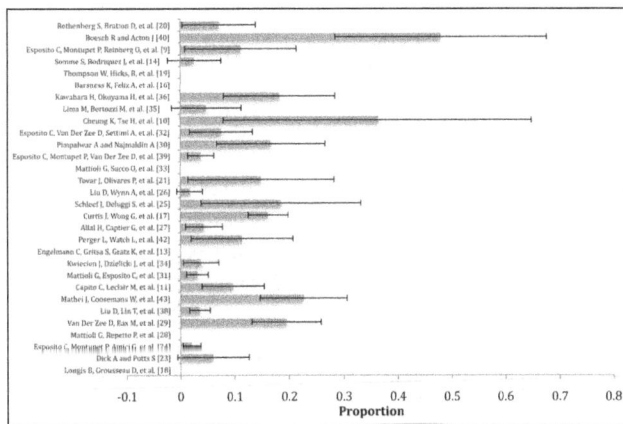

Figure 3) *Recurrence rates. Bars represent 95% CIs*

DISCUSSION

LF is the current standard surgical treatment for refractory pediatric GERD. However, little is known about the long-term outcomes of this procedure and its true effectiveness. The available literature is of extremely poor quality according to evidence-based standards. Presently, there are no randomized trials or prospective cohort studies comparing LF with medical therapy. Thus, there is no conclusive evidence that surgery is superior to medical therapy (4).

In our review, 75% of studies were case series, which are known to favour the described intervention. They lead to false inferences up to 50% of the time (45). Multiple innovative treatments, once believed to be effective based on case series, were subsequently found to be no better than standard treatments when rigorously studied (45). Although nine of the included studies were comparative, none were randomized and three used historical controls. The use of historical controls is often confounded by changes in management, separate from the intervention in question, leading to false inferences in 40% to 60% of cases (45).

Studies frequently failed to adequately describe their study populations, diagnostic criteria, follow-up protocols and outcome measures. The majority of studies indicated the proportion of the study population that was neurologically impaired. However, most failed to analyze this population separately, despite its association with worse outcomes (46). We found a statistically significant difference in reoperation rates between these two groups in our study. Similar concerns exist over studies including patients with esophageal atresia (3). Mixed populations were reported by 57% of reviewed studies. The failure to report and control for underlying comorbidities makes it difficult to apply results to a given patient population (3).

There was also a consistent failure to explicitly outline the diagnostic criteria of GERD, the selection criteria for intervention and the outcome measures used. The lack of criteria for diagnosis and treatment likely relates to the lack of a standard definition of GERD in the pediatric population. An international panel of experts created guidelines in 2009 (1); however, most studies were published before 2009. Furthermore, these guidelines have yet to be universally adopted; therefore, recent studies fail to apply them (1,47). Comparing studies was further hindered by the lack of clear, a priori outcomes and standardized follow-up protocols. Many have called for the use of standardized outcome measures when reporting the efficacy of GERD treatments (3,17 19). However, as noted by Gold et al (49), validated outcome measures do not currently exist. Finally, patient- and parent-reported outcomes were heavily used in this body of literature, increasing the risk of a placebo effect, especially given the subjective nature of many of the reported outcomes. This is compounded by a potential second placebo response due to the natural history of GERD in children, the efficacy of nonpharmacological methods and expectation bias (50). All of these factors likely overestimate the true effectiveness of LF.

The biases present in the analyzed studies further limit the conclusions that can be drawn from them. Selection bias was present because clear inclusion and exclusion criteria were lacking from the majority of the studies. Thus, surgeons were likely to include patients they believed would benefit most from LF, and exclude those considered to be at increased risk of complications. The lack of clear a priori follow-up protocols means that many complications were likely not detected, not reported or both. Significant attrition bias existed due to the failure to account for patients lost to follow-up. The proportion lost to follow-up, as well as the reasons for that loss, was not reported by any of the reviewed studies.

Recurrence rates varied widely. The largest study of open fundoplication, a multicentre retrospective series of 7467 cases (51), reported a recurrence rate of 7%. However, this was probably a gross underestimation because the study was poorly designed to detect recurrence. Objective testing for GERD using esophagogastroduodenoscopy or pH probe was only performed in 54% and 26%, respectively, and the results of this objective testing were not reported (51). The study presented no standard follow-up, no standard assessment of outcomes and no quality of life measures (51). The wide range of recurrences in the current review are likely due to variations in the definition of recurrence and generally poor follow-up data. Studies with very high recurrence rates may have erroneously implicated GERD as the reason for the patient's symptoms (5,52). For example, a recurrence rate of 48±19.6% was found in a population with respiratory disease attributed to GERD (40). The link between respiratory disease and GERD is not firmly established, and several studies have shown no benefit to LF when performed for respiratory indications (48,53,54).

Reoperation was required in all 18 studies reporting this outcome. The indications for reoperation varied among studies and included recurrence, wrap failure, esophageal stenosis, recurrent hiatal hernia and pyloroplasty for postoperative delayed gastric emptying. The pooled estimate of reoperation rate in neurologically impaired patients was 15.4±4.2% versus 7.0±3.3% in neurologically normal patients. Neurologically impaired patients also had the highest mortality rates, along with patients undergoing fundoplication before their first birthday (19,36). These differences support the notion that neurologically impaired patients experience worse outcomes after LF (55). LF should be considered a palliative procedure for many of these patients and the surgeon should openly share the outcome information to provide the family with realistic expectations.

Prospective studies comparing LF with medical therapies are needed. Although, a randomized controlled trial would be optimal, it is unlikely to occur due to the wide adoption of LF by surgeons and parents alike as a common treatment option for pediatric GERD. A well-designed multicentre prospective cohort study using matched controls is a more realistic option. Such a study should aim to provide long-term follow-up and provide subgroup analysis to determine the long-term effects of LF in different populations. In the meantime, adoption of a universal definition of GERD may allow more objective selection of patients for LF (47). The use of standard outcome measures, as suggested by Gold et al (49), can create uniformity in the literature, allowing meaningful comparisons among studies. The enthusiasm for LF in children should be tempered until higher-quality evidence is available to support its long-term efficacy.

SUMMARY

Pediatric LF is one of the most common operative procedures performed in children. Multiple case series and several reviews of pediatric LF have been published over the past 15 years. However, none of the reviews critically evaluated the quality of the literature from an evidence-based perspective. We performed a critical review of the literature on pediatric LF outcomes over a 15-year period. Our results indicate that the level and quality of the evidence supporting LF are extremely poor. Higher-quality data are required before the procedure can be considered to be an effective intervention for the treatment of pediatric GERD.

REFERENCES

1. Vandenplas Y, Rudolph C, Di Lorenzo C, et al. Pediatric gastroesophageal reflux clinical practice guidelines: Joint recommendations of the North American Society for Pediatric Hastroenterology, Hepatology, and Nutrition (NASPGHAN) and the European Society for Pediatric Gastroenterology, Hepatology, and Nutrition (ESPGHAN). J Pediatr Gastroenterol Nutr 2009;49:498-547.
2. Hassall E. Step-up and step-down approaches to treatment of gastroesophageal reflux disease in children. Curr Gastroenterol Rep 2008;10:324-31.
3. Hassall E. Outcomes of fundoplication: Causes for concern, newer options. Arch Dis Child 2005;90:1047-52.
4. Kumar Y, Sarvananthan R. GORD in children. Clin Evid 2008;10:310.
5. Lobe T. The current role of laparoscopic surgery for gastroesophageal reflux disease in infants and children. Surg Endosc 2007;21:167-74.
6. Kane T, Brown M, Chen M, et al. Position paper on laparoscopic antireflux operations in infants and children for gastroesophageal reflux disease. J Pediatr Surg 2009;44:1034-40.
7. Rafay M, Siddiqui S, Abdulaal Y, et al. A meta-analysis of outcomes after open and laparoscopic Nissen's fundoplication for gastroesophageal reflux disease in children. Pediatr Surg Int 2011;27:359-66.
8. IPEG guidelines for the surgical treatment of pediatric gastroesophageal reflux disease (GERD). J Laparoendosc Adv Surg Tech 2008;18:x-xiii.
9. Esposito C, Montupet P, Reinberg O. Laparoscopic surgery for gastroesophageal reflux disease during the first year of life. J Pediatr Surg 2001;36:715-7.
10. Cheung KM, Tse HW, Tse PW, et al. Nissen fundoplication and gastrostomy in severely neurologically impaired children with gastroesophageal reflux. Hong Kong Med J 2006;12:282-8.
11. Capito C, Leclair MD, Piloquet H, et al. Long-term outcome of laparoscopic Nissen-Rossetti fundoplication for neurologically impaired and normal children. Surg Endosc 2008;22:875-80.
12. Engelmann C, Gritsa S, Ure BM. Impact of laparoscopic anterior 270 degrees fundoplication on the quality of life and symptoms profile of neurodevelopmentally delayed versus neurologically unimpaired children and their parents. Surg Endosc 2010;24:1287-95.
13. Engelmann C, Gritsa S, Gratz KF, et al. Laparoscopic anterior hemifundoplication improves key symptoms without impact on GE in children with and children without neurodevelopmental delays. J Pediatr Gastroenterol Nutr 2010;51:437-42.
14. Somme S, Rodriguez JA, Kirsch DG, et al. Laparoscopic versus open fundoplication in infants. Surg Endosc 2002;16:54-6.
15. Diaz DM, Gibbons TE, Heiss K, et al. Antireflux surgery outcomes in pediatric gastroesophageal reflux disease. Am J Gastroenterol 2005;100:1844-52.
16. Barsness KA, Feliz A, Potoka DA, et al. Laparoscopic versus open Nissen fundoplication in infants after neonatal laparotomy. JSLS 2007;11:461-5.
17. Curtis JL, Wong G, Gutierrez I, et al. Pledgeted mattress sutures reduce recurrent reflux after laparoscopic Nissen fundoplication. J Pediatr Surg 2010;45:1159-64.
18. Longis B, Grousseau D, Alain JL, et al. Laparoscopic fundoplication in children: Our first 30 cases. J Laparoendosc Surg Adv Surg Tech 1996;6:S21-S29.
19. Thompson WR, Hicks BA, Guzzetta PC. Laparoscopic Nissen fundoplication in the infant. J Laparoendosc Surg Adv Surg Tech 1996;6:S5-7.
20. Rothenberg SS, Bratton D, Larsen G, et al. Laparoscopic fundoplication to enhance pulmonary function in children with severe reactive airway disease and gastroesophageal reflux disease. Surg Endosc 1997;11:1088-90.
21. Tovar JA, Olivares P, Diaz M, et al. Functional results of laparoscopic fundoplication in children. J Pediatr Gastroenterol Nutr 1998;26:429-31.
22. Hopkins MA, Stringel G. Laparoscopic Nissen fundoplication in children: A single surgeon's experience. JSLS. 1999;3:261-6.
23. Dick AC, Potts SR. Laparoscopic fundoplication in children – an audit of fifty cases. Eur J Pediatr Surg 1999;9:286-8.
24. Esposito C, Montupet P, Amici G, et al. Complications of laparoscopic antireflux surgery in childhood. Surg Endosc 2000;14:622-4.
25. Schleef J, Deluggi S, Schaarschmidt K, et al. Multi-institutional experience in laparoscopic surgery for gastroesophageal reflux: A five-year experience with 30 children. Pediatr Endosurg Innov Tech 2000;4:265-70.
26. Liu DC, Wynn AR, Rodriguez JA, et al. Laparoscopic Nissen-Rossetti fundoplication in children. Pediatr Endosurg Innov Tech 2001;5:19-22.
27. Allal H, Captier G, Lopez M, et al. Evaluation of 142 consecutive laparoscopic fundoplications in children: Effects of the learning curve and technical choice. J Pediatr Surg 2001;36:921-6.
28. Mattioli G, Repetto P, Leggio S, et al. Laparoscopic Nissen-Rossetti fundoplication in children. Semin Laparosc Surg 2002;9:153-62.
29. van der Zee DC, Bax KN, Ure BM, et al. Long-term results after laparoscopic Thal procedure in children. Semin Laparosc Surg 2002;9:168-71.
30. Pimpalwar A, Najmaldin A. Results of laparoscopic antireflux procedures in neurologically impaired children. Semin Laparosc Surg 2002;9:190-6.
31. Mattioli G, Esposito C, Lima M, et al. Italian multicenter survey on laparoscopic treatment of gastro-esophageal reflux disease in children. Surg Endosc 2002;16:1666-8.
32. Esposito C, van der Zee DC, Settimi A, et al. Risks and benefits of surgical management of gastroesophageal reflux in neurologically impaired children. Surg Endosc 2003;17:708-10.
33. Mattioli G, Sacco O, Gentilino V, et al. Outcome of laparoscopic Nissen-Rossetti fundoplication in children with gastroesophageal reflux disease and supraesophageal symptoms. Surg Endosc 2004;18:463-5.
34. Kwiecien J, Dzielicki J, Korlacki W, et al. Long-term effects of laparoscopic antireflux surgery in children with gastroesophageal reflux disease. Pediatria Wspolczesna 2004;6:249-53.

35. Lima M, Bertozzi M, Ruggeri G, et al. Laparoscopic antireflux surgery in neurologically impaired children. Pediatr Surg Int 2004;20:114-7.
36. Kawahara H, Okuyama H, Kubota A, et al. Can laparoscopic antireflux surgery improve the quality of life in children with neurologic and neuromuscular handicaps? J Pediatr Surg 2004;39:1761-4.
37. Okuyama H, Kubota A, Kawahara H, et al. The efficacy and long-term outcome of laparoscopic Nissen fundoplication in neurologically impaired children. Pediatr Endosurg Innov Tech 2004;8:5-11.
38. Liu DC, Lin T, Statter MB, et al. Laparoscopic Nissen fundoplication without division of short gastric vessels in children. J Pediatr Surg 2006;41:120-5.
39. Esposito C, Montupet P, van der Zee D, et al. Long-term outcome of laparoscopic Nissen, Toupet, and Thal antireflux procedures for neurologically normal children with gastroesophageal reflux disease. Surg Endosc 2006;20:855-8.
40. Boesch RP, Acton JD. Outcomes of fundoplication in children with cystic fibrosis. J Pediatr Surg 2007;42:1341-4.
41. Tannuri AC, Tannuri U, Mathias AL, et al. Gastroesophageal reflux disease in children: Efficacy of Nissen fundoplication in treating digestive and respiratory symptoms. Experience of a single center. Dis Esophagus 2008;21:746-50.
42. Perger L, Watch L, Weinsheimer R, et al. Laparoscopically supervised PEG at time of Nissen fundoplication: A safe option. J Laparoendosc Adv Surg Tech 2008;18:136-9.
43. Mathei J, Coosemans W, Nafteux P, et al. Laparoscopic Nissen fundoplication in infants and children: Analysis of 106 consecutive patients with special emphasis in neurologically impaired vs. neurologically normal patients. Surg Endosc 2008;22:1054-9.
44. Shariff F, Kiely E, Curry J, et al. Outcome after laparoscopic fundoplication in children under 1 year. J Laparoendosc Adv Surg Tech 2010;20:661-4.
45. Frader JE, Flanagan-Klygis E. Innovation and research in pediatric surgery. Semin Pediatr Surg 2001;10:198-203.
46. Pearl R, Robie D, Ein S, et al. Complications of gastroesophageal antireflux surgery in neurologically impaired versus neurologically normal children. J Pediatr Surg 1990;25:1169-73.
47. Sherman P, Hassall E, Fagundes-Neto U, et al. A global, evidence-based consensus on the definition of gastroesophageal reflux disease in the pediatric population. Am J Gastroenterol 2009;104:1278-95.
48. Tolia V, Vandenplas Y. Systematic review: The extra-oesophageal symptoms of gastro-oesophageal reflux disease in children. Aliment Pharmacol Ther 2009;29:258-72.
49. Gold B, Co J, Colletti R, et al. What outcome measures are needed to assess gastroesophageal reflux disease in chidlren? What study design is appropriate? What new knowledge is needed? J Pediatr Gastroenterol Nutr 2003;37:S72-75.
50. Orenstein S, Hassall E, Furmaga-Jablonska W, et al. Multicenter, double-blind, randomized, placebo-controlled trial assessing the efficacy and safety of proton pump inhibitor lansoprazole in infants with symptoms of gastroesophageal reflux disease. J Pediatr 2009;154:514-20.
51. Fonkalsrud EW, Ashcraft KW, Coran AG, et al. Surgical treatment of gastroesophageal reflux in children: A combined hospital study of 7467 patients. Pediatrics 1998;10:419-22.
52. Di Lorenzo C, Orenstein S. Fundoplication: Friend or foe? J Pediatr Gastroenterol Nutr 2002;34:117-24.
53. Thakkar K, Boatright R, Gilger M, et al. Gastroesophageal reflux and asthma in children: A systematic review. Pediatrics 2010;125:e925-e930.
54. Lee S, Shabatian H, Hsu J, et al. Hospital admissions for respiratory symptoms and failure to thrive before and after Nissen fundoplication. J Pediatr Surg 2008;43:59-65.
55. de Veer A, Bos J, Niezen-de Boer R, et al. Symptoms of gastroesophageal reflux disease in severely mentally retarded people: A systematic review. BMC Gastroenterol 2008;8:23.

22

Geographical variation and factors associated with colorectal cancer mortality in a universal health care system

Mahmoud Torabi PhD[1], Christopher Green PhD[1], Zoann Nugent PhD[1,2,3], Salaheddin M Mahmud PhD[1,3],

Alain A Demers PhD[1,3], Jane Griffith PhD[1,3], Harminder Singh MD MPH FACG[1,2,4,5]

M Torabi, C Green, Z Nugent, et al. Geographical variation and factors associated with colorectal cancer mortality in a universal health care system. Can J Gastroenterol Hepatol 2014;28(4): 191-197.

OBJECTIVE: To investigate the geographical variation and small geographical area level factors associated with colorectal cancer (CRC) mortality.
METHODS: Information regarding CRC mortality was obtained from the population-based Manitoba Cancer Registry, population counts were obtained from Manitoba's universal health care plan Registry and characteristics of the area of residence were obtained from the 2001 Canadian census. Bayesian spatial Poisson mixed models were used to evaluate the geographical variation of CRC mortality and Poisson regression models for determining associations with CRC mortality. Time trends of CRC mortality according to income group were plotted using joinpoint regression.
RESULTS: The southeast (mortality rate ratio [MRR] 1.31 [95% CI 1.12 to 1.54]) and southcentral (MRR 1.62 [95% CI 1.35 to 1.92]) regions of Manitoba had higher CRC mortality rates than suburban Winnipeg (Manitoba's capital city). Between 1985 and 1996, CRC mortality did not vary according to household income; however, between 1997 and 2009, individuals residing in the highest-income areas were less likely to die from CRC (MRR 0.77 [95% CI 0.65 to 0.89]). Divergence in CRC mortality among individuals residing in different income areas increased over time, with rising CRC mortality observed in the lowest income areas and declining CRC mortality observed in the higher income areas.
CONCLUSIONS: Individuals residing in lower income neighbourhoods experienced rising CRC mortality despite residing in a jurisdiction with universal health care and should receive increased efforts to reduce CRC mortality. These findings should be of particular interest to the provincial CRC screening programs, which may be able to reduce the disparities in CRC mortality by reducing the disparities in CRC screening participation.

Key Words: *Colorectal cancer mortality; Spatial patterns; Universal health care; Worsening socioeconomic disparities*

La variation géographique et les facteurs associés à la mortalité causée par le cancer colorectal dans un système de santé universel

OBJECTIF : Examiner la variation géographique et les facteurs liés à une petite région géographique associés à la mortalité causée par le cancer colorectal (CCR).
MÉTHODOLOGIE : Les chercheurs ont obtenu l'information relative à la mortalité causée par le CCR dans le Registre du cancer du Manitoba (un registre en population), le décompte de la population dans le registre d'assurance-maladie universelle du Manitoba et les caractéristiques des régions de résidence dans le recensement du Canada de 2001. Ils ont utilisé des modèles bayésiens mixtes de Poisson avec généralisation spatiale pour évaluer la variation géographique de la mortalité causée par le CCR et des modèles de régression de Poisson pour déterminer les associations avec la mortalité causée par le CCR. Ils ont consigné les tendances de la mortalité causée par le CCR dans le temps selon le groupe de revenu d'après la régression Joinpoint.
RÉSULTATS : Les régions du sud-est (ratio des taux de mortalité [RTM] 1,31 [95 % IC 1,12 à 1,54]) et du centre-sud (RTM 1,62 [95 % IC 1,35 à 1,92]) du Manitoba présentaient des taux de mortalité causée par le CCR plus élevés que la région suburbaine de Winnipeg (capitale du Manitoba). Entre 1985 et 1996, le taux de mortalité causée par le CCR ne variait pas selon le revenu familial, mais entre 1997 et 2009, les personnes qui habitaient dans les régions au revenu le plus élevé étaient moins susceptibles de mourir d'un CCR (RTM 0,77 [95 % IC 0,65 à 0,89]). La divergence du taux de mortalité causée par le CCR chez les personnes qui habitent dans des régions aux revenus variés augmentait au fil du temps, le taux de mortalité causée par le CCR s'accroissant dans les régions à faible revenu et diminuant dans les régions au revenu le plus élevé.
CONCLUSIONS : Les personnes qui habitaient dans des quartiers à faible revenu présentaient un taux de mortalité croissant causée par le CCR, même si le système de santé universel était offert dans leur territoire de compétence et aurait dû s'associer à plus d'efforts pour réduire la mortalité causée par le CCR. Ces observations devraient susciter l'intérêt des programmes provinciaux de dépistage du CCR, qui pourront peut-être réduire les disparités en matière de mortalité causée par le CCR en atténuant les écarts de participation au dépistage du CCR.

Colorectal cancer (CRC) continues to be the second most common cause of cancer deaths in North America (1), although many of these deaths could be prevented by removal of precancerous precursor lesions or by detection of CRC at early and curable stages (2,3). Although there has been a recent emphasis on lowering the incidence of CRC, reduction in CRC mortality is the primary objective of CRC screening activities. An apparent increase in incidence is witnessed after the initiation of screening programs due to the identification of prevalent cases and, subsequently, due to overdiagnosis of indolent cases, inherent in most screening activities (4). Hence, CRC mortality remains the primary outcome of interest for public health programs aiming to reduce the burden of CRC and, accordingly, was the focus of the present study.

Exploring geographical variation in CRC mortality and predictors of CRC mortality could help in developing risk-tailored approaches for CRC screening by rapidly expanding CRC screening programs. Several studies have investigated the variation in CRC mortality among small geographical areas, but few explored the effect of socioeconomic factors in jurisdictions with universal health care systems such as Canada (5,6). Universal health care systems are expected to

[1]*Department of Community Health Sciences;* [2]*University of Manitoba IBD Clinical and Research Centre, University of Manitoba;* [3]*Department of Epidemiology and Cancer Registry;* [4]*Department of Hematology and Oncology, CancerCare Manitoba;* [5]*Department of Internal Medicine, University of Manitoba, Winnipeg, Manitoba*
Correspondence: Dr Harminder Singh, Section of Gastroenterology, University of Manitoba, 805-715 McDermot Avenue, Winnipeg, Manitoba R3E 3P4. e-mail harminder.singh@med.umanitoba.ca

provide equitable access to health care services to different sections of the population and, thereby, reduce disparities in disease outcomes such as CRC mortality. Review of outcomes in such health care systems is of increasing relevance, even to the jurisdictions without such systems (such as the United States) because they are initiating programs aiming to increase health care coverage in their populations.

Manitoba, a central Canadian province, has a universal health care plan without premiums that covers all residents irrespective of their age or socioeconomic status (SES) (7). In addition, efforts are continuously made to reduce any potential disparities in access to health care services across the province (eg, providing diagnostic imaging such as computed tomography scanning and onsite chemotherapy at remote areas in the province). We hypothesized that CRC mortality rates would be comparable across the different socioeconomic strata in the province and would change at a comparable rate over time.

The objectives of the current study were to determine the geographical and temporal variation in CRC mortality in Manitoba and to identify population-level factors associated with CRC mortality.

METHODS

Data sources and study measures

Manitoba is a central Canadian province with a relatively stable population (1.11 million in 1985 and 1.21 million in 2009). Manitoba Health is the publicly funded health insurance agency providing comprehensive universal health insurance to all residents of Manitoba (except inmates, and members of the Armed Forces and Royal Canadian Mounted Police) and maintains a population registry of permanent residents in the province. The population registry is a demographic, vital status and migration status database, and was used to determine the population size and distribution across the province.

Information regarding deaths from CRC was obtained from the Manitoba Cancer Registry (MCR), a population-based database actively recording all cancers diagnosed in residents of the province since 1956. Reporting to the MCR is mandated by law. The coding and capture of cancer data are audited regularly by the North American Association of Central Cancer Registries and the Canadian Cancer Registry. The quality of the MCR data is high, with consistently high levels of reporting completeness and histological verification (8,9). The MCR receives reports from Manitoba Vital Statistics on cause of death and investigates and documents all cases in which the reported cause of death is cancer.

Information regarding cause and date of death was obtained from the MCR for all Manitoba residents who died from CRC between 1985 and 2009, and who had a diagnosis of CRC. Cases of CRC were identified using *International Classification of Diseases, Ninth Revision,* Clinical Modification (ICD-9-CM) codes 153.0-153.4, 153.6-154.1 and 159.0 (for cases diagnosed before 2002) and ICD-10-CA codes C18.0, C18.2-C18.9, C19, C20 and C26.0 (from 2002 onward). Also included were CRC patients whose cause of death was listed as another cancer (lung, liver, primary unknown) but had no record of diagnosis of a cancer other than CRC.

There are differences in the biology and phenotype of CRC occurring in the proximal (upper/right) part of the colon compared with those occurring in the distal (lower/left) colon (10,11). Several recent studies suggest that in routine clinical practice, all commonly used CRC screening tests are less effective in reducing proximal CRC incidence and mortality (12-15). The incidence of CRC occurring in the proximal part of the colon has been increasing in Canada (16). Therefore, geographical variation in mortality due to proximal colon CRCs (cancers occurring in and proximal to the splenic flexure) and distal colon CRCs (cancers distal to the splenic flexure) were determined separately. To determine the CRC subsite, the subsite at the time of cancer diagnosis as recorded in the MCR was used.

A combination of the six-digit postal code and the municipal code of residence at time of diagnosis was used to geocode each CRC death to one of the 230 neighbourhoods in Winnipeg (average population during the study years 653,100) or to one of the 268 municipalities in

rural Manitoba (average population during the study years 500,977). For the population included in the denominator, the residential codes used were those recorded on July 1 of each year. These 498 areas were the geographical units used in the analyses. Areas within Winnipeg – the only urban centre in Manitoba with a population >50,000 – were considered to be urban. All other areas were considered to be rural. Sociodemographic characteristics, such as mean household income, proportion of recent immigrants, Jewish ethnicity (increased CRC incidence has been reported in some studies among those of Jewish ethnicity [17]), visible minority status and unemployment status, were obtained for each area from the 2001 Canadian census microdata files.

Statistical analysis

To visualize geographical variation in CRC mortality, a spatial Poisson mixed model was used to calculate age- and sex-standardized rates, using the 1991 general Canadian population as the standard. To control for potentially unstable rate estimates resulting from small case counts in areas with small populations, rate estimates were smoothed using Bayesian spatial Poisson hierarchical models incorporating two random variables indicating geographical variation and any other unspecified variation across study areas (15). Using hierarchical models, the mortality rate in each area is smoothed by pooling information from the neighbouring areas to generate stable rate estimates (18). Details of the Bayesian models used in this analysis are discussed elsewhere (19). The deviance information criterion was used for model diagnostics. ArcGIS version 10.0 (Environmental Systems Research Institute, USA) was used to produce choropleth maps of rates.

To model the relationship between CRC mortality and the characteristics of the geographical units, two approaches were taken, both using age- and sex-adjusted Poisson regression models. First, a series of Bayesian Poisson regression models were implemented for each characteristic with adjustment for age and sex to control for differences in demographic structures. Second, a saturated Bayesian Poisson regression model containing multiple predictor variables was developed. All models were fitted to individual cases, whereby cases were assigned the ecological characteristics (eg, average income level) of the geographical unit to which they were geocoded. Variables were categorized using Jenks natural breaks classification method, which attempts to find natural break points in the data when identifying category cut-offs (20). In the saturated model, a variable for the region of residence in the province (Winnipeg urban core; Winnipeg areas outside the urban core [suburban]; Northern Manitoba, Southwestern Manitoba, Southcentral Manitoba; and Southeastern Manitoba) was included. Some of the ecological variables, such as the proportion of Jewish or visible minorities and urban/rural residence, were not included in the saturated model to avoid multicollinearity. Potential overdispersion in the models was managed by incorporating a random variable to capture unspecified variation across small areas. The results are based on posterior probability and presented as mortality rate ratios (MRR) and corresponding 95% credible intervals (equivalent to confidence intervals in non-Bayesian analyses). The WinBUGS software package (MRC Biostatistics unit, Institute of Public Health, United Kingdom) was used for all Bayesian analyses.

All analyses (choropleth maps and regression models) were separately repeated for proximal and distal colon CRC mortality and for two different periods (1985 to 1996; 1997 to 2009). The year 1997 has been previously noted to be the year with potentially sharper increase in CRC screening in the province (16) and the year at which CRC mortality started decreasing in Canada (21).

To further explore the findings of the main Bayesian analyses, the linear time trends of CRC mortality in the different income groups were assessed by the Joinpoint Regression program developed by SEER (Surveillance Epidemiology and End Results, National Cancer Institute, USA). The average annual percentage changes (APC) in CRC mortality were calculated. The APC gives the estimated average annual rate of change in the rates and is equal to $100*(e^{m}-1)$, in which m is the slope of the corresponding regression line. The P value

TABLE 1
Colorectal cancer mortality counts and rates (per 100,000) according to site, sex and age, 1985 to 2009

Age group, years	Overall mortality				Distal colon				Proximal colon			
	Female		Male		Female		Male		Female		Male	
	Count	Rate	Count	Rate	Count	Rate	Count	Rate	Count	Rate	Count	Rate
Overall	3411	23.4	3838	26.9	1695	11.6	2313	16.2	1262	8.6	1146	8.0
<50	139	1.4	169	1.6	84	0.8	106	1.0	44	0.4	47	0.4
50–69	906	32.1	1348	49.7	515	18.2	863	31.8	317	11.2	369	13.6
≥70	2366	155.7	2321	228.8	1096	72.1	1344	132.5	901	59.3	730	72.0

TABLE 2
Time trends in overall colorectal cancer mortality rate according to sex and income

Annual income, $	Time period	APC (P)	Pairwise comparisons	P for pairwise comparisons*	
				Coincident	Parallel
Men					
All	1985–2009	−0.41 (0.48)			
<47,000 (low)	1985–2009	+0.95 (0.03)	Low versus high	<0.01	0.01
47,000 to 85,000 (average)	1985–2009	−0.44 (0.19)	Low versus average	<0.01	<0.01
>85,000 (high)	1985–2009	−1.83 (0.03)	Average versus high	0.04	0.15
Women					
All	1985–2009	−0.24 (0.37)			
<47,000 (low)	1985–1992	+8.07 (0.01)	Low versus high	0.01	0.02
	1992–2009	+0.04 (0.94)			
47,000 to 85,000 (average)	1985–2009	−0.63 (0.05)	Low versus average	<0.01	<0.01
>85,000 (high)	1985–2009	−1.86 (0.07)	Average versus high	0.38	0.20

The test of coincidence assesses whether two Joinpoint regression functions are identical and the test of parallelism assesses whether the two regression mean functions are parallel

presented with the APC estimates assesses the statistical significance of the estimates slope derived from the log-linear regression model. Pairwise comparability tests were performed to compare the different sets of trend data (22).

RESULTS

The number of deaths from CRC totalled 7249 between 1985 and 2009, with an average of 25.1 fatalities per 100,000 population per year (Table 1). The number of deaths from distal and proximal colon CRCs was 4008 and 2408, respectively. The annual mortality rates (per 100,000) from distal colon CRC ranged from 10.5 in 1989 to 16.8 in 2004, and for proximal colon CRC from 5.4 in 1986 to 10.9 in 2007. Men ≥70 years of age had the highest CRC mortality rates, regardless of the site of CRC in the colon (Table 1). The differences in rates between men and women were smaller for deaths due to proximal colon CRC than for distal colon CRC.

The choropleth maps depict the smoothed rates of CRC mortality across Manitoba, which ranged between 8.1 to 43.2 (per 100,000) in 1985 to 2009 (Figure 1). The highest CRC mortality rates were observed in the Northcentral part of Winnipeg and in rural areas in Southwestern and Eastern Manitoba, while Northern Manitoba had the lowest CRC mortality rates. Mortality rates from distal colon CRC ranged from 4.1 to 23.3 (per 100,000), with the highest distal colon CRC mortality rates in the northern part of Winnipeg and in discrete rural areas in eastern Manitoba (data not shown). The mortality rates from proximal colon CRC (1985 to 2009) ranged from 1.6 to 14.6 (per 100,000), with the highest rates observed in discrete areas of southern Winnipeg (data not shown). The mortality rates (overall, proximal colon and distal colon CRC) across Manitoba for the two different time periods 1985 to 1996 and 1997 to 2009 suggested that in the second time period of the study, there was an increase in the CRC mortality in the northern part of the province and in the northern part of Winnipeg (an area with higher proportion of immigrants from Southeast Asia and Indian subcontinent).

Overall, CRC mortality rates tended to decrease for both men and women over the study period (Table 2). However, changes in rates differed substantially depending on the mean household income of the

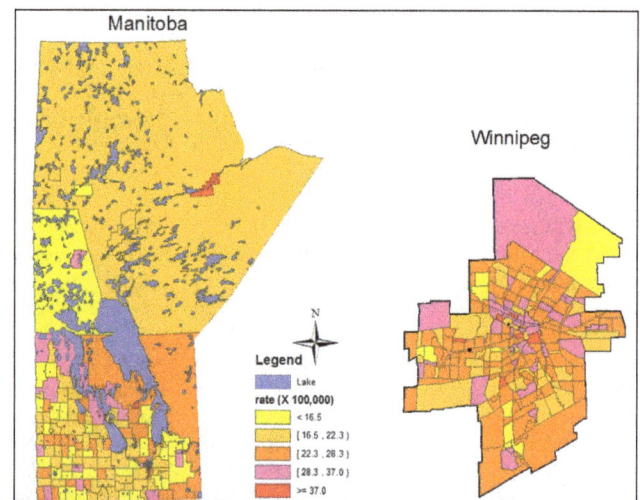

Figure 1) *Smoothed colorectal cancer mortality rates (per 100,000) (all sites combined), province of Manitoba and city of Winnipeg, Manitoba, 1985 to 2009, age- and sex-adjusted to the 1991 Canadian population*

area where individuals resided. Although men and women residing in areas with the highest annual income (>$85,000) had higher CRC mortality in the 1980s than those residing in the other neighbourhoods, they had a significant decrease in CRC mortality between 1985 and 2009 (APC approximately −1.8%), while those residing in areas with the lowest annual income (<$47,000) experienced an increase (APC men 1985 to 2009: +0.95; APC women 1985 to 1992: +8.07 and 1992 to 2009: +0.04) (Table 2; Figures 2A and 2B). The pairwise comparability tests suggest that the trend for the lowest income group was statistically significantly different than that of the other two income groups.

In the age- and sex-adjusted Poisson regression models for CRC mortality 1985 to 2009, the overall, proximal colon and distal colon CRC mortality rates among those living in the highest-income areas

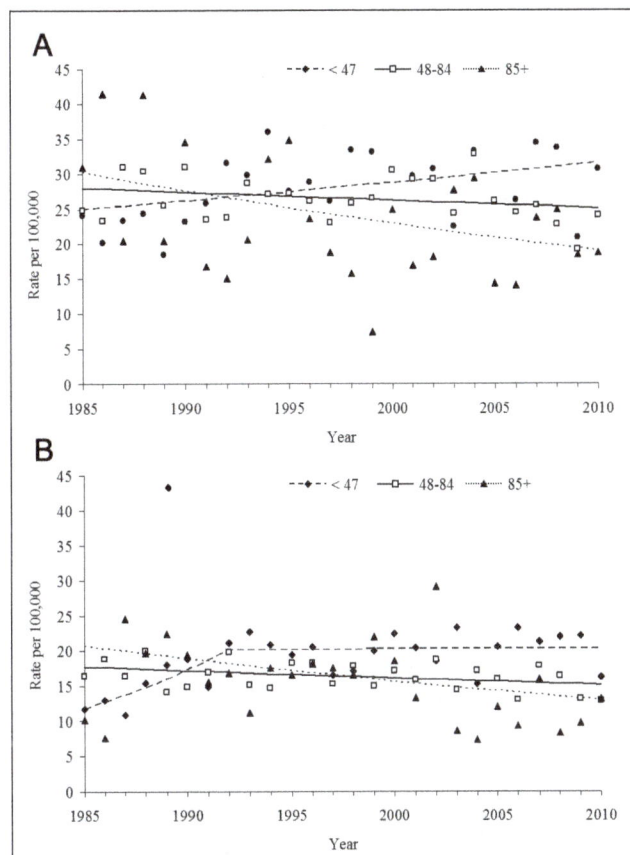

Figure 2) A *Time trends of overall colorectal cancer mortality among men in different income groups (1985 to 2009), joinpoint regression analysis.* **B** *Time trends of overall colorectal cancer mortality among women in different income groups (1985 to 2009); joinpoint regression analysis*

TABLE 3
Age- and sex-adjusted Poisson regression analyses of colorectal cancer (CRC) mortality, 1985 to 2009

	All CRC	Distal colon	Proximal colon
Region (Manitoba)			
Urban*	1.03 (0.98–1.0)	1.02 (0.95–1.09)	1.07 (0.98–1.17)
Rural	1.00 (–)	1.00 (–)	1.00 (–)
Winnipeg (excl core)	1.00 (–)	1.00 (–)	1.00 (–)
Winnipeg core	0.95 (0.85–1.06)	0.82 (0.71–0.95)	1.21 (0.96–1.51)
Northern	0.89 (0.78–1.01)	0.80 (0.68–0.94)	1.12 (0.86–1.44)
Southwestern	1.09 (0.97–1.21)	0.94 (0.81–1.08)	1.43 (1.14–1.78)
Southcentral	1.19 (1.07–1.34)	1.04 (0.89–1.19)	1.54 (1.23–1.93)
Southeastern	0.98 (0.88–1.08)	0.86 (0.76–0.98)	1.27 (1.03–1.56)
Annual income, $			
<47,000	1.00 (–)	1.00 (–)	1.00 (–)
47,000 to 85,000	0.89 (0.84–0.94)	0.84 (0.78–0.90)	0.96 (0.87–1.06)
>85,000	0.80 (0.72–0.88)	0.79 (0.69–0.90)	0.79 (0.65–0.93)
Unemployment rate, %			
<9	1.00 (–)	1.00 (–)	1.00 (–)
9 to <19	1.12 (1.05–1.21)	1.22 (1.11–1.33)	1.00 (0.88–1.14)
19 to 35	1.09 (0.97–1.21)	1.28 (1.11–1.46)	0.69 (0.54–0.88)
Recent immigrants, %			
<9	1.00 (–)	1.00 (–)	1.00 (–)
9 to <20	0.97 (0.92–1.02)	0.94 (0.87–1.00)	1.06 (0.97–1.16)
20 to <40	0.95 (0.88–1.01)	0.93 (0.85–1.02)	1.06 (0.93–1.19)
Jewish ethnicity, %			
<4	1.00 (–)	1.00 (–)	1.00 (–)
4 to <13	1.01 (0.90–1.13)	0.87 (0.73–1.02)	1.20 (0.98–1.43)
13 to <30	0.84 (0.72–0.88)	0.85 (0.68–1.04)	0.87 (0.65–1.12)
Visible minorities, %			
<6	1.00 (–)	1.00 (–)	1.00 (–)
6 to <19	1.06 (1.00–1.11)	1.04 (0.97–1.11)	1.12 (1.02–1.23)
19 to <48	0.98 (0.91–1.05)	0.99 (0.90–1.09)	1.01 (0.89–1.14)

*Data presented as mortality rate ratio (95% CI). *Urban-rural differences were evaluated in a separate model. excl Excluding*

were approximately 20% lower than those residing in the lowest-income areas (Table 3). There was no relationship to recent immigrant status or higher visible minorities' status. Areas with higher proportion of individuals of Jewish ethnicity did not experience increased CRC mortality. Individuals residing in the southern parts of the province had higher rates of death from proximal colon CRC.

The saturated Poisson regression analysis suggested that between 1985 and 2009, the highest CRC mortality rates occurred in Southcentral Manitoba (MRR 1.62) and Southeastern Manitoba (MRR 1.31) (regions of the province with higher proportion of individuals of Dutch-German Mennonite ethnic descent and farming communities) (Table 4). While the mean household income was not associated with CRC mortality rate in 1985 to 1996, areas with higher income experienced lower CRC mortality in 1997 to 2009. The impact of income was similar for deaths due to distal colon CRC and deaths due to proximal colon CRC. Geographical areas with a higher proportion of recent immigrants had lower CRC mortality; this reduction was essentially related to lower mortality due to distal colon CRC.

DISCUSSION

The present analysis highlights that individuals residing in higher-income areas in Manitoba experienced a decrease in CRC mortality over the study period while people residing in lower income areas experienced an increase. In the mid-1980s, individuals residing in lower income areas had lower mortality rates from CRC than people in higher income areas, which reversed over time.

We are not aware of a similar analysis in Canada, but comparable observations have been reported from the United States (5). Saldana-Ruiz et al (5) reported that before 1980, people living in counties with higher average SES were at greater risk for dying from CRC than

individuals living in counties with lower SES. In that study, the gradient also reversed direction over time. Our initial hypothesis was that income would not be significantly associated with the risk of dying from CRC in Manitoba because of the universal health care system and because of efforts to diminish social inequity in the province. Far from supporting that notion, our results suggest a disconcerting scenario of widening SES gap in CRC mortality over time. In their study, Saldana-Ruiz et al (5) suggest that a framework of fundamental social causes ("resources that can be used to avoid risks or to minimize the consequences of disease once it occurs" [23]), including "money, knowledge, status and availability of social support" (5) may be used to understand gaps in health outcomes such as CRC mortality. The framework predicts that when a new resource becomes available (eg, screening for cancer), it will be more readily accessed by people who already have resources, leading to earlier and more rapid reduction in disease incidence and mortality in that group. Our results suggest that this framework could also be applicable to a jurisdiction with a universal health care system. The widening gap in CRC mortality among socioeconomic groups could be due to earlier access to knowledge regarding screening among the higher income groups. A recent report from Ontario (24) suggests that the inequities in CRC screening participation according to SES in Ontario may have increased between 2005 and 2011, despite the launch of province-wide CRC screening program in 2008.

Our observation that the differences with income were no more marked for deaths from distal colon CRC suggests there may be additional contributing factors because CRC screening in usual clinical

TABLE 4
Adjusted saturated Poisson regression analysis of colorectal cancer (CRC) mortality

Time period	Parameter	All CRC		Distal colon		Proximal colon	
		MRR	95% CI	MRR	95% CI	MRR	95% CI
1985–2009	Region (Manitoba)						
	Winnipeg excluding core	1.00	–	1.00	–	1.00	–
	Winnipeg core	1.03	0.90–1.18	0.96	0.81–1.13	1.04	0.82–1.32
	Northern	1.00	0.86–1.16	0.99	0.81–1.18	0.96	0.73–1.24
	Southwestern	1.13	0.99–1.30	1.04	0.87–1.22	1.22	0.95–1.54
	Southcentral	1.62	1.35–1.92	1.50	1.19–1.87	1.39	1.01–1.87
	Southeastern	1.31	1.12–1.54	1.33	1.08–1.63	1.11	0.84–1.46
	Annual income, $						
	<47,000	1.00	–	1.00	–	1.00	–
	47,000 to 85,000	0.95	0.89–1.01	0.91	0.83–1.00	0.95	0.85–1.07
	>85,000	0.84	0.75–0.94	0.85	0.73–0.99	0.76	0.61–0.92
	Unemployment rate, %						
	<9	1.00	–	1.00	–	1.00	–
	9 to <19	1.00	0.92–1.09	1.10	0.98–1.22	0.89	0.76–1.03
	19 to 35	1.06	0.92–1.23	1.17	0.96–1.40	0.71	0.52–0.94
	Recent immigrants, %						
	<9	1.00	–	1.00	–	1.00	–
	9 to <20	0.82	0.74–0.91	0.76	0.66–0.87	1.04	0.86–1.24
	20 to <40	0.71	0.62–0.80	0.68	0.57–0.79	0.93	0.74–1.15
1985–1996	Region (Manitoba)						
	Winnipeg excluding core	1.00	–	1.00	–	1.00	–
	Winnipeg core	1.11	0.89–1.36	1.25	0.92–1.67	1.03	0.68–1.52
	Northern	1.15	0.90–1.44	1.51	1.09–2.07	0.95	0.59–1.47
	Southwestern	1.33	1.08–1.64	1.56	1.15–2.09	1.39	0.93–2.02
	Southcentral	1.94	1.46–2.50	2.20	1.47–3.10	1.47	0.85–2.40
	Southeastern	1.55	1.21–1.97	2.02	1.41–2.77	1.08	0.66–1.69
	Annual income, $						
	<47,000	1.00	–	1.00	–	1.00	–
	47,000 to 85,000	1.04	0.94–1.15	1.00	0.88–1.15	0.99	0.83–1.19
	>85,000	1.03	0.86–1.21	1.04	0.81–1.29	1.00	0.73–1.33
	Unemployment rate, %						
	<9	1.00	–	1.00	–	1.00	–
	9 to <19	1.02	0.90–1.16	1.17	0.98–1.38	0.87	0.68–1.09
	19 to 35	0.86	0.66–1.08	0.91	0.63–1.25	0.27	0.13–0.48
	Recent immigrants, %						
	<9	1.00	–	1.00	–	1.00	–
	9 to <20	0.82	0.70–0.95	0.77	0.61–0.94	1.07	0.79–1.40
	20 to <40	0.71	0.58–0.85	0.70	0.54–0.88	0.90	0.63–1.26
1997–2009	Region (Manitoba)						
	Winnipeg excluding core	1.00	–	1.00	–	1.00	–
	Winnipeg core	1.06	0.90–1.25	0.94	0.76–1.17	1.04	0.76–1.13
	Northern	0.98	0.81–1.17	0.88	0.69–1.11	0.91	0.64–1.28
	Southwestern	1.11	0.93–1.30	0.93	0.74–1.16	1.10	0.80–1.50
	Southcentral	1.48	1.19–1.83	1.34	0.98–1.79	1.28	0.83–1.87
	Southeastern	1.23	1.01–1.48	1.16	0.88–1.50	1.07	0.73–1.53
	Annual income, $						
	<47,000	1.00	–	1.00	–	1.00	–
	47,000 to 85,000	0.88	0.81–0.96	0.83	0.74–0.94	0.92	0.79–1.08
	>85,000	0.77	0.65–0.89	0.77	0.63–0.94	0.68	0.52–0.87
	Unemployment rate, %						
	<9%	1.00	–	1.00	–	1.00	–
	9 to <19	0.99	0.88–1.11	1.05	0.91–1.22	0.92	0.75–1.13
	19 to 35	1.34	1.12–1.60	1.41	1.11–1.77	1.07	0.75–1.47
	Recent immigrants, %						
	<9	1.00	–	1.00	–	1.00	–
	9 to <20	0.84	0.73–0.95	0.76	0.63–0.91	1.06	0.84–1.33
	20 to <40	0.74	0.63–0.89	0.98	0.55–0.84	1.00	0.75–1.30

CI Credible interval; MRR Mortality rate ratio

practice is more effective in preventing deaths from distal colon CRC (12). These factors may include changes over time in CRC lifestyle risk factors (eg, obesity), receipt of treatment and survival after CRC diagnosis, and should be investigated. The important implication of the fundamental social causes framework for policy makers includes significantly more emphasis when introducing new organized screening programs and treatments on ensuring equal uptake among lower socioeconomic groups. To the best of our knowledge, the Canadian provincial CRC screening programs have not, to date, made extra efforts to encourage CRC screening among lower SES groups. Our results, combined with that from the recent study from Ontario (24), emphasize the urgent need for such efforts. We suggest that all recently established Canadian provincial CRC screening should investigate the SES inequities in CRC screening participation in their jurisdictions and develop measures to reduce any such disparities.

In the saturated regression models, we found that southcentral and southeastern regions in the province had a higher CRC mortality rate. Differences in the ethnic composition of the populations could be contributing to this pattern. There are a higher proportion of individuals of Dutch-German Mennonite ethnic descent in these regions. A specific genetic mutation has been described in several families of Mennonite background in Manitoba (25), which has been associated with Lynch syndrome, a hereditary syndrome with very high risk for developing CRC. Although a 40% to 60% lifetime risk of CRC has been suspected in families with this mutation (26), we do not know the prevalence of this mutation in our population. Additional studies should investigate the reasons for the regional variations in CRC mortality and assess whether there are variations in CRC incidence, stage at presentation and survival after CRC diagnosis.

It is interesting to note that areas with higher proportions of recent immigrants had lower mortality rates from CRC in the analysis adjusted for income, but not in the analysis adjusted for age and sex only. This finding may have some implications for the CRC screening programs, which may be concerned about potentially lower rates of CRC screening among the immigrant populations. Our results suggest the focus should be on areas with lower income, irrespective of the proportion of recent immigrants among their inhabitants.

The results of our study should be interpreted in the context of its strengths and limitations. We used Bayesian Poisson mixed models to obtain stable rate estimates for areas with small case counts. We used the population-based MCR, which has been found to have very high data quality (8,9). We accessed the Manitoba Population Registry, which is regularly updated and, hence, had comprehensive follow-up. Our multiple regression analysis to determine the effect of average household income included variables indicating different regions of the province, thereby adjusting for potential regional variations in delivery of health care. The cause-of-death data from Manitoba Vital Statistics was supplemented by the data on CRC mortality by an algorithm to identify additional cases of CRC mortality. The routine, careful evaluation of each cancer death by the Manitoba Cancer Registry has enabled us to develop and use such an algorithm in this and previous studies (12).

On the other hand, the present study was an ecological analysis and additional studies are needed to confirm its findings. Although previous studies from Manitoba have shown a substantial correlation between self-reported household income and an individual's neighbourhood average income (27), the increase in CRC mortality among those residing in the lowest income neighbourhood found in the present study should be interpreted in the context of average neighbourhood household income and suggests the potential importance of focusing on lower-income neighbourhoods. The present study was observational in nature, a study design that has the potential for residual confounding by unmeasured or unrecognized factors. We were not able to evaluate the effect of ethnicity independent of income. We used the data from a single census year (2001) to determine the ecological characteristics. However, most important variables, such as relative average neighbourhood income, have not changed over time.

We did not adjust our analyses for CRC stage at diagnosis because for most of the study, period stage information was not collected reliably by the Registry (routinely collected from 2004 onward). However, stage is likely a mediator of the effects of SES differences on mortality; therefore, adjusting for it will only serve to explain at least some of the differences, but will not change the conclusions.

CONCLUSION
We identified regional variations in CRC mortality in Manitoba and widening SES gap in CRC mortality between income groups. The results suggest that SES disparities in CRC mortality could exist or even increase over time, even in jurisdictions with a universal health care system. The results also suggest that lower income areas should be a focus of CRC screening programs and other health care programs aiming to reduce the health burden of CRC.

DISCLOSURES: Dr Torabi was supported by an establishment grant from Manitoba Health Research Council (MHRC). Dr Mahmud holds a Canada Research Chair in Pharmacoepidemiology and Vaccine Research, and was supported by an establishment grant from the MHRC and by the Great-West Life, London Life and Canada Life Junior Investigator Award from the Canadian Cancer Society. The results and conclusions are those of the authors, and no official endorsement by CancerCare Manitoba or Manitoba Health is intended or should be inferred. There are no conflicts of interest. The analyses were performed by Drs Torabi and Nugent. All of the authors were involved in the study concept and design; acquisition of data, interpretation of data and critical revision of the manuscript for important intellectual content.

REFERENCES
1. Canadian Cancer Society's Steering Committee. Canadian Cancer Statistics 2012. Toronto: Canadian Cancer Society, 2012.
2. Zauber AG, Winawer SJ, O'Brien MJ, et al. Colonoscopic polypectomy and long-term prevention of colorectal-cancer deaths. N Engl J Med 2012;366:687-96.
3. Hewitson P, Glasziou P, Watson E, et al. Cochrane systematic review of colorectal cancer screening using the fecal occult blood test (hemoccult): An update. Am J Gastroenterol 2008;103:1541-9.
4. Moynihan R, Doust J, Henry D. Preventing overdiagnosis: How to stop harming the healthy. BMJ 2012;344:e3502.
5. Saldana-Ruiz N, Clouston SA, Rubin MS, Colen CG, Link BG. Fundamental causes of colorectal cancer mortality in the United States: Understanding the importance of socioeconomic status in creating inequality in mortality. Am J Public Health 2013;103:99.
6. Steinbrecher A, Fish K, Clarke CA, et al. Examining the association between socioeconomic status and invasive colorectal cancer incidence and mortality in California. Cancer Epidemiol Biomarkers Prev 2012;21:1814-22.
7. Roos LL, Walld R, Uhanova J, et al. Physician visits, hospitalizations, and socioeconomic status: Ambulatory care sensitive conditions in a Canadian setting. Health Services Res 2005;40:1167-85.
8. Hotes Ellison J, Wu XC, McLaughlin C, et al, eds. Cancer in North America: 1999-2003. Vol 1: Incidence: North American Asociation of Central Cancer Registries Inc, 2006:II-325.
9. Chen VW, Wu XC. Incidence, cancer in North America, 1991-1995. In: Andrews PA, ed. North American Association of Cancer Registries. Sacramento, 1999.
10. Iacopetta B. Are there two sides to colorectal cancer? Int J Cancer 2002;101:403-8.
11. Nawa T, Kato J, Kawamoto H, et al. Differences between right- and left-sided colon cancer in patient characteristics, cancer morphology and histology. J Gastroenterol Hepatol 2008;23:418-23.
12. Singh H, Nugent Z, Demers AA, et al. The reduction in colorectal cancer mortality after colonoscopy varies by site of the cancer. Gastroenterology 2010;139:1128-37.
13. Baxter NN, Goldwasser MA, Paszat LF, et al. Association of colonoscopy and death from colorectal cancer. Ann Intern Med 2009;150:1-8.
14. Atkin WS, Edwards R, Kralj-Hans I, et al. Once-only flexible sigmoidoscopy screening in prevention of colorectal cancer: A multicentre randomised controlled trial. Lancet 2010;375:1624-33.

15. Haug U, Knudsen AB, Brenner H, et al. Is fecal occult blood testing more sensitive for left- versus right-sided colorectal neoplasia? A systematic literature review. Exp Rev Molecul Diagnos 2011;11:605-16.

16. Singh H, Demers AA, Xue L, et al. Time trends in colon cancer incidence and distribution and lower gastrointestinal endoscopy utilization in Manitoba. Am J Gastroenterol 2008;103:1249-56.

17. Locker GY, Lynch HT. Genetic factors and colorectal cancer in Ashkenazi Jews. Fam Cancer 2004;3:215-21.

18. Torabi M, Rosychuk RJ. Hierarchical Bayesian spatiotemporal analysis of childhood cancer trends. Geogr Anal 2012;44:109-20.

19. Torabi M. Hierarchical Bayes estimation of spatial statistics for rates. J Statist Planning Inference 2012;142:358-65.

20. Jenks GF. The Data Model Concept in Statistical Mapping. International Yearbook of Cartography 1967;7:186-90.

21. Canadian Cancer Society's Steering Committee. Canadian Cancer Statistics 2011. Toronto: 2011.

22. Kim H-J, Fay MP, Yu B, et al. Comparability of segmented line regression models. Biometrics 2004;60:1005-14.

23. Link BG, Phelan J. Social conditions as fundamental causes of disease. J Health Soc Behav 1995;Spec No:80-94.

24. Honein-AbouHaidar GN, Baxter NN, Moineddin R, et al. Trends and inequities in colorectal cancer screening participation in Ontario, Canada, 2005-2011. Cancer Epidemiol 2013;37:946-56.

25. Lwiwski N, Greenberg CR, Mhanni AA. Genetic testing of children at risk for adult onset conditions: When is testing indicated? J Gen Counsel 2008;17:523-5.

26. Orton NC, Innes AM, Chudley AE, et al. Unique disease heritage of the Dutch-German Mennonite population. Am J Med Gen 2008;146A:1072-87.

27. Mustard CA, Derksen S, Berthelot J-M, et al. Assessing ecologic proxies for household income: A comparison of household and neighbourhood level income measures in the study of population health status. Health Place 1999;5:157-71.

23

Registered nurse-performed flexible sigmoidoscopy in Ontario: Development and implementation of the curriculum and program

Mary Anne Cooper MSc MD MEd FRCPC[1,2,3],

Jill Margaret Tinmouth MD PhD FRCPC[2,3,4], Linda Rabeneck MD MPH FRCPC[3,5]

MA Cooper, JM Tinmouth, L Rabeneck. Registered nurse-performed flexible sigmoidoscopy in Ontario: Development and implementation of the curriculum and program. Can J Gastroenterol Hepatol 2014;28(1):13-18.

Although colorectal cancer is a leading cause of death in Canada, it is curable if detected in the early stages. Flexible sigmoidoscopy has been shown to reduce the incidence and mortality of colorectal cancer in patients who are at average risk for this disease and, therefore, is an appropriate screening intervention. Moreover, it may be performed by nonphysicians. A program to enable registered nurses to perform flexible sigmoidoscopy to increase colorectal cancer screening capacity in Ontario was developed. This program incorporated practical elements learned from other jurisdictions as well as specific regional considerations to fit within the health care system of Ontario. The nurses received structured didactic and simulation training before performing sigmoidoscopies on patients under physician supervision. After training, nurses were evaluated by two assessors for their ability to perform complete sigmoidoscopies safely and independently. To date, 17 nurses have achieved independence in performing flexible sigmoidoscopy at 14 sites. In total, nurses have screened >7000 Ontarians, with a cancer detection rate of 5.1 per 1000 screened, which is comparable with rates in other jurisdictions and with sigmoidoscopy performed by gastroenterologists, surgeons and other trained nonphysicians. We have shown, therefore, that with proper training and program structure, registered nurses are able to perform flexible sigmoidoscopy in a safe and thorough manner resulting in a significant increase in access to colorectal cancer screening.

Key Words: *Colorectal cancer screening; Flexible sigmoidoscopy; Registered nurses*

Les infirmières autorisées effectuant des sigmoïdoscopies flexibles en Ontario : l'élaboration et la mise en œuvre du cursus et du programme

Même si le cancer colorectal est une cause majeure de cancer au Canada, on peut le guérir s'il est décelé au stade précoce. Il est démontré que la sigmoïdoscopie flexible réduit l'incidence de cancer colorectal et la mortalité y étant associée chez les patients qui courent un risque moyen de cette maladie et, par conséquent, qu'elle constitue une intervention de dépistage pertinente. De plus, elle peut être effectuée par des non-médecins. Un programme visant à faire exécuter des sigmoïdoscopies flexibles par des infirmières autorisées afin d'accroître la capacité de dépistage du cancer colorectal a été élaboré en Ontario. Ce programme incluait des éléments pratiques tirés d'autres territoires de compétence et tenant compte de considérations régionales précises pour fonctionner dans le système de santé de l'Ontario. Les infirmières recevaient une formation didactique et en simulation structurée avant d'effectuer des sigmoïdoscopies sur des patients sous la supervision d'un médecin. Après la formation, les infirmières étaient notées par deux évaluateurs pour leur capacité d'exécuter des sigmoïdoscopies complètes seules et de manière autonome. Jusqu'à présent, 17 infirmières se sont mises à faire des sigmoïdoscopies flexibles en toute autonomie dans 14 établissements. Au total, les infirmières ont fait le test de dépistage auprès de plus de 7 000 Ontariens et obtenu un taux de dépistage du cancer de 5,1 cas sur 1 000 personnes faisant l'objet du test, ces taux étant comparables à ceux d'autres territoires de compétence et aux sigmoïdoscopies exécutées par des gastroentérologues, des chirurgiens et d'autres non-médecins formés. Nous avons donc démontré qu'en possédant une formation et une structure de programme convenables, les infirmières autorisées sont en mesure d'effectuer des sigmoïdoscopies flexibles de manière sécuritaire et détaillée, ce qui entraîne une augmentation importante de l'accès au dépistage du cancer colorectal.

Colorectal cancer (CRC) is the second leading cause of cancer deaths in Canada. It is estimated that approximately 8700 individuals in Ontario were diagnosed with CRC in 2013 and that 3350 died from the disease (1). If detected sufficiently early, however, >90% of CRCs can be cured.

Several screening modalities for CRC exist, enabling early detection or even prevention. Importantly, it has been shown that flexible sigmoidoscopy (FS), a procedure associated with minimal risk, cost and patient inconvenience, is one such intervention that can reduce the risk of CRC (2,3). Compared with colonoscopy, FS requires less onerous preparation and has a lower procedural risk. It is also typically performed without sedation so that the time required for FS is much less than that for a colonoscopy (4). As such, FS is considered to be an appropriate screening method for CRC in several jurisdictions including Canada. The Canadian Association of Gastroenterology position statement cites FS as a viable option for screening persons who are at average risk for CRC (5).

Additionally, it has been shown that nonphysicians can perform FS, which allows flexibility in the distribution of the procedure to maximize patient access. In particular, registered nurses (RNs) have been shown to be able to perform FS as proficiently as physicians in terms of depths of insertion of the endoscope and in polyp detection rates (6).

It is imperative that there is access to effective screening to benefit from the impact such interventions can offer to reduce the morbidity and mortality of CRC. To provide adequate CRC screening capacity in Ontario, we developed a program to train RNs to perform FS. To achieve this, several hurdles had to be overcome, requiring the coordination of multiple organizations. Issues included ensuring malpractice insurance coverage for both nurses and physician trainers, developing institution-specific medical directives, developing physician remuneration packages, developing participant recruitment plans for each centre involved, and creating and delivering an appropriate curriculum and evaluation process. Support was obtained from the Registered Nurses Association of Ontario, the Ontario Nursing

---

[1]*RNFS Program, Cancer Care Ontario;* [2]*Department of Gastroenterology, Sunnybrook Health Sciences Centre;* [3]*Department of Medicine, University of Toronto;* [4]*ColonCancerCheck Program, Cancer Care Ontario;* [5]*Cancer Care Ontario and the University of Toronto, Toronto, Ontario*
Correspondence: Dr Mary Anne Cooper, Department of Medicine, Sunnybrook Health Sciences Centre, 2075 Bayview Avenue, Room HG64, Toronto, Ontario M4N 3M5. e-mail maryanne.cooper@sunnybrook.ca

Secretariat, the College of Physicians and Surgeons of Ontario, the Canadian Medical Protective Agency, the Michener Institute of Applied Health Sciences, Cancer Care Ontario (CCO), and the Ministry of Health and Long-term Care. Much of the groundwork and the solutions to the hurdles we encountered have been reported elsewhere (7).

The objective of the present report is to describe the training and education component of the Ontario Registered Nurse-performed Flexible Sigmoidoscopy (RNFS) initiative, outlining the curriculum and the pedagogical principles used in training the nurses and certifying them for independent practice.

METHODS

The first formal RNFS training program began in Ontario in 2005, after a year of planning and research of similar programs in other jurisdictions. Since then, there have been four additional training programs conducted as part of this CRC screening initiative. The Ontario program has evolved with each iteration as lessons learned became incorporated. This section describes considerations made and research performed as preparatory work in advance of the first implementation of the training program and the subsequent refinements incorporated over time. These factors included research and site visits to other jurisdictions, investigation into the legal parameters in which medical professionals work in Ontario and consideration of the large geographical area that constitutes this province.

Lessons from other jurisdictions – Kaiser Permanente, California, USA

It was acknowledged at the outset that other jurisdictions had successfully developed nurse FS programs to screen patients for CRC. Most notably, Kaiser Permanente in California (USA) had developed a program in the early 1990s to help them achieve acceptable screening rates for the patient population within their health maintenance organization (HMO). Their nurse-performed FS program was fundamental in achieving a screening participation rate of 80% of eligible HMO members (8). The lead educator (MAC) of the Ontario RNFS program received an education travel grant from the Professional Association of Internes and Residents of Ontario to visit three Kaiser Permanente sites in 2004 to assess their program for its applicability in Ontario.

Significant lessons learned during these visits included the observation that a model of a strong physician-nurse dyad was critical for essential mentorship to occur so that the nurse always felt supported and able to approach his/her physician mentor with all questions. It was also necessary for the trust to be reflected back to the physician who needed to be comfortable in transferring patient care to the nurse.

By extension, the Kaiser Permanente program had observed that the nurses who performed best had at least two years of experience as endoscopy assistants before commencing training in performing FS. By this point in their careers, the nurses had determined whether they enjoyed gastrointestinal endoscopy and, therefore, were likely to remain in this field for a reasonable length of time. This improved the return-on-investment made in training, increased the likelihood that the nurses were truly content in this vocation and that the pool of trained nurses could be maintained, both for the sustained functioning of the program and for nursing collegiality. Importantly, the physicians already had a foundation of trust with the nurses who trained in FS.

It was also noted that all of the nurses interviewed in the Kaiser Permanente program emphasized several key elements in their practice. They believed that there was significant professional benefit in having nurse coworkers who were engaged in the program work with them so that they did not perform FS without the support of their colleagues. This was particularly noted among the nurses who had been with the program when it began and when they were changing their practice profile from endoscopy assistants to endoscopists.

All of the nurses interviewed during the site visits to California and who performed FS also commented on the significant role change from supporter to service provider that performing FS had brought to their careers. This specifically included the notion that they had been accustomed to comforting patients who experienced discomfort during the procedure and had become the ones who caused patient discomfort as they performed the procedures. They emphasized the need for support with this professional practice change.

Lessons from other jurisdictions – National Health Service, United Kingdom

It was recognized that there was also the need to provide standardization among the physician leads at each site who would train the nurses to perform FS. Some centres had experience in training endoscopy learners if they were associated with resident physician training. Not all centres, however, had such experience and, therefore, there was a need to be sure all physician trainers were aware of approaches to teaching endoscopy, the related pedagogy and the particular issues related to the scope of practice of the RN endoscopists in Ontario. The education lead (MAC) received financial support from CCO to travel to the United Kingdom to participate in their well-developed 'Train-the Endoscopic-Trainer' program to learn the pedagogical principles involved in teaching endoscopy trainers.

In addition to the practical element of training, it was observed that physician leads and physician trainers required an orientation to the role of the RN as an endoscopist and the scope of practice they could follow within the parameters of the Public Hospitals Act of Ontario (9). With these considerations in mind, a 'Train-the-Trainer' element and RNFS program orientation for physicians was incorporated into the Ontario RNFS training program in 2007.

Ontario requirements

Successful implementation of our RNFS program required that the nurses be able to perform FS and to decide appropriate follow-up based on the results of the procedure. This required that a nurse assume some autonomy in interpreting the results of the sigmoidoscopy. It was the responsibility of the nurse to follow-up results of any tissue samples taken during the FS, review with the physician trainer and ensure appropriate actions were pursued. The nurses, therefore, had to be educated on the pertinent physiology and pathophysiology of polyps and CRC, and be able to communicate this information appropriately to their patients. This communication of information had to occur within the bounds of the Public Hospitals Act of Ontario that precludes nurses from giving diagnoses (9). The nurse endoscopists, therefore, were educated on how to relay this information appropriately. For example, nurses could not give a diagnosis of 'diverticulosis' and, therefore, were required to present findings to patients as 'You appear to have diverticulosis'.

The nurses were also an important link in communicating the results of the FS, not only to their supervising physician, but also to the patients' primary care physicians. They ensured that appropriate correspondence about the procedure and any subsequent results were transmitted to the primary care physicians according to site-specific protocols.

Once trained, nurses worked with some independence, although the formal assignation of a physician mentor still applied. The efficiency of the functioning of this dyad reflected the trust that needed to exist between the nurse and the physician and underpinned the success of the program.

Finally, the Ontario program had to be designed such that not only did the curriculum cover the necessary didactic material and practical training but that it could be implemented over the large geographical area of Ontario (1,076,00 km^2 [larger than France and Spain combined]) (10).

After considering the work performed at Kaiser Permanente and the training expertise from the United Kingdom, and considering the specific geographical challenges faced in Ontario, a curriculum was developed that would bring the nurses together for basic training but obtain their experiences in performing FS on patients at their home hospitals. The following section describes how this program has manifested in Ontario.

RESULTS

The training program

Given the background research performed and the particular needs of Ontario, a program was developed that included the following elements:

1. Pretraining observation at the nurses' home hospital sites;
2. Didactic curriculum and simulator training course at a central training site;
3. Train-the-endoscopic trainer for physicians at a central training site;
4. Clinical experience at the home hospital site with physician trainers; and
5. Home hospital site evaluation.

A detailed syllabus was prepared to encompass all elements of the training program. It included space for journaling, tables to record progress on simulators (see below), all of the required didactic material and a log for on-site training. It was provided to the nurses several weeks before attending the central course so that they could familiarize themselves with the entire course curriculum.

Pretraining observations at the nurses' home hospital sites: One of the first principles considered in the training was that the RNs would assume a role that traditionally had been in the domain of the physician. This role change required that nurses accept both the change in the physical requirements of the task and the philosophical change from supporter to provider. One of the ways in which this challenge was met in the program was to require that the nurses undergo a formal pretraining process of observing a physician perform FS. The purpose of this was to provide the specific opportunity for them to view the difference in the technical aspects of the procedure between the one performing the FS compared with the traditional perspective of the RN assisting. The nurses were also instructed to observe and comment on the role difference from the individual who may cause discomfort during the performance of the procedure compared with one who comforts the patient. They had the opportunity during this period of observation to discuss with the physician technical aspects of the procedure they neither had observed nor with which they previously had had concerns as an assistant.

Didactic curriculum and simulator training at a central training site: The next phase in training was to teach the nurses the theoretical and practical basics of performing FS. The nurses were brought together from around the province to Toronto (Ontario) for one week. The program was conducted at the Michener Institute for Applied Health Sciences in a setting that allowed classroom and practical training. The classroom curriculum included discussions on basic anatomy, physiology and pathophysiology as they applied to the performance of flexible sigmoidoscopy, the polyp-to-cancer sequence, and role of FS in cancer prevention and early detection. Other material covered during this week included a discussion of the nurses' practice limitations, how to obtain consent, and how to dictate and/or report the procedures.

Throughout the one-week course, the nurses participated in a professional practice assessment led by a nursing faculty member. This involved journaling, a review of nursing principles, a dialogue regarding the medical directives and a discussion of their evolving role. It included a reflection of their observations made before the course and of those made during the week.

The nurses began their practical training on the first day of the week with an orientation to a real endoscope to learn about its various functions. The nurses were then introduced to the simulators. Considerable time was scheduled for the nurses to practice on the simulators during the week. Two instructors circulated among the learners to provide instruction and feedback but the nurses also had ample time for independent practice.

The nurses were introduced to the practical aspects of performing FS using two types of simulators. A box simulator was available for basic training to allow the nurses to develop facility with the endoscopes, which was built for this course (11) based on a previously developed 'choose-the-hole' fibre-optic intubation simulator (12). It consisted of an open box with a series of panels in which numbered holes were drilled and through which an endoscope could be passed. A list was developed that outlined the appropriate series of numbered holes through which the nurse would direct the endoscope. The series of numbers were listed in order of difficulty to guide training.

The training course also used a high-fidelity simulator (EndoVR endoscopy simulator, CAE Healthcare, Canada) to provide a sense of realism and haptic feedback (13). Programmed cases were also presented to the nurses in terms of increasing difficulty to guide their training.

For all of the skills of the course to coalesce, a session with standardized patients was held in the latter half of the week. For this encounter, a standardized patient was interviewed by the trainee to obtain a focused history and consent for the procedure. The standardized patient then lay on a stretcher in the left decubitus position in close proximity to the simulator. The sounds of the simulator were transmitted to the standardized patient by an earphone and the standardized patient then vocalized the sounds as cued by the simulator so that the nurse would have to respond to the patient while performing the procedure. On completion of this simulated FS, the nurse was required to dictate a report of the procedure. The report was transcribed and reviewed to provide feedback to the nurses.

Train-the-endoscopic trainer for physicians at a central training site: On completion of the one-week course, the nurses returned to their home hospital sites to commence practical training under the supervision of physicians with experience in endoscopy, typically gastroenterologists and general surgeons. To provide consistency in performance across the province and to expose the site trainers to the concepts of teaching endoscopy if they came from sites not affiliated with a university teaching program that already trained resident doctors, a lead physician from each site attended the course in Toronto for a day of training that overlapped with the nurses at the end of their week-long course. A representative of CCO met with the physicians to review administrative details and discuss the provincial screening plan. The physicians were oriented to the program, including the limits of the nurses' scope of practice, and reviewed basic pedagogical principles of teaching endoscopy. The physicians then had an opportunity to explore these principles and practice teaching endoscopy in training exercises with the nurses in the course. In addition to providing the physicians with essential information and creating a provincial standard in the expected performance of the RN endoscopists, the interactive session with nurses was an excellent interprofessional experience.

Coordination of the one-week course elements was critical in accomplishing all the training goals. Figure 1 represents a typical schedule for a course within the program.

Clinical experience at the home hospital site with physician trainers: After returning to their home hospital sites from the central training course, the nurses performed FS on real patients enrolled into the program for screening, which included patients 50 to 75 years of age who had no symptoms and who did not have a family history of CRC. To help ease their transition into performing procedures on patients, the nurses first completed 25 procedures by simply withdrawing the endoscope under supervision. Following this, they then performed 50 full procedures, still under supervision of the physician trainer. The nurses were required to perform these procedures before being considered for evaluation. If, in the opinion of the nurse and the trainer, more experience was needed, the nurse continued to perform more procedures under supervision until prepared.

Home hospital site evaluations: Once ready for independent practice, two evaluators travelled to the nurse's site to assess her/him. It was decided a priori that each nurse would perform five flexible sigmoidoscopies on which she/he would be evaluated. Each site typically scheduled six patients, however, in case one patient was unable to make the appointment or a bowel preparation was particularly poor. The evaluators used both a checklist and a global rating scale to guide their assessments of the candidates (14). The physician trainer from the home hospital site was required to be in the room for all of the cases because the assessors were visitors to the institutions and did not have privileges at any of the sites. The physician trainer was also asked to complete the checklists and global rating scales to assist in the evaluation of the nurse.

	MON	TUES	WED	THUR	FRI-RN	FRI - MD	
7	FLEX SIG WEEK						7
8	Breakfast	Breakfast	Breakfast	Breakfast	Joint RN/MD Breakfast		8
		Dictation	Didactic Review	Written Exam			
9	Intro Background Course outline	Endo Training II	Endo Training IV	Endo Training VI	Prof Practice Issues	CCO Info	9
						Program Review	
10	Prof Prac Issues					Teaching Theory & Tips	10
	Break	Break	Nutrition Break		Break		
11	Anatomy	Physiology/ Pathology			Teaching Drills - MD trainers teaching RN endoscopists		11
12			Lunch	Lunch			12
	Lunch	Lunch	Endo Training V -	Q&A with	Debriefing		
1	Anatomy of the Endoscope	Review of screening prot	SP* ENDO WITH DICTATIONS	Nurse Endoscopist	Lunch		1
	Intro to Simulators	Endo Training III		Exam Review			
2				Endo Training VI			2
	Break	Nutrition Break					
3	Endo Training I						3
4		Didactic Review		Dictation Review, Course Review & Evaluations			4
5							5
			Didactic Review				

Figure 1) *An example of a schedule for the one-week registered nurse (RN)-performed flexible sigmoidoscopy training course. CCO CancerCareOntario; Endo Endoscope; MD Medical doctor; Prac Practice; Prof Professional; Q&A Question and answer*

Independent practice

Once approved for independent practice, the nurses were then able to continue performing FS on appropriate patients according to site-specific guidelines and medical directives. A physician trainer was no longer required to be in the endoscopy room while the nurse performed the procedures but one was required to be accessible if the nurse encountered difficulties, either with technical issues in performing the FS or with interpretation of findings. Each facility determined a schedule that would best work for that site. If a physician's outpatient office was located near the endoscopy suite, he/she might see outpatients while the nurses performed FS in the suite. In most instances, however, the nurses were scheduled to perform FS while a physician trainer worked in another room in the endoscopy unit.

Additional considerations

In some cases, it took considerable time for nurses to achieve the skills necessary to be evaluated and deemed competent for individual practice. As such, refresher courses were run for the nurses and they came to Toronto for two days of review as deemed necessary by the nurses themselves and the site coordinators. Didactic material that had been covered in the course was reviewed, and the nurses also spent time on both the box and high-fidelity simulators. The nurses were encouraged to bring forward any questions they had about the theoretical material and practice issues after having acquired some practical experience.

Evaluations by the nurse endoscopists

The nurses' experience in the one-week central course has been critical to the success of the overall training because it provided the foundation for the theoretical knowledge and practical skills, and firmly established a rapport among the nurses and their physician trainers who returned to work at sites broadly distributed throughout the province. These courses and the nurses' involvement in the program as a whole have been evaluated and met with a high level of satisfaction by the nurses. They have felt valued in that they have

been able to expand their scope of practice, lead in a new initiative for nurses and participate more directly in CRC screening in Ontario.

Typical comments from anonymized evaluations of the courses included the following:

- The course was above my expectations. Fantastic support and encouragement by teachers and colleagues.
- The course was amazing. [I] learned so much.
- Got great basic skills to build on.
- Use of the simulators [was] excellent.
- For one week the knowledge and skill that was obtained was excellent. I felt confident leaving here. I know I still have lots of skill and knowledge to gain but look forward to the challenge and look forward to the future.
- It was a wonderful week. Everyone was very friendly; went out of their way to make us feel comfortable!!! Thoroughly enjoyed – would recommend the program to others.

Program results and impact

To date, 17 RNs have achieved independence in performing FS at 14 sites. An additional nine nurses at existing and new sites remain to be evaluated. In total, RNs performing FS, either under supervision or independently, have screened >7000 Ontarians. Data from the first 5000 cases have shown a cancer detection rate of 5.1 per 1000 screened.

DISCUSSION

We described the development of a comprehensive training program to prepare RNs to perform FS in an independent clinical setting, as has been accomplished in other jurisdictions. Nurses have been performing FS in California within the Kaiser Permanente HMO for approximately 20 years. The nurses in the United Kingdom perform both sigmoidoscopy and colonoscopy. As well, an independent clinician in Ontario had reported previously on nurse-performed FS in a single-centre community (15).

Nursing considerations

To date, five iterations of the training program of the RNFS curriculum have been conducted and many practical aspects have been learned in each implementation. In the first iteration of the program, two large Toronto teaching hospitals were chosen as the sites. Because of resource issues related to maintenance of provision of existing endoscopy services, endoscopy nurses were not available to participate in the training. Despite the recommendations from the Kaiser Permanente system that nurses have at least two years endoscopy experience, we attempted to train nurses from a range of backgrounds, but none who had worked in endoscopy. From a pedagogical perspective, it was believed that if nonendoscopy nurses could be trained, then the training principles could be transferred easily to nurses with endoscopy experience. While the nurses were enthusiastic and interested in adding a new dimension to their career, some simply did not enjoy this type of work. This, combined with logistical issues at sites without significant endoscopy resources, prevented this cohort of nurses from gaining practice independence. In subsequent iterations, sites were chosen that had the reserve in human resources to enable endoscopy nurses to participate in the training.

It must also be recognized that the nurses work within union structures. It has been observed that union rules have required nurses in endoscopy to be transferred to other departments outside of endoscopy within an institution. In one specific instance, an RN who was already performing FS independently was transferred to another unit outside of endoscopy to accommodate a nurse with greater union seniority. The RN trained to perform FS, therefore, had to withdraw from the program and could no longer perform procedures. Not only was she unable to contribute to the provincial screening program, her nursing colleague who was also trained to perform FS no longer had her much-valued support and assistance. Such realities must be considered when choosing which nurses should be trained to promote sustainability of the program as a whole and at individual sites.

It has also been observed within our program and, as recommended from the Kaiser Permanente program, that it is best if at least two nurses are involved at each site. Because sites are so geographically distant from one another and because there remains the need to consolidate the acceptance of the nurses performing this role in Ontario, there was a significant benefit to a nurse having a local colleague with whom she/he could train and discuss program issues. As the program has matured, we have observed that the implementation at each site worked better with three nurses trained in performing FS. Ongoing program development, therefore, has included a concerted effort to increase the numbers of nurses trained at each site.

To help build camaraderie on a provincial basis, we also learned that regularly scheduled teleconferences with the nurses and the site administrative support staff have been extremely beneficial. The nurses are able to discuss implementation and practice issues to learn additional insights and approaches and the site administrators can confer with others to find solutions to specific concerns such as patient recruitment, site scheduling, medical directives and other practical issues.

Training considerations
Within the actual training course held centrally in Toronto, practical issues emerged that were addressed to optimize training. It was observed that the nurses were excellent self-directed learners and did well using the simulators independently, with occasional input from the instructors. They diligently worked through the proscribed lists of series on the box simulator and case sequences of the high-fidelity simulator. Once instructions regarding use of the simulators and basic endoscopy principles were given, the instructors would circulate to assist the nurses as needed. The number of simulators, therefore, was a key determinant in the maximum number of learners who could be accommodated during each program. Typically, three box simulators and three high-fidelity simulators were available so that the maximum number of learners was capped at 12. This allowed nurses to work in pairs at each simulation station and obtain considerable hands-on experience during the one-week training. Having the same equipment but fewer attendees allowed the nurses even more practical training during the week. Such physical arrangements were met with more positive course reviews by the nurses.

The benefits of simulator training have been shown to be of the greatest benefit in learners at early stages (16). We also have observed significant improvements in the nurses' technical ability throughout the one-week training (14,17). Importantly, however, we believe that the simulator also played a significant role in helping the nurses' transition in their professional role from supporter to provider. In particular, the audible and haptic feedback from the high-fidelity simulator and the use of standardized patients to mimic a real environment as much as possible helped the nurses with this transition, having provided them with a sense about the impact of performing this procedure on a patient before their home site clinical training began.

Patient considerations
It was apparent from the inception of the program that considerable effort and coordination was required to ensure adequate enrollment of patients for RNFS-performed FS. As such, the role of a site coordinator was developed and financed by CCO. The site coordinator's primary role was to contact and inform family physicians and family practice groups in the region of the nurses' home hospital about the program and to encourage patient enrollment for an RN-performed FS as a CRC screening modality in the community.

One of the challenges of this program has been the recruitment of patients to be screened for colonic polyps by RN-performed FS. There were many reasons for this (6) but recruitment has had a significant impact on the training of the nurses because it has hampered their ability to gain experience in a proficient and timely manner, causing delays in the time in which it was expected some nurses would have achieved competence to work independently. Over time, experience showed that a strong network with the community family doctors and the presence of a physician champion at each site were required to

establish and maintain momentum in patient recruitment. As noted above, another of the ways this issue was addressed was with the creation of the role of site coordinator to promote the program in local communities. Additionally, it was learned that meeting with the site coordinator's administrative leads for the program for a one-day workshop held in advance of the one-week central course helped in having a recruitment plan in place to which the nurses would return. The regularly scheduled teleconferences with involvement of all sites also helped with recruitment because they shared their specific recruitment challenges and solutions.

Impact of the funding model
Some of the issues with patient recruitment and site involvement have related to the funding model that was required during the pilot phase of this project. As a project of the Ministry of Health and Long-term Care of Ontario, funding was provided annually through recurrent one-time funding. This hampered the ability of the program organizers to reach out to communities until funding was assured. The consequences of this was that site involvement, selection of nurses to be candidates for training, the running of the actual complete training program (observation, didactic and simulator learning, clinical training and evaluations) and patient recruitment for the specific site all had to be conducted within a period of ≤12 months. The constraints induced by this process contributed to some of the difficulties in patient recruitment. It also led to some short-cuts being taken, specifically, reducing or eliminating the observation component of the training program. We observed, however, that when time allowed for the full observation portion of the program to occur, the nurses were more comfortable when they arrived for the one-week course and had already begun to make the intellectual transition from supporter to provider.

Train-the-endoscopic trainer
The earliest iterations of training did not directly involve the doctors who would train the nurses. It became apparent that this was a key element of a successful program for several reasons. The nurses must work within the limitations of the Public Hospitals Act of Ontario (9). It was extremely important that the physicians were made explicitly aware of these limitations so that they would know what they could ask of their nurses. The doctors also needed to be informed what the nurses' curriculum contained and the rationale for the inclusions (or exclusion) of material. It was also recognized that while some hospitals were sites for resident training, this was not the case for all. Some element of training-the-endoscopy trainer was deemed essential, therefore, to provide a pedagogical foundation for skills training and consistency across all sites of the province for the nurses in their practical training. There were also administrative issues in the program that were specific to the doctors such as remuneration. Finally, the doctors also needed to know where the RNFS program fit within the provincial screening philosophy. For all of these reasons, it was imperative to incorporate a component in the one-week training course for physician trainers. They were able to obtain the necessary information about the course, learn basic principles of teaching endoscopy and discuss with one another the practical implementation details at their sites. This was incorporated in such a way as to minimize the physician's time required in Toronto and overlap with the nurses. The resultant session has been very successful, particularly the interactive session with the physicians and nurses.

Licenses and hospital privileges
The design of this program from the outset allowed implementation across many provincial sites without limitations conferred by licenses and hospital privileges by the trainers. The nurses received all of their clinical training involving patients at their sites with physician trainers who held the necessary privileges. The introduction to practical training was conducted on simulators and, therefore, did not require exposure to real patients. When the evaluators travelled to the sites to assess the nurses, the physician trainers at the sites remained present in the room and were able to provide technical intervention when required.

The fact that the evaluators did not have privileges at any of the distributed sites, therefore, was not of practical concern.

Evaluations

As the program has grown, a need for more evaluators has emerged. The evaluations are conducted at each site necessitating that the evaluators travel there. Not all nurses at each site attain competence at the same rate and, therefore, to maintain a positive momentum for the site program and the enthusiasm of the nurses, individuals were sometimes evaluated at different times at the same site so that a prepared nurse was not held back if it was believed that the time for her/his colleague to achieve the same level of competence was going to be excessive. The consequence of this has been that evaluators have needed to make multiple trips to some sites. There have been times, therefore, when the demands on the evaluators' time have been high and they have not been able to get to all sites in a timely manner. It is expected that more evaluators will be trained to conduct these site visits to enable nurses to progress to independence as soon as they are able. This will both reduce the demands on the time of the doctors supervising the nurses who must continue to be supervised directly by the physician trainer until certified for independence, and increase the number of patients being screened.

Project impact

As discussed above, the RNs have contributed to CRC screening in Ontario by performing FS on >7000 individuals. The cancer detection rate of 5.1 per 1000 screened is comparable with rates in other jurisdictions and with FS performed by gastroenterologists, surgeons, nurses, and other trained nonphysicians (8,18-20).

Summary

The Ontario RNFS initiative has become established at multiple sites across the province. It has been successful in training RNs to perform FS to screen for CRC. The nurses have been able to assume a new professional role while respecting the legal framework in which they must practice. Patient recruitment to this program has been a challenge since its inception. This has been a factor in the training of some

nurses who were limited at times by the low numbers of patients. Once this problem was overcome at each site, the nurses have had no difficulty in completing their training. We have been able to create a program distributed throughout the province in a coordinated and organized manner using a structure that has allowed a broad implementation unencumbered by license and hospital privilege issues. A professional network of trained nurses has been created by bringing them together for a core course with relationships maintained by regular tele- and videoconferencing. All of the features of this program make it portable and able to be implemented in most jurisdictions.

CONCLUSION

Since 2005, the program developed in Ontario to train RNs to perform FS to increase CRC screening has matured. The next step will be to incorporate RNFS into Ontario's organized province-wide CRC screening program. We have shown that, with proper training, RNs are able to perform FS in a safe and thorough manner, resulting in increased access to CRC screening. We continue to expand the program by increasing both the number of sites where the nurses perform screening FS and the number of nurses at each site. Because the structure of the program does not rely on the need for licenses and hospital privileges for the trainers, it has the potential either to be an anchor for a national training program for Canada or to serve as a model that can be implemented in other jurisdictions.

DISCLOSURES: The authors have no financial disclosures or conflicts of interest to declare.

ACKNOWLEDGEMENT: The authors acknowledge Dr Catharine M Walsh MD MEd FRCPC, Division of Gastroenterology, Hepatology and Nutrition, Hospital for Sick Children and The Wilson Centre, University of Toronto, for her contribution in design and inclusion of the box simulator in the program and for her participation in training and evaluation of the nurses.

REFERENCES

1. Canadian Cancer Society's Steering Committee on Cancer Statistics. Canadian Cancer Statistics 2013. Toronto: Canadian Cancer Society; 2013.
2. Atkin WS, Edwards R, Kralj-Hans I, et al. Once-only flexible sigmoidoscopy screening in prevention of colorectal cancer: A multicentre randomised controlled trial. Lancet 2010;375:1624-33.
3. Schoen RE, Pinsky PF, Weissfeld JL, et al. Colorectal-cancer incidence and mortality with screening flexible sigmoidoscopy. N Engl J Med 2012;366:2345-57.
4. Ransohoff DF and Sandler RS. Screening for colorectal cancer. N Engl J Med 2002;346:40-4.
5. Leddin DJ, Enns R, Hilsden R, et al. Canadian Association of Gastroenterology position statement on screening individiuals at average risk for developing colorectal cancer: 2010. Can J Gastroenterol 2010;24:705-14.
6. Ho C, Jacobs P, Sandha G, et al. Non-physicians performing screening flexible sigmoidoscopy: Clinical efficacy and cost-effectiveness [Technology report no 60]. Ottawa: Canadian Coordinating Office for Health Technology Asessment, 2006. <www.cadth.ca/media/pdf/277_endoscopist_model_tr_e.pdf> (Accessed April 30, 2013).
7. Dobrow MJ, Cooper MA, Gayman K, et al. Referring patients to nurses: Outcomes and evaluation of a nurse flexible sigmoidoscopy training program for colorectal cancer screening. Can J Gastroenterol 2007;21:301-8.
8. Palitz AM, Selby JV, Grossman S. The Colon Cancer Prevention Program (CoCaP): Rationale, implementation and preliminary results. HMO Pract 1997;11:5-12.
9. Public Hospitals Act R.S.O. 1990, CHAPTER P.40 Consolidation Period: From January 1, 2011 to the e-Laws currency date. Last amendment: 2010, c. 25, s. 27. (Accessed April 30, 2013).
10. About Ontario: Geography <www.ontario.ca/trave-and-recreation/about-ontario> (Accessed October 25, 2013).
11. Walsh CM, Cooper MA, Rabeneck L, et al. High versus low fidelity simulation training in gastroenterology: Expertise discrimination. Can J Gastroenterol 2008;22(Suppl A):164A. (Abst)
12. Naik VN, Matsumoto ED, Houston PL, et al. Fiberoptic orotracheal intubation on anesthetize patients: Do manipulation skills learned on a simple model transfer into the operating groom? Anesthesiology 2001;95:343-8.
13. EndoVR <http://caehealthcare.com/eng/surgical-simulators/endovr> (Accessed October 25, 2013)
14. Walsh CM, Cooper MA, Rabeneck L, et al. Flexible Sigmoidoscopy Simulation Training: Task Trainers and Virtual Reality Simulators Both Show Benefit. Research in Medical Education, San Antonio, November 2008.
15. Shapero TF, Alexander PE, Hoover J, et al. Colorectal cancer screening: Video-reviewed flexible sigmoidoscopy by nurse endoscopists – a Canadian community-based perspective. Can J Gastroenterol 2001;15:441-5.
16. Datta V, Mandalia M, Mackay S, Darzi A. The PreOp flexible sigmoidoscopy trainer. Validation and early evaluation of a virtual reality based system. Surg Endosc 2002;16:1459-63.
17. Walsh CM, Cooper MA, Rabeneck L, et al. Task trainers and virtual reality simulators both show benefit in training gastrointestinal endoscopy skills. Association for Medical Education in Europe. Prague, Czechoslovakia, August 2008.
18. UK Flexible Sigmoidoscopy Screening Trial Investigators. Single flexible sigmoidoscopy screeng to prevent colorectal cancer: Baseline findings of a UK multicenter randomized trial. Lancet 2002;359:1291-300.
19. Segnan N, Senore C, Andreoni B, et al. Baseline findings of the Italian multicenter randomized controlled trial of "once-only sigmoidoscopy": SCORE. J Natl Cancer Inst 2002;94:1763-72.
20. Weissfeld JL, Schoen RE, Pinsky PF, et al. Flexible sigmoidoscopy in the PLCO cancer screening trial: Results from the baseline screening examination of a randomized trial. J Natl Cancer Inst 2005;97:989-97.

24

Hepatocellular carcinoma in a large Canadian urban centre: Stage at treatment and its potential determinants

Korosh Khalili MD[1], Ravi Menezes PhD[1], Leyla Kochak Yazdi MD[1], Hyun-Jung Jang MD[1], Tae Kyoung Kim MD[1], Suraj Sharma MD[2], Jordan Feld MD[2], Morris Sherman MD[2]

K Khalili, R Menezes, LK Yazdi, et al. Hepatocellular carcinoma in a large Canadian urban centre: Stage at treatment and its potential determinants. Can J Gastroenterol Hepatol 2014;28(3):150-154.

OBJECTIVE: To determine whether there is a significant difference in tumour stage between patients initially found with hepatocellular carcinoma (HCC) at a tertiary hepatobiliary centre and patients referred with tumours detected elsewhere; and to determine variables associated with referral in a palliative stage.

METHODS: A retrospective review of 12,199 patients seen at a liver clinic over a 10.5-year period revealed 236 patients with HCC first detected internally (internal) and 163 who were referred with a known mass (referred). All patients were staged at the time of treatment using the Milan criteria for transplantation and Barcelona Clinic Liver Cancer (BCLC) staging system. Curative disease was defined as BCLC stages 0 and A. In the referred group, univariate and multivariate analyses were used to determine which of the following factors were significantly associated with presentation in a palliative stage: age, sex, ethnicity, cause of liver disease, presence of cirrhosis, location of residence and quintile of neighbourhood income.

RESULTS: In comparing the internal versus referred patients, significant differences were found in the proportion of patients fulfilling Milan criteria (72% versus 36%), those with curative disease (75% versus 49%) and those with very early stage tumour (BCLC stage 0, 23% versus 7%); all differences were statistically significant (P<0.001). In patients referred for treatment of HCC from an outside institution, none of the variables tested were associated with presentation in a palliative stage.

CONCLUSION: Patients with HCC referred to a liver treatment centre were more likely to be in palliative stages than those whose tumour was detected internally.

Key Words: Cirrhosis; Hepatitis; Hepatocellular carcinoma; Surveillance

Le carcinome hépatocellulaire dans un grand centre urbain canadien : le stade de traitement et ses déterminants potentiels

OBJECTIF : Déterminer si le stade de tumeur présente une différence importante entre les patients qui se font diagnostiquer un carcinome hépatocellulaire (CHC) dans un centre hépatobiliaire de soins tertiaires et ceux qui sont aiguillés parce que leur tumeur a été décelée ailleurs; déterminer les variables associées à l'aiguillage en phase palliative.

MÉTHODOLOGIE : Une analyse rétrospective de 12 199 patients vus à une clinique hépatique pendant une période de 10,5 ans a révélé que 236 patients ayant un CHC avaient été dépistés à l'hôpital (à l'interne) et 163 avaient été aiguillés parce qu'ils avaient une masse connue (aiguillés). Le stade des patients était établi au moment du traitement au moyen des critères de transplantation de Milan et du système de classification de la clinique de cancer hépatique de Barcelone (CCHB). Une maladie curative était définie comme les stades 0 et A de la CCHB. Dans le groupe aiguillé, les analyses univariées et multivariées ont permis de déterminer lesquels des facteurs suivants s'associaient de manière significative à la présentation en phase palliative : âge, sexe, ethnie, cause de maladie hépatique, présence de cirrhose, lieu de résidence et quintile du revenu du quartier.

RÉSULTATS : En comparant les patients à l'interne aux patients aiguillés, les chercheurs ont constaté des différences importantes dans la proportion de patients qui respectaient les critères de Milan (72 % par rapport à 36 %), qui avaient une maladie curative (75 % par rapport à 49 %) ou qui avaient une tumeur de stade précoce (stade 0 de la CCHB, 23 % par rapport à 7 %). Toutes les différences étaient statistiquement significatives (P<0,001). Chez les patients aiguillés pour le traitement d'un CHC à partir d'un établissement externe, aucune des variables examinées ne s'associait à une présentation en phase palliative.

CONCLUSION : Les patients ayant un CHC qui étaient aiguillés vers un centre de traitement hépatique étaient plus susceptibles d'être en phase palliative que ceux dont la tumeur avait été décelée à l'interne.

Of the 25 most common cancers in Canada, liver cancer is the only cancer with a statistically significant rise in mortality rate; the Canadian age-adjusted incidence of hepatocellular carcinoma (HCC) was projected to rise by 73% in males and 28% in females from 1996 to 2015 (1,2). Ultrasound surveillance of populations at risk for HCC has not been promoted by Canadian governmental health agencies but has been considered to be the standard of care by the hepatology community both in Canada and internationally (3-7). Supporting surveillance are its cost effectiveness and reported decreased mortality in a randomized controlled trial (8-10). Despite a universal health care system, survival data suggest that the identification and/or treatment of patients with HCC are lagging in Canada. The latest statistics reveal that the highest reported survival rate of patients with HCC is in Japan, where the five-year survival rate is 39% to 44%, whereas it is 26% in British Columbia and 22% in Ontario (11-14). While the

Canadian urban population contains a unique mix of ethnicities and risk factors for HCC, there have been no previous studies investigating HCC stage at presentation in Canada.

Approximately 3000 patients undergo annual HCC surveillance within the University Hospital Network (Toronto, Ontario). We have anecdotally noted that patients with HCC referred to our centre for treatment are more often in palliative stages of disease than those within our own surveillance group who develop HCC. Our hospital network is the only designated regional treatment centre for HCC and, therefore, nearly all HCCs discovered in the region, regardless of the stage, are referred to our centre for treatment, minimizing referral bias. Therefore, we undertook a study to establish whether patients referred to us with HCC were significantly more likely to present in a palliative stage compared with those whose HCC was discovered through our own hospital. Furthermore, we aimed to determine which

[1]Department of Medical Imaging; [2]Department of Gastroenterology, University of Toronto, Toronto, Ontario
Correspondence: Dr Korosh Khalili, Department of Medical Imaging, University Health Network, Princess Margaret Hospital, 610 University Avenue, Room 3-964, Toronto, Ontario M5G 2M9. e-mail korosh.khalili@uhn.ca

independent variables were associated with referral in the palliative stage among patients referred to our centre for treatment.

METHODS

A retrospective review of charts of 12,199 patients seen at the liver clinic at one of the authors' hospitals (Toronto Western Hospital, Toronto, Ontario) from January 2000 to June 2010 revealed 475 patients with a diagnosis of HCC. This single hospital was selected because the records of the liver clinic were in electronic fromat. Patients with a history of HCC or without available contrast-enhanced computed tomography/ magnetic resonance imaging data were excluded (Figure 1). Patients were divided into 'internal' (tumour first discovered in the authors' institution) or 'referred' (patient referred with a known hepatic mass) groups based on chart review and cross-confirmed by reviewing the indication for imaging at the authors' institution. Of the 236 internal patients, 201 (85.1%) were undergoing ultrasound surveillance at the authors' institution and distributed as follows: regular surveillance (≤12 months interval between last two surveillance scans [n=109]), irregular surveillance (>12 months [n=38]) or first surveillance (tumour detected on first scan [n=54]).

The diagnosis of HCC was confirmed for all patients using the following criteria: updated American Association for Study of Liver Disease (AASLD) HCC management guidelines' imaging diagnostic criteria of one positive contrast-enhanced imaging scan in at-risk patients (5); positive histopathology from core biopsy or explant specimens; or recurrence after treatment of tumour. All relevant imaging data were directly and retrospectively reviewed by a fellowship-trained abdominal imager to ensure compliance with the latest imaging criteria and to confirm staging.

Outcome measures

The stage of disease based on the Barcelona Clinic Liver Cancer (BCLC) staging classification was used as an outcome measure (15). Curative disease was defined as early BCLC stages 0 (one nodule <2 cm) or A (one resectable nodule of any size or three nodules <3 cm). Palliative disease was defined in patients with the advanced stages B to D. The Milan criteria for treatment of HCC by transplantation were used as an additional outcome measure, with early disease defined as fulfilling the criteria of one nodule <5 cm or three nodules <3 cm without venous invasion or distant metastases (16). To ensure a fair comparison of tumour stage among referred and internal surveillance patients, the imaging available on assessment for treatment at multidisciplinary tumour board was used for all patients. Therefore, if a tumour had been discovered earlier by surveillance but had been followed, the tumour stage at time of treatment rather than time of discovery was used.

Variables potentially associated with presentation in a palliative stage

In the referred group of patients, the following variables were tested for an association with presentation in a palliative stage: age, sex, ethnicity, cause of liver disease, presence of cirrhosis, location of residence and quintile of neighbourhood income. Due to the limited number of patients in some subcategories, certain variables were grouped for the analysis. The surveillance history of the referred patients was unavailable due to the retrospective nature of the study.

Ethnicity was divided into two groups: Caucasian (European descent) and others (including East and Southeast Asians, African, Middle-Eastern, South-Asian, Caribbean and Latin American). Causes of liver disease included chronic hepatitis B virus (HBV) infection, chronic hepatitis C virus (HCV) infection, other causes and multiple causes (patients with more than one cause of disease). The Child-Pugh score was used for severity of liver disease with noncirrhotic patients grouped with Child-Pugh A versus patients with Child-Pugh B and C scores. Year of detection was divided into two groups – 2000 to 2005 and 2006 to 2010 – to determine the effect of implementation of the first AASLD HCC guidelines (in 2005) along with installation of the latest generation of scanners at the authors' institution (in 2006). Patients were divided based on their residence in

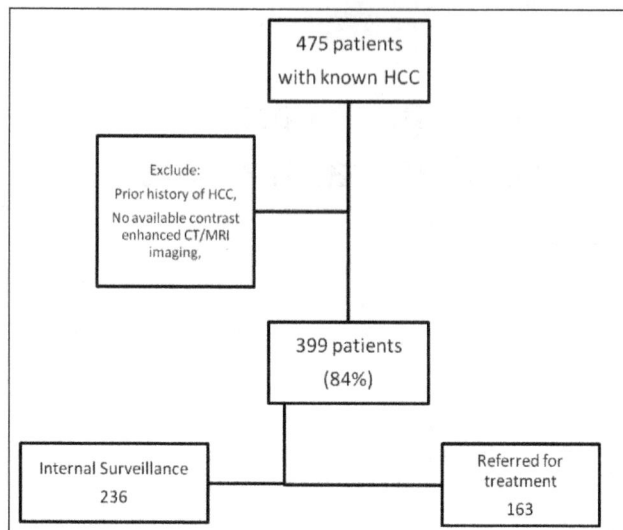

Figure 1) *Flowchart of patient population. CT Computed tomography; HCC Hepatocellular carcinoma; MRI Magnetic resonance imaging*

metropolitan (greater Toronto [Ontario] area) versus beyond metropolitan groups to determine whether there was a difference in urban versus rural populations. Finally, surveillance frequency was grouped into ≤12 months (adequate) and >12 months (inadequate) based on the interval between last and immediately previous surveillance scans. Table 1 summarizes the patient characteristics.

Statistical methods

Associations with referral status were examined using the Fisher's exact test (for cirrhosis), t test (for age) and χ^2 test (for all other variables). χ^2 and logistic regression analyses were used to examine associations with presentation in a palliative stage. For the latter analysis, two outcome measures were used, as described (BCLC stage 0/A versus B/C/D; fulfill Milan criteria yes versus no). Patients' quintile of neighbourhood income and region of residence were derived using the Postal Code Conversion File + Version 5 (PCCF+) (17). PCCF+ is a series of files created by Statistics Canada based on the most recent Canadian census data and assigns geographical identifiers based on postal codes. For the purposes of the present study, patients' quintile of neighbourhood income was used as a proxy measure of personal income of study participants, while region of residence was classified as within or beyond the metropolitan area (greater Toronto area).

Analyses were performed using SAS version 9.2 (SAS Institute, USA) and SPSS version 17.0 (IBM Corporation, USA) for Windows 2008 (Microsoft Corporation, USA); $P<0.05$ was considered to indicate statistically significant associations.

RESULTS

Comparison of referred and internal patients

Table 2 summarizes the characteristics of internal versus referred patients. Significant differences were apparent between referred and internal patients in the proportion of Caucasian patients (61% versus 37%; $P<0.001$), of those fulfilling Milan criteria (36% versus 72%; $P<0.001$) and those with curative BCLC stages 0 and A (49% versus 75%; $P<0.001$). In addition, a significantly lower proportion of referred patients (12 of 163 [7%]) had their tumour discovered at the very early BCLC stage (ie, stage 0, <2 cm) compared with internal patients (55 of 236 [23%]; $P<0.001$, data not shown in Table 1). Figure 2 illustrates the differences between internal and referred patients.

Potential determinants of early stage presentation in referred patients.

Tables 3 and 4 summarize the results of univariate analyses in predicting presentation in an early stage among referred patients using

TABLE 1
Patient demographics

	Patients	
	Internal (n=236)	Referred (n=163)
Age, years		
Mean ± SD	61.6±10.8	61.2±11.3
Median (range)	61 (26–86)	61 (31–85)
Ethnicity		
African	7 (3)	3 (2)
Asian, East/Southeast	63 (27)	81 (50)
Asian, South	11 (5)	8 (5)
Caribbean	3 (1)	3 (2)
Caucasian	143 (61)	61 (37)
Latin American	3 (1)	1 (0.6)
Middle Eastern	5 (2)	5 (3)
North American Natives	1 (0.4)	1 (0.6)
Cause(s) of liver disease		
Hepatitis C virus	105 (44)	51 (31)
Hepatitis B virus	58 (25)	82 (50)
More than one cause	36 (15)	14 (9)
Alcohol	22 (9)	5 (3)
Nonalcoholic fatty liver disease	8 (3)	2 (1)
Primary biliary cirrhosis	2 (1)	–
Hemochromatosis	–	1 (0.6)
Alagille syndrome	1 (0.4)	–
Autoimmune hepatitis	1 (0.4)	–
Budd-Chiari syndrome	1 (0.4)	–
Unknown	2 (1)	0 (0)
Cirrhosis		
Yes	229 (97)	150 (92)
Symptomatic presentation		
Yes	12 (5)	7 (4)

Data presented as n (%) unless otherwise indicated

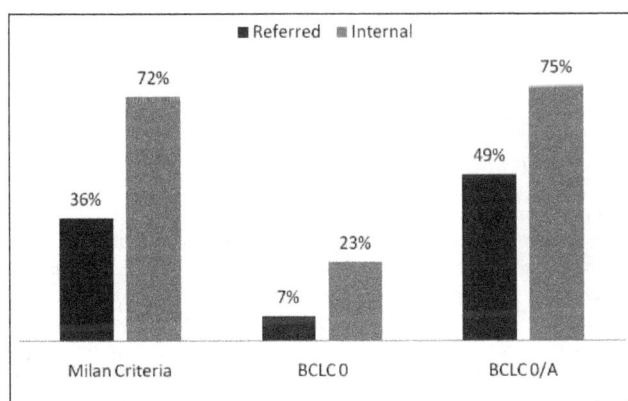

Figure 2) *Comparison of heaptocellular carcinoma stage in referred versus internal patients (all differences are statististically significant [P<0.001]). BCLC Barcelona Clinic Liver Cancer*

BCLC staging (Table 3) and Milan criteria (Table 4). Multivariate analysis was not performed because none of the variables reached significance in univariate analysis (unadjusted). There was a trend among non-Caucasian patients to present in curable stages using both BCLC and Milan criteria, but this did not reach statistical significance (P=0.11 and P=0.09, respectively).

DISCUSSION

The present study yielded two key findings. The first was that there was a significantly higher proportion of patients with incurable HCC

TABLE 2
Comparison of internal and referred patients

	Internal (n=236)	Referred (n=163)	P	Unadjusted OR (95% CI)
Sex				
Female	44 (19)	35 (21)	0.486	1.19 (0.73–1.96)
Male	192 (81)	128 (79)		1.00
Ethnicity				
Caucasian	143 (61)	61 (37)	<0.001	1.00
Other	93 (39)	102 (63)		2.57 (1.71–3.88)
Cirrhosis				
No	7 (3)	13 (8)	0.024	2.83 (1.11–7.27)
Yes	229 (97)	150 (92)		1.00
BCLC stage at treatment				
0/A	178 (75)	80 (49)	<0.001	1.00
B/C/D	58 (25)	83 (51)		3.18 (2.08–4.88)
Milan criteria				
No	65 (28)	104 (64)	<0.001	4.64 (3.02–7.12)
Yes	171 (72)	59 (36)		1.00
Income quintile (postal code)				
1 (lowest)	56 (24)	37 (23)	0.734	1.00
2	53 (22)	42 (26)		1.20 (0.67–2.14)
3	41 (17)	32 (20)		1.18 (0.64–2.20)
4	39 (17)	32 (20)		1.24 (0.67–2.32)
5 (highest)	36 (15)	19 (12)		0.80 (0.40–1.60)
Unmatchable	11 (5)	1 (0.6)		0.14 (0.02–1.11)
Cause(s) of liver disease				
Hepatitis B virus	58 (25)	82 (50)	<0.001	2.90 (1.53–5.52)
Hepatitis C virus	105 (44)	51 (31)		1.00 (0.52–1.90)
Combined	34 (14)	11 (7)		0.66 (0.28–1.59)
Other/unknown	39 (17)	19 (12)		1.00
Age, years				
Mean ± SD	61.6±10.8	61.2±11.3	0.627	1.00 (0.98–1.01)
Median (range)	61 (26–86)	61 (31–85)		
Residence				
Beyond metropolitan*	32 (14)	26 (16)	0.505	1.21 (0.69–2.12)
Metropolitan*	204 (86)	137 (84)		1.00

*Data presented as n (%) unless otherwise indicated. *Greater Toronto (Ontario) area. BCLC Barcelona Clinic Liver Cancer*

among those whose tumours were discovered elsewhere compared with those whose cancer was discovered at our institution. The second is that cause of liver disease, ethnicity nor any of the other variables tested appeared to be a significant determinant of this late presentation in the referred group.

The differences between the tumour stage of referred versus internal group of patients is striking. The proportion of those who fulfilled the Milan criteria – so called 'early stage cancers' – among the internal patients (72%) was double that of the referred patients (36%). Patients had a 4.6 times higher odds of having a tumour discovered according to Milan criteria when they were undergoing care in our hospital. The odds were less (OR 3.18 [95% CI 2.08 to 4.88]) when using the BCLC staging system as an end point, but this is because BCLC stage A includes single operable tumours >5 cm in addition to those meeting the Milan criteria.

Which factors are associated with the relatively late presentation in most of the referred patients? Among the seven variables tested, none showed a significant association with presentation with advanced HCC (Tables 3 and 4). Interestingly, neither residence in the greater

TABLE 3
Predicting presentation of hepatocellular carcinoma at an early stage using the Barcelona Clinic Liver Cancer (BCLC) staging system

	BCLC		P	Unadjusted OR (95% CI)
	0/A (n=80)	B/C/D (n=83)		
Sex				
Female	16 (20)	19 (23)	0.653	0.84 (0.40–1.78)
Male	64 (80)	64 (77)		1.00
Ethnicity				
Caucasian	25 (31)	36 (43)	0.110	1.00
Other	55 (69)	47 (57)		1.69 (0.89–3.20)
Cirrhosis				
No	9 (11)	5 (6)	0.349	1.73 (0.54–5.54)
Yes	72 (90)	78 (94)		1.00
Income quintile (postal code)				
1 (lowest)	16 (20)	21 (25)	0.948	1.00
2	22 (28)	20 (24)		1.44 (0.59–3.51)
3	16 (20)	16 (19)		1.31 (0.51–3.40)
4	16 (20)	16 (19)		1.31 (0.51–3.40)
5 (highest)	9 (11)	10 (12)		1.18 (0.39–3.59)
Unmatchable	1 (1)	0 (0)		
Cause(s) of liver disease				
Hepatitis B virus	41 (51)	41 (49)	0.991	1.11 (0.41–3.02)
Hepatitis C virus	25 (31)	26 (31)		1.07 (0.37–3.07)
Combined	5 (6)	6 (7)		0.93 (0.21–4.11)
Other/unknown	9 (11)	10 (12)		1.00
Age, years				
Mean ± SD	60.8±12	61.6± 10.7	0.638	0.99 (0.97–1.02)
Median (range)	60 (31–85)	61 (34–83)		
Residence				
Beyond metropolitan*	13 (16)	13 (16)	0.918	1.05 (0.45–2.42)
Metropolitan*	67 (84)	70 (84)		1.00

Data presented as n (%) unless otherwise indicated. *Greater Toronto (Ontario) area

TABLE 4
Predicting presentation of hepatocellular carcinoma at an early stage using the Milan criteria for transplantation

	Milan criteria		P	Unadjusted OR (95% CI)
	Yes (n=59)	No (n=104)		
Sex				
Female	14 (24)	21 (20)	0.597	1.23 (0.57–2.65)
Male	45 (76)	83 (80)		1.00
Ethnicity				
Caucasian	17 (29)	44 (42)	0.087	1.00
Other	42 (71)	60 (58)		1.81 (0.91–3.59)
Asian	31 (53)	50 (48)	0.699	1.00
Non-Asian	28 (47)	54 (52)		0.84 (0.44–1.59)
Cirrhosis				
No	2 (3)	11 (11)	0.137	0.30 (0.06–1.39)
Yes	57 (97)	93 (89)		1.00
Income quintile (postal code)				
1 (lowest)	9 (15)	28 (27)	0.570*	1.00
2	17 (29)	25 (24)		2.12 (0.80–5.59)
3	12 (20)	20 (19)		1.87 (0.66–5.27)
4	12 (20)	20 (19)		1.87 (0.66–5.27)
5 (highest)	8 (14)	11 (11)		2.26 (0.70–7.37)
Unmatchable	1 (2)	0 (0)		
Cause(s) of liver disease				
Hepatitis B virus	30 (51)	52 (50)	0.977	1.25 (0.43–3.63)
Hepatitis C virus	19 (32)	32 (31)		1.29 (0.42–3.95)
Combined	4 (7)	7 (7)		1.24 (0.26–5.91)
Other/unknown	6 (10)	13 (13)		1.00
Age, years				
Mean ± SD	61.5±12.1	61.0±10.9	0.810	1.00 (0.97–1.03)
Median (range)	60 (31–85)	61 (34–83)		
Residence				
Beyond metropolitan*	8 (14)	18 (17)	0.530	0.75 (0.30–1.85)
Metropolitan*	51 (86)	86 (83)		1.00

Data presented as n (%) unless otherwise indicated. *Greater Toronto (Ontario) area

Toronto area nor quintile of neighbourhood income (a marker of personal income) correlated with this late presentation. Caucasians and East/Southeast Asians comprised the two largest ethnic groups in the present study, accounting for 87% of the referred patient group. Neither ethnic group had any advantage in early presentation fulfilling the Milan criteria (Table 4). Therefore, ethnicity was also not significantly associated with the stage of presentation.

The one variable that could not be examined was the referred patients' HCC surveillance history; this is the most likely difference between the internal and referred populations. The internal patient population included everyone whose HCC was discovered at our institution, also counting those who presented symptomatically or with terminal liver failure (BCLC stage D). However, most of the internal patients were undergoing some surveillance. A low rate of HCC surveillance and/or its low effectiveness among referred patients are the most likely causes of the differences in the two populations. This assertion is supported by other international studies that have described a similar difference in presenting tumour stage of patients referred for treatment compared with those within a surveillance population (18-21). The present study was the first to assess the Canadian experience with its unique mix of risk factors. Ineffective surveillance may be due to low sensitivity, incorrect method (ie, not by ultrasound) or improper management. The incidence and mortality rates of HCC are diluted in provincial and national statistics but much of the HCC at-risk population reside in the few large Canadian urban centres (22). This concentration also renders targeted interventions potentially more cost effective. By identifying individuals at risk and making effective surveillance widespread, we believe that stage migration is achievable.

Strengths and limitations
Because our hospital is the only designated regional centre for HCC treatment, referral bias is likely to be small, especially because nearly all potentially curative therapies, including all liver transplants in the region, are performed here. Nevertheless, a small but unknown volume of surgical interventions are performed outside our institution, raising the possibility that the referred population would have a higher proportion of more advanced tumours. Counteracting this bias is the fact that external patients presenting with end-stage HCC are less likely to be referred because their survival is <3 months and some would have died before staging at our institution (15). As part of the internal group of patients, we included all newly discovered HCCs found in our hospital, even if the patients were not part of our surveillance group and presented symptomatically with an end-stage HCC (ie, BCLC stage D). Retrospective studies assessing survival in a surveillance setting are subject to both lead-time and length-time biases. By using tumour stage at the time of treatment rather than survival as an end point, we hoped to diminish both of these. Finally, the surveillance history of referred patients could not be examined in the present retrospective study; therefore, we cannot determine whether the cause of the late presentation for treatment was related to a lack of surveillance, its ineffectiveness or improper management once a nodule was found.

CONCLUSION

The present study shows a significant worsening of HCC stage at time of treatment in patients not undergoing care in a health care centre specialized in liver diseases. Lack of, or ineffective surveillance practice in the community setting is the likely cause of this discrepancy. Targeted public-health interventions are needed to address this growing problem.

DISCLOSURES: This study was not funded by grants or other financial support.

REFERENCES

1. Canadian Cancer Society's Steering Committee on Cancer Statistics. Canadian Cancer Statistics 2012. Toronto: Canadian Cancer Society; 2012.
2. Pocobelli G, Cook LS, Brant R, Lee SS. Hepatocellular carcinoma incidence trends in Canada: Analysis by birth cohort and period of diagnosis. Liver Int 2008;28:1272-9.
3. Asmis T, Balaa F, Scully L, et al. Diagnosis and management of hepatocellular carcinoma: Results of a consensus meeting of The Ottawa Hospital Cancer Centre. Curr Oncol 2010;17:6-12.
4. Sherman M, Bain V, Villeneuve JP, et al. The management of chronic viral hepatitis: A Canadian consensus conference 2004. Can J Gastroenterol 2004;18:715-28.
5. Bruix J, Sherman M. Management of hepatocellular carcinoma: An update. Hepatology 2011;53:1020-2.
6. EASL-EORTC clinical practice guidelines: Management of hepatocellular carcinoma. J Hepatol 2012;56:908-43.
7. Omata M, Lesmana LA, Tateishi R, et al. Asian Pacific Association for the Study of the Liver consensus recommendations on hepatocellular carcinoma. Hepatol Int 2010;4:439-74.
8. Zhang BH, Yang BH, Tang ZY. Randomized controlled trial of screening for hepatocellular carcinoma. J Cancer Res Clin Oncol 2004;130:417-22.
9. Andersson KL, Salomon JA, Goldie SJ, Chung RT. Cost effectiveness of alternative surveillance strategies for hepatocellular carcinoma in patients with cirrhosis. Clin Gastroenterol Hepatol 2008;6:1418-24.
10. Ruggeri M. Hepatocellular carcinoma: Cost-effectiveness of screening. A systematic review. Risk Manag Healthc Policy 2012;5:49-54.
11. Ikai I, Kudo M, Arii S, et al. Report of the 18th follow-up survey of primary liver cancer in Japan. Hepatol Res 2010;40:1043-59.
12. BCCA. Survival Statistics 2007: BC Cancer Agency; 2007.
13. Cancer Care Ontario. Cancer Fact: The most fatal cancers in Ontario. April 2011. <www.cancercare.on.ca/cancerfacts/> (Accessed January 14, 2013).
14. Saito H, Masuda T, Tada S, et al. Hepatocellular carcinoma in Keio affiliated hospitals – diagnosis, treatment, and prognosis of this disease. Keio J Med 2009;58:161-75.
15. Forner A, Hessheimer AJ, Isabel Real M, Bruix J. Treatment of hepatocellular carcinoma. Crit Rev Oncol Hematol 2006;60:89-98.
16. Mazzaferro V, Regalia E, Doci R, et al. Liver transplantation for the treatment of small hepatocellular carcinomas in patients with cirrhosis. N Engl J Med 1996;334:693-9.
17. Statistics Canada. Geography Division. Postal code conversion file. 2011 <www5.statcan.gc.ca/bsolc/olc-cel/olc-cel?lang=eng&catno=82F0086X> (Accessed January 14, 2013).
18. Stravitz RT, Heuman DM, Chand N, et al. Surveillance for hepatocellular carcinoma in patients with cirrhosis improves outcome. Am J Med 2008;121:119-26.
19. Kuo YH, Lu SN, Chen CL, et al. Hepatocellular carcinoma surveillance and appropriate treatment options improve survival for patients with liver cirrhosis. Eur J Cancer 2010;46:744-51.
20. Noda I, Kitamoto M, Nakahara H, et al. Regular surveillance by imaging for early detection and better prognosis of hepatocellular carcinoma in patients infected with hepatitis C virus. J Gastroenterol 2010;45:105-12.
21. Qian MY, Yuwei JR, Angus P, Schelleman T, Johnson L, Gow P. Efficacy and cost of a hepatocellular carcinoma screening program at an Australian teaching hospital. J Gastroenterol Hepatol 2010;25:951-6.
22. Chen Y, Yi Q, Mao Y. Cluster of liver cancer and immigration: A geographic analysis of incidence data for Ontario 1998-2002. Int J Health Geogr 2008;7:28.

25

Invasive amoebiasis: A review of *Entamoeba* infections highlighted with case reports

Christopher Skappak PhD[1], Sarah Akierman BSc BA[2], Sara Belga MD[3], Kerri Novak MD FRCPC[1,4], Kris Chadee PhD[1], Stefan J Urbanski MD FRCPC[5], Deirdre Church MD PhD FRCPC[1], Paul L Beck PhD MD FRCPC[1,4]

C Skappak, S Akierman, S Belga, et al. Invasive amoebiasis: A review of *Entamoeba* infections highlighted with case reports. Can J Gastroenterol Hepatol 2014;28(7):355-359.

Entamoeba histolytica infections of the gastrointestinal tract are common in the developing world but rare in North America. The authors present two cases: one involving an individual who had not travelled to an endemic area and another involving an individual who was born in Bulgaria. Both presented with severe abdominal pain and diarrhea. Endoscopic assessment revealed scattered colonic ulcerations and one patient was found to have a liver abscess on imaging. Stool ova and parasite studies were negative in both cases and both were diagnosed on review of colonic biopsies. On review of all *Entamoeba* cases in the Calgary Health Zone (Alberta), ova and parasite analysis found an average of 63.7 *Entamoeba* cases per year and a pathology database review revealed a total of seven cases of invasive *E histolytica* (2001 to 2011). Both patients responded well to antibiotic therapy. *E histolytica* should be considered in new-onset colitis, especially in individuals from endemic areas.

Key Words: *Amoebic colitis*; Entamoeba histolytica; *Extraintestinal abscesses*

L'amibiase invasive : une analyse des infections à *Entamoeba* mise en évidence par des rapports de cas

Les infections à *Entamoeba histolytica* des voies digestives sont courantes dans les pays en développement, mais rares en Amérique du Nord. Les auteurs présentent deux cas : l'un d'une personne qui ne s'était pas rendue dans une région endémique et l'autre, d'une personne née en Bulgarie. Toutes deux avaient eu des crampes abdominales importantes et de la diarrhée. L'évaluation endoscopique a révélé des ulcérations diffuses dans le colon, et l'imagerie a démontré la présence d'un abcès hépatique chez l'une d'entre elles. Les examens parasitologiques dans les selles étaient négatifs dans les deux cas, et tous deux ont été diagnostiqués à l'analyse des biopsies du côlon. À l'examen de tous les cas d'*Entamoeba* dans la zone de santé de Calgary, en Alberta, les examens parasitologiques ont permis de déterminer une moyenne de 63,7 cas d'*Entamoeba* par année et une analyse de la base de données pathologiques a révélé un total de sept cas d'*E histolytica* invasive entre 2001 et 2011. Les deux patients ont bien réagi à l'antibiothérapie. L'*E histolytica* devrait être envisagé en cas de colite *de novo*, particulièrement chez des personnes provenant de régions endémiques.

*E*ntamoeba histolytica infections of the gastrointestinal (GI) tract are common in the developing world; however, in first-world countries, they are typically found in first-generation immigrant populations and returning international travellers. *E histolytica* is a parasitic protozoa that primarily infects the human bowel (1). It exists in two forms, a short-lived mobile trophozoite (10 μm to 20 μm in length) that can invade multiple organ systems, and a long-surviving cyst form that can colonize a patient (1). Diagnosis of a non-travel-related *E histolytica* infection in Canada is rare, with the most recent reported studies investigating cases in Inuit communities in Northern Labrador (2) and sexually transmitted cases in the homosexual population of Toronto, Ontario (3). Herein, we describe two cases of *E histolytica* colitis that presented to the Foothills Medical Centre, a large urban tertiary care centre located in Calgary, Alberta.

METHODS

The Calgary Zone, Alberta Health Services (CZ-AHS) serves a population of 1.2 million residents of Calgary and surrounding communities. All laboratory and pathology services for CZ-AHS are centralized and have searchable databases. The pathology database was searched for all reports containing the words "*Entamoeba histolytica*", "*Entamoeba*" and "*E. histolytica*", from 2001 to 2011. The microbiology database was searched for all positive stool studies consistent with *Entamoeba*. The microbiology database was searched from 2006 to 2011 for all positive stool ova and parasite (O&P) microscopic examinations that reported the presence of *Entamoeba*; data were only available from this period of time. Age (2007 to 2011) and sex (2006 to 2011), however, were the only variables that could be assessed due to privacy and ethics regulations. Unfortunately, *E histolytica* cannot be

morphologically differentiated from *Entamoeba dispar* (a common noninvasive parasite) and *Entamoeba moshkovskii* (considered primarily to be a free-living amoeba); however, *E dispar* and E *moshkovskii* are generally believed to be nonpathogenic. Commercial ELISAs and molecular biological testing, such as polymerase chain reaction (PCR), are available to differentiate *E histolytica* from *E dispar* but they are not routinely used in the CZ-AHS due to the rarity of these infections in the region. *Entamoeba* serology testing can diagnose infection with *E histolytica* (both *E dispar* and *E moshkovskii* do not elicit an antibody response), although it also is not routinely ordered because it takes up to 12 weeks before results are available from the reference laboratory. Serology test results for most of the patients were, therefore, not available. No commercial molecular methods are currently available for distinguishing *E moshkovskii*, although PCR has been used to detect this parasite directly in stool samples during surveillance studies (4). Because serology testing is sent to a reference laboratory, these data were not searchable.

The CZ-AHS pathology database was searched from 2001 to 2011 to identify all cases of invasive *E histolytica*. Data are presented as mean ± SEM. Statistical analysis was performed using Graph Pad Prism (GraphPad, USA) using a parametric unpaired *t* test for age and nonparametric Mann-Whitney for sex. Ethics approval was obtained from the CZ-AHS for a limited data recovery as above. Permission to present the cases was obtained from both individuals.

RESULTS

Data were available for stool O&P analysis in the CZ-AHS from January 2006 to December 31, 2011. From 2006 to 2011, a mean (± SEM) of 63.7±2.3 cases of *Entamoeba* were diagnosed according to stool O&P

[1]*Department of Medicine;* [2]*Department of Biological Sciences, University of Calgary, Calgary;* [3]*Department of Medicine, University of Alberta, Edmonton;* [4]*Department of Medicine, Division of Gastroenterology;* [5]*Department of Pathology, University of Calgary, Calgary, Alberta*
Correspondence: Dr Paul Beck, Room 1865, Foothills Hospital – Health Sciences Centre, 1403 – 29 Street Northwest, Calgary, Alberta T2N 2T9.
e-mail plbeck@ucalgary.ca

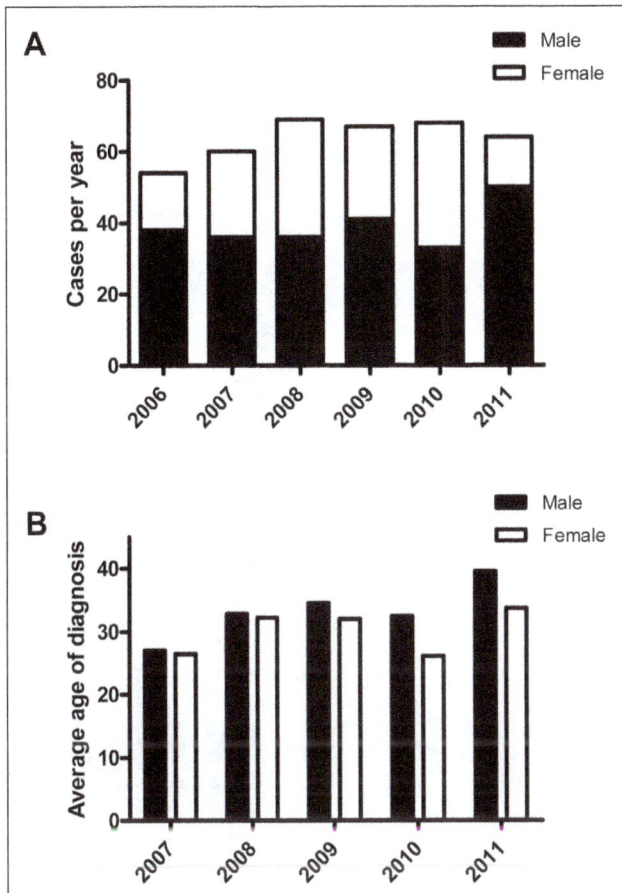

Figure 1) *Cases of* Entamoeba *from stool ova and parasite analysis in the Calgary Health Region (Alberta) according to year (A) and age (B)*

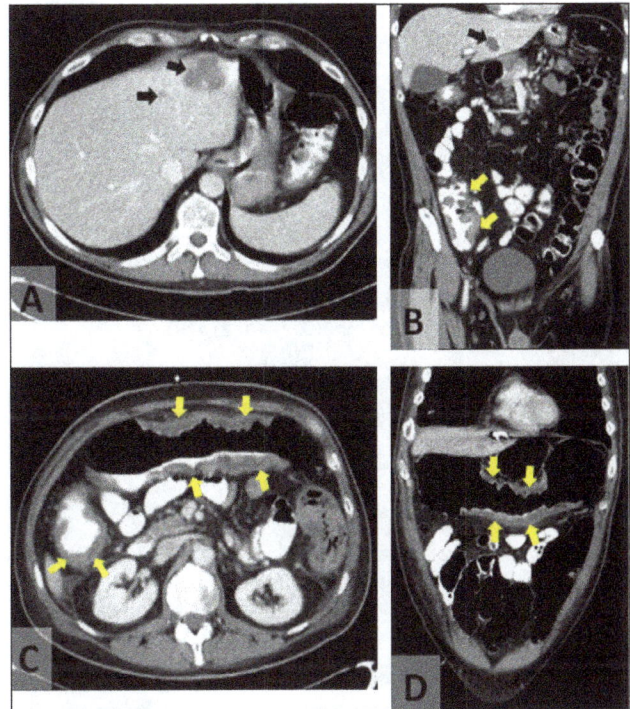

Figure 2) *Transverse (A) and coronal (B) computed tomography images of the abdomen demonstrating liver abscesses (black arrows) and colonic wall thickening (yellow arrows) on initial presentation of patient 1. Computed tomography images of the abdomen demonstrating worsening colitis (arrows), pericolic stranding and fluid on day 6 of hospital admission of patient 1 (C and D)*

examination (Figure 1A). Again, this would include *E histolytica*, *E dispar* and *E moshkovskii*. During the time period assessed, *Entamoeba* was more commonly diagnosed in men (39.0 ± 2.4 cases/year) versus women (24.7 ± 3.4 cases/year) ($P<0.01$). The average age of diagnosis was 31.7 years, with men being slightly older (33.2 years) than females (30.1 years) ($P=0.25$ [not significant]) (Figure 1B).

The CZ-AHS pathology database search from 2001 to 2011 revealed a total of seven cases, with three females and a mean age of 55 ± 7.4 years (this includes the two cases reported below). In six cases, colitis with invasive *E histolytica* was only noted in the cecum and ascending colon and, in one case (patient 1 below), there was evidence of *E histolytica* throughout the colon involving the rectum to the cecum. Again, no further details of these cases could be obtained except for the two cases decribed below.

Patient 1

A 56-year-old heterosexual man presented to the emergency department with a 10-day history of abdominal pain, nausea and vomiting, and diarrhea. The patient denied taking any medication and had no history of recent travel. His medical history was also unremarkable and he denied having any previous homosexual partners. On physical examination, the patient had a temperature of 38.4°C, a heart rate of 110 beats/min and a blood pressure of 95/55 mmHg. Head and neck, respiratory and cardiovascular, and musculoskeletal examinations were all normal. The patient had a distended abdomen and identified marked right lower quadrant tenderness with guarding. Laboratory results revealed a hemoglobin level of 127 g/L (normal 127 g/L to 165 g/L), an increased white blood cell count of 18.2×10^9/L (normal 4.0×10^9/L to 11.0×10^9/L), lactate level of 8.2 mmol/L (normal 0.5 mmol/L to 2.2 mmol/L) and increased levels of alkaline

phosphatase (232 U/L [normal 30 U/L to 145 U/L]) and gamma glutamyl-transferase (176 U/L [normal 11 U/L to 63 U/L]).

Computed tomography (CT) imaging of the abdomen and pelvis revealed severe colitis involving the cecum and ascending colon, and liver abscesses (Figures 2A and 2B). The liver abscesses were drained and the fluid was analyzed. Although microscopic examination of the fluid revealed an increased number of neutrophils, no organisms were visualized on Gram stain and the fluid cultures were negative. At this point, the differential diagnosis included infection, ischemia and new-onset inflammatory bowel disease (IBD). Blood and stool cultures, stool testing for O&P and *Clostridium difficile* were all negative. Serology for *Entamoeba* and *Yersinia* were also sent to the reference laboratory. The patient was initially treated with broad-spectrum antibiotics and conservative management.

Despite broad-spectrum antibiotics and conservative management, the patient deteriorated, developing more severe abdominal pain, with guarding and nausea. A repeat CT scan revealed worsening of colitis with increased bowel wall thickening, pericolic stranding and free fluid (Figures 2C and 2D). A colonoscopy was performed and classic amoebic ulcers were visualized (Figures 3A and 3B) and biopsies were collected. Histological examination revealed classic features of *E histolytica* (Figures 4A and 4B). The patient was treated with 14 days of metronidazole (750 mg per oral three times per day) followed by seven days of paromomycin (500 mg per oral three times per day). His symptoms resolved rapidly; however, a colonoscopy performed three months later showed normal colonic mucosa with a mid-transverse colonic stricture. After six weeks, his serology result was available and was positive for *E histolytica* and negative for *Yersinia*. This stricture did not cause symptoms and it has gradually improved over three years of follow-up.

Patient 2

A 24-year-old heterosexual man presented to the outpatient gastroenterology clinic with a three-month history of intermittent diarrhea

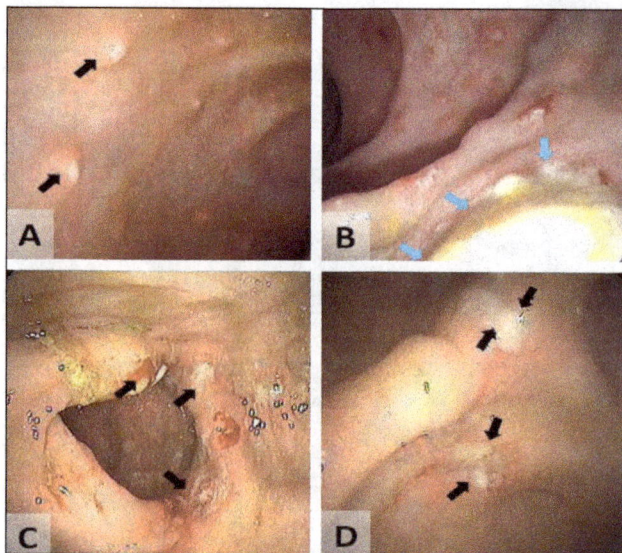

Figure 3) *Colonoscopic imaging of patient 1 (A and B) and patient 2 (C and D) demonstrating classic amoebic ulceration in both patients (arrows)*

and rectal bleeding. He lived in Bulgaria until eight years of age before immigrating to Canada. The patient had returned to Bulgaria for five months approximately one year previously. He was never sick nor did he experience any GI issues during his stay. Approximately four months after his visit to Bulgaria, he developed bloody diarrhea (at most six bowel motions per day) and lost 5.85 kg (13 lbs), which was associated with abdominal pain, bloating and tenesmus. At that time, his hemoglobin level was normal but his platelet count was slightly elevated (408×10^9/L [normal 150×10^9/L to 400×10^9/L]), as was his white blood cell count (11.9×10^9/L [normal 4.0×10^9/L to 11.0×10^9/L]) and erythrocyte sedimentation rate (13 mm [normal 0 mm to 10 mm]). His electrolyte and thyroid stimulating hormone levels, liver function studies, celiac serology, HIV serology and stool studies (O&P, *C difficile* toxin, culture and sensitivities) were all normal. A colonoscopy was performed (Figures 3C and 3D) and biopsies were collected. There were many endoscopic features consistent with Crohn disease including skip segments, deep ulcers and some linear ulcers. The ileum was normal. Biopsies again revealed classic features of *E histolytica* (Figures 4C and 4D). A CT scan was performed after the diagnosis and revealed colonic inflammation but no liver abscesses (not shown). The patient had a complete and rapid response to a 10-day course of metronidazole (750 mg per oral three times per day) followed by seven days of paromomycin (500 mg per oral three times per day). Serology was not performed.

DISCUSSION

Locally acquired *E histolytica* infections are a very rare occurrence in urban Canada aside from travellers, recent immigrants and the male homosexual population (5). A recent study investigating the prevalence of intestinal parasites in the United States demonstrated that for individuals infected with a single GI parasite, <5% were caused by *E histolytica* or a similar asymptomatic species (*E dispar*) (6). In the United States, the annual incidence of amoebic liver abscess (occurring in <1% of *E histolytica* colitis cases) was 1.38 per million population and mostly occurred in Hispanic men in the western and southern states (7). Similar studies have not been undertaken across Canada; however, *E histolytica* infections have been reported in both humans and canines in Canadian northern Aboriginal communities (2,8). A recent study from Ontario (9) reported 29 cases of amoebic liver abscesses that presented to seven hospitals in Toronto over a 30-year period. Of these cases, 86% had recent travel to endemic areas and some patients were born in endemic areas (9). They did not report any cases that developed in Canada without recent travel, foreign birth or

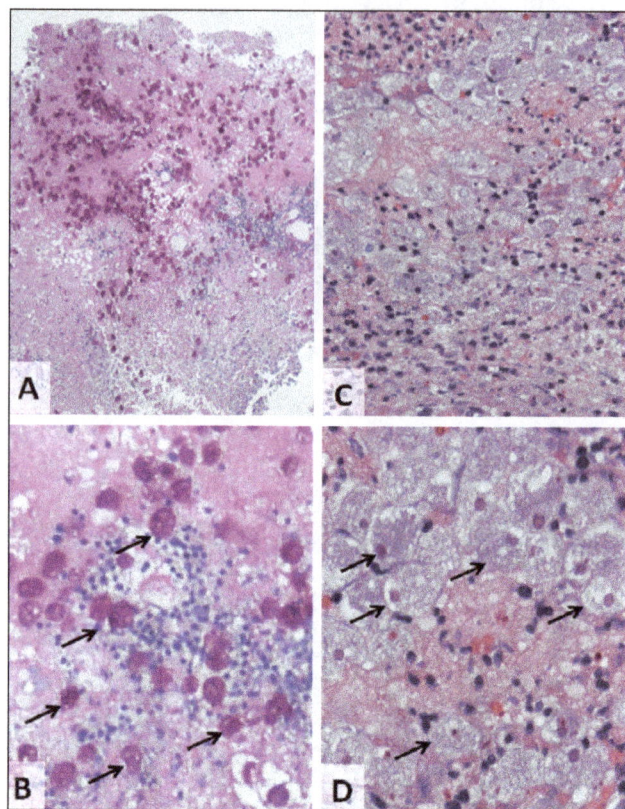

Figure 4) *A and B Colon biopsies of patient 1. Alcian blue periodic acid Shiff (PAS) stain (A: original magnification ×40, B: higher magnification of A), arrows indicate* Entamoeba histolytica *trophozoites (many do not have arrows). C and D Patient 2 (hematoxylin and eosin stain C: original magnification ×100, D: higher magnification C, arrows indicate PAS-positive E histolytica* trophozoites *(many do not have arrows)*

other risk factors (9). Because most studies from endemic areas report that <1% of individuals with *E histolytica* colitis develop a liver abscess and only 10% with *E histolytica* in their stool develop invasive disease, one could estimate that in the Toronto area (based on one *E histolytica* abscess per year) there are >100 cases of *E histolytica* colitis per year and approximately 1000 without invasive disease (carriers).

Our two sources of review of the CZ-AHS databases consisted of identifying positive stool studies and intestinal pathology. On average, 63.7 cases of *Entamoeba* were identified by stool studies per year (Figure 1). As noted above, these are based on light microscopy assessment of morphology and cannot differentiate *E histolytica* from the nonpathogenic *E dispar* and *E moshkovskii*. This is likely an underestimate of the incidence/prevalence of *Entamoeba* in the CZ-AHS due to the low sensitivity and specificity (discussed further below). In the Ontario study above, only 24% of cases of proven *E histolytica* were found to have positive stool studies (9). Seven (including our two cases) were identified on review of pathology over a 10-year period.

There are several risk factors for acquiring *E histolytica* infection other than recent travel to an endemic area, including men who have sex with men (MSM). In a study from Los Angeles (USA), 6% of MSM were seropositive for *E histolytica*; however, significantly higher rates have been reported in MSM populations in other parts of the world including Rome, Italy (21%), Mexico City, Mexico (25% of HIV-positive MSM) and South Africa (43% in HIV positive and 15% in HIV negative, and 69% in those 50 to 59 years of age) (10,11). Both individuals in our study denied ever engaging in sex with men.

E histolytica is a parasite that is transmissible by the oral-fecal route. Infections can range from asymptomatic to severe or fatal invasions of multiple organ systems. Asymptomatic infections are responsible for the continuous transmission of the parasite because numerous cysts are produced and passed in feces. If exocystation occurs, E histolytica trophozoites are produced and invade the intestinal wall leading to amoebic dysentery and resulting in amoebic ulcers (1). Trophozoites are capable of penetrating the intestinal wall and can lead to more severe complications including liver abscesses (the most common) and, in rare cases, can spread to the brain and/or lungs, which is often fatal (12). A typical treatment regimen for E histolytica infection is metronidazole for 10 to 14 days (500 mg to 750 mg three times per day) followed by a seven-day treatment of paromomycin (25 mg/kg to 35 mg/kg daily in three divided doses) to eliminate colonization (13).

Amoebic liver abscesses usually present with fever and pain in the right upper quadrant (13,14). Diagnosis of E histolytica is based on the patient's history, imaging modalities, serological findings, stool studies, fecal antigen testing (via ELISA) as well as real-time PCR (9,14). Stool microscopic assessment (which is the most common test used in Canada) has a low sensitivity (10% to 50%) and cannot differentiate E histolytica from the noninvasive, nonpathogenic E dispar and E moshkovskii (both of our cases had negative stool O&P studies) (9,14,15). Typically, a patient's history reveals recent travel from an endemic area or other risk factors; however, this was not the case in either of our two cases. Serological testing can differentiate E histolytica from E dispar and E moshkovskii (the latter two do not induce antibody responses) (9); the sensitivity and specificity ranges from 85% to 95% (9-11,15). It is important to differentiate E histolytica from E dispar because, even in asymptomatic individuals, E histolytica should be treated to prevent spread and invasive disease. Unfortunately, most diagnostic laboratories in most centres in Canada refer serological testing to an external site, which can take several weeks before results are available. Stool antigen and DNA tests are generally not available 'in house' at most Canadian centres and are discussed further below.

Our first case was unique because it occurred in an individual who was born in Alberta, had not recently travelled to endemic areas and had no other identifiable risk factors. Furthermore, the differential for both cases included IBD. Corticosteroids are contraindicated in E histolytica because, not surprisingly, it has been associated with more adverse outcomes (16). The second case could also have been locally acquired; however, because of his history of travel to Bulgaria for five months in the past year, it is highly possible that he acquired E histolytica infection abroad because Eastern Europe has significantly higher prevalence rates than North America (17). As noted above, many individuals who are infected with E histolytica are asymptomatic and only approximately 10% develop invasive disease. Thus, although this entity is rare in Canada, one should consider this diagnosis in patients with new symptoms of colitis, especially in those with recent travel to endemic areas.

It can be difficult to differentiate E histolytica-associated colitis from IBD and invasive bacterial dysentery. In general, those who present with E histolytica-associated colitis have a duration of symptoms >7 days, most will be fecal occult blood positive whereas only approximately 40% of those with invasive bacterial dysentery will be fecal occult positive and generally experience a shorter disease duration (18). Fever (>38°C) is common in invasive bacterial dysentery but is less common in individuals with uncomplicated IBD or E histolytica-associated colitis (<40%) (1) (although those with E histolytica liver abscesses are commonly febrile) (18). E histolytica-associated colitis more commonly presents with weight loss compared with those with invasive bacterial dysentery (18). More than 90% of patients with E histolytica-associated colitis present with diarrhea and tenesmus whereas frank blood in stools and fever are rare (18). In short, the history, stool studies and colonic biopsy assessment play critical roles in differentiating E histolytica-associated colitis from IBD and invasive bacterial dysentery. Unfortunately, E histolytica antigen and antibody tests are not readily available in most North American centres; most laboratories outsource these tests, with results taking seven to 21 days. These ELISA-based antibody tests have a sensitivity and specificity of 85% to 95% but are less useful in patients from endemic areas because they

may have antibodies from previous exposure (15). Again, stool studies (microscopy and culture) can miss cases, with studies reporting 10% to 50% sensitivity. Because E histolytica trophozoites degenerate rapidly in unfixed fresh samples, fixation and multiple collections increase the yield (18,19). Again, microscopy cannot differentiate E histolytica from other Entamoeba species. The best tests at present are the PCR- and ELISA-based assays that detect E histolytica DNA or antigens in stool, and have sensitivities and specificities of 90% to 95% and 95% to 100%, respectively (15,18,20,21). With the increase in world travel and emigration, we may have to consider increasing our use of more rapid and accurate DNA/antigen-based stool studies.

Because E histolytica-associated colitis can be localized to the cecum and right colon, a sigmoidoscopy can miss cases (18). Endoscopically, E histolytica colitis is associated with mucosal thickening, multiple discrete ulcers separated by regions of normal-appearing mucosa, diffuse inflammation and erythema and, rarely, necrosis and perforation (18). Recently, Upadhyay et al (22) described E histolytica ulcers as having a 'poached egg' appearance. They describe a patient who had multiple large irregular ulcers with a white slough and yellowish necrotic material on the top of the white slough, giving a 'poached egg' appearance. Both of our cases had irregular ulcers with white slough but neither patient had ulcers with the 'poached egg' appearance (they were missing the yellowish necrotic material). The most feared complication of E histolytica-associated colitis is acute necrotizing colitis and the development of toxic megacolon. This is rare but has been reported in approximately 0.5% of cases and is associated with high mortality (18). E histolytica colitis can also rarely be associated with penetrating disease, causing enterocutaneous, rectovaginal and enterovesicular fistulas (18). E histolytica can also cause inflammation of the appendix and present as appendicitis; in addition, it can cause pronounced granulomatous inflammation resulting in a pseudotumour that can lead to bowel obstruction (18). Fewer than 1% of individuals with E histolytica infections develop extraintestinal features that can include pericarditis, lung abscesses, peritonitis and skin lesions; however, the most common is hepatic abscesses (18). Hepatic abscesses are more common in men (male:female ratio 3.3:1 [23], 7.2:1 [24]), with a peak age of incidence between 30 and 50 years (25), and appears to be associated with increased alcohol consumption (18). Interestingly, a laboratory-based study (26) found that testosterone increased the susceptibility of mice to E histolytica liver abscesses by decreasing interferon-gamma secretion by natural killer T cells (26).

SUMMARY

With increased travel and emigration, we must keep E histolytica-associated colitis in our differential diagnosis list. Because one of our patients had no risk factors for E histolytica, we should entertain this diagnosis when we encounter new cases of colitis and wait for biopsies and stool studies before starting corticosteroids for presumed IBD.

ACKNOWLEDGEMENTS: Dr Beck is an Alberta Innovates Health Solutions Clinical Scholar and has research grants from Canadian Institute of Health Research and Crohn's and Colitis Foundation of Canada.

DISCLOSURES: The authors have no financial disclosures or conflicts of interest to declare.

REFERENCES

1. Adams EB, MacLeod IN. Invasive amebiasis. I. Amebic dysentery and its complications. Medicine (Baltimore) 1977;56:315-23.
2. Sole TD, Croll NA. Intestinal parasites in man in Labrador, Canada. Am J Trop Med Hyg 1980;29:364-8.
3. Keystone JS, Keystone DL, Proctor EM. Intestinal parasitic infections in homosexual men: Prevalence, symptoms and factors in transmission. Can Med Assoc J 1980;123:512-4.
4. Ali IK, Hossain MB, Roy S, et al. Entamoeba moshkovskii infections in children, Bangladesh. Emerg Infect Dis 2003;9:580-4.

5. Marcus VA, Ward BJ, Jutras P. Intestinal amebiasis: A diagnosis not to be missed. Pathol Res Pract 2001;197:271-4; discussion 275-8.

6. Amin OM. Evaluation of a new system for the fixation, concentration, and staining of intestinal parasites in fecal specimens, with critical observations on the trichrome stain. J Microbiol Methods 2000;39:127-32.

7. Congly SE, Shaheen AA, Meddings L, Kaplan GG, Myers RP. Amoebic liver abscess in USA: A population-based study of incidence, temporal trends and mortality. Liver Int 2011;31:1191-8.

8. Unruh DH, King JE, Eaton RD, Allen JR. Parasites of dogs from Indian settlements in northwestern Canada: A survey with public health implications. Can J Comp Med 1973;37:25-32.

9. Wuerz T, Kane JB, Boggild AK, et al. A review of amoebic liver abscess for clinicians in a nonendemic setting. Can J Gastroenterol 2012;26:729-33.

10. Hung CC, Chang SY, Ji DD. *Entamoeba histolytica* infection in men who have sex with men. Lancet Infect Dis 2012;12:729-36.

11. Samie A, Barrett LJ, Bessong PO, et al. Seroprevalence of *Entamoeba histolytica* in the context of HIV and AIDS: The case of Vhembe district, in South Africa's Limpopo province. Ann Trop Med Parasitol 2010;104:55-63.

12. Stanley SL Jr. Amoebiasis. Lancet 2003;361:1025-34.

13. Li E, Stanley SL Jr. Protozoa. Amebiasis. Gastroenterol Clin North Am 1996;25:471-92.

14. Marn H, Ignatius R, Tannich E, Harms G, Schurmann M, Dieckmann S. Amoebic liver abscess with negative serologic markers for *Entamoeba histolytica*: Mind the gap! Infection 2012;40:87-91.

15. Fotedar R, Stark D, Beebe N, Marriott D, Ellis J, Harkness J. Laboratory diagnostic techniques for *Entamoeba* species. Clin Microbiol Rev 2007;20:511-32.

16. Kobayashi CI, Yamamoto G, Hayashi A, et al. Fatal amebic colitis after high-dose dexamethasone therapy for newly diagnosed multiple myeloma. Ann Hematol 2011;90:225-6.

17. Nowak P, Jochymek M, Pietrzyk A. [Occurrence of human intestinal parasites in selected populations of Cracow region in the years 2000-2006 on the basis of parasitological stool examinations performed in the Laboratory of Parasitology of the District Sanitary-Epidemiological Center]. Wiad Parazytol 2007;53:285-93.

18. Choudhuri G, Rangan M. Amebic infection in humans. Indian J Gastroenterol 2012;31:153-62.

19. Proctor EM. Laboratory diagnosis of amebiasis. Clin Lab Med 1991;11:829-59.

20. Mirelman D, Nuchamowitz Y, Stolarsky T. Comparison of use of enzyme-linked immunosorbent assay-based kits and PCR amplification of rRNA genes for simultaneous detection of *Entamoeba histolytica* and *E. dispar*. J Clin Microbiol 1997;35:2405-7.

21. Haque R, Ali IK, Akther S, Petri WA Jr. Comparison of PCR, isoenzyme analysis, and antigen detection for diagnosis of *Entamoeba histolytica* infection. J Clin Microbiol 1998;36:449-52.

22. Upadhyay R, Gupta N, Gogia P, Chandra S. Poached egg appearance in intestinal amebiasis. Gastrointest Endosc 2012;76:189-90.

23. Acuna-Soto R, Maguire JH, Wirth DF. Gender distribution in asymptomatic and invasive amebiasis. Am J Gastroenterol 2000;95:1277-83.

24. Shandera WX, Bollam P, Hashmey RH, Athey PA, Greenberg SB, White AC Jr. Hepatic amebiasis among patients in a public teaching hospital. South Med J 1998;91:829-37.

25. Blessmann J, Van Linh P, Nu PA, et al. Epidemiology of amebiasis in a region of high incidence of amebic liver abscess in central Vietnam. Am J Trop Med Hyg 2002;66:578-83.

26. Lotter H, Helk E, Bernin H, et al. Testosterone increases susceptibility to amebic liver abscess in mice and mediates inhibition of IFNgamma secretion in natural killer T cells. PLoS One 2013;8:e55694.

26

Physician global assessments or blood tests do not predict mucosal disease activity in ulcerative colitis

Mayur Brahmania MD, Charles N Bernstein MD

M Brahmania, CN Bernstein. Physician global assessments or blood tests do not predict mucosal disease activity in ulcerative colitis. Can J Gastroenterol Hepatol 2014;28(6):325-329.

BACKGROUND: Mucosal healing has been proposed as the therapeutic end point in the treatment of patients with ulcerative colitis (UC).

OBJECTIVE: To investigate the relationship between physician global assessment (PGA) and laboratory blood tests (complete blood count, ferritin, C-reactive protein, albumin) and endoscopic findings in UC to determine whether they could be adequate surrogates for endoscopy.

METHODS: A retrospective chart review of patients known to have UC from July 2008 to November 2012 was performed at the Health Sciences Centre, Winnipeg, Manitoba. Patients included individuals with UC who underwent colonoscopy within one month of clinic assessment. Blood tests were standard at the time of colonoscopy. Patients presenting through the emergency department, those with colonoscopies performed outside the authors' institution, or whose colonoscopies and clinical assessments were undertaken more than one month apart were excluded. The PGA was used to determine disease activity in patients before colonoscopy. The Ulcerative Colitis Endoscopic Index of Severity, a validated scoring system to rate endoscopic disease severity in ulcerative colitis, was adapted.

RESULTS: A total of 154 patients (mean [± SD] age 44±15.7 years) with UC were identified including 82 (53%) men. Mean hemoglobin level was 139 g/L, mean platelet level was $296×10^9$/L, mean ferritin level was 102 µg/L, mean C-reactive protein level was 10 mg/L and mean albumin level was 40 g/L. Using endoscopy as the 'gold standard' for assessing UC activity (moderate-severe), abnormalities in laboratory parameters and PGA were both highly specific but not sensitive for identifying individuals with at least moderately active endoscopic disease. The PGA had higher positive and negative predictive values than the laboratory parameters.

CONCLUSION: Neither blood tests nor PGA could replace endoscopy for assessing mucosal healing. When patients experienced active symptoms and abnormal serum markers, they were highly likely to have abnormal endoscopy. However, inactive symptoms or normal laboratory values did not preclude having active endoscopic disease.

Key Words: *Mucosal healing; Physician global assessment; Ulcerative colitis; Ulcerative Colitis Endoscopic Index of Severity (UCEIS)*

Les évaluations globales des médecins ou les hémocultures ne prédisent pas l'activité de la colite ulcéreuse sur les muqueuses

HISTORIQUE : La guérison des muqueuses est proposée comme indicateur de résultat thérapeutique pour le traitement des patients atteints d'une colite ulcéreuse (CU).

OBJECTIF : Examiner la relation entre l'évaluation globale du médecin (ÉGM), ainsi que les analyses sanguines en laboratoire (hémogramme, ferritine, protéine C-réactive, albumine), et les résultats endoscopiques de la CU pour déterminer si elles peuvent remplacer convenablement l'endoscopie.

MÉTHODOLOGIE: Entre juillet 2008 et novembre 2012, les chercheurs ont effectué un examen rétrospectif des dossiers des patients qu'on savait atteints de CU au *Health Sciences Centre* de Winnipeg, au Manitoba. Les patients incluaient des personnes atteintes de CU qui avaient subi une coloscopie dans le mois suivant l'évaluation clinique. Les hémocultures étaient standards au moment de la coloscopie. Les patients qui s'étaient présentés par l'urgence et ceux qui avaient subi une coloscopie à l'extérieur de l'établissement des auteurs ou dont la coloscopie et l'évaluation clinique avaient été effectuées à plus d'un mois d'écart étaient exclus. L'ÉGM a permis de déterminer l'activité de la maladie chez les patients avant la coloscopie. Les chercheurs ont adopté l'indice endoscopique de gravité de la CU, un système de pointage validé pour évaluer la gravité endoscopique de la CU.

RÉSULTATS : Au total, 154 patients (âge moyen [± ÉT] de 44±15,7 ans) atteints de CU ont été retenus, y compris 82 hommes (53 %). Le taux d'hémoglobine moyen s'établissait à 139 g/L, le taux plaquettaire moyen, à $296×10^9$/L, le taux de ferritine moyen, à 102 µg/L, le taux de protéine C-réactive moyen, à 10 mg/L et le taux d'albumine moyen, à 40 g/L. Si on utilise l'endoscopie comme norme de référence pour évaluer l'activité de la CU (modérée à grave), les anomalies dans les paramètres de laboratoire et l'ÉGM étaient tous deux hautement spécifiques, mais pas sensibles pour déterminer les individus atteints d'une maladie au moins modérément active à l'endoscopie. L'ÉGM avait des valeurs prédictives positives et négatives plus élevées que les paramètres de laboratoire.

CONCLUSION : Ni les hémocultures ni les ÉGM ne pouvaient remplacer l'endoscopie pour évaluer la guérison des muqueuses. Lorsque les patients ressentaient des symptômes actifs et présentaient des marqueurs sériques anormaux, ils étaient hautement susceptibles d'obtenir une endoscopie anormale. Cependant, les symptômes inactifs ou les valeurs de laboratoire normales n'excluaient pas une maladie active à l'endoscopie.

Ulcerative colitis (UC) is an inflammatory disorder of the gastrointestinal tract characterized by radiological, endoscopic and histological changes. An assessment of disease activity and extent can help direct therapy and, potentially, also assess for dysplasia (1). For Crohn disease, the Crohn's Disease Activity Index, a predominately subjective index, remains the main outcome measure used to assess disease activity in clinical trials. For UC, there has been increasing interest in using endoscopic scoring scales to assess endoscopic activity as the critical outcome in clinical trials. Currently, there is no consensus on a validated scale to define disease activity in UC; however, the Mayo score, which is a combination of clinical and endoscopic disease

parameters (or the modified Mayo score, which only uses clinical parameters), has been widely adopted for clinical trials (2). However, clinicians have not adopted these indexes or scores for routine clinical use. Blood tests, such as C-reactive protein (CRP), hemoglobin (Hg), platelet (plt) count, and ferritin and albumin levels, are also used as markers of disease activity; however, abnormalities in these measures may also indicate other medical problems and have been shown to correlate poorly with disease activity (3,4). Endoscopy is currently the gold standard to assess for inflammatory changes in the colonic mucosa. However, with resource constraints, risks with invasive procedures and the discomfort with colonoscopy, physicians often rely on

Department of Internal Medicine, Division of Gastroenterology, University of Manitoba Inflammatory Bowel Disease Clinical and Research Centre, Winnipeg, Manitoba

Correspondence: Dr Charles N Bernstein, 804F-175 McDermot Avenue, Winnipeg, Manitoba R3E 3P4. e-mail charles.bernstein@med.umanitoba.ca

TABLE 1
Ulcerative Colitis Endoscopic Index of Severity (UCEIS)

Descriptor (score of most severe lesions)	Scale anchor points	Definition
Vascular pattern	Normal (1)	Normal vascular pattern with arborization of capillaries clearly defined, or with blurring or patchy loss of capillary margins
	Patchy obliteration (2)	Patchy obliteration of vascular pattern
	Obliterated (3)	Complete obliteration of vascular pattern
Bleeding	None (1)	No visible blood
	Mucosal (2)	Some spots or streaks of coagulated blood on the surface of the mucosa ahead of the scope, which can be washed away
	Luminal mild (3)	Some free liquid blood in the lumen
	Luminal moderate or severe (4)	Frank blood in the lumen ahead of endoscope or visible oozing from mucosa after washing intraluminal blood, or visible oozing from a hemorrhagic mucosa
Erosions and ulcers	None (1)	Normal mucosa, no visible erosions or ulcers
	Erosions (2)	Tiny (≤5 mm) defects in the mucosa, of a white or yellow colour with a flat edge
	Superficial ulcer (3)	Larger (>5 mm) defects in the mucosa, which are discrete fibrin-covered ulcers when compared with erosions, but remain superficial
	Deep ulcer (4)	Deeper excavated defects in the mucosa, with a slightly raised edge

UCEIS = sum of scores, which accounts for 92% of the variance between observers in the overall assessment of endoscopic severity

clinical acumen (ie, a physician global assessment [PGA]) along with laboratory markers to determine disease activity. It has been proposed that endoscopic mucosal healing (MH) be used as the primary end point in the treatment of UC to judge response to medical treatment, to predict the course of the disease and to prevent complications (5-10). How to optimally achieve MH or the necessity for achieving MH in asymptomatic patients is currently unclear. In the present study, we investigated the relationship between PGA and readily available blood tests (complete blood count, ferritin, CRP, albumin) to endoscopic findings in UC. We hypothesized the PGA or usual blood tests would highly correlate with endoscopic findings and, hence, would be sufficient to guide clinicians in patient management.

METHODS

Colonoscopy reports of all patients known to have UC from July 2008 to November 2012 from a single gastroenterology practice at the Health Sciences Centre, Winnipeg, Manitoba, a tertiary care referral centre for inflammatory bowel disease (IBD), were retrospectively reviewed. Patients included individuals with UC having bloodwork (complete blood count, CRP, ferritin, albumin) within one week of visit and undergoing colonoscopy after clinic assessment (within one month). Cut-off values for bloodwork in the analysis included Hg levels <120 g/L for females and <140 g/L for males, plt count >4.0×10⁹/L, albumin <33g/L, ferritin <20 μg/mL and CRP >8 mg/L, which represented abnormal values at the authors' institution. No deviations from standard care were taken (ie, patients being expedited to endoscopy). Patients presenting through the emergency room, those with colonoscopies performed outside the authors' institution, or whose colonoscopies and clinical assessments were undertaken more than one month apart were excluded. The PGA was used to determine disease activity in patients before colonoscopy and was performed at time of clinic visit. Currently, no validated PGA exists; therefore, an assessment tool based on routine questions gastroenterologists use during interviews to gauge disease activity was created. To determine a global assessment, patients were queried at each clinic visit as to the number of bowel movements, presence or absence of abdominal pain, presence of blood with defecation and objective weight loss (as determined by the clinic scale). These criteria used in the PGA are documented in all patient encounters at the authors' centre. The assessment was rated as:

1. Remission: no abdominal pain, ≤2 bowel movements/day, absence of blood with defecation, and stable/no weight loss.
2. Mildly active disease: mild to moderate abdominal pain, ≤4 bowel movements/day, occasional blood with defecation and objective weight loss.

3. Active symptoms: moderate to severe abdominal pain, >4 bowel movements/day, bloody defecation with most bowel movements and objective weight loss.

Patient disease activity was categorized based on having at least two of the four symptoms identified with each category. If they had only one symptom that moved them to a higher, more active category, it would not have changed their categorization. For example, an individual with one mild symptom and three symptoms that would have been considered to be in remission were categorized as remission. If at least two mild symptoms were present and zero or one active symptom, then they were considered to be mild. If there were at least two active symptoms they were categorized as active. For example, if a patient had mild abdominal pain (mild symptom), six bowel movements/day (active symptom), minimal blood with defecation (mild symptom) and no weight loss, they would be categorized as having 'mildly active' disease. Patients were identified through an electronic database of all persons presenting to the IBD clinic and their charts were systematically reviewed. Demographic data including age, sex and blood tests (serum Hg, plt count, CRP, ferritin and albumin level) were collected. Patients were grouped as active (active symptoms) or mild to inactive (remission, mild) for the PGA. A total of 154 patients met the inclusion criteria for the study. An adapted form of the Ulcerative Colitis Endoscopic Index of Severity (UCEIS), a validated scoring system to rate endoscopic disease activity in UC (Table 1), was used because the UCEIS was not available during the study period. Evaluating the most diseased area on endoscopy, the following parameters were used and categorized patients into:

1. Remission: complete MH that could include 'footprints' of past disease such as pseudopolyps or white scars.
2. Mild disease: vascular blush or loss of vascular pattern, minimal exudates or friability.
3. Moderate disease: friability, granularity, scattered erosions and ulcers.
4. Severe disease: contiguous or deep ulcers and frank bleeding.

Similar to the PGA, the authors use a standard reporting format with all UC patients and include these elements in their colonoscopy reports in addition to pictures documenting diseased areas. Because the authors evaluated the most diseased areas, every endoscopic report included information regarding the most diseased area; the reports at their centre included the necessary variables to report a UCEIS. If there was insufficient information on the endoscopy report, the subject was excluded. The primary end point was to assess how well the PGA could assess MH as defined by features on endoscopy. Secondary end points included a correlation of blood tests (Hg, plt count, CRP,

TABLE 2
Patient characteristics

Variable	Mean outcome (except for sex)
Male sex, %	53
Age, years	44
Hemoglobin, g/L	139
Platelet count, ×10⁹/L	296
C-reactive protein, mg/L	10
Ferritin, µg/L	102
Albumin, g/L	40
Disease duration, years	15

TABLE 3
Ulcerative colitis characteristics

Variable	Ulcerative colitis (n=154)
Reason for colonoscopy (dysplasia surveillance)	76
Disease extent at diagnosis (pancolitis)	82
Medication use	
None	22
5-aminosalicylic acid	46
Immunomodulator (AZA/6-MP)	13
Biologic (infliximab/adalimunab)	8
Combination (AZA/infliximab)	1
Other*	10
Endoscopic severity	
Remission	42
Mild	26
Moderate	26
Severe	6

*Data presented as %. *Combination of 5-aminosalicylic acid/azathioprine (AZA), infliximab/methotrexate, methotrexate. 6-MP 6-Mercaptopurine*

ferritin and albumin) with endoscopic features. Because the present analysis was a retrospective observational study, results are presented with descriptive statistics. Mean and SD are used to report continuous variables following a normal distribution and median (range) are used to report non-normal continuous variables.

RESULTS

A total of 154 patients with UC were identified. Males comprised 53% (n=82) of the total population. The mean (± SD) age of patients was 44±15.7 years. The mean Hg level was 139 g/L, mean platelet level was 296×10⁹/L, mean ferritin level was 102 µg/L, mean CRP level was 10 mg/L and mean albumin level was 40 g/L (Table 2). The average disease duration was 15 years (range two to 42 years), with 82% having pancolitis and 18% having left-sided colitis (including proctosigmoiditis) as the predominant disease extent at time of diagnosis. Of the colonoscopies, 76% were performed as routine dysplasia surveillance and 24% were performed due to patient experiencing symptoms such as abdominal pain, diarrhea or bright red blood per rectum. In terms of medications used, 46% were using 5-aminosalicylic acid products with varying doses as their predominant maintenance regimen, 22% were not on any medications, 13% were on immunomodulator therapy (azathioprine or 6-mercaptopurine), 8% were on anti-tumour necrosis factor (Remicade [Janssen Inc, USA] or Humira [Abbott Laboratories, USA]), 2% were on methotrexate and 9% were on combination therapy (Table 3). Using endoscopy as the 'gold standard' for assessing UC activity (moderate-severe), abnormalities in laboratory parameters were highly specific (Hg 88%; albumin 97%, ferritin 91%, plt count 89%, CRP 72%) but not sensitive (Hg 34%; albumin 7%, ferritin 23%, plt count 16%, CRP 28%) for identifying individuals with at least moderately active endoscopy. The PGA was comparably sensitive (30%) and specific (97%) as laboratory parameters but with higher positive (83%) and negative (74%) predictive values (Table 4). Also conducted was a subgroup analysis of patients experiencing symptoms, either 'mild' or 'active' according to the PGA, excluding those considered to be in remission, and found similarly high specificities for laboratory parameters (Hg 91%, albumin 92%, ferritin 72%, plt count 84%, CRP 86%) but still low sensitivities (Hg 45%, albumin 12%, ferritin 24%, plt count 23%, CRP 36%). The PGA also had comparable sensitivity (48%) and specificity (86%) but with higher positive (83%) and lower negative (54%) predictive values than the when analyzing all persons including those in remission (Table 5).

DISCUSSION

Traditionally, initiation and escalation of therapy in UC has been based on severity of symptoms with the goal of alleviating those symptoms using a variety of medications (5-aminosalicylic acid, steroids, immunomodulators and biologics). However, treating symptoms alone may not be sufficient to achieve optimal long-term outcomes (eg, fewer complications and hospitalizations, and better quality of life), and targeting mucosal inflammation and associated tissue damage may be equally important. MH has been proposed as an optimal goal of treatment because it can correlate with hospitalizations and colectomy rates (7-10). The exact definition of MH is unclear and has not been

validated; however, the International Organization for the Study of Inflammatory Bowel Disease has proposed defining MH in UC as the absence of friability, blood, erosions and ulcers in all visualized segments of gut mucosa (12). Whether MH should represent the complete absence of any characteristic endoscopic lesions or simply marked improvement in the severity of previously noted lesions is an issue that is evolving. Currently, no guidelines have been developed to determine the optimal timing for follow-up endoscopy to identify MH (13). Endoscopic evaluation can be time consuming and costly, while incurring small but real risks for adverse events. Froslie et al (7) documented the important role of MH in monitoring treatment effectiveness and long-term disease outcome during a five-year follow-up period. In their study, 50% of patients with UC had confirmed MH after one year and had a significantly lower risk of future colectomy than patients without MH (P=0.02). Several other long-term benefits of MH have been identified, including decreased need for surgery and hospitalization, lower steroid use, decreased risk of colorectal cancer and higher remission rates (5-10).

The PGA or, less formally, a clinician's impression of the patient's disease status, is typically used to guide therapeutic decisions. Many activity indexes have been used indirectly to assess clinical status. Common indexes, such as Truelove and Witts, Powell-Tuck, Ulcerative Colitis Disease Activity Index and Mayo Disease Activity Index, use a combination of symptoms, signs and sigmoidoscopy to assess clinical disease; however, none of these scales have been validated specifically for MH (14-20). Attempts are now underway to develop a validated endoscopic score that may be universally adopted such as the UCEIS developed by Travis et al (11). In our study, we found the PGA to correlate poorly with active endoscopic disease; however, it was marginally better than the blood tests routinely ordered by gastroenterologists to estimate disease activity status. When the PGA or any of the blood tests are abnormal, there was a high likelihood the endoscopic findings were at least moderately active. When the PGA or blood tests were normal, however, they missed many subjects who had active endoscopic disease.

Noninvasive quantitative indexes have been developed in UC based on symptoms and blood tests (Hg, albumin and erythrocyte sedimentation rate) that have correlated well with the Truelove and Witts classification (mild, moderate, severe) (21). However, a previous study involving 82 patients showed that CRP is only raised 50% of the time in active UC but does aid in differentiating IBD from chronic abdominal pain (22,23). In addition, blood tests such as Hg, plt

TABLE 4

Association of abnormal laboratory data with endoscopy as the gold standard (moderate-severe disease)

	Hemoglobin (<120 g/L females, <140 g/L males)	Albumin (<33 g/L)	Ferritin (<20 μg/mL)	Platelet count (>4.0×10^9/L)	C-reative protein (>8 mg/L)	Physician global assessment
Sensitivity	34	7	23	16	28	30
Specificity	88	97	91	89	72	97
Positive predictive value	57	60	63	44	47	83
Negative predictive value	73	62	65	66	53	74

Data presented as %

TABLE 5

Association of abnormal laboratory data with endoscopy as the gold standard (moderate-severe disease) excluding patients in remission according to physician global assessment

	Hemoglobin (<120 g/L females, <140 g/L males)	Albumin (<33 g/L)	Ferritin (<20 μg/mL)	Platelet count (>4.0×10^9/L)	C-reative protein (>8 mg/L)	Physician global assessment
Sensitivity	45	12	24	23	36	48
Specificity	91	92	72	84	75	86
Positive predictive value	88	75	67	70	78	83
Negative predictive value	54	33	30	40	33	54

Data presented as %

counts, ferritin levels and CRP can serve as markers to assess disease activity, but in the case of a hospitalized or sick patient, low or high laboratory markers can reflect an acute or chronic inflammatory process such as infection, malabsorption, trauma, cancer or the disease itself giving false positive/negative results. Unfortunately, none of these disease activity indexes, invasive or noninvasive, endoscopic or histological, has been formally well validated in terms of reflecting the evolution of the disease in the long term.

Our analysis highlights a few key points. First, physicians are not adequately able to predict endoscopic disease with reasonable sensitivity for UC based on their PGA or the 'usual' blood tests that are ordered. However, abnormal PGA or laboratory parameters do signal active endoscopic disease. The main limitation of our study was that it was retrospective in design, with all of the biases of retrospectively grading endoscopy scores and PGA. That a single physician performed all of the endoscopy and had a uniform pattern of assessment, including clinical details during the assessment, was a strength of the study; however, a single physician's practice limits the external validity of the results. Additionally, most patients underwent routine screening endoscopy (76%) and were not being assessed for acutely active symptoms.

CONCLUSION

A combination of serum markers (Hg, plt count, and ferritin, albumin and CRP levels), and clinical symptoms (PGA) in a comprehensive activity index may be a promising, noninvasive and, possibly, cost-effective approach to evaluate patients with UC; however, individually cannot replace endoscopy for assessing MH. Nonetheless, when patients experienced active symptoms and abnormal serum markers, they were highly likely to have abnormal endoscopy in our study. However, inactive symptoms or normal laboratory values did not preclude having active endoscopic disease. It is possible that other blood markers or fecal markers of inflammation may add to the PGA to serve as better surrogate markers of MH in future prospective studies involving adult patients with UC.

DISCLOSURES: The authors have no financial disclosures or conflicts of interest to declare.

REFERENCES

1. Danese S, Fiocchi C. Ulcerative colitis. N Engl J Med 2011;365:1713-25.
2. Stange EF, Travis SP, Vermeire S, et al. European evidence-based consensus on the diagnosis and management of ulcerative colitis: Definitions and diagnosis. J Crohns Colitis 2008;2:1-23.
3. Fagan EA, Dyck RF, Maton PN, et al. Serum levels of C-reactive protein in Crohn's disease and ulcerative colitis. Eur J Clin Invest 1982;12:351-9.
4. Lewis JD. The utility of biomarkers in the diagnosis and therapy of inflammatory bowel disease. Gastroeterology 2011;140:1817-26.
5. Rutgeerts P, Vermeire S, Van Assche G. Mucosal healing in inflammatory bowel disease: impossible ideal or therapeutic target? Gut 2007;56:453-5.
6. Peyrin-Biroulet L, Ferrante M, Magro F, et al. Results from the 2nd scientific workshop of the ECCO. I: Impact of mucosal healing on the course of inflammatory bowel disease. J Crohns Colitis 2011;5:477-83.
7. Froslie KF, Jahnsen J, Moum BA, et al. Mucosal healing in inflammatory bowel disease: Results from a Norwegian population-based cohort. Gastroenterology 2007;133:412-22.
8. Ardizzone S, Cassinotti A, Duca P, et al. Mucosal healing predicts late outcomes after the first course of corticosteroids for newly diagnosed ulcerative colitis. Clin Gastroenterol Hepatol 2011;9:483-9.
9. Parente F, Molteni M, Marino B, et al. Are colonoscopy and bowel ultrasound useful for assessing response to short-term therapy and predicting disease outcome of moderate-to-severe forms of ulcerative colitis? A prospective study. Am J Gastroenterol 2010;105:1150-7.
10. Colombel JF, Rutgeerts P, Reinisch W, et al. Early mucosal healing with infliximab is associated with improved long-term clinical outcomes in ulcerative colitis. Gastroenterology 2011;141:1194-201.
11. Travis SP, Schnell D, Krzeski P, et al. Developing an instrument to assess the endoscopic severity of ulcerative colitis: The Ulcerative Colitis Endoscopic Index of Severity (UCEIS). Gut 2012;61:535-42.
12. D'Haens G, Sandborn WJ, Feagan BG, et al. A review of activity indices and efficacy end points for clinical trials of medical therapy in adults with ulcerative colitis. Gastroenterology 2007;132:763-86.
13. Fefferman DS, Farrell RJ. Endoscopy in inflammatory bowel disease: Indications, surveillance, and use in clinical practice. Clin Gastroenterol Hepatol 2005;3:11-24.
14. Truelove SC, Witts LJ. Cortisone in ulcerative colitis: Final report on a therapeutic trial. Br Med J 1955;2:1041-8.
15. Baron JH, Connell AM, Lennard-Jones JE. Variation between observers in describing mucosal appearances in proctocolitis. Br Med J 1964;1:89-92.

16. Powell-Tuck J, Bown RL, Lennard-Jones JE. A comparison of oral prednisolone given as single or multiple daily doses for active proctocolitis. Scand J Gastroenterol 1978;13:833-7.

17. Sutherland LR, Martin F, Greer S, et al. 5-aminosalicylic acid enema in the treatment of distal ulcerative colitis, proctosigmoiditis, and proctitis. Gastroenterology 1987;92:1894-8.

18. Schroeder KW, Tremaine WJ, Ilstrup DM. Coated oral 5-aminosalicylic acid therapy for mildly to moderately active ulcerative colitis. A randomized study. N Engl J Med 1987;317:1625-9.

19. Rachmilewitz D. Coated mesalazine (5-aminosalicylic acid) versus sulphasalazine in the treatment of active ulcerative colitis: A randomised trial. Br Med J 1989;298:82-6.

20. Feagan BG, Greenberg GR, Wild G, et al. Treatment of ulcerative colitis with a humanized antibody to the alpha4beta7 integrin. N Engl J Med 2005;352:2499-507.

21. Seo M, Okada M, Yao T, Ueki M, Arima S, Okumura M. An index of disease activity in patients with ulcerative colitis. Am J Gastroenterol 1992; 87:971-6.

22. Shine B, Berghouse L, Jones JE. et al C-reactive protein as an aid in the differentiation of functional and inflammatory bowel disorders. Clin Chim Acta 1985;148:105-9.

23. Vermeire S, Van Assche G, Rutgeers P. Laboratory markers in IBD: Useful, magic, or unnecessary toys? Gut 2006;55:426-43.

27

Management of thrombocytopenia in advanced liver disease

VGR Gangireddy MBBS[1], PC Kanneganti MBBS[2], S Sridhar MBBS MPH FRCP FACP[1], S Talla MBBS[3], T Coleman MD FACP[4]

VGR Gangireddy, PC Kanneganti, S Sridhar, S Talla, T Coleman. Management of thrombocytopenia in advanced liver disease. Can J Gastroenterol Hepatol 2014;28(10):558-564.

Thrombocytopenia (defined as a platelet count <150×10⁹/L) is a well-known complication in patients with liver cirrhosis and has been observed in 76% to 85% of patients. Significant thrombocytopenia (platelet count <50×10⁹/L to 75×10⁹/L) occurs in approximately 13% of patients with cirrhosis. Thrombocytopenia can negatively impact the care of patients with severe liver disease by potentially interfering with diagnostic and therapeutic procedures. Multiple factors can contribute to the development of thrombocytopenia including splenic platelet sequestration, immunological processes, bone marrow suppression by chronic viral infection, and reduced levels or activity of the hematopoietic growth factor thrombopoietin. The present review focuses on the etiologies and management options for severe thrombocytopenia in the setting of advanced liver disease.

Key Words: *Advanced liver disease; Cirrhosis; Splenectomy; Splenic artery embolization; Thrombocytopenia; Thrombopoietin stimulators*

La prise en charge de la thrombocytopénie en cas de maladie hépatique avancée

La thrombocytopénie (définie comme une numération plaquettaire inférieure à 150×10⁹/L) est une complication bien connue chez les patients atteints de cirrhose du foie, qui s'observe chez 76 % à 85 % des patients. Une thrombocytopénie importante (numération plaquettaire de moins de à 50×10⁹/L à 75×10⁹/L) se déclare chez environ 13 % des patients atteints de cirrhose. La thrombocytopénie peut nuire aux soins des patients atteints d'une maladie hépatique grave et compromettre les interventions diagnostiques et thérapeutiques. De nombreux facteurs peuvent contribuer à l'apparition d'une thrombocytopénie, y compris la séquestration des plaquettes spléniques, les processus immunologiques, la suppression de la moelle épinière par une infection virale chronique et le ralentissement de la thrombopoïétine, un facteur de croissance hématopoïétique. La présente analyse porte sur les étiologies et les options de prise en charge de la thrombocytopénie grave en cas de maladie hépatique avancée.

Thrombocytopenia is a well-known complication in advanced liver disease, with an incidence of 77% to 85% in patients with cirrhosis (1). Patients with chronic liver disease and thrombocytopenia are at increased risk for bleeding, requiring recurrent platelet transfusions, increased ambulatory visits and inpatient hospital stays compared with individuals without thrombocytopenia (2). It has been estimated that the annual health care costs of a patient with hepatitis C virus (HCV) infection with and without thrombocytopenia is $37,924 and $12,174, respectively (2). Thrombocytopenia can also interfere with diagnostic and therapeutic procedures in patients with advanced liver disease. For example, patients with chronic HCV-related cirrhosis, who are not candidates for liver transplantation, often cannot be treated with interferon (IFN) therapy because of low platelet counts. This is clinically important because successful therapy for HCV infection may reduce the progression to hepatocellular carcinoma (3). Liver transplantation can be safely avoided if timely IFN therapy is provided to HCV patients. Repetitive platelet transfusions are not a practical solution to thrombocytopenia because of the short half-life of platelets and the associated alloimmunization that ultimately develops. The risk of transfusion-associated complications also significantly increases with repeated transfusions. The characterization of thrombocytopenia in these patient populations in the literature is sparse; accordingly, the present review concentrates on the etiology and management of thrombocytopenia in 'advanced liver disease' as a whole and HCV infection when mentioned.

ETIOLOGY

Thrombocytopenia in patients with advanced liver disease is secondary to hypersplenism, possible immune-mediated mechanisms, direct viral suppression of platelet production and decreased thrombopoietin (TPO) production from the diseased liver. The general approach to the diagnosis and major mechanisms of thrombocytopenia is highlighted in Figure 1.

Hypersplenism

Most cases of thrombocytopenia in the setting of liver disease are associated with splenomegaly (4). Splenomegaly is defined as enlargement of the spleen, diagnosed either on physical examination or imaging studies. In general, splenic enlargement to approximately 285 g is palpable (5). Normal splenic size on ultrasound is <13 cm in length and ≤15 cm in thickness and, on computed tomography scan is <10 cm (6). Hepatic diseases account for 36% of cases of splenomegaly; 35% are attributed to hematological conditions, 16% to infectious diseases (50% in AIDS/HIV), 4% to primary spleen disorders, 5% to inflammatory conditions and 4% to other causes (7). Splenomegaly is a common finding in patients with cirrhosis and portal hypertension. Conversely, not all patients with cirrhosis and portal hypertension have splenomegaly (8). To date, the reasons behind this discordance are unclear. It has also been noted that portal venous pressure only increases to a certain level, after which portal venous pressure decreases with an increase in total portal systemic shunt and splenic shunt (9). This may partially explain the occasional lack of correlation between portal venous pressure and splenic size. The etiology of splenomegaly in patients with liver cirrhosis is multifactorial and may be a congestive or hyperplastic phenomenon (10). In most cases, increases in portal venous pressure cause splenic congestion, thereby leading to the development of splenomegaly with resulting increased platelet sequestration and subsequent thrombocytopenia.

Immunological mechanisms of thrombocytopenia in cirrhosis and HCV patients

Noting a variable response in thrombocytopenia after portal vein decompression in cirrhotic patients, Jabbour et al (11) questioned whether other mechanisms of thrombocytopenia may be occurring in specific patient populations. It has been long observed that HCV

[1]*Georgia Regents University, Augusta, Georgia;* [2]*Helena Regional Medical Center, Helena, Arkansas, USA;* [3]*Luzhou Medical College, Luzhou, China;* [4]*Archbold Medical Center, Thomasville, Georgia, USA*
Correspondence: Dr VGR Gangireddy, Georgia Regents University, 1120 15th Street, Augusta, Georgia 30912, USA. e-mail venureddy82@gmail.com

patients are prone to several autoimmune disorders, suggesting the possibility of an autoimmune etiology for thrombocytopenia in this patient population (12-14). A recent study by Olariu et al (15) investigating thrombocytopenia in HCV patients found that both decreased platelet production by bone marrow suppression (the 'central' mechanism) and increased destruction by autoimmune processes (the 'peripheral' mechanism) was present in approximately 93.3% of patients with severe thrombocytopenia and 64% of patients with moderate thrombocytopenia. However, these conclusions should be viewed with caution because there were several limitations to the study, such as excluding patients with cirrhosis and, thereby, potentially excluding the majority of patients with splenomegaly. Moreover, there was no mention of the bone marrow biopsy or megakaryocyte quantification methods used. It was also noted that only dual-colour immunoflorescence and flow cytometry could identify both mature and immature megakaryocytes as opposed to light microscopy, which may exclude immature megakaryocytes (16).

The role of the spleen in the autoimmune process of immune thrombocytopenic purpura (ITP) has been extensively studied (17). The etiology of thrombocytopenia in liver cirrhosis may have some similarities with ITP. Autoimmune antibodies possibly contribute to the immunological destruction of platelets in both; however, the severity of thrombocytopenia in liver cirrhosis is typically less than that found in ITP. This may be explained by impaired functioning of the reticuloendothelial system, thereby decreasing platelet opsonizing capacity acting via Fc receptors in cirrhotic patients (18). Other explanations may be differences in the subclass activation of immunoglobulin (Ig) G isotypes in cirrhotic patients. Both platelet-associated antibodies (PAIgG and anti-GP antibodies) and serum circulating antiplatelet antibodies are found in patients with cirrhosis (19,20). Increased PAIgG autoimmune antibodies in cirrhosis patients were first noted by Landolfi et al (21). Subsequent studies have also shown an inverse correlation between platelet counts and PAIgG levels (22-24). PAIgG is also increased in many nonimmune causes of thrombocytopenia and hypergammaglobulinemia. The PAIgG assay is not regarded to be an appropriate test for the diagnosis of ITP by the American Society of Hematology; hence, its diagnostic role in HCV or cirrhotic patients is also questionable (25).

The role of other antiplatelet antibodies (anti-GP antibodies) in cirrhosis patients was first studied by Pereira et al (26) in 1995. Anti-GPIIb-IIIa antibody-producing B cells are present in approximately 99% of patients with liver cirrhosis irrespective of the etiology of cirrhosis (19,26). They are found to be the strongest independent factor associated with thrombocytopenia and inversely correlated with platelet count (19). The glycocalicin index, which measures platelet turnover rate, is abnormally high in liver cirrhosis patients. Reticulated platelets, which reflect the rate of bone marrow platelet production, is increased in all patients with alcoholic cirrhosis, hepatitis B virus cirrhosis and ITP patients (20,27-29). This, in addition to the presence of anti-GPIIb-IIIa autoantibodies, suggests at least some immunological component of platelet destruction and thrombocytopenia in some advanced liver disease patients (20). The low reticulated platelet count in the HCV subgroups may be explained by the central effect of HCV in bone marrow suppression (20).

The role of TPO

Immunological processes may partially explain thrombocytopenia in cirrhotic patients in whom portal vein congestion has not been demonstrated; however, in some cases, immune complexes cannot be implicated. There is mounting evidence that impaired hepatic production of TPO may be a major cause of thrombocytopenia in liver disease. TPO is synthesized in the liver and is the principle physiological regulator of platelet production (30). Thrombocytopenic patients with advanced liver disease have inappropriately low levels of TPO (31-33). Patients with splenomegaly and normal platelet counts have significantly higher TPO levels than those with thrombocytopenia, which suggests that higher TPO levels result in a compensatory

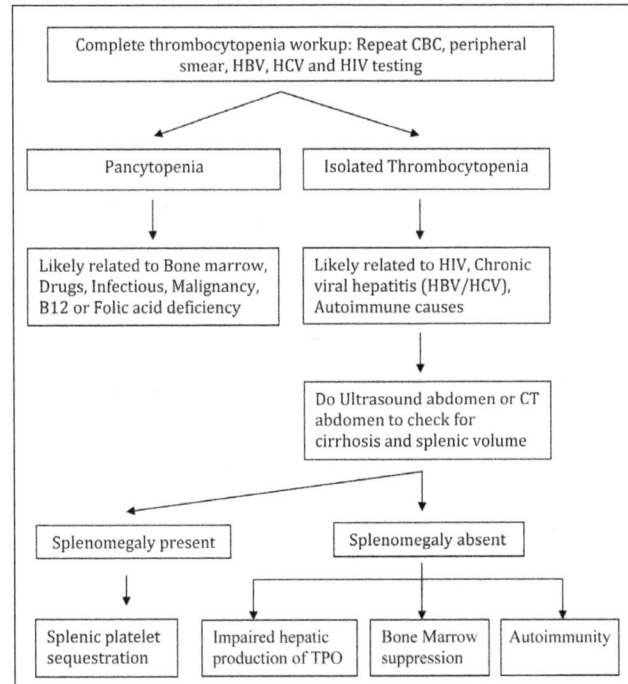

Figure 1) *General approach and mechanism to the diagnosis of thrombocytopenia in liver disease. CBC Complete blood count; CT Computed tomography; HBV Hepatitis B virus; HCV Hepatitis C virus; TPO Thrombopoietin*

increase in platelet production (34). Serum TPO levels correlate inversely with the severity of liver disease as reflected by the degree of fibrosis, Child-Pugh class and other synthetic measures of liver function (35,36). TPO levels and platelet counts increase after orthotopic liver transplantation, strongly supporting impaired TPO production as a primary cause of thrombocytopenia in at least some patients (37,38).

MANAGEMENT: OVERVIEW

The management of thrombocytopenia in cirrhotic patients has been a challenging problem for many years. Splenorenal shunts were developed in the 1960s but later abandoned due to a high mortality rate from liver failure (39,40). Splenectomy and, later, partial splenectomy (PS), gained popularity because of fewer complications associated with the procedure. With refined laparoscopic techniques, splenectomies have been performed since the late 1990s with minimal complications and better resolution of thrombocytopenia compared with PS. Splenic embolization has been successfully performed since the 1970s. Now, partial splenic embolization (PSE) is gaining in popularity. Newer techniques, such as radiofrequency ablation (RFA) and TPO stimulators, are currently being investigated to treat the thrombocytopenia associated with liver disease. Here, we discuss the merits and drawbacks of each intervention, with a special emphasis on recent advances in the management of thrombocytopenia in chronic liver disease patients (Table 1). Figures 2 and 3 summarize the general approach to management.

Splenectomy

Splenomegaly is a common complication in patients with cirrhosis, with portal hypertension being the primary mechanism of pathogenesis. Splenectomy is a common surgical strategy for correcting thrombocytopenia due to hypersplenism. Open splenectomy and laparoscopic splenectomy are the two most widely available procedures commonly performed for severe thrombocytopenia.

Since the 1950s, open splenectomies were primarily performed in cirrhotic patients with splenomegaly to relieve portal hypertension and reduce variceal bleeding (41,42). Due to the high risk for bleeding,

TABLE 1
Summary of management of thrombocytopenia in liver disease

Procedure	Advantages	Disadvantages	Comments
Laparoscopic splenectomy	• Most effective in improving thrombocytopenia • Can be performed in patients with low splenic volumes (<400 mL) • Lower complication rates compared with open splenectomy.	• Overall complication rates ranges from 2.5% to 17% • Increased risk for intra- and postoperative bleeding • Increased risk for portal vein thrombosis and splenic vein thrombosis (19% to 55%)	• Extensively studied
Partial splenic artery embolization	• Decreased postprocedure bleeding rate • Lower morbidity rates compared with laparoscopic splenectomy	• Reported complications were pneumonia, peritonitis, splenic abscess and portal vein thrombosis	• Comparable with laparoscopic splenectomy in improving the platelet counts
Radiofrequency splenic ablation	• Lower complication rates, better cost effectiveness and convenience compared with PSE • >70% RFA showed sustained platelet counts similar to splenectomized patients • Additional improvement in liver function	• Suboptimal ablation can result in unsustained platelet counts	• Newer technique • Further randomized control studies and clinical trials are needed to evaluate its effectiveness
Shunt procedures		• Unsustained improvement in thrombocytopenia • More complications (eg, hepatic encephalopathy, hepatic failure)	• Currently obsolete • TIPS for the treatment of hypersplenism are currently discouraged by AASLD
Antiviral therapy	• No procedure-related complications	• Unsustained improvement in thrombocytopenia • Only shown to improve mild thrombocytopenia	• Only case reports and case series • Further randomized control studies and clinical trials are needed to evaluate its effectiveness
Immune suppression	• No procedure-related complications	• Not used for thrombocytopenia related to liver diseases or HCV • Shown to increase chances of recurrence and viral load in post transplant HCV patients	• Used in patients with ITP • Not be recommended to improve thrombocytopenia associated with liver disease
Thrombopoietin stimulators	• No procedure-related complications • Can be considered in patients who are poor surgical candidates	• Portal vein thrombosis	• Eltrombopag is approved for treatment of thrombocytopenia in chronic HCV patients who are considered for HCV therapy

AASLD American Association for the Study of Liver Diseases; HCV Hepatitis C virus; ITP Immune thrombocytopenic purpura; PSE Partial splenic embolization; RFA Radiofrequency ablation; TIPS Transjugular intrahepatic portosystemic shunts

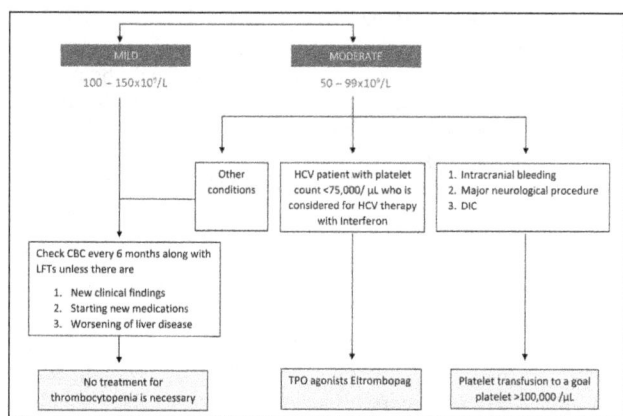

Figure 2) *Cirrhosis and thrombocytopenia. CBC Complete blood count; HCV Hepatitis C virus; DIC Disseminated intravascular coagulation; LFTs Liver function tests; TPO Thrombopoietin*

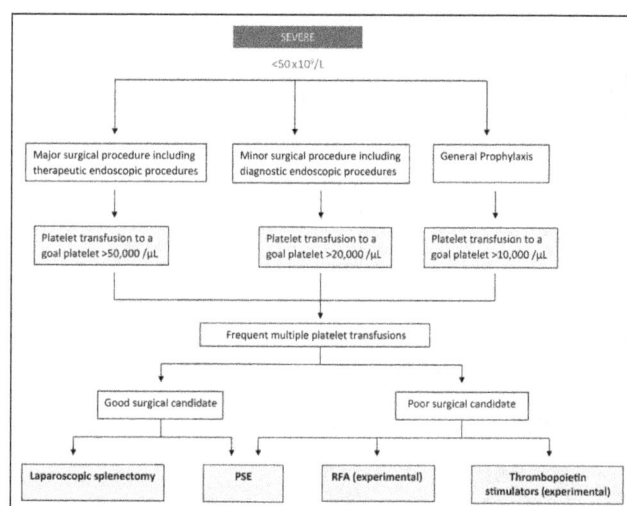

Figure 3) *Cirrhosis and thrombocytopenia. PSE Partial splenic embolization; RFA Radiofrequency ablation*

some studies preferred shunt procedures to open splenectomy (43,44). Additional complications reported after open splenectomy include portal vein thrombosis (8% to 10%) and wound pain (45,46). Due to advances in laparoscopic surgical techniques, laparoscopic splenectomies have been performed since the early 1990s on patients who were initially not considered for this procedure (47,48). Comparative studies investigating open versus laproscopic splenectomy in cirrhosis patients to improve platelet counts were largely missing in the literature until recently, when Hayashi et al (49) first published a case

series involving HCV patients. In this study, the mean hospital stay, significant complication rate and transfusion rate were nine days, 14% and 71% for open splenectomy compared with 2.6 days, 0% and 0%, respectively, for laparoscopic splenectomy. Other recent studies have favoured laparoscopic approaches to decrease complication rates. Compared with open splenectomy, laparoscopic splenectomy has resulted in less blood loss and shorter hospital stays (50). Currently,

TABLE 2
Management of thrombocytopenia due to cirrhosis at a single centre

Preoperative splenic volume	Procedure	Target
<400 mL	Left splenectomy	
400 mL to 700 mL	Single partial splenic embolization or laparoscopic splenectomy (in selective cases)	Infarcted splenic area (Infarcted splenic volume <540 mL)
>700 mL	Repeated partial splenic embolization (two-month interval) or laparoscopic splenectomy (in selective cases)	Noninfarcted splenic area (Noninfarcted splenic ratio <20% and noninfarcted splenic volume <170 mL)

Data adapted from reference 64

due to lack of strong supportive evidence of efficacy and a high associated complication rate, open splenectomy to improve thrombocytopenia is not commonly practiced or recommended.

Portal and splenic vein thrombosis are the main complications of laparoscopic splenectomy (19% to 55%) compared with open splenectomy (8% to 10%) (45,46,51-54). Risk factors for thrombosis include larger spleen size and large splenic vein diameter (55). The most significant complication following laparoscopic splenectomy is bleeding. The amount of bleeding in laparoscopic splenectomy groups is significantly less compared with open splenectomy groups (51,56-58). The conversion rate from laparoscopic to open splenectomy due to bleeding ranges from 0% to 9.6% (56,58). Overall complication rates in cirrhotic patients range from 2.5% to 17% (57,59). However, in patients with massive splenomegaly, the complication rate can be as high as 56% (60). The indication of laparoscopic splenectomy in the management of thrombocytopenia is largely limited because of the associated surgical complications with the procedure, as mentioned above.

Splenic artery embolization
The use of splenic artery embolization (SAE) in the management of thrombocytopenia was first reported by Maddison (61) in 1973 as a proposed alternative to splenectomy in surgically unfit patients. The two types of SAE techniques widely published in the literature include total embolization and partial embolization. Due to an increased risk for splenic abscess from total splenic embolization, partial SAE (PSE) is now the preferred option in patients who are candidates (62,63). Embolization occludes the arterial supply of the spleen peripherally with ischemic necrosis of functional splenic tissue followed by a decrease in spleen size. Partial embolization allows the preservation of some normal splenic tissue and thereby avoids the theoretical risk of overwhelming postembolization sepsis. The role of preoperative splenic volume in the management of thrombocytopenia in patients with cirrhosis is a matter of significant debate. Unfortunately, there were no clear guidelines to direct splenectomy or PSE based on splenic volume. The recommended splenic infarct volume to effectively increase the platelet counts (at one year) and decrease the post-PSE complication is between 388 mL and 540 mL (64). One institution's approach is shown in Table 2; however, this approach needs to be further validated (65). In patients with cirrhosis and splenic volume <400 mL, splenectomy is mainly preferred because PSE can cause significant inflammatory reactions and preclude further splenectomy if needed. In patients with splenic volume <700 mL, the infarcted splenic volume is shown to correlate (r=0.53; P≤0.001) with the long-term (one year) increase in platelet counts; however, in patients with splenic volume ≥700 mL, noninfarcted splenic volume (r=−0.71; P=0.003) and splenic infarction ratio (r=0.72; P=0.002) were shown to correlate (65).

The extent and sustainability of improvements in platelet counts appears to be dependent on the extent of SAE. It has been reported that embolization of <30% of splenic mass results in an unsustained improvement in platelet counts, but embolization of >50% is associated with an increased risk for complications (66,67). Complication rates are reported to be approximately 28% with <50% embolization, 56% with 50% to 70% embolization, and 95% with >70% embolization (68). The complications reported with PSE are pneumonia,

peritonitis, splenic abscess and portal vein thrombosis (67). Laparoscopic splenectomy has a higher morbidity rate compared with PSE (16% to 36% versus 0% to 16%, respectively) (69,70). Splenic abscess is a severe complication of PSE, with a reported incidence of up to 16%; death may occur in 6% of cases (69,70). Retrospective series suggest that PSE can control cytopenias in nearly all patients (70,71). In a randomized trial, PSE was comparable with splenectomy with regard to increasing platelet counts (211×10^9/L versus 240×10^9/L at two weeks, and 146×10^9/L versus 322×10^9/L at six months). The patients in the PSE group also experienced fewer episodes of portal vein thrombosis (72).

It should be noted that in other studies, patients with HCV infection had a poorer response rate to PSE, which was believed to be secondary to possible immunological mechanisms contributing to the thrombocytopenia, which PSE could not correct (73,74).

RFA of the spleen
RFA of the spleen is a minimally invasive, relatively new procedure that has shown promising results in patients with cirrhosis and splenomegaly (75). In a randomized controlled trial comparing RFA with laparoscopic splenectomy, platelet counts improved after RFA but were not sustained after 12 months and 24 months of follow-up (76). Suboptimal ablation was likely the reason for the unsustained platelet counts. Patients with >70% ablation showed sustained platelet counts similar to splenectomized patients. The other benefits of RFA were improved liver function secondary to improved hepatic artery blood flow to the liver, increased oxygenation and decreased liver sinusoidal congestion (77). The main advantages of RFA over PSE were lower complication rates, cost effectiveness and convenience. The major complications in this group of patients included hemorrhagic shock and intra-abdominal bleeding. Complications such as hyperpyrexia, splenic rupture or abscess, which are commonly observed in patients with PS, were absent in patients treated with RFA (76). Further clinical trials with longer follow-up studies are needed to definitively elucidate its effectiveness.

Shunt procedures
Splenic congestion is believed to be the primary mechanism of thrombocytopenia in patients with cirrhosis. After the success of surgical splenectomy in improving thrombocytopenia, the focus shifted to shunt procedures. Shunt procedures decompress the spleen and decrease portal pressures, thereby creating a 'physiological splenectomy'. The types of shunts widely published in the literature for these purposes are portocaval shunts, splenorenal shunts and transjugular intrahepatic portosystemic shunts (TIPS). When compared with a control group, patients with portocaval shunts and distal splenorenal shunts have experienced more complications, such as hepatic encephalopathy and hepatic failure, and minimal improvements in hypersplenism and thrombocytopenia (78,79). These approaches have now been largely abandoned. TIPS has been in use for >20 years to treat the complications of portal hypertension. Several case series suggested an improvement in the platelet count within a few days of TIPS placement (80-82). However, prospective series do not support this because the mean platelet counts appear to remain unchanged after TIPS (83,84). Complications include encephalopathy (up to 45%) and

portal vein thrombosis (15%) (85). Recent practice guidelines update the use of TIPS in cirrhosis. TIPS for the treatment of hypersplenism are currently discouraged by the American Association for the Study of Liver Diseases (85).

Antiviral therapy to improve thrombocytopenia

The role of antiviral therapy in the management of thrombocytopenia is a much-debated topic. Direct viral suppression of megakaryocytes and, therefore, TPO deficiency causing thrombocytopenia, has been proposed. New questions have arisen as to whether the eradication of HCV would itself improve thrombocytopenia.

In one of the earlier case series investigasting the treatment of HCV to improve thrombocytopenia with or without cirrhosis, Rajan and Liebman (86) showed that IFN therapy can improve platelet counts in severely thrombocytopenic patients (range 16×10^9/L to 48×10^9/L) (86). In a study involving eight patients, 63% (five of eight) of patients experienced improvement in their platelet counts to >50×10^9/L. Two patients had neither an improvement in platelet count nor an antiviral response to IFN. The most significant response (one of one) was observed in a patient who achieved a sustained virological response (SVR). In patients with cirrhosis (three of eight), platelet counts improved in two. Patients who had improved platelet counts also had decreased rheumatoid factor antibodies and cryoglobulins, as well as improved transaminase levels. In another study (74), the authors showed that all of the patients (n=5) with thrombocytopenia (<150×10^9/L) who achieved an SVR with IFN improved their platelet counts at least by 5% (two patients between 5% and 15%, one between 15% and 25%, and two >25%). The limitations of this study were small sample size, the majority of the patients treated with IFN in the thrombocytopenia group were mildly thrombocytopenic (80% of the patient's platelets counts >100×10^9/L) (74). Further randomized control studies and clinical trials are needed to evaluate the role of antiviral therapy in the management of thrombocytopenia.

Immune suppression for the treatment of thrombocytopenia

The role of autoantibodies in thrombocytopenia, especially in HCV, is well known. Steroids and other immunosuppressive agents have been used for the treatment of ITP. The treatment of HCV in patients with liver transplantation shows that immunosuppression increases the viral load and recurrence of HCV infection even after achieving an SVR (87-90). Presently, immunosuppression cannot be recommended to improve thrombocytopenia in this patient population.

TPO stimulators

Clinical studies investigating thrombopoietic growth factors showed that they were effective in increasing the platelet count in several clinical settings including myelodysplastic syndromes, nonmyeloablative chemotherapy and ITP. The development of first-generation thrombopoietic growth factors (recombinant human TPO and pegylated recombinant human megakaryocyte growth and development factor [PEG-rHuMGDF]) was stopped due to development of antibodies to PEG-rHuMGDF (91). Of the second-generation thrombopoietic growth factors, only romiplostim and eltrombopag have been extensively tested in human diseases. Both increased platelet counts in patients with ITP and could do so for a prolonged time without apparent untoward effects. Both drugs are now United States Food & Drug Administration-approved for the treatment of patients with chronic ITP. Studies are ongoing in patients with thrombocytopenia related to chemotherapy, hepatitis C and myelodysplastic syndromes. McHutchinson et al (92) conducted a phase II randomized controlled trial involving 74 patients with HCV-related cirrhosis. Only 6% of patients in the placebo group completed the 12-week antiviral course. In contrast, 36%, 53% and 65% of patients receiving 30 mg, 50 mg and 75 mg of eltrombopag completed the same antiviral course, respectively. Moreover, 75% to 95% of patients in the eltrombopag group achieved the primary end point (platelet count 100×10^9/L at week 4) in a dose-dependent manner (92). The Eltrombopag Evaluated for Its Ability

to Overcome Thrombocytopenia and Enable Procedures (ELEVATE) study is a randomized, double-blind, placebo-controlled, multinational follow-up study in patients with thrombocytopenia and chronic liver disease (93). It was terminated following the identification of an imbalance of thrombosis of the portal venous system in the patients treated with eltrombopag versus matching placebo. Six patients (4%) in the eltrombopag group and one (1%) in the placebo group experienced a thrombotic event of the portal venous system. Of note, five of the six patients treated with eltrombopag experienced the portal venous thrombosis at platelet counts >200×10^9/L (93). Eltrombopag was recently United States Food & Drug Administration-approved for thrombocytopenia in patients with HCV who are eligible for antiviral therapy with IFN and ribavirin (94). Its effects on newer antiviral medications, such as sofosbuvir and semepivir, is yet to be determined. Phase III studies of romiplostim treatment in HCV-associated thrombocytopenia are currently ongoing. Some of the risk for thrombosis in these patients is dose related, although portal vein thrombosis has also been reported with this agent (95). TPO stimulators may play an important role in the management of thrombocytopenia in patients with advanced liver disease, primarily in patients who are poor surgical candidates.

CONCLUSIONS

Hypersplenism in patients with advanced liver disease remains a challenging issue and thrombocytopenia is a multifactorial problem. Currently available therapeutic solutions are not without significant complications. Intuitively, it would appear that correcting the underlying liver disease with immune therapy, use of immunosuppressives or liver transplantation would provide the best solution with fewest complications. Less is known about the impact of platelet autoantibodies and direct viral suppression of megakaryocytes. Management of thrombocytopenia in patients with cirrhosis should be a goal-oriented and team approach. In HCV patients with high viral loads and mild thrombocytopenia without accompanying cirrhosis, IFN therapy can be safely considered in the hope of improving platelet counts. Combination therapy consisting of pegylated IFN and TPO stimulators, such as eltrombopag, can also be considered in these patients. In patients with splenomegaly, PSE and laparoscopic splenectomy can be considered as therapeutic options. The role of immune suppression and TPO stimulators in patients with massive splenomegaly in whom these interventions are considered unsafe is an area for ongoing investigation.

DISCLOSURES: The authors have no financial disclosures or conflicts of interest to declare.

REFERENCES

1. Qamar AA, Grace ND, Groszmann RJ, et al; Portal Hypertension Collaborative Group. Incidence, prevalence, and clinical significance of abnormal hematologic indices in compensated cirrhosis. Clin Gastroenterol Hepatol 2009;7:689-95.
2. Poordad F, Theodore D, Sullivan J, Grotzinger K. Medical resource utilisation and healthcare costs in patients with chronic hepatitis C viral infection and thrombocytopenia. J Med Econ 2011;14:194-206.
3. Morihara D, Kobayashi M, Ikeda K, et al. Effectiveness of combination therapy of splenectomy and long-term interferon in patients with hepatitis C virus-related cirrhosis and thrombocytopenia. Hepatol Res 2009;39:439-47.
4. Sakai K, Iwao T, Oho K, Toyonaga A, Sata M. Propranolol ameliorates thrombocytopenia in patients with cirrhosis. J Gastroenterol 2002;37:112-8.
5. Aito H. The estimation of the size of the spleen by radiological methods. A comparative radiographic, gamma imaging and ultrasonic study. Ann Clin Res 1974;(6 Suppl):1-54.
6. Tamayo SG, Rickman LS, Mathews WC, et al. Examiner dependence on physical diagnostic tests for the detection of splenomegaly: A prospective study with multiple observers. J Gen Intern Med 1993;8:69-75.

7. O'Reilly RA. Splenomegaly in 2,505 patients at a large university medical center from 1913 to 1995. 1963 to 1995: 449 patients. West J Med 1998;169:88-97.

8. Gibson PR, Gibson RN, Ditchfield MR, Donlan JD. Splenomegaly – an insensitive sign of portal hypertension. Aust N Z J Med 1990;20:771-4.

9. Ohnishi K, Nakayama T, Saito M, et al. Effects of propranolol on portal hemodynamics in patients with chronic liver disease. Am J Gastroenterol 1985;80:132-5.

10. Bolognesi M, Merkel C, Sacerdoti D, Nava V, Gatta A. Role of spleen enlargement in cirrhosis with portal hypertension. Dig Liver Dis 2002;34:144-50.

11. Jabbour N, Zajko A, Orons P, Irish W, Fung JJ, Selby RR. Does transjugular intrahepatic portosystemic shunt (TIPS) resolve thrombocytopenia associated with cirrhosis? Dig Dis Sci 1998;43:2459-62.

12. Clifford BD, Donahue D, Smith L, et al. High prevalence of serological markers of autoimmunity in patients with chronic hepatitis C. Hepatology 1995;2:613-9.

13. Hadziyannis SJ. Nonhepatic manifestations and combined diseases in HCV infection. Dig Dis Sci 1996;41(12 Suppl):63S-74S.

14. Tran A, Benzaken S, Yang G, et al. Chronic hepatitis C and autoimmunity: Good response to immunosuppressive treatment. Dig Dis Sci 1997;42:778-80.

15. Olariu M, Olariu C, Olteanu D. Thrombocytopenia in chronic hepatitis C. J Gastrointest Liver Dis 2010;19:381-5.

16. Law HK, Bol SJ, Palatsides M, Williams NT. Analysis of human megakaryocytic cells using dual-color immunofluorescence labeling. Cytometry 2000;41:308-15.

17. Kuwana M, Okazaki Y, Kaburaki J, Kawakami Y, Ikeda Y. Spleen is a primary site for activation of platelet-reactive T and B cells in patients with immune thrombocytopenic purpura. J Immunol 2002;168:3675-82.

18. Rimola A, Soto R, Bory F, Arroyo V, Piera C, Rodes J. Reticuloendothelial system phagocytic activity in cirrhosis and its relation to bacterial infections and prognosis. Hepatology 1984;4:53-8.

19. Kajihara M, Kato S, Okazaki Y, et al. A role of autoantibody-mediated platelet destruction in thrombocytopenia in patients with cirrhosis. Hepatology 2003;37:1267-76.

20. Pradella P, Bonetto S, Turchetto S, et al. Platelet production and destruction in liver cirrhosis. J Hepatol 2011;54:894-900.

21. Landolfi R, Leone G, Fedeli G, Storti S, Laghi F, Bizzi B. Platelet-associated IgG in acute and chronic hepatic diseases. Scand J Haematol 1980;25:417-22.

22. Barrison IG, Knight ID, Viola L, Boots MA, Murray-Lion IM, Mitchell TR. Platelet associated immunoglobulins on chronic liver disease. Br J Haematol 1981;48:347-50.

23. Graber D, Giuliani D, Leevy CM, Morse BS. Platelet-associated IgG in hepatitis and cirrhosis. J Clin Immunol 1984;4:108-11.

24. de Noronha R, Taylor BA, Wild G, Triger DR, Greaves M. Inter-relationships between platelet count, platelet IgG, serum IgG, immune complexes and severity of liver disease. Clin Lab Haematol 1991;13:127-35.

25. George JN, Woolf SH, Raskob GE, et al. Idiopathic thrombocytopenic purpura: A practice guideline developed by explicit methods for the American Society of Hematology. Blood 1996;88:3-40.

26. Pereira J, Accatino L, Alfaro J, Brahm J, Hidalgo P, Mezzano D. Platelet autoantibodies in patients with chronic liver disease. Am J Hematol 1995;50:173-8.

27. Michur H, Maślanka K, Szczepiński A, Mariańska B. Reticulated platelets as a marker of platelet recovery after allogeneic stem cell transplantation. Int J Lab Hematol 2008;30:519-25.

28. Thomas-Kaskel AK, Mattern D, Köhler G, Finke J, Behringer D. Reticulated platelet counts correlate with treatment response in patients with idiopathic thrombocytopenic purpura and help identify the complex causes of thrombocytopenia in patients after allogeneic hematopoietic stem cell transplantation. Cytometry B Clin Cytom 2007;72:241-8.

29. Harrison P, Robinson MS, Mackie IJ, Machin SJ. Reticulated platelets. Platelets 1997;8:379-83.

30. Kuter DJ, Begley CG. Recombinant human thrombopoietin: Basic biology and evaluation of clinical studies. Blood 2002;100:3457-69.

31. Martin III TG, Somberg KA, Meng YG, et al. Thrombopoietin levels in patients with cirrhosis before and after orthotopic liver transplantation. Ann Intern Med 1997;127:285-8.

32. Ishikawa T, Ichida T, Matsuda Y, et al. Reduced expression of thrombopoietin is involved in thrombocytopenia in human and rat liver cirrhosis. J Gastroenterol Hepatol 1998;13:907-13.

33. Peck-Radosavljevic M, Zacherl J, Meng YG, et al. Is inadequate thrombopoietin production a major cause of thrombocytopenia in cirrhosis of the liver? J Hepatol 1997;27:127-31.

34. Giannini E, Botta F, Borro P, et al. Relationship between thrombopoietin serum levels and liver function in patients with chronic liver disease related to hepatitis C virus infection. Am J Gastroenterol 2003;98:2516-20.

35. Kawasaki T, Takeshita A, Souda K, et al. Serum thrombopoietin levels in patients with chronic hepatitis and liver cirrhosis. Am J Gastroenterol 1999;94:1918-22.

36. Giannini E, Borro P, Botta F, et al. Serum thrombopoietin levels are linked to liver function in untreated patients with hepatitis C virus-related chronic hepatitis. J Hepatol 2002;37:572-7.

37. Peck-Radosavljevic M, Wichlas M, Zacherl J, et al. Thrombopoietin induces rapid resolution of thrombocytopenia after orthotopic liver transplantation through increased platelet production. Blood 2000;95:795-801.

38. Yanaga K, Tzakis AG, Shimada M, et al. Reversal of hypersplenism following orthotopic liver transplantation. Ann Surg 1989;210:180-3.

39. Mutchnick MG, Lerner E, Conn HO. Portal-systemic encephalopathy and portacaval anastomosis: A prospective, controlled investigation. Gastroenterology 1974;66:1005-19.

40. Vang J, Simert G, Hansson JA, Thylen U, Bengmark TS. Results of a modified distal spleno-renal shunt for portal hypertension. Ann Surg 1977;185:224-8.

41. Lord JW Jr. The surgical management of secondary hypersplenism. Surgery 1951;29:407-18.

42. Linton RR, Ellis DS, Geary JE. Critical comparative analysis of early and late results of splenorenal and direct portacaval shunts performed in 169 patients with portal cirrhosis. Ann Surg 1961;154:446-59.

43. Yamamoto S, Hidemura R. Surgical treatment of portal hypertension with special reference to the feature of intrahepatic circulatory disturbances. Jpn Circ J 1964;28:178-80.

44. El-Khishen MA, Henderson JM, Millikan WJ Jr, Kutner MH, Warren WD. Splenectomy is contraindicated for thrombocytopenia secondary to portal hypertension. Surg Gynecol Obstet 1985;160:233-8.

45. Hassn AM, Al-Fallouji MA, Ouf TI, Saad R. Portal vein thrombosis following splenectomy. Br J Surg 2000;87:362-73.

46. Winslow ER, Brunt LM, Drebin JA, Soper NJ, Klingensmith ME. Portal vein thrombosis after splenectomy. Am J Surg 2002;184:631-5.

47. Carroll BJ, Phillips EH, Semel CJ, Fallas M, Morgenstern L. Laparoscopic splenectomy. Surg Endosc 1992;6:183-5.

48. Delaitre B, Maignien B, Icard P. Laparoscopic splenectomy. Br J Surg 1992;79:1334.

49. Hayashi PH, Mehia C, Joachim Reimers H, Solomon HS, Bacon BR. Splenectomy for thrombocytopenia in patients with hepatitis C cirrhosis. J Clin Gastroenterol 2006;40:740-4.

50. Shigekawa Y, Uchiyama K, Takifuji K, et al. A laparoscopic splenectomy allows the induction of antiviral therapy for patients with cirrhosis associated with hepatitis C virus. Am Surg 2011;77:174-9.

51. Watanabe Y, Horiuchi A, Yoshida M, et al. Significance of laparoscopic splenectomy in patients with hypersplenism. World J Surg 2007;31:549-55.

52. Ushitora Y, Tashiro H, Takahashi S, et al. Splenectomy in chronic hepatic disorders: Portal vein thrombosis and improvement of liver function. Dig Surg 2011;28:9-14.

53. Ikeda M, Sekimoto M, Takiguchi S, et al. High incidence of thrombosis of the portal venous system after laparoscopic splenectomy: A prospective study with contrast-enhanced CT scan. Ann Surg 2005;241:208-16.

54. Harris W, Marcaccio M. Incidence of portal vein thrombosis after laparoscopic splenectomy. Can J Surg 2005;48:352-4.

55. Kinjo N, Kawanaka H, Akahoshi T, et al. Risk factors for portal venous thrombosis after splenectomy in patients with cirrhosis and portal hypertension. Br J Surg 2010;97:910-6.

56. Hashizume M, Tomikawa M, Akahoshi T, et al. Laparoscopic splenectomy for portal hypertension. Hepatogastroenterology 2002;49:847-52.

57. Zhu JH, Wang YD, Ye ZY, et al. Laparoscopic versus open splenectomy for hypersplenism secondary to liver cirrhosis. Surg Laparosc Endosc Percutan Tech 2009;19:258-62.

58. Kercher KW, Carbonell AM, Heniford BT, Matthews BD, Cunningham DM, Reindollar RW. Laparoscopic splenectomy reverses thrombocytopenia in patients with hepatitis C cirrhosis and portal hypertension. J Gastrointest Surg 2004;8:120-6.

59. Wang Y, Zhan X, Zhu Y, Xie Z, Zhu J, Ye Z. Laparoscopic splenectomy in portal hypertension: A single-surgeon 13-year experience. Surg Endosc 2010;24:1164-9.

60. Patel AG, Parker JE, Wallwork B, et al. Massive splenomegaly is associated with significant morbidity after laparoscopic splenectomy. Ann Surg 2003;238:235-40.

61. Maddison EF. Embolic therapy of hypersplenism. Invest Radiol 1973;8:280-1.

62. Witte CL, Ovitt TW, Van Wyck DB, Witte MH, O'Mara RE, Woolfenden JM. Ischemic therapy in thrombocytopenia from hypersplenism. Arch Surg 1976;111:1115-21.

63. Wholey MH, Chamorro HA, Rao G, Chapman W. Splenic infarction and spontaneous rupture of the spleen after therapeutic embolization. Cardiovasc Radiol 1978;1:249-53.

64. Hayashi H1, Beppu T, Okabe K, et al. Therapeutic factors considered according to the preoperative splenic volume for a prolonged increase in platelet count after partial splenic embolization for liver cirrhosis. J Gastroenterol 2010;45:554-9.

65. Hayashi H, Beppu T, Okabe K, Masuda T, Okabe H, Baba H. Risk factors for complications after partial splenic embolization for liver cirrhosis. Br J Surg 2008;95:744-50.

66. Lee CM, Leung TK, Wang HJ, et al. Evaluation of the effect of partial splenic embolization on platelet values for liver cirrhosis patients with thrombocytopenia. World J Gastroenterol 2007;28:619-22.

67. Zhu K, Meng X, Qian J, et al. Partial splenic embolization for hypersplenism in cirrhosis: A long-term outcome in 62 patients. Dig Liver Dis 2009;41:411-6.

68. Mukaiya M, Hirata K, Yamashiro K, Katsuramaki T, Kimura H, Denno R. Changes in portal hemodynamics and hepatic function after partial splenic embolization (PSE) and percutaneous transhepatic obliteration (PTO). Cancer Chemother Pharmacol 1994;(33 Suppl):S37-S41.

69. Sakai T, Shiraki K, Inoue H et al. Complications of partial splenic embolization in cirrhotic patients. Dig Dis Sci 2002;47:388-91.

70. N'Kontchou G, Seror O, Bourcier V, et al. Partial splenic embolization in patients with cirrhosis: Efficacy, tolerance and long-term outcome in 32 patients. Eur J Gastroenterol Hepatol 2005;17:179-84.

71. Romano M, Giojelli A, Capuano G, Pomponi D, Salvatore M. Partial splenic embolization in patients with idiopathic portal hypertension. Eur J Radiol 2004;49:268-73.

72. Amin MA, el-Gendy MM, Dawoud IE, Shoma A, Negm AM, Amer TA. Partial splenic embolization versus splenectomy for the management of hypersplenism in cirrhotic patients. World J Surg 2009;33:1702-10.

73. Hernandez F, Blanquer A, Linares M, Lopez A, Tarin F, Cervero A. Autoimmune thrombocytopenia associated with hepatitis C virus infection. Acta Haematol 1998;99:217-20.

74. Pockros PJ, Duchini A, McMillan R, Nyberg LM, McHutchison J, Viernes E. Immune thrombocytopenic purpura in patients with chronic hepatitis C virus infection. Am J Gastroenterol 2002;97:2040-5.

75. Liu Q, Ma K, He Z, et al. Radiofrequency ablation for hypersplenism in patients with liver cirrhosis: A pilot study. J Gastrointest Surg 2005;9:648-57.

76. Feng K, Ma K, Liu Q, Wu Q, Dong J, Bie P. Randomized clinical trial of splenic radiofrequency ablation versus splenectomy for severe hypersplenism. Br J Surg 2011;98:354-61.

77. Liu Q, Ma K, Song Y, Zhou N, He Z. Two-year follow-up of splenic radiofrequency ablation in patients with cirrhotic hypersplenism: Does increased hepatic arterial flow induce liver regeneration? Surgery 2008;143:509-18.

78. Mutchnick MG, Lerner E, Conn HO. Portal-systemic encephalopathy and portacaval anastomosis: A prospective, controlled investigation. Gastroenterology 1974;66:1005-19.

79. Vang J, Simert G, Hansson JA, Thylen U, Bengmark TS. Results of a modified distal spleno-renal shunt for portal hypertension. Ann Surg 1977;185:224-8.

80. Alvarez OA, Lopera GA, Patel V, Encarnacion CE, Palmaz JC, Lee M. Improvement of thrombocytopenia due to hypersplenism after transjugular intrahepatic portosystemic shunt placement in cirrhotic patients. Am J Gastroenterol 1996;91:134.

81. Lawrence SP, Lezotte DC, Durham JD, et al. Course of thrombocytopenia of chronic liver disease after transjugular intrahepatic portosystemic shunts (TIPS). A retrospective analysis. Dig Dis Sci 1995;40:1575.

82. Pursnani KG, Sillin LF, Kaplan DS. Effect of transjugular intrahepatic portosystemic shunt on secondary hypersplenism. Am J Surg 1997;173:169.

83. Sanyal AJ, Freedman AM, Purdum PP, et al. The hematologic consequences of transjugular intrahepatic portosystemic shunts. Hepatology 1996;23:32.

84. Jabbour N, Zajko A, Orons P, Irish W, Fung JJ, Selby RR. Does transjugular intrahepatic portosystemic shunt (TIPS) resolve thrombocytopenia associated with cirrhosis? Dig Dis Sci 1998;43:2459-62.

85. Boyer TD, Haskal Z. AASLD Practice Guidelines: The role of transjugular intrahepatic portosystemic shunt in the management of portal hypertension. Hepatology 2010;51:1-16.

86. Rajan S, Liebman HA. Treatment of hepatitis C related thrombocytopenia with interferon alpha. Am J Hematol 2001;68:202-9.

87. Iga D, Tomimatsu M, Endo H, Ohkawa S, Yamada O. Improvement of thrombocytopenia with disappearance of HCV RNA in patients treated by interferon-alpha therapy: Possible etiology of HCV-associated immune thrombocytopenia. Eur J Haematol 2005;75:417-23

88. Lin A, Thadareddy A, Goldstein MJ, Lake-Bakaar G. Immune suppression leading to hepatitis C virus re-emergence after sustained virological response. J Med Virol 2008;80:1720-2.

89. Lladó L, Fabregat J, Castellote J, et al; THOSIN Study Group. Impact of immunosuppression without steroids on rejection and hepatitis C virus evolution after liver transplantation: Results of a prospective randomized study. Liver Transpl 2008;14:1752-60.

90. Lake JR. The role of immunosuppression in recurrence of hepatitis C. Liver Transpl 2003;9:S63-6.

91. Li J, Yang C, Xia Y, et al. Thrombocytopenia caused by the development of antibodies to thrombopoietin. Blood 2001;98:3241-8.

92. McHutchison JG, Dusheiko G, Shiffman ML, et al; TPL102357 Study Group. Eltrombopag for thrombocytopenia in patients with cirrhosis associated with hepatitis C. N Engl J Med 2007;29:2227-36.

93. The ELEVATE study. <www.clinicaltrials.gov> TPL104054. Clincal Trial.gov NCT00678587 (Accesed March 1, 2013).

94. Afdhal NH, Dusheiko GM, Theodore D, et al. Eltrombopag increases platelet numbers in thrombocytopenic patients with HCV infection andcirrhosis, allowing for effective antiviral therapy. Gastroenterology 2014;146:442-52.

95. Dultz G, Kronenberger B, Azizi A, et al. Portal vein thrombosis as complication of romiplostim treatment in a cirrhotic patient with hepatitis C-associated immune thrombocytopenic purpura. J Hepatol 2011;55:229-32.

28

Management of the pregnant inflammatory bowel disease patient on antitumour necrosis factor therapy: State of the art and future directions

Yvette PY Leung MD FRCPC[1], Remo Panaccione MD FRCPC[1],

Subrata Ghosh MBBS MD FRCPC FRCPE[1], Cynthia H Seow MBBS MSc FRACP[1,2]

YPY Leung, R Panaccione, S Ghosh, CH Seow. Management of the pregnant inflammatory bowel disease patient on antitumour necrosis factor therapy: State of the art and future directions. Can J Gastroenterol Hepatol 2014;28(9):505-509.

Antitumour necrosis factor (anti-TNF) therapy has been a major advance in the treatment of inflammatory bowel disease (IBD) by improving rates of mucosal healing, steroid-free remission, and decreasing rates of hospitalization and surgery. Because IBD affects women in their reproductive years, clinicians have and will continue to be asked in the future about the safety profile of these agents and their potential impact on pregnancy, the developing fetus and newborn. Immunoglobulin G transfer from the mother to fetus begins in the second trimester, with an elevation starting at 22 weeks of gestation and the largest amount transferred in the third trimester. Although research investigating the long-term outcomes of children exposed to anti-TNF therapy in utero is limited, there is no known adverse effect on either pregnancy or newborn outcomes including infectious complications with this class of drugs. The World Congress of Gastroenterology consensus statement on biological therapy for IBD considered infliximab and adalimumab to be low risk and compatible with use during conception and during pregnancy in at least the first two trimesters. Based on a clinical algorithm used at the University of Calgary Pregnancy and IBD clinic (Calgary, Alberta), recommendations have been provided on the management of pregnant patients on anti-TNF therapy, particularly with regard to third-trimester dosing, taking into account disease characteristics of individual patients. When educated about the safety of anti-TNF therapy during pregnancy, patients often choose to continue on therapy during the third trimester.

Key Words: *Antitumour necrosis factor therapy; Inflammatory bowel disease; Pregnancy*

La prise en charge de la patiente enceinte atteinte d'une maladie inflammatoire de l'intestin traitée par un inhibiteur du facteur de nécrose tumorale : mesures de pointe et futures orientations

L'inhibiteur du facteur de nécrose tumorale (anti-TNF) est un progrès important dans le traitement des maladies inflammatoires de l'intestin (MII), car il améliore le taux de guérison des muqueuses et de rémission sans stéroïdes et réduit le taux d'hospitalisations et d'opérations. Puisque les MII touchent des femmes en âge de procréer, les cliniciens doivent connaître le profil d'innocuité de ce traitement et ses répercussions possibles sur la grossesse, le fœtus et le nouveau-né. Le transfert d'immunoglobuline G de la mère au fœtus s'amorce au deuxième trimestre, l'élévation commençant à 22 semaines de grossesse et le transfert le plus important s'observant au troisième trimestre. Même si les recherches sur les effets à long terme du traitement anti-TNF *in utero* chez les enfants qui y sont exposés sont limitées, cette catégorie de médicaments ne s'associe à aucun effet indésirable connu sur la grossesse ou le nouveau-né, y compris les complications infectieuses. D'après la déclaration consensuelle du Congrès mondial de gastroentérologie sur le traitement biologique des MII, l'infliximab et l'adalimumab sont peu à risque et peuvent être utilisés pendant la période périconceptionnelle et au moins les deux premiers trimestres de la grossesse. Selon un algorithme clinique utilisé à la clinique de grossesse et de MII de l'université de Calgary, en Alberta, des recommandations ont été formulées sur la prise en charge des patientes enceintes sous traitement anti-TNF, notamment la posologie au troisième trimestre, compte tenu des caractéristiques de la maladie de chaque patiente. Lorsqu'elles sont informées de l'innocuité du traitement anti-TNF pendant la grossesse, les patientes choisissent souvent de le poursuivre au troisième trimestre.

The impact of antitumour necrosis factor (anti-TNF) therapy in the treatment of inflammatory bowel disease (IBD) has changed our concept of disease remission from that of purely symptomatic remission to endoscopic healing, with a corresponding reduction in hospitalizations and surgeries for IBD. In Canada, the available anti-TNF agents for Crohn disease and ulcerative colitis are infliximab (IFX; Remicade, Janssen, USA), a chimeric immunoglobulin (Ig) G1 monoclonal antibody and adalimumab (ADA; Humira, Abbvie, USA), a recombinant human IgG1 monoclonal antibody; and, for ulcerative colitis, golimumab (Simponi, Janssen, USA), a recombinant human IgG1 monoclonal antibody. With the exception of certolizumab (not available in Canada), all Food and Drug Administration (FDA)-approved anti-TNF agents for IBD are IgG1 antibodies with an Fc portion (IFX, ADA and golimumab).

Because IBD affects women in their reproductive years, clinicians have and will continue to be asked in the future about the safety profile of these agents and their potential impact on the developing fetus and newborn. While experiments involving nonhuman primates suggest that TNF-α is not required for normal development of the immune system (1), there are limited data regarding the long-term impact of these drugs on children beyond the first year of life. Both IFX and ADA are FDA category B drugs, meaning there is no evidence of risk in humans. However, due to concerns of the potential implications of TNF blockade in the fetus' developing immune system, uncertainty from both patients and physicians exist on how to best manage patients undergoing anti-TNF therapy during pregnancy.

According to the World Congress of Gastroenterology on biological therapy for IBD, IFX and ADA are considered to be low risk and compatible with use during conception and during pregnancy in at least the first two trimesters (2). However, the second trimester of pregnancy ends at gestational week 27. With a full-term pregnancy duration spanning approximately 40 weeks, this poses a clinical dilemma for gastroenterologists and patients. Withholding an anti-TNF agent for the entire third trimester equates to a significant drug holiday, and has risks for disease flare and the development of anti-drug antibodies.

[1]*Department of Medicine;* [2]*Department of Community Health Sciences, University of Calgary, Calgary, Alberta*
Correspondence: Dr Yvette Leung, Department of Medicine, University of Calgary, 3280 Hospital Drive Northwest, Calgary, Alberta T2N 4N1.
e-mail yvette.leung@albertahealthservices.ca

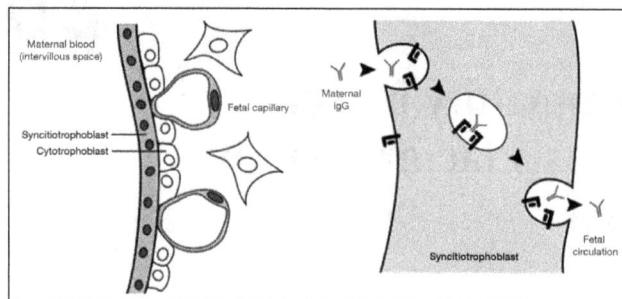

Figure 1) *Active transplacental transport of immunoglobulin G (IgG). Reproduced with permission, Oxford University Press (http://creativecommons.org/licenses/by-nc/2.5), Hazes JMW. Rheumatoid Am J Reprod Immunol 2011;50(11):1955-68*

The present review focuses on the latest research investigating transplacental passage of anti-TNF agents, the safety data on anti-TNF therapy during pregnancy, the optimal use of anti-TNF agents during pregnancy and highlight future areas requiring research.

HOW DO IGs CROSS THE PLACENTA IN A NORMAL PREGNANCY?

IgG is the only antibody class that significantly crosses the human placenta and, by doing so, provides short-term passive immunity to the newborn. This crossing is mediated by the neonatal Fc receptor (FcRn) that is expressed on syncytiotrophoblast cells of the placenta (3). Syncytiotrophoblasts on the maternal side of the placenta internalize IgG in endosomes (Figure 1). FcRn is expressed on the internal surface of endosomes. The endosomes then fuse with the fetal side of the syncytiotrophoblast, where the IgG dissociates from the FcRn to the fetal circulation (4). Preferential transport occurs for IgG1, followed by IgG4, then IgG3, with IgG2 having the lowest affinity for binding. IgG transfer from the mother to fetus begins in the second trimester, with an elevation starting at 22 weeks' gestation, with the largest amount transferred in the third trimester (Figure 2) (4-6). Accordingly, there are significantly lower levels of IgG and corresponding seroprotection to diphtheria, tetanus, pertussis, *Haemophilus influenza* type b and *Neisseria meningitides* serogroup C in preterm compared with full-term infants (7).

PLACENTAL TRANSFER OF ANTI-TNF AGENTS

Placental transfer of IFX was first published as a case report in 2006 (8). An infant born to a mother receiving IFX 10 mg/kg with the last infusion two weeks before delivery was found to have higher than expected levels at six weeks of age. Because IFX was not detected in the breast milk, this case provided the first evidence in humans of transplacental transfer of an anti-TNF agent. The authors of this case report and subsequent reviews and guidelines suggested terminating IFX at gestational week 30 (9,10). Zelinkova et al (11) then tested this guideline by determining the IFX levels in cord blood at delivery and the mothers' peripheral blood at delivery in four patients. All four patients received IFX between gestational weeks 21 and 30. Of the four infants, three had IFX levels in cord blood that were two- to threefold higher than in the peripheral blood of their mothers (mothers received IFX at gestational weeks 26, 26 and 30). The patient who received IFX at gestational week 21 gave birth to a newborn with no detectable IFX in the cord blood.

Mahadevan et al (12) studied maternal peripheral blood, and newborn cord and peripheral blood of 11 IFX-treated patients and 10 ADA-treated patients. The median time from the last dose of IFX to delivery was 35 days (range two to 91 days). In every case, the cord or infant level of IFX was higher than the mother's at the time of delivery, and took two to seven months to become undetectable. The median cord drug level was 160% of the maternal drug level (range 87% to 400%). The median time from the last dose of ADA to delivery was 5.5 weeks

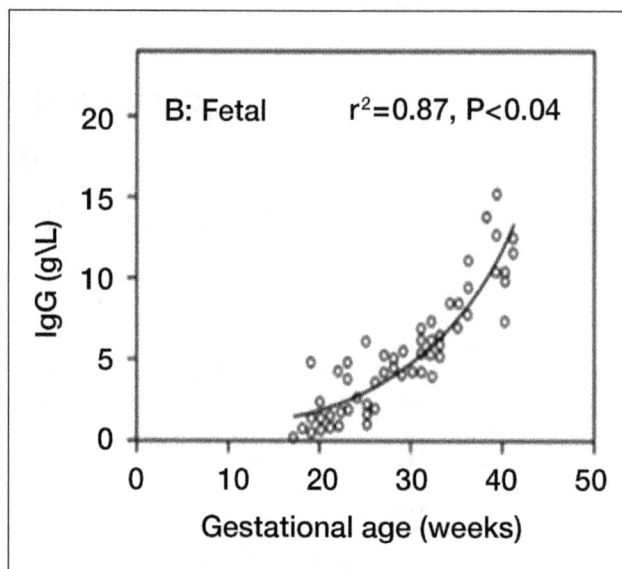

Figure 2) *Immunoglobulin G (IgG) placental transport over time. Reproduced with permission, Wiley-Blackwell Publishing Ltd, Malek A. Evolution of maternofetal transport of immunoglobulins during human pregnancy. Am J Reprod Immunol 1996;36:248-55*

(range 0.14 to 8 weeks). Again, in every case, the cord or infant level of ADA was higher than the mother's at the time of delivery, with the median cord drug level 179% of the maternal drug level (range 98% to 293%). Levels in newborns were detectable for at least 11 weeks from birth. There were no significant complications to newborns during the follow-up period in both IFX and ADA groups.

Zelinkova et al (13) further published on 31 pregnancies in 28 women with IBD: 17 IFX-treated patients and 11 ADA-treated patients. In 12 of 17 IFX-treated patients, and all 11 ADA-treated patients, anti-TNF therapy was intentionally discontinued during pregnancy before week 30 (range, gestational weeks 18 to 27). In the IFX group, they compared the cord blood of the newborn between the group that had ≤10 weeks compared with >10 weeks (the group that discontinued) from the last infusion to delivery. In the early discontinuation group the drug was stopped on average at week 23. The mean cord blood concentration of IFX was significantly lower in the early discontinuation group (13). The study was not powered to detect clinical differences in newborn outcomes and, presently, there are no published data regarding the effects of early versus late discontinuation of anti-TNF therapy on the neonatal immune system. The authors of the study recommended discontinuation of the anti-TNF agent in the second trimester, although this has been met with some controversy.

WHAT HAPPENS WHEN PATIENTS DISCONTINUE ANTI-TNF THERAPY DURING PREGNANCY?

In the same study published by Zelinkova et al (13), data regarding discontinuation of anti-TNF therapy during pregnancy demonstrated the risk for disease relapse. In the ADA group, therapy was discontinued between gestational weeks 21 and 26 in 11 patients. Two patients relapsed: one flared at gestational week 30 and required corticosteroids; the second flared at gestational week 36 and underwent an elective Caesarean section at week 37. In the IFX group, of 12 patients with early discontinuation of the therapy, one developed an allergic reaction postpartum on resumption of IFX. In total, this patient had a drug holiday of 22 weeks because of postpartum concerns about mastitis. In Leuven (Belgium), of patients taken off anti-TNF by week 22 of pregnancy, 12.5% of patients flared in the third trimester and 20.6% flared postpartum (14). In the series published by Mahadevan et al (12), 60% of patients flared when ADA was stopped >35 days before delivery.

More importantly, there are no prospective controlled data to demonstrate that corticosteroid use is safer for maternal and neonatal outcomes in the third trimester than anti-TNF therapy. Reddy et al (15) published a case control study demonstrating that pregnant women with IBD requiring hospitalization for active disease were at significant risk for preterm delivery compared with pregnant IBD patients with stable disease (mean 35.0 weeks versus 38.7 weeks; P<0.05) and were also at risk for delivering a low birthweight infant (mean 2001 g versus 3018 g; P<0.05) (15). This highlights the importance of stringent disease control during pregnancy.

SAFETY OF ANTI-TNF AGENTS DURING PREGNANCY

Although there is evidence that newborns exposed to anti-TNF therapy during gestation are born with higher levels of IFX and ADA than the mother, there are no data that these agents are associated with short-term adverse newborn outcomes. To put risks into perspective, in the general Canadian population, the rate of congenital anomalies is 6.0%, preterm birth is 7.7% and Caesarean section is 27.1% (16).

The largest prospective registry of 1052 pregnant women with IBD is the Pregnancy and Neonatal Outcomes in Women with Inflammatory Bowel Disease (PIANO) registry. In an abstract presented at Digestive Diseases Week in 2012, 797 patients had completed their pregnancy with no reported increase in congenital anomalies by drug exposure (17). Of these patients, 337 were unexposed to a biologic or a thiopurine, 265 were thiopurine exposed, 102 were biologic (IFX, ADA or certolizumab) exposed, and 59 exposed to combination biologic and thiopurine therapy. The proportion of congenital anomalies overall was 4.6%. There was no increase in preterm birth, intrauterine growth retardation, Caesarean section or neonatal intensive care unit associated with drug exposure.

Gisbert and Chaparro (18) systematically reviewed data from 21 studies involving 462 women with IBD exposed to anti-TNF agents during pregnancy and also concluded that these therapies are low risk in the short term. The overall proportion of spontaneous abortions (11%) and congenital anomalies (1.7%) were similar to the control groups. There was no increase in rates of preterm birth, intrauterine growth retardation or Caesarean section associated with drug exposure. Nielsen et al (19) published a similar systematic review, with the inclusion of 58 studies. Due to the heterogeneity of studies, results could not be meta-analyzed; however, there were four studies with a control population that reported nonsignificant ORs or relative risks for spontaneous abortion, preterm delivery, low birth weight and or congenital anomalies in patients exposed to anti-TNF therapy during pregnancy to those without anti-TNF drug exposure.

The infliximab safety database and the The Crohn's Therapy, Resource, Evaluation, and Assessment Tool Registry (TREAT) were also included in these two recent systematic reviews. The infliximab safety database is a retrospective registry maintained by the manufacturers of IFX and relies on voluntary reporting of pregnancies of women with rheumatoid arthritis (RA) or Crohn disease (20). There were 96 pregnancies that resulted in 100 births. Only two major structural anomalies were reported: one Tetralogy of Fallot and one intestinal malrotation with no differences from the observed outcomes to expected outcomes from the general population. The TREAT registry is an ongoing, prospective, observational, multicentre, long-term registry of North American patients with Crohn disease. In the TREAT registry, there were 142 IFX-exposed pregnancies with no differences in the rate of live births or congenital anomalies compared with IFX versus non-IFX-treated patients (21). A review of the FDA database of adverse events with etanercept (not used in IBD), IFX and ADA from 1999 to 2005 found a total of 61 congenital anomalies in 41 children born to mothers taking anti-TNF agents (22). Fifty-nine percent of the children had one or more congenital anomalies that were part of the VACTERL spectrum (vertebral abnormalities, anal atresia, cardiac defect, tracheoesophageal defects, renal defects, and limb defects). However, there was no denominator available for the calculation of incidence, and no child exhibited the full VACTERL syndrome, which requires a minimum of three of the seven defects to be present.

SAFETY OF ANTI-TNF THERAPY IN LONG-TERM OUTCOMES OF EXPOSED CHILDREN

Apart from data on congenital anomalies and data from PIANO on outcomes up to one year, there are little long-term data regarding outcomes of children exposed to anti-TNF therapy in utero. Bortlik et al (23) published outcomes on a series of 25 children with a median age of 34 months at the last follow-up (range 14 to 70 months) exposed to IFX or ADA. The mean gestational age of exposure to the anti-TNF agent was 26 weeks (range 17 to 37 weeks). There was one case of psychomotor delay in a boy born as a dizygotic twin and four cases of serious infections requiring hospitalization. While circulating levels of anti-TNF drug in the child were not measured, the infections occurred between 10 and 29 months of age when, according to existing pharmacokinetic data, the anti-TNF agent would likely have been cleared from the infant's circulation. There were no clinical signs of immunodeficiency or impaired cellular immunity. Mildly low levels of IgA and/or IgG were observed in seven of 17 infants. In the absence of a control group, the authors attributed the findings to transient hypogammaglobulinemia of infancy. In the same study, 15 infants exposed to IFX received the live Bacille Calmette-Guerin vaccine. Three of these children experienced local skin reactions. Despite the absence of systemic adverse effects in this study, there was a previous case report of disseminated Bacille Calmette-Guerin in an infant exposed to anti-TNF therapy in utero after receiving the live vaccine (24). Therefore, we would strongly recommend avoidance of all live vaccines in children who have had in utero exposure to anti-TNF therapy until at least six months of age.

Both the infliximab safety database (20) and the study by Carter et al (22) included patients with RA. The British Society for Rheumatology Biologics Register reported on 130 pregnancies to women with RA exposed to anti-TNF therapy during conception and or/pregnancy (25). In the subgroup of patients exposed to anti-TNF monotherapy, the rate of spontaneous abortion was 25% compared with 10% in the never-exposed group; however, the cohort was small and results were only presented descriptively. Reports of anti-TNF exposure in patients with psoriasis have been limited to case reports/series (26,27).

HOW DO WE MANAGE PATIENTS ON ANTI-TNF AGENTS DURING PREGNANCY?

At the University of Calgary (Calgary, Alberta), patients are seen preconception to discuss the benefits and potential risks of continuing therapy during pregnancy up to and including the third trimester. The decision to continue or stop a treatment during pregnancy represents a very difficult decision for gastroenterologists and patients. Given the known half-lives of IFX (9.5 days) and ADA (10 to 20 days) and the incremental rise in transplacental transfer of immunoglobulins after gestational week 22, we aim to minimize anti-TNF exposure in the final one-half of the third trimester because the results of studies investigating the long-term outcomes of children exposed to anti-TNF therapy in utero are lacking. At this time, there are insufficient data to support complete anti-TNF therapy cessation in the third trimester for the reasons outlined above, namely increased risk for disease flare. Therefore, our approach is to minimize both disease flare and neonatal exposure by modifying the timing of the last dose of anti-TNF therapy, giving it earlier in the third trimester where possible. This decision needs to be individualized, taking into consideration the disease characteristics of the patient (Figure 3).

The decision to stop anti-TNF treatment partway through pregnancy only applies to patients in stable, steroid-free remission with objective markers to confirm remission
The priority for any patient is induction and maintenance of steroid-free remission, regardless of pregnancy status. Due to the risk of flare with cessation of anti-TNF therapy, we also recommend that an

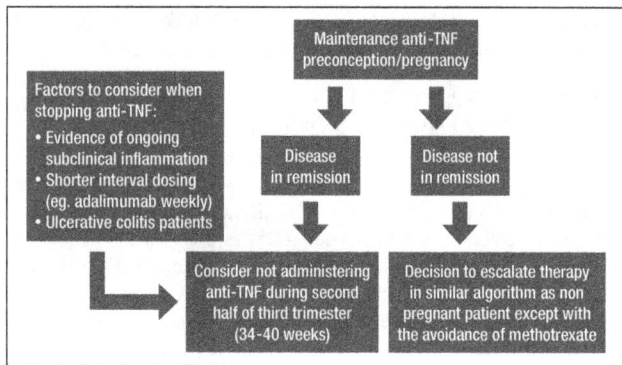

Figure 3) *Algorithm for management of patients on maintenance antitumour necrosis factor (anti-TNF) therapy*

objective measure of activity should be performed to confirm that the disease is in deep remission such as small bowel ultrasound, flexible sigmoidoscopy or fecal calprotectin.

Patients in steroid-free clinical remission who may be at risk for flare if there is a missed dose should continue therapy
Patients who are at risk for flare if there is a missed dose include individuals who feel clinically well, but are not in deep remission based on imaging (for example, patients at risk of ileal obstruction) or who have elevated biomarker levels such as fecal calprotectin.

Other factors to consider include the current dosing interval. For example, if a patient is on weekly ADA, withholding a dose in early third trimester would equate to eight to 10 missed doses, increasing the risk for flare. Finally, there is evidence that patients with ulcerative colitis are at higher risk for disease flare during pregnancy; therefore, missing multiple doses in this disease phenotype may increase their risk for flare (28).

Patients initiating anti-TNF therapy during pregnancy require special consideration
Patients initiating anti-TNF therapy while pregnant are very different from patients who enter pregnancy already on maintenance therapy. Depending on the disease severity at presentation and response to steroids, patients who are diagnosed with IBD during pregnancy may require initiation of anti-TNF therapy. Even in patients with known IBD, there is still a risk for disease flare during pregnancy (28) that may require initiation of anti-TNF therapy. Induction dosing of anti-TNF therapy depends on the stage of pregnancy (Figure 4). In patients who are at gestational week <22, anti-TNF therapy can be prescribed at standard induction-dose intervals similar to nonpregnant patients. Subsequent maintenance dosing should not be withheld in the third trimester. For patients who require anti-TNF therapy after 22 weeks' gestation, the decision to initiate anti-TNF will depend on the patient's disease activity and phenotype (similar to how nonpregnant patients are managed) with the added consideration of time to delivery. For example, in patients who are likely to imminently deliver, anti-TNF therapy can likely be delayed until after pregnancy. We recommend that all patients with a new diagnosis of IBD during pregnancy are comanaged with specialists from the high-risk obstetrics group and internists from the maternal fetal medicine group.

Patients with a well-documented history of stable remission confirmed by objective markers, on anti-TNF therapy, may discontinue therapy earlier during the pregnancy to reduce transplacental transfer of drug to the fetus
In our clinic, patients are informed that transplacental passage of anti-TNF agents begins in early second trimester, with the largest amount transferred in the third trimester. Discontinuing therapy at the start of the third trimester can represent a significant drug holiday for IFX and ADA patients, and often it is the patients themselves who are hesitant to stop the drug this early given concerns of disease flare and its impact on

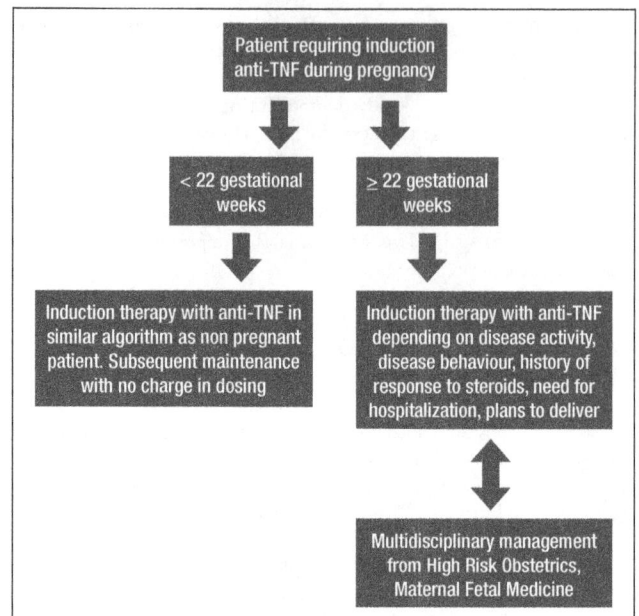

Figure 4) *Algorithm for management of patients who need antitumour necrosis factor (anti-TNF) induction during pregnancy and subsequent maintenance*

both mother and child. Ongoing and open dialogue between physician and patient is fundamental and, when presented with the data, the majority of our patients choose to accept anti-TNF therapy during early third trimester. The majority of our patients on eight-weekly dosing for IFX and bi-weekly dosing of ADA receive their last dose of anti-TNF therapy at gestational week 32 for IFX and gestational week 34 for ADA.

Monotherapy or combination therapy in pregnancy and issues of immunogenicity
Studies investigating anti-TNF levels and antidrug antibody levels during pregnancy are not available at this time. Immunogenicity or the presence of antidrug antibodies are associated with adverse reactions and reduced efficacy of therapy (29,30). Therefore, in our practice, we do not routinely discontinue thiopurines that are used in combination with anti-TNF therapy if the patient was on the thiopurine during preconception. In the case of a patient who wants to stop concomitant thiopurine therapy, we discuss the benefits and risks of monotherapy and combination therapy. Additionally, we discuss the extensive data on the safety of thiopurines in pregnancy (31-33). However, due to its FDA rating of D, despite education of its excellent safety profile during pregnancy, many patients are inclined to stop this class of drugs during pregnancy when used as a concomitant immunomodulator. For patients who are initiating anti-TNF therapy during pregnancy, we tend not to start thiopurines for the first time during pregnancy (as the concomitant immunomodulator) due to the small but possible risk of thiopurine-associated pancreatitis and hepatitis, and side effects such as nausea and malaise.

Methotrexate is a well known teratogen in women and should be stopped a minimum of six months before conception.

Role of therapeutic drug monitoring in pregnancy
Presently, there are no data on anti-TNF therapy therapeutic drug monitoring in pregnancy to guide or optimize dosing. Therefore, we recommend that clinicians use the same decision making in pregnant patients as they would in their nonpregnant patients.

Unanswered questions
1. What are the long-term effects on the immune system of children born to mothers on anti-TNF agents? If there are implications for the immune system of children, does this change depending on trimester exposure?

2. Can anti-TNF therapeutic drug monitoring in the first trimester with subsequent modification of dose and dosing interval be used to optimize disease course for the remainder of the pregnancy and postpartum?

3. Can we individualize anti-TNF therapy based on an understanding of an individual's pharmacokinetics and, therefore, tailor dosing during pregnancy to minimize placental transfer? In other words, change the dose but not stop therapy.

FUTURE DIRECTIONS

With the introduction of new therapeutic molecules on the market for the treatment of IBD, the uptake of anti-TNF therapy and other biologics will likely continue to increase and, therefore, an increasing number of patients in their reproductive years will be on these agents. In response to the abovementioned clinical and research needs, a Maternofetal Outcomes Research in IBD – Canadian Registry (MORe CaRe) has been started with two fundamental goals. The first goal is to optimize the clinical care of pregnant IBD patients through education, continuing medical education of physicians (family physicians, obstetricians and fertility experts, and gastroenterologists), and establishment of clinical care pathways and guidelines that apply to Canadian practitioners. The second goal is to establish a national biorepository with biospecimens from mother's peripheral blood, breastmilk, cord blood and infant peripheral blood to answer additional questions regarding the long-term safety and optimal use of biologics in pregnancy.

REFERENCES

1. Arsenescu R, Arsenescu V, de Villiers WJ. TNF-alpha and the development of the neonatal immune system: Implications for inhibitor use in pregnancy. Am J Gastroenterol 2011;106:559-62.
2. Mahadevan U, Cucchiara S, Hyams JS, et al. The London position statement of the World Congress of Gastroenterology on Biological Therapy for IBD with the European Crohn's and Colitis Organisation: Pregnancy and pediatrics. Am J Gastroenterol 2011;106:214-23; quiz 24.
3. Firan M, Bawdon R, Radu C, et al. The MHC class I-related receptor, FcRn, plays an essential role in the maternofetal transfer of gamma-globulin in humans. Int Immunol 2001;13:993-1002.
4. Palmeira P, Quinello C, Silveira-Lessa AL, Zago CA, Carneiro-Sampaio M. IgG placental transfer in healthy and pathological pregnancies. Clin Developmental Immunol 2012;2012:985646.
5. Saji F, Samejima Y, Kamiura S, Koyama M. Dynamics of immunoglobulins at the feto-maternal interface. Rev Reproduction 1999;4:81-9.
6. Malek A, Sager R, Kuhn P, Nicolaides KH, Schneider H. Evolution of maternofetal transport of immunoglobulins during human pregnancy. Am J Reproductive Immunol 1996;36:248-55.
7. van den Berg JP, Westerbeek EA, Berbers GA, van Gageldonk PG, van der Klis FR, van Elburg RM. Transplacental transport of IgG antibodies specific for pertussis, diphtheria, tetanus, Haemophilus influenzae type b, and Neisseria meningitidis serogroup C is lower in preterm compared with term infants. Pediatr Infect Dis J 2010;29:801-5.
8. Vasiliauskas EA, Church JA, Silverman N, Barry M, Targan SR, Dubinsky MC. Case report: Evidence for transplacental transfer of maternally administered infliximab to the newborn. Clin Gastroenterol Hepatol 2006;4:1255-8.
9. Gisbert JP. Safety of immunomodulators and biologics for the treatment of inflammatory bowel disease during pregnancy and breast-feeding. Inflamm Bowel Dis 2010;16:881-95.
10. Van Assche G, Dignass A, Reinisch W, et al. The second European evidence-based consensus on the diagnosis and management of Crohn's disease: Special situations. J Crohn's Colitis. 2010;4:63-101.
11. Zelinkova Z, de Haar C, de Ridder L, et al. High intra-uterine exposure to infliximab following maternal anti-TNF treatment during pregnancy. Aliment Pharmacol Ther 2011;33:1053-8.
12. Mahadevan U, Wolf DC, Dubinsky M, et al. Placental transfer of anti-tumor necrosis factor agents in pregnant patients with inflammatory bowel disease. Clin Gastroenterol Hepatol 2013;11:286-92

13. Zelinkova Z, van der Ent C, Bruin KF, et al; Dutch Delta IBD Group. Effects of discontinuing anti-tumor necrosis factor therapy during pregnancy on the course of inflammatory bowel disease and neonatal exposure. Clin Gastroenterol Hepatol 2013;11:318-21.
14. Schnitzler F, Fidder H, Ferrante M, et al. Outcome of pregnancy in women with inflammatory bowel disease treated with antitumor necrosis factor therapy. Inflamm Bowel Dis 2011;17:1846-54.
15. Reddy D, Murphy SJ, Kane SV, Present DH, Kornbluth AA. Relapses of inflammatory bowel disease during pregnancy: In-hospital management and birth outcomes. Am J Gastroenterol 2008;103:1203-9.
16. Information CIfH. In due time, why maternal age matters 2011. <https://secure.cihi.ca/free_products/AIB_InDueTime_WhyMaternalAgeMatters_E.pdf> (Accessed February 17, 2014).
17. Mahadevan U, Martin C, Sandler RS, et al. PIANO: A 1000 patient prospective registry of pregnancy outcomes in women with IBD exposed to immunomodulators and biologic. Gastroenterology 2012;142:S-149. (Abst)
18. Gisbert JP, Chaparro M. Safety of anti-TNF agents during pregnancy and breastfeeding in women with inflammatory bowel disease. Am J Gastroenterol 2013;108:1426-38.
19. Nielsen OH, Loftus EV Jr, Jess T. Safety of TNF-alpha inhibitors during IBD pregnancy: A systematic review. BMC Med 2013;11:174.
20. Katz JA, Antoni C, Keenan GF, Smith DE, Jacobs SJ, Lichtenstein GR. Outcome of pregnancy in women receiving infliximab for the treatment of Crohn's disease and rheumatoid arthritis. Am J Gastroenterol 2004;99:2385-92.
21. Lichtenstein GR, Feagan BG, Cohen RD, et al. Serious infection and mortality in patients with Crohn's disease: More than 5 years of follow-up in the TREAT registry. Am J Gastroenterol 2012;107:1409-22.
22. Carter JD, Ladhani A, Ricca LR, Valeriano J, Vasey FB. A safety assessment of tumor necrosis factor antagonists during pregnancy: A review of the Food and Drug Administration database. J Rheumatol 2009;36:635-41.
23. Bortlik M, Duricova D, Machkova N, et al. Impact of anti-tumor necrosis factor alpha antibodies administered to pregnant women with inflammatory bowel disease on long-term outcome of exposed children. Inflamm Bowel Dis 2014;20:495-501.
24. Cheent K, Nolan J, Shariq S, Kiho L, Pal A, Arnold J. Case report: Fatal case of disseminated BCG infection in an infant born to a mother taking infliximab for Crohn's disease. J Crohn's Colitis 2010;4:603-5.
25. Verstappen SM, King Y, Watson KD, Symmons DP, Hyrich KL; BSRBR Control Centre Consortium. Anti-TNF therapies and pregnancy: Outcome of 130 pregnancies in the British Society for Rheumatology Biologics Register. Ann Rheumatic Dis 2011;70:823-6.
26. Puig L, Barco D, Alomar A. Treatment of psoriasis with anti-TNF drugs during pregnancy: Case report and review of the literature. Dermatology 2010;220:71-6.
27. Berthelot JM, De Bandt M, Goupille P, et al. Exposition to anti-TNF drugs during pregnancy: Outcome of 15 cases and review of the literature. Joint Bone Spine 2009;76:28-34.
28. Pedersen N, Bortoli A, Duricova D, et al. The course of inflammatory bowel disease during pregnancy and postpartum: A prospective European ECCO-EpiCom Study of 209 pregnant women. Aliment Pharmacol Ther 2013;38:501-12.
29. Karmiris K, Paintaud G, Noman M, et al. Influence of trough serum levels and immunogenicity on long-term outcome of adalimumab therapy in Crohn's disease. Gastroenterology 2009;137:1628-40.
30. Baert F, Noman M, Vermeire S, et al. Influence of immunogenicity on the long-term efficacy of infliximab in Crohn's disease. N Engl J Med 2003;348:601-8.
31. de Meij TG, Jharap B, Kneepkens CM, van Bodegraven AA, de Boer NK; Dutch Initiative on Crohn and Colitis. Long-term follow-up of children exposed intrauterine to maternal thiopurine therapy during pregnancy in females with inflammatory bowel disease. Aliment Pharmacol Ther 2013;38:38-43.
32. Coelho J, Beaugerie L, Colombel JF, et al. Pregnancy outcome in patients with inflammatory bowel disease treated with thiopurines: Cohort from the CESAME Study. Gut 2011;60:198-203.
33. Casanova MJ, Chaparro M, Domenech E, et al. Safety of thiopurines and anti-TNF-alpha drugs during pregnancy in patients with inflammatory bowel disease. Am J Gastroenterol 2013;108:433-40.

29

Gastroesophageal reflux symptoms not responding to proton pump inhibitor: GERD, NERD, NARD, esophageal hypersensitivity or dyspepsia?

Mohammad Bashashati MD[1], Reza A Hejazi MD[2], Christopher N Andrews MD[3], Martin A Storr MD[1,4]

M Bashashati, RA Hejazi, CN Andrews, MA Storr. Gastroesophageal reflux symptoms not responding to proton pump inhibitor: GERD, NERD, NARD, esophageal hypersensitivity or dyspepsia? Can J Gastroenterol Hepatol 2014;28(6):335-341.

Gastroesophageal reflux (GER) is a common gastrointestinal process that can generate symptoms of heartburn and chest pain. Proton pump inhibitors (PPIs) are the gold standard for the treatment of GER; however, a substantial group of GER patients fail to respond to PPIs. In the past, it was believed that acid reflux into the esophagus causes all, or at least the majority, of symptoms attributed to GER, with both erosive esophagitis and nonerosive outcomes. However, with modern testing techniques it has been shown that, in addition to acid reflux, the reflux of nonacid gastric and duodenal contents into the esophagus may also induce GER symptoms. It remains unknown how weakly acidic or alkaline refluxate with a pH similar to a normal diet induces GER symptoms. Esophageal hypersensitivity or functional dyspepsia with superimposed heartburn may be other mechanisms of symptom generation, often completely unrelated to GER. Detailed studies investigating the pathophysiology of esophageal hypersensitivity are not conclusive, and definitions of the various disease states may overlap and are often confusing. The authors aim to clarify the pathophysiology, definition, diagnostic techniques and medical treatment of patients with heartburn symptoms who fail PPI therapy.

Key Words: *Gastroesophageal reflux disease; Heartburn; Proton pump inhibitor*

Les symptômes de reflux gastro-œsophagien ne répondant pas aux inhibiteurs de la pompe à protons : RGO, RNE, RNA, hypersensibilité œsophagienne ou dyspepsie?

Le reflux gastro-œsophagien (RGO) est un processus gastro-intestinal fréquent qui peut provoquer des symptômes de brûlures d'estomac et de douleurs thoraciques. Les inhibiteurs de la pompe à protons (IPP) représentent la norme du traitement du RGO, mais un groupe important de patients qui en sont atteints n'y répondent pas. Par le passé, on pensait que le reflux acide dans l'œsophage était responsable de la totalité, ou du moins de la majorité, des symptômes attribués au RGO, y compris une œsophagite érosive et des manifestations non érosives. Cependant, les techniques d'examen modernes démontrent qu'en plus du reflux acide, le reflux de contenu gastrique et duodénal non gastrique dans l'œsophage peut également produire des symptômes de RGO. On ne sait pas si le liquide de reflux peu acide ou alcalin, au pH similaire à celui d'une alimentation normale, produit des symptômes de RGO. L'hypersensibilité œsophagienne ou la dyspepsie fonctionnelle accompagnée de brûlures d'estomac peuvent constituer d'autres mécanismes de production des symptômes, qui n'ont souvent rien à voir avec le RGO. Des études détaillées portant sur la physiopathologie de l'hypersensibilité œsophagienne ne sont pas concluantes, et les définitions des divers états de la maladie peuvent se chevaucher et prêtent souvent à confusion. Les auteurs cherchent à présenter clairement la physiopathologie, la définition, les techniques diagnostiques et les traitements médicaux des patients ayant des symptômes de brûlures d'estomac qui ne répondent pas aux IPP.

Symptoms suggestive of gastroesophageal reflux (GER; eg, heartburn, reflux or chest pain) affect up to 30% of the population in Western countries and their prevalence continues to increase (1-3). Management of patients with GER symptoms is one of the most expensive among chronic gastrointestinal disorders, with direct and indirect costs in the United States estimated to be $10 billion annually (4). Proton pump inhibitors (PPIs) are the gold standard treatment for GER and account for two of the top-five selling drugs in the United States (5).

Recent studies have shown that approximately 10% to 40% of patients with GER symptoms fail to respond to standard-dose PPIs. Although PPI factors may play a role (such as inadequate dosing or nonadherence to treatment), other factors such as visceral hypersensitivity, upper gut dysmotility or inflammatory disorders, may underlie PPI failure (6,7). Based on a recent study (8), up to 35% of patients with PPI failure had an underlying pathology other than acid reflux.

Considering the economic burden of GER and PPI use on one hand and the substantial PPI failure rate on the other, it must be questioned whether acid suppression with PPIs is always being

used optimally for the treatment of GER symptoms. Thus, a better understanding of the underlying etiologies of these symptoms may help to optimize treatment. In the present review, we discuss the potential mechanisms involved in the genesis of symptoms in patients with GER, possible causes of PPI failure, diagnostic tests and available treatments for PPI failure.

DEFINITION AND ETIOLOGIES OF GER SYMPTOMS

Gastroesophageal reflux disease, nonerosive reflux disease, nonacid reflux disease, functional esophageal disorders and noncardiac chest pain

GER symptoms include the classic definition of reflux – a rising retrosternal burning sensation. In English, the terms 'reflux' and 'heartburn' are generally used interchangeably. Chest pain (typically after cardiac evaluation rules out cardiac sources and, thus, termed 'noncardiac chest pain' [NCCP]) is also commonly included as a GER symptom but dysphagia is not. GER symptoms may result from acid reflux, esophageal hypersensitivity, sustained esophageal contractions or

[1]*Gastrointestinal Research Group, University of Calgary, Calgary, Alberta;* [2]*Department of Internal Medicine, Texas Tech University Health Sciences Center, Paul L Foster School of Medicine, El Paso, Texas, USA;* [3]*Division of Gastroenterology, Department of Medicine, University of Calgary, Calgary, Alberta;* [4]*Division of Gastroenterology, Ludwig Maximilians University of Munich, Munich, Germany*
Correspondence: Dr Martin A Storr, Department of Medicine, Division of Gastroenterology, Ludwig Maximilians University of Munich, Munich, Germany. e-mail martin.storr@med.uni-muenchen.de

abnormal tissue resistance (9). The nomenclature for etiologies of GER symptoms can be confusing and the definitions may overlap.

GER disease (GERD) is caused by the reflux of gastric contents into the esophagus and may or may not induce esophageal injury, although the original definition (in the pre-PPI era) usually meant erosive esophagitis (10,11). The mechanisms underlying GERD remain debatable (12); however, transient lower esophageal sphincter relaxation (TLESR), hypotensive lower esophageal sphincter (LES) and retrograde movement of gastric or duodenal contents into the esophagus are the accepted major pathologies in GERD (13).

Nonerosive reflux disease (NERD) refers to the presence of GER symptoms attributed to the (typically acidic) reflux of gastric contents into the esophagus but without endoscopically visible esophageal inflammation.

Esophageal hypersensitivity may be an independent phenomenon or may overlap with GERD. It describes a condition in which an esophageal stimulus that does not lead to any esophageal injury induces symptoms such as heartburn and chest pain. In other words, patients with esophageal hypersensitivity have a lower threshold for the perception of physiologically nonpainful stimuli (14). According to the American Gastroenterological Association consensus on GERD (15), hypersensitivity symptoms are attributable to reflux events, whereas functional heartburn is not associated with reflux events. Despite this definition, esophageal hypersensitivity may be apparent in GERD, nonacid reflux disease or weakly acid reflux disease, and functional esophageal disorders.

Esophageal hypersensitivity has overlap with functional esophageal disorders including functional heartburn, functional chest pain of presumed esophageal origin or NCCP. Functional heartburn is a controversial issue from both the diagnostic and pathophysiological perspectives. According to the Rome III criteria, burning retrosternal discomfort or pain without any evidence of gastroesophageal acid reflux or esophageal motility disorder for the past three months and with symptom onset at least six months before the diagnosis is defined as functional heartburn. The symptoms of these patients are often indistinguishable from GERD. The Rome committee suggested that histopathology and a gastroesophageal acid reflux work-up should be performed to rule out acid reflux and eosinophilic esophagitis in these patients (16,17). Based on the Rome III criteria, chest pain without evidence of GERD or esophageal motility disorder is known as functional chest pain of presumed esophageal origin. Acidity, mechanical distension, osmolality, temperature, as well as esophageal muscular contractions have been considered to be potential causes of the chest pain in this group. Finally, NCCP is defined as angina-like chest pain in patients in whom a cardiac pathology is ruled out (18,19).

Esophageal motility disorders and eosinophilic esophagitis

Esophageal motility disorders, such as diffuse esophageal spasm, may also present with GER symptoms (eg, reflux and chest pain), but patients rarely complain about reflux as the sole symptom (20). Eosinophilic esophagitis is an increasingly common cause of GER symptoms and dysphagia. Because esophageal intramucosal eosinophilia is a frequent finding associated with GERD, lack of histological response to high-dose PPIs should be considered before making the final diagnosis (21-23). On the other hand, in recent years, a form of esophageal eosinophilia has been recognized that responds to PPI therapy. The recognition of PPI-responsive esophageal eosinophilia (PPI-REE) has made the diagnosis of eosinophilic esophagitis more difficult because lack of response to PPI therapy was a previously important diagnostic criterion for eosinophilic esophagitis. As a result, based on recent guidelines, exclusion of PPI-REE with a PPI is required for the diagnosis of eosinophilic esophagitis. Whether PPI-REE is a form of GERD-induced esophageal eosinophilia is not clear. To determine whether reflux is the underlying cause of eosinophila, further evaluation for NERD may be necessary (24,25).

GERD not only presents with esophageal symptoms but also may manifest with symptoms of dyspepsia (26). Therefore, it is wise to test for acid reflux in dyspeptic patients with dominant esophageal symptoms.

In summary, symptoms of GER (eg, heartburn or chest pain) may occur with acid reflux, nonacidic or weakly acidic reflux, functional esophageal disorders, esophageal motility disorders, eosinophilic esophagitis or other organic/anatomical disorders of the esophagus. All of these etiologies should be considered in patients with GER symptoms. Moreover, drugs, such as nonsteroidal anti-inflammatory drugs, tetracyclines and bisphosphonates, may induce esophagitis and GER symptoms (27).

CURRENT APPROACH TO PATIENTS WITH GER SYMPTOMS

Taking an appropriate history is an important step in diagnosis. Accompanying symptoms and a drug history are two important parameters that must be included. Review of eating habits and diet may be helpful in some patients (ie, avoiding large meals just before bed or raising the head of the bed); however, there is little evidence to support these interventions. Weight loss may appreciably improve GER symptoms (28). Urgent upper endoscopy is required for evaluation of patients with alarm symptoms (dysphagia, vomiting, weight loss, anemia or an abnormal physical examination). In patients with GER symptoms and no alarm features, acid suppression therapy using a regular dose of PPI for at least eight weeks should be started (Table 1).

DIAGNOSTIC APPROACH TO REFRACTORY PATIENTS

Initial response to PPI therapy should be assessed clinically after four to eight weeks. Failure to respond to a regular dose of PPI is defined as refractory GERD (6,15). In patients with persistent symptoms, assessment of the method of administration of PPI is important because patients frequently perform it incorrectly. Doubling the dose of PPI or switching to another PPI may also be beneficial, although the evidence for these manoeuvres is weak. In refractory patients or those with new or worsening symptoms on high-dose PPIs, endoscopy and biopsy are indicated (10). The current approach to PPI failure is summarized in Figure 1. Although the majority of patients with GERD are adherent to PPI therapy (29), PPI failure may occur in patients who take PPIs incorrectly. Failing to take doses 30 min to 60 min before a meal will lead to lower effectiveness because gastric acid production is stimulated by food, and the proton pumps are inactivated by PPI during acid production. A common example is taking PPI at bedtime for night-time symptoms, which is less effective than taking the dose before the evening meal. This is a more important issue for an immediate-release PPIs but less so for a PPI with a dual-dose (combined immediate release/slow-release) formulation such as dexlansoprazole. Similarly, failing to take the medication at all or infrequent, as-needed use will significantly reduce the overall benefit from PPI.

Variability in PPI metabolism is another possible cause of PPI failure that is less well understood. Cytochrome P450 is the major enzyme involved in the metabolic degradation of PPIs, with CYP2C19 and CYP3A4 isoenzymes being the most important (30). Patients with the CYP2C19 wild-type allele are considered to be rapid metabolizers and those who possess the CYP2C19*17 allele are ultrarapid metabolizers. Rapid metabolizers will have lower serum levels of PPI, leading to less effect. The clinical benefit of CYP2C19 genotype testing in GERD, and especially in PPI failure, is unclear (31), particularly because it is easier to empirically increase the dose than to perform genotypic analysis. The potential causes of PPI failure are summarized in Table 2.

Insufficient response to high-dose PPIs in patients with normal endoscopy and biopsy is an indication for esophageal manometry and esophageal pH monitoring (6,15). Manometry is generally required to document the location of the lower esophageal sphincter for suitable pH probe placement. In certain cases, significant primary esophageal motility disorders that may lead to symptoms of reflux or regurgitation (such as achalasia or scleroderma) may also be diagnosed on manometry.

TABLE 1
Potential medications for gastroesophageal reflux symptoms

Class	Mechanism	Medication	Standard dose	Double-dose (refractory)
Proton pump inhibitors	Inhibition of gastric acid secretion through blocking (H+, K+)-ATPase enzyme	Omeprazole	20 mg daily	20 mg twice daily
		Pantoprazole	40 mg daily	40 mg twice daily
		Esomeprazole	40 mg daily	40mg twice daily
		Rabeprazole	20 mg daily	20 mg twice daily
		Lansoprazole	30 mg daily	30 mg twice daily
Prokinetics/TLESR inhibitors	D2 receptor antagonist	Metoclopramide	10–15 mg up to 4 times daily	
	Peripherally acting D2 receptor antagonist	Domperidone*	10 mg 3 times daily	
	Gamma-aminobutyric acid-B receptor agonists	Baclofen	10–20 mg 2–3 times daily	
Antinociceptives	Tricyclic antidepressants	Imipramine	10–50 mg at bedtime	
		Nortriptyline	10–25 mg at bedtime	
	Serotonin reuptake inhibitors	Trazodone	100–150 mg at bedtime	
	Selective serotonin reuptake inhibitors	Sertraline	50–200 mg at bedtime	
		Paroxetine	10–40 mg daily	
	Serotonin and norepinephrine reuptake inhibitors	Venlafaxine	75 mg daily	
	Inhibiting excitatory neurotransmitter release	Pregabalin	50 mg 3 times daily	

*Data adapted from references 60, 85-87. *In patients with dyspepsia and delayed gastric emptying. TLESR Transient lower esophageal sphincter relaxation*

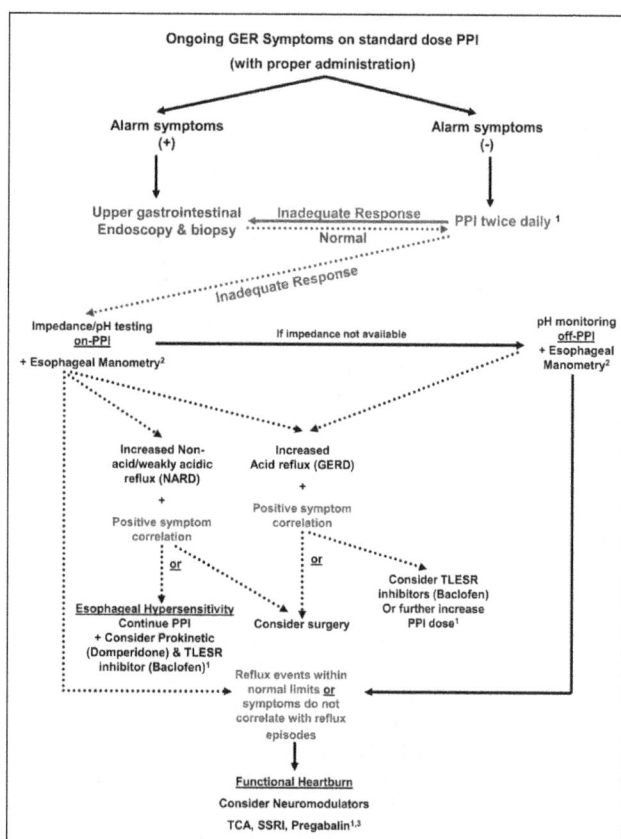

Figure 1) *Approach to proton pump inhibitor (PPI) failure in patients with gastroesophageal reflux (GER) symptoms. Alarm symptoms: weight loss, dysphagia, gastrointestinal bleeding, age >55 years, etc. [1]If additional dyspeptic symptoms, treat as functional dyspepsia; [2]If esophageal manometry shows specific diagnosis (eg, achalasia or spastic disorder), treat as appropriate, if only nonspecific, abnormalites are apparent (eg, ineffectual esophageal motility), continue on pathway; [3]Consider transient lower esophageal sphincter relaxation (TLESR) inhibitors if the diagnosis is based on pH monitoring and not impedance testing. TCA Tricyclic antidepressant; SSRI Selective serotonin reuptake inhibitor*

TABLE 2
Causes of proton pump inhibitor (PPI) failure

PPI related	Insufficient dose
	Nonadherence
	Genetical/pharmacological rapid/ultra-rapid metabolism
Reflux related	Nonacid/weakly acidic reflux
Esophageal	Esophageal hypersensitivity
	Esophageal motility disorders
	Eosinophilic esophagitis
	Anatomical abnormality (eg, hiatal hernia, malignancy)
Gastric	Dyspepsia
	Gastroparesis

Esophageal pH testing

Esophageal pH testing has been used for decades to measure the degree of acid exposure in the esophagus. Transnasal catheter-based methods remain the most commonly used in Canada and are typically left in situ for 24 h. Wireless, capsule-based pH testing methods that are fixed to the esophageal mucosa (Bravo system, Given Imaging Inc, Israel) are also available and are typically measured over 48 h. Patients push a button on a pH recorder when they experience symptoms so that the symptom event may be correlated with the presence or absence of a reflux event. Acid reflux is defined as a pH <4 in the esophagus.

The sensitivity of pH testing for acid reflux is obviously optimal with patients off PPIs. Thus, a pH study used to document the severity and extent of acid reflux in the natural state (eg, for preoperative work-up for a fundoplication) should be performed with the patient off PPIs for five to seven days before the study. However, if a patient continues to experience symptoms on PPIs, performing a standard pH study with the patient on PPIs may only yield information about acid breakthrough and will not provide any information about nonacidic reflux events. A normal pH study on PPIs suggests either nonacid reflux or esophageal hypersensitivity, but will not be able to differentiate between the two (32).

Esophageal impedance testing

Esophageal multichannel intraluminal impedance (MII) testing is a catheter-based method similar to catheter-based pH testing. By recording changes in resistance to electrical currents, numerous impedance sensors on the catheter can measure both bolus type (liquid or gas) and direction (aboral or oral), regardless of pH in the esophagus. The catheter also contains standard pH sensor(s) so that boluses can be characterized as acidic or otherwise. In patients with refractory symptoms, MII is recommended (6); however, consensus has not yet implemented this as a routine approach (10,15). Using this technique, it was discovered that nonacidic reflux from the stomach into the esophagus was common. Using combined pH/impedance testing, GER is generally grouped into classical acid reflux (pH <4) or nonacid reflux (pH >4). The latter can be categorized into weakly acid (4 <pH <7) and weakly alkaline reflux (pH ≥7) (33,34).

Based on a study using pH/MII monitoring, the majority of symptomatic reflux episodes in patients who failed to respond to a PPI were weakly acidic (35). This study, along with others, suggests high proximal extent of the refluxate and sensitization of the esophagus by preceding acid exposure as the most probable causes of sustained symptoms in patients treated with a PPI (35-37). Another study revealed that impedance testing of patients with NERD for possible underlying nonacid reflux decreased the number of patients diagnosed with functional heartburn (38). Accordingly, we can speculate that patients who were diagnosed with functional heartburn in the preimpedance testing era should now be retested, and grouped into patients experiencing either nonacid reflux or nonreflux disorders. Because there may be a substantial overlap between functional heartburn and nonacid reflux, esophageal impedance testing may help in clarifying it to some extent (33).

In patients with inadequate response to PPI treatment, it is important to assess the relationship between patients' reported symptoms and esophageal acid or nonacid reflux events. For this, indexes, such as the symptom index and symptom association probability, are used. These indexes and their value and limitations are clearly discussed elsewhere (39).

Testing for esophageal hypersensitivity

Because esophageal hypersensitivity represents a lowered threshold of perception and symptoms in response to the same degree of chemical, mechanical, emotional or unidentified stimuli (14), lack of diagnostic methods and variability of the stimuli make the diagnosis of this condition challenging.

A convenient diagnostic test for esophageal hypersensitivity in the presence of acid reflux is not available. In the 1950s, Bernstein and Baker (40), and Berstein et al (41) introduced a test for the diagnosis of esophagitis using mild hydrochloric acid infusion into the esophagus to induce esophageal pain in patients with GERD. A positive test result was defined as the generation of typical GERD symptoms. At that time, Bernstein and Baker could not perform esophageal pH monitoring to define a clear association between acid reflux and GERD symptoms. Subsequently, Jung et al (42) performed both esophageal pH monitoring and a Bernstein test simultaneously in patients with heartburn, and no correlation between positive symptom indexes and positive Bernstein results was apparent. Esophageal hypersensitivity to acid stimulation may be a distinct category that may not be related to acid reflux; the benefit of a Bernstein test within the diagnostic approach to GERD or functional esophageal disorders is undefined.

The potential role of esophageal hypersensitivity in nonacid reflux is not known. It is not clear what induces symptoms in patients with weakly acidic or alkaline reflux. A previous study showed that patients with GERD, and especially those with NERD, are hypersensitive to esophageal perfusion with acid as well as with saline (43). This finding also supports the non-acid-dependent role of esophageal hypersensitivity in the presentation of reflux symptoms (43). Interestingly, another study showed that infusion of bile salts into the esophagus can induce pain in 100% of patients previously diagnosed with functional heartburn and also induced pain in some of the healthy controls (44).

In a previous study, despite negative endoscopy and pH monitoring, approximately 30% of individuals who were chronically using antacids for heartburn experienced esophageal hypersensitivity to both acid and mechanical stimuli (45). Another study showed that patients with a history of functional heartburn with negative pH monitoring and PPI failure were more sensitive to both esophageal balloon distention and acid perfusion compared with patients with NERD (46). It was also shown that patients with normal acid exposure but symptom-associated reflux events ≥50% had a lower threshold for both initial perception and discomfort in response to esophageal balloon distension compared with healthy controls or patients with acid reflux (47). Based on studies using a balloon-distension test, approximately 80% of patients with functional chest pain have a hypersensitive esophagus with lower thresholds for perception, discomfort and pain (48,49). Moreover, studies showed no symptoms after acid perfusion in up to 90% of patients with NCCP (50) and hypersensitivity to acid is not a general phenomenon in patients with functional heartburn because these patients have more somatization features, reports of chest pain and changes in autonomic function compared with NERD patients with abnormal pH recordings (51).

The above-mentioned studies indicate that esophageal exposure to high or low pH, as well as mechanical stimulation, may induce symptoms in patients with GERD and/or functional esophageal disorders. Regardless of the reflux contents, it should be emphasized that esophageal hypersensitivity may play a critical role in the development of heartburn. In patients with GER symptoms, visceral hypersensitivity may occur as a consequence of long-term exposure to acid or nonacid reflux, or may even be present without exposure to erosive substances. However, it remains unclear whether esophageal hypersensitivity is a primary or secondary phenomenon. The concept of hypersensitivity following a previous insult has been suggested to play a major role in other hypersensitivity disorders (eg, irritable bowel syndrome) in which a previous infection triggers visceral hypersensitivity (52). Exposure to acid may, thus, be the initial insult inducing esophageal hypersensitivity later in life. Whether and how weakly acidic or weakly alkaline reflux potentially induce hypersensitivity has yet to be studied. One previous study showed that experimental short exposure of rabbit esophageal mucosa to bile acids in acidic, weakly acidic or neutral conditions may change mucosal permeability and, in some conditions, may impair esophageal mucosal integrity (53). Other potential underlying mechanisms include activation of acid-sensitive ion channels or esophageal mechanoreceptors, changes in afferent sensory neuron conductivity, as well as alterations in central processing; all of these warrant further investigation (46,54). Dilation of intercellular spaces has also been reported in patients with GERD (55,56).

Collectively, GER symptoms may be apparent in patients with acid reflux, nonacid reflux, esophageal hypersensitivity, esophageal dysmotility, eosinophilic esophagitis and other organic diseases. Therefore, in patients with GER symptoms and PPI failure, a comprehensive evaluation may often be required including endoscopy with biopsy, esophageal manometry and combined pH/impedance testing.

Tests in patients with refractory GERD with dyspepsia

Patients with dyspepsia present with epigastric pain or burning, early satiety and postprandial fullness. The differential diagnosis of dyspepsia is broad and because it has substantial overlap with GERD, a work-up is essential to differentiate GER symptoms with an underlying esophageal pathology from dyspeptic patients with additional GERD-suggesting symptoms. Studies have shown that 10% to 33% of patients with GERD have some form of delayed gastric emptying. It appears that delayed gastric emptying correlates with less acidic but more voluminous refluxate to the proximal esophagus (57,58). Most patients with refractory GERD do not require gastric emptying testing unless they also have symptoms of severe dyspepsia, vomiting or gastroparesis.

MEDICAL TREATMENT OF REFRACTORY GER SYMPTOMS

Current medications

As mentioned, GER symptoms may be caused by acid reflux, nonacid reflux, motility disorders of the esophagus, esophageal hypersensitivity, eosinophilic esophagitis or other organic diseases. After ruling out alarm symptoms, treatment of patients with GER symptoms primarily consists of avoiding culprit foods and exacerbating behaviours, losing weight and acid suppression with a regular-dose PPI (Table 1).

In refractory GER symptoms and in the absence of alarm symptoms, patients are treated with double-dose PPI (6). In rapid metabolizers, giving even higher doses of PPI (quadruple dose) may be beneficial (31). Because genotype testing for metabolism alleles is generally not available, the rationale for giving more than double-dose PPI would have to be based on a pH study that shows persisting significant acid reflux despite correctly administered PPI use.

By including esophageal hypersensitivity as a possible cause of patients' symptoms, visceral analgesics can be beneficial in the treatment of patients with GER symptoms who do not respond to double-dose PPI treatment. Pain modulators, such as tricyclic antidepressants, selective serotonin reuptake inhibitors (SSRIs) and serotonin-norepinephrine reuptake inhibitors (SNRIs) all improve esophageal pain in patients with NCCP and are helpful in patients with refractory GERD (59). Based on a systematic review of antidepressants in patients with NCCP, which included six randomized trials studying SSRIs (paroxetine and sertraline), tricyclic antidepressants (impramine), SNRI (venlafaxine) and a triazolopyridine (trazodone), the percentage reduction in chest pain with venlafaxine, sertraline and imipramine was 50% to 63%, while it was 1% to 15% in the placebo group. This improvement was independent of improvement of depression scores. On the other hand, the adverse effects were relatively high in the treated groups and were the reported reason for discontinuation of trials in 53% of patients from the antidepressant groups (60). The effective doses of these antidepressants are summarized in Table 1.

Moreover, we know that TLESRs play a crucial role in the pathophysiology of GERD. Prokinetics, such as dopamine-2 receptor antagonists (eg, metoclopramide and domperidone), and TLESR inhibitors such as gamma-aminobutyric acid-B receptor agonists (eg, baclofen), are helpful in patients with refractory GERD. Although baclofen decreases the symptoms in some patients, the symptomatic benefit remains poor in others (61-63).

All potential medications, including antinociceptives and TLESR inhibitors, should be given in combination with PPIs because given alone, their effect on patients symptoms is poor (33).

Potential medications for the treatment of GERD symptoms are summarized in Table 1. In addition, a trial of antidyspeptic drugs including phytotherapeutics (such as STW5) could be considered.

Future treatments

Reflux inhibitors: Novel TLESR inhibitors, such as metabotropic glutamate receptor 5 antagonists (eg, AZD2066) are potential treatments for patients with refractory symptoms (64). Cannabinoid receptor agonists potentially inhibit TLESR; therefore, they may be potential treatment for patients with GER symptoms (65,66).

Antinociceptives: One possible future direction in the therapeutic area of esophageal hypersensitivity is the development of analgesic medications that specifically target receptors such as transient receptor potential cation channel subfamily V member 1 (TRPV1), a receptor that was shown to be crucially involved in the pain sensation pathways of the esophagus (54,67,68). To support this, a recent study has shown that a TRPV1 antagonist (AZD1386) increases esophageal pain thresholds in human (69). Targeting protease-activated receptors (eg, PAR-2), which are involved in both nociception and LES relaxation, or cholecystokinin with their antagonists would be potential treatments in patients with GER symptoms(36,70,71).

Mucosal protection with medications such as sucralfate (72) or those which affect esophageal bicarbonate/mucin secretion (73) are other possible treatments that should be considered in patients with refractory symptoms.

Cannabinoids with both central and peripheral antinociceptive effects are potential treatments for esophageal hypersensitivity (65).

Surgical and endoluminal therapies

Interventional strategies for the treatment of GERD are primarily based on mechanical blocking of the LES and, therefore, decreasing the episodes/amounts of gastric reflux into the esophagus. The real indications of interventional treatments of GERD are not well defined. Regurgitation, respiratory symptoms, acid reflux and nonacid/ weakly acidic reflux both with positive symptom correlation are potential indications of interventional treatment of patients with GER symptoms; however, more studies are needed to define the actual therapeutic effect of these interventional methods (74-76).

PPI FAILURE DUE TO PPI SIDE EFFECTS

Studies have shown acid-related symptoms and rebound acid hypersecretion may occur after PPI treatment (77-79). Aside from rebound acid hypersecretion, rare side effects that have been associated with long-term PPI treatment include hypomagnesemia, abdominal symptoms (cramps, pain or diarrhea), *Clostridium difficile* infection, small intestinal bacterial overgrowth and spontaneous bacterial peritonitis (80-82). Moreover, PPIs may delay gastric emptying and cause dyspepsia in certain patients (83). In general, PPIs are safe and well-tolerated medications, but it is important to be aware of their rare side effects that may mimic PPI failure.

RECOMMENDATIONS AND CONCLUSIONS

Nonacid reflux and esophageal hypersensitivity are not sufficiently considered in the management of patients with heartburn or NCCP, especially when the patients fail to respond to a PPI treatment. The definitions of 'functional heartburn' and 'functional chest pain of presumed esophageal origin' need to be re-evaluated because heartburn or chest pain are clearly more than just a consequence of acid reflux.

A failure of PPI, after exclusion of organic (eg, eosinophilic esophagitis) or drug (eg, nonsteroidal anti-inflammatory drugs) -related reasons may occur under three major possible conditions: nonacid esophageal reflux; esophageal hypersensitivity; and CYP2C19 polymorphisms. Esophageal hypersensitivity occurs with or without reflux, independent of the pH of the refluxate.

Considering the potential overlap among esophageal hypersensitivity, acid and nonacid reflux, functional heartburn and dyspepsia, esophageal impedance testing is valuable in both the clinic and in research. In this regard, the importance of esophageal impedance testing is clear, especially in the management of patients with refractory symptoms; however, the role of provocative and sensory assessments needs to be further elucidated.

CONCLUSION

Patients with GERD, functional heartburn or NCCP may experience esophageal hypersensitivity to chemical, mechanical or other stimuli. Studying esophageal hypersensitivity in patients with GERD-indicating symptoms may change our understanding of GERD and other functional esophageal diseases. Therefore, one potential future direction in the diagnosis of patients with refractory heartburn or NCCP may be sensory assessment with multimodal probes integrating electrical, mechanical, thermal and chemical stimuli (84) in addition to esophageal impedance, pH and motility testing. Additionally, pharmacogenomics may help us in selecting sufficient doses of PPIs and predicting response to therapy.

While response to PPIs in patients with GER symptoms is promising, antinociceptive medications and TLESR inhibitors are beneficial in refractory cases.

DISCLOSURES: The authors have no financial disclosures or conflicts of interest to declare.

REFERENCES

1. Dent J, El-Serag HB, Wallander MA, Johansson S. Epidemiology of gastro-oesophageal reflux disease: A systematic review. Gut 2005;54:710-7.
2. El-Serag HB. Time trends of gastroesophageal reflux disease: A systematic review. Clin Gastroenterol Hepatol 2007;5:17-26.
3. El-Serag HB, Sweet S, Winchester CC, Dent J. Update on the epidemiology of gastro-oesophageal reflux disease: A systematic review. Gut 2013, July 13 (Epub ahead of print).
4. American Gastroenterological Association. The burden of chronic gastrointestinal diseases study. 2001. AGA; Bethesda: Pamphlet.
5. Shaheen NJ, Hansen RA, Morgan DR, et al. The burden of gastrointestinal and liver diseases, 2006. Am J Gastroenterol 2006;101:2128-38.
6. Hershcovici T, Fass R. An algorithm for diagnosis and treatment of refractory GERD. Best Pract Res Clin Gastroenterol 2010;24:923-36.
7. Kohata Y, Fujiwara Y, Machida H, et al. Pathogenesis of proton-pump inhibitor-refractory non-erosive reflux disease according to multichannel intraluminal impedance-pH monitoring. J Gastroenterol Hepatol 2012;27 Suppl 3:58-62.
8. Galindo G, Vassalle J, Marcus SN, Triadafilopoulos G. Multimodality evaluation of patients with gastroesophageal reflux disease symptoms who have failed empiric proton pump inhibitor therapy. Dis Esophagus 2013;26:443-50.
9. Barlow WJ, Orlando RC. The pathogenesis of heartburn in nonerosive reflux disease: A unifying hypothesis. Gastroenterology 2005;128:771-8.
10. Armstrong D, Marshall JK, Chiba N, et al. Canadian Consensus Conference on the management of gastroesophageal reflux disease in adults – update 2004. Can J Gastroenterol 2005;19:15-35.
11. Moraes-Filho J, Cecconello I, Gama-Rodrigues J et al. Brazilian consensus on gastroesophageal reflux disease: Proposals for assessment, classification, and management. Am J Gastroenterol 2002;97:241-8.
12. Diamant NE. Pathophysiology of gastroesophageal reflux disease. GI Motility Online, May 16, 2011.
13. Orlando RC. Pathophysiology of gastroesophageal reflux disease. J Clin Gastroenterol 2008;42:584-8.
14. Prakash GC. Esophageal hypersensitivity. Gastroenterol Hepatol (N Y) 2010;6:497-500.
15. Kahrilas PJ, Shaheen NJ, Vaezi MF et al. American Gastroenterological Association Medical Position Statement on the management of gastroesophageal reflux disease. Gastroenterology 2008;135:1383-91.
16. Galmiche JP, Clouse RE, Balint A, et al. Functional esophageal disorders. Gastroenterology 2006;130:1459-65
17. Fass R. Functional heartburn: What it is and how to treat it. Gastrointest Endosc Clin N Am 2009;19:23-33.
18. Sifrim D, Blondeau K. New techniques to evaluate esophageal function. Dig Dis 2006;24:243-51.
19. Galmiche JP, Clouse RE, Balint A, et al. Functional esophageal disorders. Gastroenterology 2006;130:1459-65.
20. Sifrim D, Fornari F. Non-achalasic motor disorders of the oesophagus. Best Pract Res Clin Gastroenterol 2007;21:575-93.
21. Atkins D, Kramer R, Capocelli K et al. Eosinophilic esophagitis: The newest esophageal inflammatory disease. Nat Rev Gastroenterol Hepatol 2009;6:267-78.
22. Sperry SL, Shaheen NJ, Dellon ES. Toward uniformity in the diagnosis of eosinophilic esophagitis (EoE): The effect of guidelines on variability of diagnostic criteria for EoE. Am J Gastroenterol 2011;106:824-32.
23. Nonevski IT, Downs-Kelly E, Falk GW. Eosinophilic esophagitis: An increasingly recognized cause of dysphagia, food impaction, and refractory heartburn. Cleve Clin J Med 2008;75:623-33.
24. Dellon ES, Speck O, Woodward K, et al. Clinical and endoscopic characteristics do not reliably differentiate PPI-responsive esophageal eosinophilia and eosinophilic esophagitis in patients undergoing upper endoscopy: A prospective cohort study. Am J Gastroenterol 2013;108:1854-60.
25. Dellon ES, Gonsalves N, Hirano I, et al. ACG clinical guideline: Evidenced based approach to the diagnosis and management of esophageal eosinophilia and eosinophilic esophagitis (EoE). Am J Gastroenterol 2013;108:679-92.
26. Vakil N, van Zanten SV, Kahrilas P, et al. The Montreal definition and classification of gastroesophageal reflux disease: A global evidence-based consensus. Am J Gastroenterol 2006;101:1900-20.

27. Kikendall JW. Pill-induced esophagitis. Gastroenterol Hepatol (N Y) 2007;3:275-6.
28. Festi D, Scaioli E, Baldi F, et al. Body weight, lifestyle, dietary habits and gastroesophageal reflux disease. World J Gastroenterol 2009;15:1690-701.
29. Hungin AP, Hill C, Molloy-Bland M, Raghunath A. Systematic review: Patterns of proton pump inhibitor use and adherence in gastroesophageal reflux disease. Clin Gastroenterol Hepatol 2012;10:109-16.
30. Hagymasi K, Mullner K, Herszenyi L, Tulassay Z. Update on the pharmacogenomics of proton pump inhibitors. Pharmacogenomics 2011;12:873-88.
31. Furuta T, Sugimoto M, Shirai N. Individualized therapy for gastroesophageal reflux disease: Potential impact of pharmacogenetic testing based on CYP2C19. Mol Diagn Ther 2012;16:223-34.
32. Bashashati M, Andrews CN. Functional studies of the gastrointestinal tract in adult surgical clinics: When do they help? Int J Surg 2012;10:280-4.
33. Storr MA. What is nonacid reflux disease? Can J Gastroenterol 2011;25:35-8.
34. Vela MF, Camacho-Lobato L, Srinivasan R, et al. Simultaneous intraesophageal impedance and pH measurement of acid and nonacid gastroesophageal reflux: Effect of omeprazole. Gastroenterology 2001;120:1599-606.
35. Iwakiri K, Sano H, Tanaka Y, et al. Characteristics of symptomatic reflux episodes in patients with non-erosive reflux disease who have a positive symptom index on proton pump inhibitor therapy. Digestion 2010;82:156-61.
36. Zerbib F, Duriez A, Roman S, et al. Determinants of gastro-oesophageal reflux perception in patients with persistent symptoms despite proton pump inhibitors. Gut 2008;57:156-60.
37. Bredenoord AJ, Weusten BL, Timmer R, Smout AJ. Characteristics of gastroesophageal reflux in symptomatic patients with and without excessive esophageal acid exposure. Am J Gastroenterol 2006;101:2470-5.
38. Savarino E, Zentilin P, Tutuian R, et al. The role of nonacid reflux in NERD: Lessons learned from impedance-pH monitoring in 150 patients off therapy. Am J Gastroenterol 2008;103:2685-93.
39. Vaezi MF. Use of symptom indices in the management of GERD. Gastroenterol Hepatol (N Y) 2012;8:185-7.
40. Bernstein LM, Baker LA. A clinical test for esophagitis. Gastroenterology 1958;34:760-81.
41. Bernstein LM, Fruin RD, Pacini R. Differentiation of esophageal pain from angina pectoris: Role of the esophageal acid perfusion test. Medicine (Baltimore) 1962;41:143-62.
42. Jung B, Steinbach J, Beaumont C, Mittal RK. Lack of association between esophageal acid sensitivity detected by prolonged pH monitoring and Bernstein testing. Am J Gastroenterol 2004;99:410-5.
43. Nagahara A, Miwa H, Minoo T, et al. Increased esophageal sensitivity to acid and saline in patients with nonerosive gastro-esophageal reflux disease. J Clin Gastroenterol 2006;40:891-5.
44. Siddiqui A, Rodriguez-Stanley S, Zubaidi S, Miner PB Jr. Esophageal visceral sensitivity to bile salts in patients with functional heartburn and in healthy control subjects. Dig Dis Sci 2005;50:81-5.
45. Rodriguez-Stanley S, Robinson M, Earnest DL, et al. Esophageal hypersensitivity may be a major cause of heartburn. Am J Gastroenterol 1999;94:628-31.
46. Yang M, Li ZS, Chen DF, et al. Quantitative assessment and characterization of visceral hyperalgesia evoked by esophageal balloon distention and acid perfusion in patients with functional heartburn, nonerosive reflux disease, and erosive esophagitis. Clin J Pain 2010;26:326-31.
47. Trimble KC, Pryde A, Heading RC. Lowered oesophageal sensory thresholds in patients with symptomatic but not excess gastro-oesophageal reflux: Evidence for a spectrum of visceral sensitivity in GORD. Gut 1995;37:7-12.
48. Nasr I, Attaluri A, Hashmi S, et al. Investigation of esophageal sensation and biomechanical properties in functional chest pain. Neurogastroenterol Motil 2010;22:520-6, e116.
49. Rao SS, Hayek B, Summers RW. Functional chest pain of esophageal origin: Hyperalgesia or motor dysfunction. Am J Gastroenterol 2001;96:2584-9.

50. Katz PO, Dalton CB, Richter JE, et al. Esophageal testing of patients with noncardiac chest pain or dysphagia. Results of three years' experience with 1161 patients. Ann Intern Med 1987;106:593-7.

51. Shapiro M, Green C, Bautista JM, et al. Functional heartburn patients demonstrate traits of functional bowel disorder but lack a uniform increase of chemoreceptor sensitivity to acid. Am J Gastroenterol 2006;101:1084-91.

52. Spiller R, Garsed K. Postinfectious irritable bowel syndrome. Gastroenterology 2009;136:1979-88.

53. Farre R, van MH, De Vos R, et al. Short exposure of oesophageal mucosa to bile acids, both in acidic and weakly acidic conditions, can impair mucosal integrity and provoke dilated intercellular spaces. Gut 2008;57:1366-74.

54. Tack J. Is there a unifying role for visceral hypersensitivity and irritable bowel syndrome in non-erosive reflux disease? Digestion 2008;78(Suppl 1):42-5.

55. Caviglia R, Ribolsi M, Maggiano N, et al. Dilated intercellular spaces of esophageal epithelium in nonerosive reflux disease patients with physiological esophageal acid exposure. Am J Gastroenterol 2005;100:543-8.

56. Neumann H, Monkemuller K, Fry LC, et al. Intercellular space volume is mainly increased in the basal layer of esophageal squamous epithelium in patients with GERD. Dig Dis Sci 2011;56:1404-11.

57. Boeckxstaens GE. Review article: The pathophysiology of gastro-oesophageal reflux disease. Aliment Pharmacol Ther 2007 15;26:149-60.

58. Emerenziani S, Sifrim D. Gastroesophageal reflux and gastric emptying, revisited. Curr Gastroenterol Rep 2005;7:190-5.

59. Armstrong D, Sifrim D. New pharmacologic approaches in gastroesophageal reflux disease. Gastroenterol Clin North Am 2010;39:393-418.

60. Nguyen TM, Eslick GD. Systematic review: The treatment of noncardiac chest pain with antidepressants. Aliment Pharmacol Ther 2012;35:493-500.

61. Vela MF, Tutuian R, Katz PO, Castell DO. Baclofen decreases acid and non-acid post-prandial gastro-oesophageal reflux measured by combined multichannel intraluminal impedance and pH. Aliment Pharmacol Ther 2003;17:243-51.

62. Zhang Q, Lehmann A, Rigda R, et al. Control of transient lower oesophageal sphincter relaxations and reflux by the GABA(B) agonist baclofen in patients with gastro-oesophageal reflux disease. Gut 2002;50:19-24.

63. Cossentino MJ, Mann K, Armbruster SP, et al. Randomised clinical trial: The effect of baclofen in patients with gastro-oesophageal reflux – a randomised prospective study. Aliment Pharmacol Ther 2012 March 20 (Epub ahead of print).

64. Rohof WO, Lei A, Hirsch DP, et al. The effects of a novel metabotropic glutamate receptor 5 antagonist (AZD2066) on transient lower oesophageal sphincter relaxations and reflux episodes in healthy volunteers. Aliment Pharmacol Ther 2012;35:1231-42.

65. Izzo AA, Sharkey KA. Cannabinoids and the gut: New developments and emerging concepts. Pharmacol Ther 2010;126:21-38.

66. Beaumont H, Jensen J, Carlsson A, et al. Effect of delta9-tetrahydrocannabinol, a cannabinoid receptor agonist, on the triggering of transient lower oesophageal sphincter relaxations in dogs and humans. Br J Pharmacol 2009;156:153-62.

67. Bhat YM, Bielefeldt K. Capsaicin receptor (TRPV1) and non-erosive reflux disease. Eur J Gastroenterol Hepatol 2006;18:263-70.

68. Guarino MP, Cheng L, Ma J, et al. Increased *TRPV1* gene expression in esophageal mucosa of patients with non-erosive and erosive reflux disease. Neurogastroenterol Motil 2010;22:746-51, e219.

69. Krarup AL, Ny L, Astrand M, et al. Randomised clinical trial: The efficacy of a transient receptor potential vanilloid 1 antagonist AZD1386 in human oesophageal pain. Aliment Pharmacol Ther 2011;33:1113-22.

70. Yoshida N, Kuroda M, Suzuki T, et al. Role of nociceptors/neuropeptides in the pathogenesis of visceral hypersensitivity of nonerosive reflux disease. Dig Dis Sci 2013;58:2237-43.

71. Huang SC. Protease-activated receptor-1 (PAR1) and PAR2 but not PAR4 mediate relaxations in lower esophageal sphincter. Regul Pept 2007;142:37-43.

72. Simon B, Ravelli GP, Goffin H. Sucralfate gel versus placebo in patients with non-erosive gastro-oesophageal reflux disease. Aliment Pharmacol Ther 1996;10:441-6.

73. Bdulnour-Nakhoul S, Tobey NA, Nakhoul NL, et al. The effect of tegaserod on esophageal submucosal glands bicarbonate and mucin secretion. Dig Dis Sci 2008;53:2366-72.

74. Fass R. Therapeutic options for refractory gastroesophageal reflux disease. J Gastroenterol Hepatol 2012;27(Suppl 3):3-7.

75. Kahrilas PJ, Boeckxstaens G, Smout AJ. Management of the patient with incomplete response to PPI therapy. Best Pract Res Clin Gastroenterol 2013;27:401-14.

76. Pandolfino JE, Krishnan K. Clinical perspectives: Do endoscopic anti-reflux procedures fit in the current treatment paradigm of GERD? Clin Gastroenterol Hepatol 2013 June 28 (Epub ahead of print.

77. Reimer C, Sondergaard B, Hilsted L, Bytzer P. Proton-pump inhibitor therapy induces acid-related symptoms in healthy volunteers after withdrawal of therapy. Gastroenterology 2009;137:80-7.

78. McColl KE, Gillen D. Evidence that proton-pump inhibitor therapy induces the symptoms it is used to treat. Gastroenterology 2009;137:20-2.

79. Gillen D, Wirz AA, Ardill JE, McColl KE. Rebound hypersecretion after omeprazole and its relation to on-treatment acid suppression and *Helicobacter pylori* status. Gastroenterology 1999;116:239-47.

80. Hess MW, Hoenderop JG, Bindels RJ, Drenth JP. Systematic review: Hypomagnesaemia induced by proton pump inhibition. Aliment Pharmacol Ther 2012;36:405-13.

81. Cundy T, Mackay J. Proton pump inhibitors and severe hypomagnesaemia. Curr Opin Gastroenterol 2011;27:180-5.

82. Corleto VD, Festa S, Di GE, Annibale B. Proton pump inhibitor therapy and potential long-term harm. Curr Opin Endocrinol Diabetes Obes 2014;21:3-8.

83. Sanaka M, Yamamoto T, Kuyama Y. Effects of proton pump inhibitors on gastric emptying: A systematic review. Dig Dis Sci 2010;55:2431-40.

84. Krarup AL, Villadsen GE, Mejlgaard E, et al. Acid hypersensitivity in patients with eosinophilic oesophagitis. Scand J Gastroenterol 2010;45:273-81.

85. Edwards SJ, Lind T, Lundell L, DAS R. Systematic review: Standard- and double-dose proton pump inhibitors for the healing of severe erosive oesophagitis – a mixed treatment comparison of randomized controlled trials. Aliment Pharmacol Ther 2009;30:547-56.

86. Hershcovici T, Achem SR, Jha LK, Fass R. Systematic review: The treatment of noncardiac chest pain. Aliment Pharmacol Ther 2012;35:5-14.

87. Lexi-Comp Online, Hudson, Ohio: Lexi-Comp, Inc. <http://online lexi com/ 2013> (Accessed January 10, 2014).

30

Validation of the National Aeronautics and Space Administration-Task Load Index as a tool to evaluate the learning curve for endoscopy training

Rachid Mohamed MD FRCPC[1], Maitreyi Raman MD FRCPC MSc[1], John Anderson BSc FRCP(Edin) MD[2],
Kevin McLaughlin MD MRCP PhD[3], Alaa Rostom MD FRCPC MSc[1], Sylvain Coderre MD FRCPC MSc[1]

R Mohamed, M Raman, J Anderson, K McLaughlin, A Rostom, S Coderre. Validation of the National Aeronautics and Space Administration Task Load Index as a tool to evaluate the learning curve for endoscopy training. Can J Gastroenterol Hepatol 2014;28(3):155-160.

BACKGROUND: Although workplace workload assessments exist in different fields, an endoscopy-specific workload assessment tool is lacking.
OBJECTIVE: To validate such a workload tool and use it to map the progression of novice trainees in gastroenterology in performing their first endoscopies.
METHODS: The National Aeronautics and Space Administration Task Load Index (NASA-TLX) workload assessment tool was completed by eight novice trainees in gastroenterology and 10 practicing gastroenterologists/surgeons. An exploratory factor analysis was performed to construct a streamlined endoscopy-specific task load index, which was subsequently validated. The 'Endoscopy Task Load Index' was used to monitor progression of trainee exertion and self-assessed performance over their first 40 procedures.
RESULTS: From the factor analysis of the NASA-TLX, two principal components emerged: a measure of exertion and a measure of self-efficacy. These items became the components of the newly validated Endoscopy Task Load Index. There was a steady decline in self-perceived exertion over the training period, which was more rapid for gastroscopy than colonoscopy. The self-efficacy scores for gastroscopy rapidly increased over the first few procedures, reaching a plateau after this period of time. For colonoscopy, there was a progressive increase in reported self-efficacy over the first three quartiles of procedures, followed by a drop in self-efficacy scores over the final quartile.
DISCUSSION: The present study validated an Endoscopy Task Load Index that can be completed in <1 min. Practical implications of such a tool in endoscopy education include identifying periods of higher perceived exertion among novice endoscopists, facilitating appropriate levels of guidance from trainers.

Key Words: *Cognitive load; Endoscopy training; Procedural skills; Workload assessment*

La validation du *National Aeronautics and Space Administration-Task Load Index* comme outil pour évaluer la courbe d'apprentissage dans la formation à l'endoscopie

HISTORIQUE : Même si on évalue la charge de travail dans divers domaines, il n'existe pas d'outil d'évaluation de la charge de travail propre à l'endoscopie.
OBJECTIF : Valider un tel outil sur la charge de travail et l'utiliser pour cartographier la progression des apprenants novices en gastroentérologie qui effectuent leurs premières endoscopies.
MÉTHODOLOGIE : Huit apprenants novices en gastroentérologie et dix gastroentérologues ou chirurgiens en exercice ont utilisé l'outil d'évaluation de la charge de travail *National Aeronautics and Space Administration-Task Load Index* (NASA-TLX). Les chercheurs ont effectué une analyse factorielle exploratoire pour établir un indice harmonieux de charge de travail propre à l'endoscopie, qui a ensuite été validé. L'indice de charge de travail en endoscopie a permis de surveiller la progression de la fatigue et le rendement personnel des apprenants au cours des 40 premières interventions.
RÉSULTATS : Selon l'analyse factorielle du NASA-TLX, deux grands volets ont émergé : une mesure de fatigue et une mesure d'auto-efficacité, qui sont devenues des éléments de l'indice de charge de travail en endoscopie nouvellement validé. Les chercheurs ont remarqué une diminution régulière de l'autoperception de fatigue tout au long de la période de formation, plus rapide dans le cadre de la gastroscopie que de la coloscopie. Les indices d'auto-efficacité de la gastroscopie ont rapidement augmenté au fil des quelques premières interventions, pour ensuite atteindre un plateau. Pour ce qui est de la coloscopie, l'auto-efficacité déclarée s'est améliorée progressivement pendant les trois premiers quartiles d'intervention, suivie d'une baisse des indices d'auto-efficacité lors du dernier quartile.
EXPOSÉ : La présente étude validait un indice de charge de travail d'endoscopie qui peut être vérifié en moins d'une minute. Les conséquences pratiques d'un tel outil pour l'enseignement de l'endoscopie incluent la détermination des périodes de plus grande fatigue perçues par les endoscopistes novices, favorisant un degré d'orientation pertinent de la part des formateurs.

The road to acquiring competence, and at times excellence, in the performance of any skill requires a combination of innate biological capacities, dedicated teachers and many hours of training. The process of skills acquisition has been described as a sequential process involving three major phases (1). The first phase, or novice phase, involves intense concentration to fully understand the activity and avoid making mistakes. The second phase is an evolution to a more fluid, less cognitively arduous step in which trainees begin to perform at an acceptable level, with fewer major mistakes. The final phase involves a process of automation, in which the skill is precisely and smoothly performed with little or no conscious cognitive involvement. Different terminology has been used to describe a similar sequence of events. The terms 'unconscious' and 'conscious' incompetence have been used to describe the early training stage, evolving to conscious competence (akin to Ericsson's second phase) and, finally, unconscious competence for the more automated phase of skill acquisition (2).

First described in 1971, endoscopy of the entire colon, or colonoscopy, is a common diagnostic procedure performed worldwide (3). During a colonoscopy training session, a novice endoscopist must attend to myriad sensory stimuli: visual stimuli from the endoscopic image of the colon on the monitor; verbal stimuli from the patient, nurse and trainer; as well as tactile/proprioceptive stimulus from the

[1]*Department of Medicine (Division Gastroenterology), University of Calgary, Calgary, Alberta;* [2]*Department of Gastroenterology, Gloucestershire Hospitals NHS Foundation Trust Hospital, United Kingdom;* [3]*Office of Undergraduate Medical Education, University of Calgary, Calgary, Alberta*
Correspondence: Dr Sylvain Coderre, Department of Medicine (Division Gastroenterology), University of Calgary, 3500-26th Avenue Northeast, Calgary, Alberta T1Y 6J4. e-mail coderre@ucalgary.ca

instrument itself (4). In addition to these sources of cognitive load (5), colonoscopy also places physical demand on the trainee, such as the process of straightening the colonoscope or loop resolution, a technique critical to the successful, safe and comfortable advancement of the instrument through the colon (6). Examination of the upper gastrointestinal tract (ie, esophagogastroduodenoscopy [EGD]) also provides many of these workload demands, although likely to a lesser extent.

The above-mentioned sources of workload, in addition to other potential sources such as time demand and frustration/anxiety, are captured in a workload assessment tool known as the National Aeronautics and Space Administration Task Load Index (NASA-TLX) (7). This subjective assessment of workload has been used in >500 published articles worldwide (8) in several domains including medicine (9). Subjective ratings are able to tap the essence of workload, and provide a valid, sensitive and practically useful indicator (7).

The objectives of the present study were threefold. The first was to identify the principal components of the NASA-TLX tool when applied to endoscopy training and to then use these data to create an endoscopy-specific rating tool. Our second objective was to assess the construct validity of the endoscopy task load rating tool. Our final study objective was to use the endoscopy task load rating tool to map our trainees' workload and perceived performance during the early phases of their training. Such attempts to measure mental effort during deliberate practice (10) and relating these measures to the level of performance has been shown to adequately represent the efficiency of the ongoing learning processes (11). We hypothesized that as trainees progress through their initial endoscopies, a steady, gradual decrease in workload would occur, correlating with an equally steady improvement in performance.

METHODS

Participants

Participants were eight first-year gastroenterology residents at the University of Calgary (Calgary, Alberta). This gastroenterology residency training program lasts two years, during which residents perform, on average, 200 colonoscopies and 200 EGDs. Proficiency in both procedures is a requirement for graduating from the program. The study was conducted over two time periods, July 1 to September 30, 2009, and July 1 to September 30, 2010. There were four participants during each time period. This enabled data collection for the residents' procedural learning curve during the first three months of their training. Ten practicing gastroenterologists and colorectal surgeons with >5 years of experience in performing colonoscopy were asked to complete the NASA-TLX rating after two consecutive colonoscopies. Before beginning the study, ethics approval from the Conjoint Health Research Ethics Board at the University of Calgary was obtained, in addition to written informed consent from each of the participants.

Materials

A slightly modified version of the NASA-TLX rating tool was used for the present study. The unmodified NASA-TLX tool was initially piloted on three experienced gastroenterologists performing colonoscopy on two occasions. After their feedback, six items on the rating scales were kept, but some of the descriptors were modified for clarity and/or to make them more relevant to endoscopy. The final rating tool had six items: mental demand, physical demand, time demand, effort, performance, and frustration and anxiety (Appendix 1). Each of these items was rated on a visual analogue scale that was interpreted as the participant's subjective rating of each variable.

Procedure

The present analysis was a prospective observational cohort study. The participants were asked to complete the NASA-TLX rating for each of their colonoscopy and EGD procedures during the study time period. Cognizant of the effect that patient variability may have on the workload of endoscopy, the participants were asked not to rate procedures for patients with known previously difficult colonoscopies (failed or

successful), one or more pelvic surgeries, two or more abdominal surgeries, previous colonic resection, as well as patients deemed to experience excessive anxiety over the procedure. These exclusion criteria were not used for the colonoscopies rated by the practicing gastroenterologists and colorectal surgeons.

Statistical analyses

The reliability of the NASA-TLX survey was assessed using Cronbach's α coefficient. Before performing factor analysis, the Kaiser-Meyer-Olkin (KMO) test was used to assess the appropriateness of performing this analysis on this dataset (ie, to ensure KMO statistic >0.5). Using the NASA-TLX survey as the unit of analysis, an exploratory factor analysis on the individual items of this tool was performed. This technique reduces a set of items to a smaller number of underlying principal components and, in doing so, uncovers the latent structure of the set of items (12). Factor analysis can evaluate discrimination by statistically testing whether two or more items differ. Items are considered to be measuring different constructs if they load most heavily on different principal components (13). Items that load most heavily, or converge, on the same principal component are considered to be measuring the same construct.

In the analysis, a Pearson product moment correlation matrix for the NASA-TLX items was initially constructed and then used principal component analysis to extract factors. A cut-off threshold was used for factor extraction of eigenvalue ≥1 (Kaiser rule). Factor loading was then performed on the extracted factors, followed by factor rotation using the Varimax method with Kaiser normalization (12). A cut-off threshold of 0.5 was used for factor loading.

Having identified the principal components of the NASA-TLX tool, simplification this tool was sought using a data-reduction technique. For this, a weighted composite score for each component was created, on which more than one item loaded. Weighting for each item corresponded to its factor loading score. Linear regression was then used to identify the minimum number of items that would allow explanation of ≥80% of the variance (R^2) of each weighted composite score.

To compare NASA-TLX scores for colonoscopies performed by practicing gastroenterologists/surgeons and residents, a two-sample t test was used and Cohen's d as a measure of effect size. A repeated-measures ANOVA was used to evaluate whether there was a change in NASA-TLX ratings over time. For this analysis, the between-subject variable was participant and the within-subject variable was procedure number. STATA version 11.0 (StataCorp, USA) was used for the analyses.

RESULTS

Principal components of the NASA-TLX for endoscopy

In the factor analysis, all 276 surveys for colonoscopy and 128 surveys for EGD were included. The participants completed a mean of 34.5 (range 12 to 54) surveys for colonoscopy and 32 (range 13 to 45) for EGD. The alpha coefficients and KMO statistics for the colonoscopy surveys were 0.78 and 0.78, respectively, while the corresponding results for EGD were 0.90 and 0.82.

For the colonoscopy surveys, two principal components (eigenvalues of 3.0 and 1.0) were identified that explained 66% of the overall variance. Five of the six individual items loaded on the first factor, which were interpreted as 'exertion', while a single item loaded on the second factor ('self-efficacy'). Factor loading scores are shown in Table 1. For the weighted exertion score, no single variable could explain ≥80% of the variance for this score, but the combination of effort and physical demand provided an R^2 of 0.89. Therefore, the tool was simplified to include three items – a weighted combination of effort and physical demand (hereby referred to as 'exertion') and performance as an indicator of 'self-efficacy'. These two measures, exertion and self-efficacy, are based solely on endoscopists' self-assessment (via NASA-TLX) and not on any specific objective measures of achievement (such as cecal intubation, detection rates, etc).

TABLE 1
Principal components of the National Aeronautics and Space Administration Task Load Index (NASA-TLX) for colonoscopy and esophagogastroduodenoscopy (EGD)

NASA-TLX item	Colonoscopy		EGD	
	Factor 1 (Exertion)	Factor 2 (Self-efficacy)	Factor 1 (Exertion)	Factor 2 (Self-efficacy)
Mental demand	0.77		0.87	
Physical demand	0.63		0.91	
Time demand	0.62		0.76	
Effort	0.89		0.89	
Performance		0.78		0.52
Frustration and anxiety	0.79		0.79	

For analysis of the EGD surveys, the same two principal components explained 80% of the overall variance. Loading of individual items paralleled that of the colonoscopy data (Table 1), as did data reduction to simplify the rating of the exertion score. Once again, the combination of effort and physical demand provided the optimal R^2 (0.96), suggesting that the same simplified survey could be used to evaluate both colonoscopy and EGD procedures.

Comparison of exertion and self-efficacy ratings for practicing gastroenterologists/surgeons and residents
Practicing gastroenterologists/surgeons had significantly lower ratings for task load when performing colonoscopy compared with residents. The mean (± SD) task load rating for practicing gastroenterologists/surgeons was 27.8±15.3 compared with fourth quartile rating for residents of 50.2±20.0 (d=1.26; P<0.0001). Practicing gastroenterologists also had significantly higher self-efficacy ratings when performing colonoscopy (89.2±9.1 compared with fourth quartile rating for residents of 44.8±26.6 [d=2.23; P<0.0001]).

Changes in exertion and self-efficacy ratings with training
Because of the wide range of surveys completed by the trainees, procedures were broken down into quartiles (for colonoscopy: first quartile ≤9 procedures, second quartile ≤18 procedures, third quartile ≤29 procedures, fourth quartile ≤54 procedures). For both colonoscopy and EGD, there was a significant reduction in residents' ratings of exertion from the first to the fourth quartile of procedures (P<0.0001 for both). The exertion ratings for the quartiles of procedures are shown in Figure 1. Over the duration of the study, there was a slight increase in perceived self-efficacy (P=0.049) for colonoscopy and a marked increase in self-efficacy for EGD (P<0.0001). These data are also shown in Figure 1.

DISCUSSION

Our first objective was to create an endoscopy-specific rating tool by identifying the principal components of the NASA-TLX tool when applied to endoscopy training. Our factor analysis (Table 1) revealed two principal components: a measure of exertion (combination of the effort and physical demand items from NASA-TLX) and a measure of self-efficacy (performance item from NASA-TLX). Therefore, our 'Endoscopy Task Load Index' is now a simplified version of the NASA-TLX, with only three items required: effort, physical demand and performance. A comparison of the exertion and self-efficacy scores between these novice endoscopists and the practicing gastroenterologists/surgeons demonstrated evidence for construct validity of this tool.

Our final study objective was to map the evolution of exertion and self-efficacy during initial training procedures of our novice endoscopists. As shown in Figure 1, for both gastroscopy and colonoscopy there was a steady decline in self-perceived exertion over this training time period. It is notable, however, that the mean exertion score of our novices at the end of their first three months (50.2) was still substantially higher than the mean exertion score of our experts (27.8). The

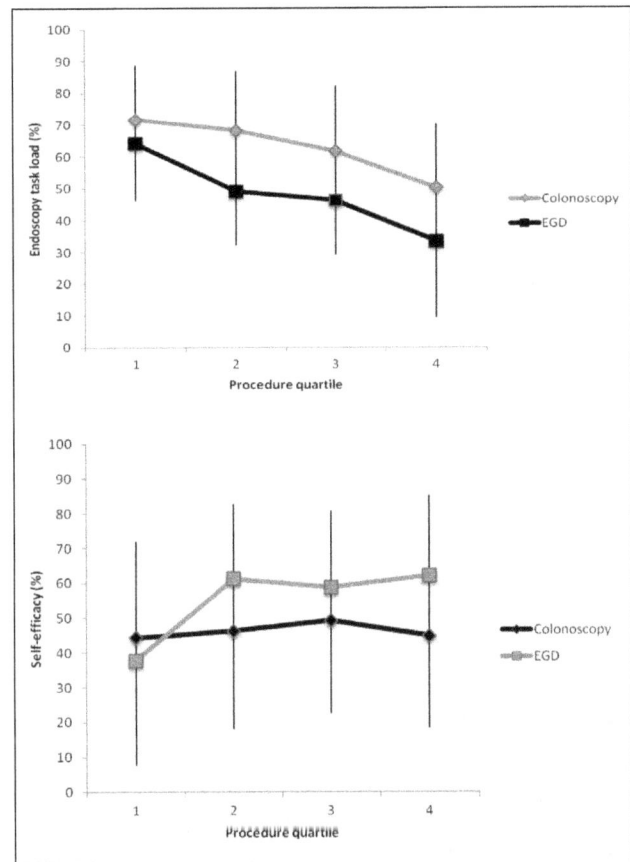

Figure 1) *Change in endoscopy task load (top) and self-efficacy with experience in performing colonoscopy and esophagogastroduodenoscopy (EGD) (with CIs)*

self-efficacy scores for gastroscopy rapidly increase over the first few procedures, reaching a plateau after this period of time. For colonoscopy, there is a progressive increase in reported self-efficacy over the first three quartiles of procedures, which is followed by a drop in self-efficacy scores over the next quartile. The final mean self-efficacy score for the novices is much lower than that for their expert counterparts.

From these findings, it appears that for gastroscopy, there is a rapid acquisition of basic skills resulting in a corresponding decrease in exertion over the first training procedures, with a rapidly increasing perception of self-efficacy that quickly reaches a plateau to a relatively stable level. This finding may reflect the ease of intubation during gastroscopy as well as the relatively consistent anatomy encountered. For the most part, once intubation of the esophagus is mastered, the manoeuvres to navigate through the esophagus into the stomach and duodenum are consistent. The higher exertion and lower self-efficacy reported in the first few procedures may represent the intubation process, which can be challenging and create a high amount of cognitive and physical demand. Once competence and experience is attained with esophageal intubation, the trainee can relax and dedicate more time and is believed to fine tune the skills necessary for the remainder of the procedure.

For colonoscopy, a similar pattern of decreasing exertion over the first training procedures emerges, although a more gradual decline in exertion scores exists compared with gastroscopy. This is perhaps not surprising because colonoscopy is generally believed to be more intrinsically challenging and demanding than gastroscopy. As well, the decline may be more gradual because novice trainees over their first few colonoscopies become more comfortable with several of the 'basic' colonoscopy manoeuvres (eg, movement of dials, torque steering), yet become aware of more advanced and challenging techniques, such as loop resolution and even possibly polypectomy.

This awareness of colonoscopy looping, and the need to resolve it, may explain the perceived drop in self-efficacy apparent in the last quartile of study colonoscopies. Learning curve theories demonstrate that learning curves, in general, do not proceed in a smooth, linear fashion, but are characterized by constant fluctuations (14). For colonoscopy training, it is quite possible that trainees spend their first training procedures acquiring the 'basics' of colonoscopy: movement of the dials, tip control and torque steering. During this time, they become increasingly adept and comfortable with these basic techniques, with a concomitant decrease in exertion and increase in self-efficacy. However, at some point (approximately 30 procedures in our study), trainees (with the advice of their trainers) become aware that more advanced techniques are required to navigate consistently and safely to the cecum.

Specifically, loop formation and the art of loop reduction became important. The majority of difficulties encountered during a colonoscopy result from lack of progression of the instrument on insertion, commonly as a consequence of looping of the colonoscope within the colon. To progress safely, effectively and with minimal patient discomfort, normally requires straightening of the instrument and resolution of the loop (6). The decreased self-efficacy scores achieved in this period may, in fact, represent loop reduction that will be interpreted by the inexperienced trainee as a shorter distance reached as less of the colonoscope is inserted into the patient when, in reality, they are in a better position to proceed.

There are several practical implications for endoscopy education that can be derived from the present study. First, the study validated a brief Endoscopy Task Load Index that can be completed in <1 min. The Endoscopy Task Load Index is easily applied and can be tracked over an entire training period, as well as applied to therapeutic interventions such as polypectomy, managing gastrointestinal bleeds and endoscopic retrograde cholangiopancreatography. It has the potential to identify periods of higher perceived exertion and facilitate appropriate levels of guidance from the trainers. Early in their training, novices will not be able to handle the additional workload imposed by questioning or verbose directions from the trainer. Verbal instruction of scope position and movement at this stage can be simplified by using a set of 12 direct, simple terms such as: tip up, tip down, tip left, tip right, clockwise torque, anticlockwise torque, insufflate, aspirate, advance/push forward, withdraw/pull back, stop and slowly (15). As the trainee becomes more comfortable and exertion decreases, the amount of direct, hands-on supervision can be gradually decreased, thereby fostering more independence.

Work has been performed on developing formal curricula encompassing both physical and cognitive aspects of procedure teaching for colonoscopy (16,17). This is a concept that is at much further stages of evolution in the surgical realm (18-20). Much of the existing work in endoscopy has largely focused on the technical skills through simulators (21-25) and with the aid of other learning tools (4). The Endoscopy Task Load Index could be a valuable guide to the potential benefit (or harm) of new educational interventions.

While it is clear that skills acquisition improves with experience, debate remains as to the necessary number of procedures required for independent competence (26-28). A tool such as the Endoscopy Task Load Index, followed longitudinally, could provide a better definition of the transition point between the intermediate and the fully automated phases of expertise development. While our study clearly showed a difference between the trainees and the experts, we did not extend it sufficiently to help determine that exact point of transition. Such knowledge may also be helpful in assessing and following expert clinicians in need of more advanced skills training.

There were several important limitations to the present study. First, the sample size was small and the study did not extend beyond the first 50 procedures; hence, other important transition points on the road to colonoscopy competence (200 procedures by some groups [29]), such as polypectomy, cannot be ascertained. In addition, we did not evaluate the trainers' hands-on involvement and degree of

supervision, which naturally varies among educators and could have influenced perceived cognitive workload of the trainee. The study used group learning curves, which can yield a misleading picture of what is occurring in individual subjects (30). Furthermore, the study did not include objective parameters, such as cecal intubation, time and detection rates, nor was repeat assessment of practicing gastroenterologists/surgeons performed. Future studies will address the impact of magnetic endoscopic imaging (6) on both novice workload and colonoscopy performance.

Colonoscopy skills training and acquisition is in an exciting state of flux and development. With increasing emphasis of quality assurance measures in endoscopy, formalizing skills training to ensure competence of those providing the service are of paramount importance. The inclusion of objective tools that encompass both the physical and cognitive components of learning will be best suited to identify the optimal methods of teaching.

DISCLOSURES: This work originated from the University of Calgary, Canada, in affiliation with Gloucestershire Hospitals NHS Foundation (United Kingdom).

APPENDIX 1: MODIFIED NASA-TLX WORKLOAD ASSESSMENT TOOL

1. Mental Demand:

How much mental and perceptual activity was required to perform the procedure (eg, thinking, decision-making, looking, listening, remembering, reasoning, etc)? Was the procedure easy or demanding, simple or complex, exacting or forgiving?

0_____100

Low   High

2. Physical Demand:

How much physical activity was required to perform the procedure (eg, pushing, pulling, turning, controlling, etc.)? Was the procedure trivial or demanding, easy or strenuous, restful or laborious?

0_____100

Low   High

3. Time Demand:

How much time pressure did you feel due to the rate or pace of the procedure? Was the pace slow and leisurely, or rapid and frantic? Were there external time pressures (eg, personal, other duties) not directly related to the procedure?

0_____100

Low   High

4. Effort:

How hard did you have to work mentally and physically to perform and learn during this procedure?

0_____100

Low   High

5. Performance:

During this procedure, how successful do you think you were in accomplishing the goals set out by the trainer or yourself? How satisfied were you with your performance in accomplishing these goals? (NOTE: Good is on left hand side of scale, poor is on right)

0_____100

Good   Poor

6. Frustration/anxiety:

How discouraged, irritated, stressed and anxious (versus gratified, content, relaxed and secure) did you feel during the procedure?

0_____100

Low   High

REFERENCES

1. Ericsson KA. Deliberate practice and the acquisition and maintenance of expert performance in medicine and related domains. Acad Med 2004;79:S70-81.
2. Coderre S, Anderson J, Rostom A, McLaughlin K. Training the endoscopy trainer: From general principles to specific concepts. Can J Gastroenterol 2010;24:700-4.
3. Thuraisingam AI, MacDonald J, Shaw IS. Insights into endoscopy training: A qualitative study of learning experience. Med Teach 2006;28:453-9.
4. Coderre S, Anderson J, Rikers R, Dunckley P, Holbrook K, McLaughlin K. Early use of magnetic endoscopic imaging in novice colonoscopists: Improved performance without increase in workload. Can J Gastroenterol 2010;24:727-32.
5. Van Gog T, Rikers RM, Paas F. Instructional design for advanced learners: Establishing connections between the theoretical frameworks of cognitive load and deliberate practice. ETR&D 2005;53:73-81.
6. Shah SG, Saunders BP, Brooker JC, Williams CB. Magnetic imaging of colonoscopy: An audit of looping, accuracy and ancillary maneuvers. Gastrointest Endosc 2000;52:1-8.
7. Hart S, Staveland L. Development of NASA-TLX (task load index): Results of empirical and theoretical Research. In: Hancock P, Meshkati N, eds. Human Mental Workload. Amsterdam: North Holland Press, 1988:239-50.
8. Hart S. NASA-task load index (NASA-TLX); 20 Years Later. NASA-TLX Home Page. <http://humansystems.arc.nasa.gov/groups/TLX/> (Accessed in 2006).
9. Young G, Zavelina L, Hooper V. Assessment of workload using NASA Task Load Index in perianesthesia. J Perianesth Nurs 2008;23:102-10.
10. Ericcson A. Deliberate practice and the acquisition and maintenance of expert performance in medicine and related domains. Acad Med 2004;(Suppl);79:570-81.
11. Rikers R, Van Gerven P, Schmidt H. Cognitive load theory as a tool for expertise development. Instr Sci 2004;32:173-82.
12. Kerlinger FN, Lee HB. Foundations of Behavioral Research, 4th edn. Toronto: Nelson Thomson Learning, 2000.
13. Straub DW. Validating instruments in MIS research. MIS Quart 1989;13:147-66.
14. The Learning Curve. <www.learningandteaching.info/learning/learning_curve.htm> (Accessed August 2010).
15. Anderson J. Teaching colonoscopy. In: Waye JD, Rex DK, Williams CB, eds. Colonoscopy: Principles and Practice, 2nd edn. New York: Wiley-Blackwell, 2009:141-53.
16. Raman M, Donnon T. Procedural skills education – colonoscopy as a model. Can J Gastroenterol 2008;22:767-70.
17. Sedlack RE. The Mayo Colonoscopy Skills Assessment Tool: Validation of a unique instrument to assess colonoscopy skills in trainees. Gastrointest Endosc 2010;72:1125-33.
18. Van Hove C, Perry KA, Spight DH, et al. Predictors of technical skill acquisition among resident trainees in a laparoscopic skills education program. World J Surg 2008;32:1917-21.
19. Boehler ML, Schwind CJ, Rogers DA, et al. A theory-based curriculum for enhancing surgical skillfulness. J Am Coll Surg 2007;204:492-7.
20. Wong JA, Matsumoto ED. Primer: Cognitive motor learning for teaching surgical skill – how are surgical skills taught and assessed? Nat Clin Pract Urol 2008;5:47-54.
21. Sedlack RE. Validation of a colonoscopy simulation model for skills assessment. Am J Gastroenterol 2007;102:64-74.
22. Lightdale JR, Newburg AR, Mahoney LB, Fredette ME, Fishman LN. Fellow perceptions of training using computer-based endoscopy simulators. Gastrointest Endosc 2010;72:13-8.
23. Haycock A, Koch AD, Familiari P, et al. Training and transfer of colonoscopy skills: A multinational, randomized, blinded, controlled trial of simulator versus bedside training. Gastrointest Endosc 2010;71:298-307.
24. Cohen J, Cohen SA, Vora KC, et al. Multicenter, randomized, controlled trial of virtual-reality simulator training in acquisition of competency in colonoscopy. Gastrointest Endosc 2006;64:361-8.
25. Sedlack RE, Kolars JC. Computer simulator training enhances the competency of gastroenterology fellows at colonoscopy: Results of a pilot study. Am J Gastroenterol 2004; 99:33-7.
26. Lee SH, Chung IK, Kim SJ, et al. An adequate level of training for technical competence in screening and diagnostic colonoscopy: A prospective multicenter evaluation of the learning curve. Gastrointest Endosc 2008;67:683-9.
27. Spier BJ, Benson M, Pfau PR, Nelligan G, Lucey MR, Gaumnitz EA. Colonoscopy training in gastroenterology fellowships: Determining competence. Gastrointest Endosc 2010;71:319-24.
28. Marshall JB. Technical proficiency of trainees performing colonoscopy: A learning curve. Gastrointest Endosc 1995;42:287-91.
29. Asfaha S, Alqahtani S, Hilsden R, MacLean A, Beck P. Assessment of endoscopic training of general surgery residents in a North American health region. Gastrointest Endosc 2008;68:1056-62.
30. Galistel CR, Fairhurst S, Balsam P. The learning curve: Implication of a quantitative analysis. PNAS 2004;101:13124-31.

The feasibility and reliability of transient elastography using Fibroscan®: A practice audit of 2335 examinations

Jack XQ Pang MD[1,2], Faruq Pradhan[1], Scott Zimmer BA[3], Sophia Niu BSc MSc[3], Pam Crotty MSc[1], Jenna Tracey BSc[1], Christopher Schneider MD[1], Steven J Heitman MD MSc[1,2], Gilaad G Kaplan MD MPH[1,2], Mark G Swain MD MSc[1], Robert P Myers MD MSc[1,2]

JXQ Pang, F Pradhan, S Zimmer, et al. The feasibility and reliability of transient elastography using Fibroscan®: A practice audit of 2335 examinations. Can J Gastroenterol Hepatol 2014;28(3):143-149.

BACKGROUND: Liver stiffness measurement (LSM) using transient elastography is widely used in the management of patients with chronic liver disease.

OBJECTIVES: To examine the feasibility and reliability of LSM, and to identify patient and operator characteristics predictive of poorly reliable results.

METHODS: The present retrospective study investigated the frequency and determinants of poorly reliable LSM (interquartile range [IQR]/median LSM [IQR/M] >30% with median liver stiffness ≥7.1 kPa) using the FibroScan (Echosens, France) over a three-year period. Two experienced operators performed all LSMs. Multiple logistic regression analyses examined potential predictors of poorly reliable LSMs including age, sex, liver disease, the operator, operator experience (<500 versus ≥500 scans), FibroScan probe (M versus XL), comorbidities and liver stiffness. In a subset of patients, medical records were reviewed to identify obesity (body mass index ≥30 kg/m²).

RESULTS: Between July 2008 and June 2011, 2335 patients with liver disease underwent LSM (86% using the M probe). LSM failure (no valid measurements) occurred in 1.6% (n=37) and was more common using the XL than the M probe (3.4% versus 1.3%; P=0.01). Excluding LSM failures, poorly reliable LSMs were observed in 4.9% (n=113) of patients. Independent predictors of poorly reliable LSM included older age (OR 1.03 [95% CI 1.01 to 1.05]), chronic pulmonary disease (OR 1.58 [95% CI 1.05 to 2.37]), coagulopathy (OR 2.22 [95% CI 1.31 to 3.76) and higher liver stiffness (OR per kPa 1.03 [95% CI 1.02 to 1.05]), including presumed cirrhosis (stiffness ≥12.5 kPa; OR 5.24 [95% CI 3.49 to 7.89]). Sex, diabetes, the underlying liver disease and FibroScan probe were not significant. Although reliability varied according to operator (P<0.0005), operator experience was not significant. In a subanalysis including 434 patients with body mass index data, obesity influenced the rate of poorly reliable results (OR 2.93 [95% CI 0.95 to 9.05]; P=0.06).

CONCLUSIONS: FibroScan failure and poorly reliable LSM are uncommon. The most important determinants of poorly reliable results are older age, obesity, higher liver stiffness and the operator, the latter emphasizing the need for adequate training.

Key Words: Biopsy; Diagnostic test; Fibrosis; Hepatitis; Stiffness

La faisabilité et la fiabilité de l'élastographie transitoire par Fibroscan® : la vérification pratique de 2 335 examens

HISTORIQUE : La mesure de rigidité du foie (MRF) par élastographie transitoire est largement utilisée dans la prise en charge des patients atteints d'une maladie hépatique chronique.

OBJECTIFS : Examiner la faisabilité et la fiabilité de la MRF et déterminer les caractéristiques des patients et des opérateurs qui prédisent des résultats peu fiables.

MÉTHODOLOGIE : La présente étude rétrospective portait sur la fréquence et les déterminants d'une MRF peu fiable (plage interquartile [PIQ]/MRF médiane [PIQ/M] >30 % et rigidité hépatique médiane ≥7,1 kPa) au moyen du FibroScan (Echosens, France) sur une période de trois ans. Deux opérateurs expérimentés ont effectué toutes les MRF. Par des analyses de régression logistique multiples, les chercheurs ont examiné les prédicteurs potentiels de MRF peu fiables, y compris l'âge, le sexe, la maladie hépatique, l'opérateur, l'expérience de l'opérateur (<500 ou ≥500 échographies), la sonde du FibroScan (moyenne plutôt que très grande), les comorbidités et la rigidité du foie. Ils ont passé en revue les dossiers médicaux d'un sous-groupe de patients pour déterminer la présence d'obésité (indice de masse corporelle ≥30 kg/m2).

RÉSULTATS : Entre juillet 2008 et juin 2011, 2 335 patients atteints d'une maladie hépatique ont subi une MRF (86 % au moyen de la sonde moyenne). Dans 1,6 % des cas (n=37), la MRF a échoué (aucune mesure valide), ce qui était plus courant avec la sonde très grande qu'avec la sonde moyenne (3,4 % par rapport à 1,3 %; P=0,01). En plus des échecs de MRF, 4,9 % des patients (n=113) ont obtenu des MRF peu fiables. Les prédicteurs indépendants de MRF peu fiables incluaient un âge plus avancé (RC 1,03 [95 % IC 1,01 à 1,05]), une maladie pulmonaire chronique (RC 1,58 [95 % IC 1,05 à 2,37]), une coagulopathie (RC 2,22 [95 % IC 1,31 à 3,76]) et une plus grande rigidité du foie (RC par kPa 1,03 [95 % IC 1,02 à 1,05]), y compris une cirrhose présumée (rigidité ≥12,5 kPa; RC 5,24 [95 % IC 3,49 à 7,89]). Le sexe, le diabète, la maladie hépatique sous-jacente et la sonde du FibroScan n'étaient pas significatifs. Même si la fiabilité dépendait de l'opérateur (P<0,0005), son expérience n'était pas significative. Dans une sous-analyse de 434 patients dont on connaissait l'indice de masse corporelle, l'obésité influait sur le taux de résultats peu fiables (RC 2,93 [95 % IC 0,95 à 9,05]; P=0,06).

CONCLUSIONS : Il est rare que le FibroScan échoue et que la MRF ne soit pas fiable. Les principaux déterminants de résultats peu fiables sont un âge plus avancé, l'obésité, une plus grande rigidité du foie et l'opérateur, cette dernière caractéristique faisant ressortir la nécessité d'une formation convenable.

The evaluation of liver fibrosis is a vital component of the management of patients with chronic liver disease, both for guiding therapy and estimating prognosis. Traditionally, liver biopsy had been used for this purpose (1); however, biopsy is limited by invasiveness, cost, variability in histological interpretation, sampling error (2,3) and difficulty of repetition for monitoring changes in fibrosis over time.

Moreover, potentially serious, albeit uncommon, complications including hemorrhage and death may occur (4). Due to these limitations, numerous, noninvasive means for staging liver fibrosis have been developed, including transient elastography (TE) (5-8) using FibroScan (Echosens, France). TE is an ultrasound-based tool for measuring liver stiffness as a surrogate of liver fibrosis. It is widely used due to its high

[1]Liver Unit, Division of Gastroenterology and Hepatology, Department of Medicine; [2]Department of Community Health Sciences, University of Calgary; [3]Medical Services, Alberta Health Services, Calgary, Alberta

Correspondence: Dr Robert P Myers, Liver Unit, University of Calgary, 6D22, Teaching, Research and Wellness Building, 3280 Hospital Drive Northwest, Calgary, Alberta T2N 4Z6. e-mail rpmyers@ucalgary.ca

accuracy for the diagnosis of advanced fibrosis, thus reducing the use of biopsy for the initial evaluation of patients with liver disease (9,10). In addition, studies have demonstrated that liver stiffness is responsive to changes in fibrosis over time (eg, attributable to treatment or disease progression), thus supporting its use for serial patient monitoring. An emerging body of literature also supports the prognostic significance of liver stiffness, suggesting that TE may be useful for guiding management strategies including the intensity of follow-up (11-17). For example, because the incidence of variceal hemorrhage is low in patients with liver stiffness <21 kPa, restriction of endoscopic screening to cirrhotic patients with higher liver stiffness has been advocated (14).

Because numerous clinical decisions are made based on the results of liver stiffness measurement (LSM) using TE, it is vital to understand the reliability of this tool and factors that influence its accuracy. Traditionally, TE examinations with <10 valid measurements, a success rate <60% and/or a ratio of the interquartile range (IQR) of liver stiffness to the median value (IQR/M) >30% have been classified as unreliable (18). According to this definition, approximately 15% of LSMs are unreliable, with higher rates among older patients, women and patients with diabetes, hypertension, and higher body mass index (BMI) and waist circumference. Limited operator experience (<500 versus ≥500 examinations) may also influence reliability (18). However, this definition has been criticized because no studies have ever demonstrated that reliable results are more accurate than unreliable results. As such, Boursier et al (19) recently proposed a new definition of poorly reliable TE results (IQR/M >30% and median liver stiffness ≥7.1 kPa). In this study, poorly reliable LSMs – which occurred in 9% of patients – were less accurate than reliable LSMs according to multiple indicators of diagnostic test performance (19). The factors that influence the rate of poorly reliable results according to this definition have not been explored.

Accordingly, the objective of the present study was to examine the feasibility and reliability of TE using this revised definition of reliability in a large cohort of patients with various liver diseases and severities to reflect routine clinical practice. We aimed to identify patient and operator characteristics associated with poorly reliable results to better inform our interpretation of LSMs using TE.

METHODS

Study population

In the present retrospective study, 2437 consecutive patients who underwent LSM using TE (FibroScan) at the University of Calgary Liver Unit (UCLU; Calgary, Alberta), between July 2008 and June 2011 were identified. The UCLU is the major referral centre for patients with liver disease who reside in Southern Alberta and serves a catchment population of approximately 1.5 million. LSM using TE is performed routinely in all patients who attend the UCLU without overt evidence of hepatic decompensation. In patients with multiple examinations, only the first LSM was considered to eliminate selection bias (ie, repeated examinations on patients who are easier to scan). For our analysis of the prevalence of FibroScan failure and reliability (see definitions below), the entire study cohort was examined. To identify predictors of poorly reliable LSM, only patients for whom linkage with Alberta administrative databases was possible (n=2335) were included to permit identification of the patients' underlying liver diseases and comorbidities. Therefore, for these analyses, 36 nonresidents of Alberta, 32 patients with invalid provincial health numbers and 34 patients for whom linkage with the administrative data were unsuccessful were excluded. These patients had demographic characteristics and liver stiffness results similar to the remainder (data not shown). The Conjoint Health Research Ethics Board at the University of Calgary approved the study protocol.

LSM

Two experienced operators (OP1 and OP2) performed all FibroScan examinations as per the manufacturer's recommendations. OP2 was employed after OP1 and performed her first LSM in September 2010. Between July 2008 and July 2009, the FibroScan M probe was used in all patients; thereafter, the FibroScan XL probe was used in obese patients (BMI ≥30 kg/m²). Briefly, with the patient lying in the dorsal decubitus position and the right arm in maximal abduction, the tip of the FibroScan transducer probe was placed on the skin between the ribs over the right lobe of the liver. Assisted by a sonographic image, a portion of the liver at least 6 cm thick and free of large vascular structures was identified, and an attempt was made to collect at least 10 valid LSMs. The median liver stiffness value (in kPa) was considered to be representative of the elastic modulus of the liver. As an indicator of LSM variability, the IQR/M was calculated.

Administrative data sources

The present study used three Alberta administrative databases to identify the underlying liver disease etiologies and comorbidities of study participants via linkage using their unique personal health number. These databases have been used to examine the epidemiology (20-22), outcomes (22,23) and coding accuracy (20,24-28) of a variety of medical conditions.

1. Physician Claims Database. This database includes claims submitted for payment by Alberta physicians for services provided to registrants of the Alberta Health Care Insurance Plan, a universal plan that covers >99% of Alberta residents (29). Each record in the database includes the service provided, the date and up to three diagnosis fields. The database was queried from April 1, 2001 to March 31, 2011.

2. Inpatient Discharge Abstract Database. This database contains diagnosis, procedure and mortality information on all discharges from hospitals within Alberta. These data are routinely transmitted to the Canadian Institute for Health Information for aggregation with nationwide hospitalization data (29). Chart validation studies have shown rates of agreement exceeding 95% for demographic data and 75% to 96% for most responsible diagnosis codes (30). The database was queried from January 1, 1991 to January 31, 2012.

3. National Ambulatory Care Reporting System (NACRS)/ Ambulatory Care Classification System (ACCS) Database. This database contains information on facility-based ambulatory care including clinic and emergency department visits, same-day surgery, day procedures and rehabilitation services (29). The database was queried from July 1, 1996 to December 31, 2011.

Outcomes and predictor variables

The primary outcome variable was poorly reliable LSM, as defined by Boursier et al (19). Specifically, poorly reliable LSMs had an IQR/M >30% and median liver stiffness ≥7.1 kPa. Very reliable LSMs had an IQR/M ≤10%, whereas reliable LSMs had an IQR/M >10% and ≤30% (regardless of liver stiffness) or an IQR/M >30% with median liver stiffness <7.1 kPa. When compared with liver biopsy as the reference standard for staging fibrosis, poorly reliable LSMs are less accurate (ie, have lower areas under the ROC curves [AUROCs] and rates of accurate patient classification for fibrosis) than very reliable and reliable scans (19). As a secondary outcome measure, LSM failure, defined as no valid measurements after at least 10 attempts, was examined. The primary predictor variables included age, sex, the underlying liver disease, median liver stiffness (examined as a continuous variable and categorized as presumed cirrhosis [liver stiffness ≥12.5 kPa]) (31), comorbidities, the FibroScan operator (OP1 versus OP2), operator experience (first 499 scans versus ≥500 scans) (18) FibroScan probe (M versus XL) and the year of the LSM (2008 to 2009 versus 2010 to 2011). The hepatic diagnosis was categorized according to a hierarchy as follows: hepatitis B virus (HBV), hepatitis C virus, autoimmune (including primary biliary cirrhosis, primary sclerosing cholangitis and autoimmune hepatitis), hereditary hemochromatosis, alcoholic liver disease, nonalcoholic fatty liver disease and other (see Appendix 1 for list of relevant International Classification of Diseases, Ninth Revision,

TABLE 1

Characteristics of the study cohort according to the reliability of liver stiffness measurement

Variable	Entire cohort* (n=2335)	FibroScan Very reliable (n=659)	Reliable (n=1526)	Poorly reliable (n=113)	OR (95% CI) for poorly reliable FibroScan
Male sex	56 (1310)	58 (381)	55 (835)	65 (73)	1.45 (0.98–2.16)
Age, years, median (IQR)	50 (40–58)	49 (40–57)	50 (40–58)	53 (48–61)	**1.04 (1.02–1.05)**
Body mass index†, kg/m², median (IQR)	25.5 (23–30)	25 (22–28)	25.5 (23–30)	32.6 (25–41)	**1.06 (1.00–1.11)**
<30	75 (332)	86 (107)	73 (211)	48 (10)	Reference
≥30	25 (112)	14 (18)	27 (77)	53 (11)	**3.68 (1.52–8.94)**
Hepatic diagnosis					
Hepatitis B	27 (638)	31 (201)	27 (413)	18 (20)	**0.55 (0.34–0.90)**
Hepatitis C	36 (840)	36 (234)	35 (541)	44 (50)	1.44 (0.99–2.11)
Autoimmune	5.5 (129)	4.3 (28)	6.0 (92)	7.1 (8)	1.31 (0.62–2.75)
Hemochromatosis	3.0 (69)	3.2 (21)	2.8 (43)	2.7 (3)	0.90 (0.28–2.92)
Alcohol	3.3 (78)	3.6 (24)	2.8 (42)	6.2 (7)	2.12 (0.95–4.73)
Nonalcoholic fatty liver disease	6.8 (158)	7.9 (52)	6.0 (92)	8.9 (10)	1.38 (0.70–2.69)
Other/unknown	18 (423)	15 (99)	20 (303)	13 (15)	0.68 (0.39–1.18)
Comorbidities‡					
Congestive heart failure	4.2 (97)	3.2 (21)	4.0 (61)	8.9 (10)	**2.49 (1.25–4.94)**
Cardiac arrhythmia	6.5 (152)	5.6 (37)	6.1 (93)	12.4 (14)	**2.24 (1.24–4.02)**
Hypertension	34 (803)	33 (218)	33 (507)	50 (56)	**1.98 (1.35–2.89)**
Paralysis	0.8 (18)	0.3 (2)	0.8 (12)	2.7 (3)	**4.23 (1.20–14.9)**
Chronic lung disease	30 (699)	29 (193)	29 (445)	40 (45)	**1.60 (1.09–2.36)**
Diabetes mellitus	12 (274)	9.4 (62)	11 (172)	23 (26)	**2.49 (1.58–3.94)**
Peptic ulcer	3.0 (69)	3.3 (22)	2.4 (37)	6.2 (7)	**2.38 (1.06–5.34)**
Coagulopathy	7.7 (179)	8.0 (53)	6.6 (100)	19 (21)	**3.03 (1.84–5.01)**
Fluid/electrolyte disorders	15 (340)	14 (94)	14 (210)	23 (26)	**1.85 (1.17–2.91)**
Alcohol abuse	13 (306)	14 (90)	12 (181)	22 (25)	**2.01 (1.26–3.18)**
Liver stiffness, kPa, median (IQR)	6.3 (4.7–10.1)	6.0 (4.6–8.8)	6.1 (4.6–9.6)	13.3 (9.0–27.0)	**1.04 (1.03–1.05)**
Cirrhosis (≥12.5 kPa)	19 (430)	17 (109)	17 (257)	57 (64)	**6.49 (4.40–9.57)**
M probe (versus XL probe)	86 (2009)	88 (582)	86 (1313)	78 (88)	**0.54 (0.34–0.85)**
Operator 2 (versus operator 1)	53 (1235)	53 (361)	54 (823)	35 (39)	**0.45 (0.30–0.66)**
Operator experience					
1–499 scans	35 (816)	38 (250)	33 (497)	37 (42)	Reference
≥500 scans	65 (1519)	62 (409)	67 (1029)	62 (71)	0.88 (0.59–1.30)
Year of FibroScan					
2008–2009	24 (550)	23 (154)	23 (334)	38 (43)	Reference
2010–2011	76 (1785)	77 (505)	78 (1192)	62 (70)	**0.47 (0.32–0.69)**

*Data presented as % (n) unless otherwise indicated. Bolded values indicate statistical significance (ie, P<0.05). *Entire cohort includes 37 FibroScan (Echosens, France) failures; †Body mass index data from medical record review available in 444 patients; ‡Only comorbidities with statistically significant associations with poorly reliable liver stiffness measurement are included. IQR Interquartile range*

Clinical Modification [ICD-9-CM] [32] and ICD-10 [33] codes). For example, according to this approach, a patient with any record of a diagnosis code for HBV with or without other hepatic diagnoses would be categorized as having HBV. Comorbid conditions occurring before the FibroScan examination were defined using the Elixhauser list of 30 comorbidities (34), a well-validated algorithm for predicting outcomes in patients with hepatic (35) and nonhepatic disorders (34,36). Liver diseases were excluded from this algorithm. Also examined were the type of FibroScan probe because use of the XL probe could be considered a surrogate marker for obesity, which is not available in the administrative databases. In a subset of patients, medical records were reviewed to extract the BMI on the day of the FibroScan examination.

Statistical analyses

Between-group comparisons were made using Fisher's exact and χ^2 tests for categorical variables, and Wilcoxon rank-sum and Kruskall-Wallis tests for continuous variables. Univariate logistic regression was used to identify predictors of poorly reliable FibroScan examinations including age, sex, underlying liver disease, liver stiffness, comorbidities, the FibroScan probe, the operator, operator experience and year. Variables that were significant in univariate analyses were included in stepwise-forward, multiple logistic regression models in which

variables with P<0.1 were retained in the models. In the subset of patients with available BMI data from medical record review, an additional multivariate analysis was performed including BMI. All analyses were performed using Stata version 11.0 (StataCorp, USA); a two-sided P<0.05 was considered to be statistically significant.

RESULTS

Patient characteristics

A total of 2335 patients underwent LSM using TE at the UCLU between July 2008 and June 2011 and met the study inclusion criteria; their characteristics are outlined in Table 1. The median age was 50 years (IQR 40 to 58 years) and 56% were male. The majority of patients had chronic hepatitis C virus (36%) or HBV (27%) infection, while 7% had nonalcoholic fatty liver disease and 6% had autoimmune liver disease. Among 444 patients with BMI data available from medical record review, the median BMI was 25.5 kg/m²; 25% of patients were obese (BMI ≥30 kg/m²). Twelve percent of the cohort had a history of diabetes mellitus, 34% had hypertension, 35% had depression, and 13% and 10% had a history of alcohol and drug abuse, respectively.

LSM results

The majority of LSMs (86%) were obtained using the FibroScan M probe, 47% were performed by OP1 and 76% were performed during

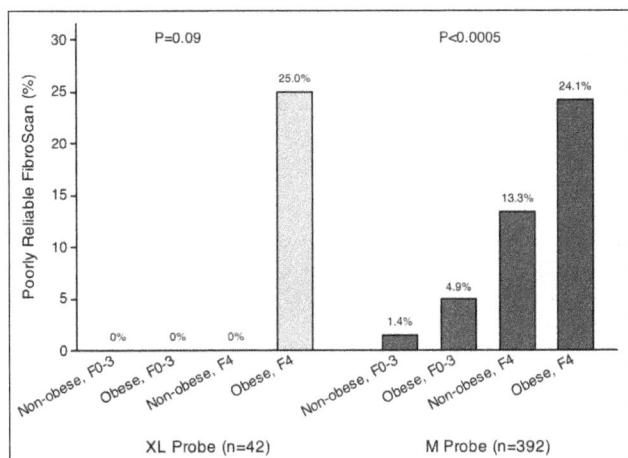

Figure 1) *Prevalence of poorly reliable FibroScan (Echosens, France) examinations according to obesity (body mass index [BMI] ≥30 kg/m², presumed cirrhosis (F4; liver stiffness ≥12.5 kPa) and FibroScan probe (M versus XL). This analysis is limited to 434 patients with available BMI data and successful liver stiffness measurement (ie, failures excluded)*

the latter part of the study (2010 to 2011). In total, LSM failure was observed in 37 (1.6%) patients. The incidence of FibroScan failure was greater with the XL probe (3.4% [11 of 326]) than the M probe (1.3% [26 of 2009]; P=0.01) and for OP1 (2.3% [25 of 1100]) compared with OP2 (1.0% [12 of 1235]; P=0.01). Among the 2335 successfully measured patients, the median LSM was 6.3 kPa (IQR 4.7 kPa to 10.1 kPa). The majority (58%) of patients were estimated to have F0 to F1 fibrosis (liver stiffness <7.1 kPa), while 19% had presumed cirrhosis (liver stiffness ≥12.5 kPa) (31).

FibroScan reliability
According to the reliability criteria of Boursier et al (19) and excluding LSM failures, FibroScan examinations were classified as very reliable in 29% (n=659), reliable in 66% (n=1526) and poorly reliable in 4.9% (n=113) of patients (Table 1). According to previously recommended criteria for reliability (18), 15% of these examinations (n=343) would have been classified as unreliable (valid shots <10, success rate <60% and/or IQR/M >30%). Based on the updated definitions of Boursier et al (19), 41% of these 'unreliable' examinations would have been classified as very reliable, 22% as reliable and 37% as poorly reliable.

Predictors of poorly reliable FibroScan results
Table 1 includes patient and procedural characteristics according to the reliability of the FibroScan examination. In univariate analysis, older age (OR per year 1.04 [95% CI 1.02 to 1.05]) was associated with an increased risk of poorly reliable LSM; male sex was of borderline significance (OR 1.45 [95% CI 0.98 to 2.16]; P=0.06). Patients with HBV were less likely to have a poorly reliable LSM (OR 0.55 [95% CI 0.34 to 0.90]). Several comorbid conditions were associated with an increased risk of poorly reliable LSM including congestive heart failure, cardiac arrhythmias, hypertension, chronic pulmonary disease, diabetes mellitus, paralysis, peptic ulcer disease, coagulopathy, fluid and electrolyte disorders, and alcohol abuse (all P<0.05; Table 1).

Patients with poorly reliable LSM had higher median liver stiffness (13.3 kPa) than those with very reliable (6.0 kPa) and reliable scans (6.1 kPa; P<0.0005). The unadjusted odds of a poorly reliable scan increased by 4% per 1 kPa increase in liver stiffness (OR 1.04 [95% CI 1.03 to 1.05]). Similarly, presumed cirrhosis was more common in patients with poorly reliable LSM (57% versus 17% in patients with very reliable and reliable LSM; P<0.0005). Among 430 patients with cirrhosis, poorly reliable scans were recorded in 15% versus only 2.6% among noncirrhotic patients (OR 6.49 [95% CI 4.40 to 9.57]). In terms of procedural characteristics, poorly reliable LSM was less frequent with the M probe than the XL probe (4.1% versus 7.6%; OR

TABLE 2
Independent predictors of poorly reliable FibroScan examinations*

Variable	OR (95% CI)	P
Age†, per year	1.03 (1.01–1.05)	**<0.0005**
Male sex†	1.32 (0.87–1.99)	0.19
Obesity‡ (body mass index ≥30 kg/m²)	2.93 (0.95–9.05)	0.06
Chronic pulmonary disease	1.58 (1.05–2.37)	**0.03**
Coagulopathy	2.22 (1.31–3.76)	**0.003**
Liver stiffness†, per kPa	1.03 (1.02–1.05)	**<0.0005**
Cirrhosis§	5.24 (3.49–7.89)	**<0.0005**
M probe (versus XL probe)	0.64 (0.38–1.06)	0.08
Operator (OP1 versus OP2)	2.58 (1.70–3.93)	**<0.0005**
Operator experience† (<500 versus ≥500 scans)	0.86 (0.67–1.10)	0.23

Data from a stepwise-forward logistic regression model (bolded values represent statistical significance) including age, sex, liver stiffness, FibroScan (Echosens, France) probe, operator (OP), OP experience, year of scan (2008 to 2009 versus 2010 to 2011), liver disease (hepatitis B versus other) and all comorbidities with P<0.05 in Table 1; †Variable forced into the model based on pre-existing literature suggesting an association with FibroScan reliability. If not shown in the Table, variables were dropped from the model due to P>0.10 (eg, liver disease, year and other comorbidties); ‡OR for obesity from a separate model including the same variables as described above in the subset of patients with available body mass index data and excluding FibroScan failures (n=434); §OR for cirrhosis from a separate model including the same variables as described above

0.54 [95% CI 0.34 to 0.85]) and in scans performed by OP2 compared with OP1 (OR 0.45 [95% CI 0.30 to 0.66]). However, operator experience (<500 versus ≥500 scans) was not a significant predictor of poorly reliable LSM. Examinations performed in the latter half of the study period were less likely to be poorly reliable than earlier scans (2010 to 2011 versus 2008 to 2009 [4.0% versus 8.1%, respectively]; OR 0.47 [95% CI 0.32 to 0.69]).

Among 434 patients with available BMI data (excluding LSM failures), the median BMI was greater in patients with poorly reliable scans (30.0 kg/m² [IQR 25.5 to 32.0 kg/m²] versus 25.4 kg/m² [IQR 22.9 to 29.0 kg/m²]; P=0.004). Poorly reliable scans were observed in 10% (11 of 106) of obese patients (BMI ≥30 kg/m²) compared with only 3.1% (10 of 328) of nonobese individuals (OR 3.68 [95% CI 1.52 to 8.94]). Using the XL probe, 5.6% (two of 36) of obese patients had poorly reliable results versus 13% (nine of 70) measured using the M probe (P=0.33). The combined influence of obesity and presumed cirrhosis on the risk of poorly reliable LSM according to FibroScan probe is illustrated in Figure 1. In patients with obesity and cirrhosis, the risk of poorly reliable results was high (24% to 25%) with both probes compared with only 0% to 13.3% in patients with none or only one of these risk factors.

Table 2 includes the results of a multivariate model for predictors of poorly reliable FibroScan examinations with adjustment for age, sex, hepatic diagnosis (HBV versus other), liver stiffness, comorbidities, FibroScan probe and operator, operator experience and year. Independent predictors of poorly reliable LSM included older age (OR 1.03 per year [95% CI 1.01 to 1.05]), OP1 (OR 2.58 [95% CI 1.70 to 3.93]), higher liver stiffness (OR 1.03 [95% CI 1.02 to 1.05]), and a history of coagulopathy (OR 2.22 [95% CI 1.31 to 3.76]) and chronic pulmonary disease (OR 1.58 [95% CI 1.05 to 2.37]). While use of the M probe was of borderline significance (OR 0.64 [95% CI 0.38 to 1.06]; P=0.08), operator experience, year of LSM and patient sex were not statistically significant. In a supplementary analysis, in which liver stiffness was categorized rather than examined as a continuous variable, presumed cirrhosis was associated with a fivefold higher risk of poorly reliable results (OR 5.28 [95% CI 3.50 to 7.95]); the remainder of the results were largely unchanged (data not shown). Finally, in an analysis including BMI from medical record review, obesity was associated with nearly threefold odds of poorly reliable results (OR 2.93 [95% CI 0.95 to 9.05]; P=0.06) after adjustment for FibroScan probe and the other factors described above.

DISCUSSION

In the present large practice audit of >2300 FibroScan examinations, poorly reliable results – as defined by the revised definition of Boursier et al (19) – were uncommon, occurring in approximately 5% of individuals. In contrast, unreliable results according to a previously recommended definition (valid shots <10, success rate <60% and/or IQR/M >30% [18]) were observed in 15% of patients. This difference is relevant because the latter 'unreliable' results have never been shown to be less accurate than reliable results. In fact, use of this outdated definition of reliability may have led to the needless discarding of approximately 10% of Fibroscan results, with potentially important implications in clinical practice and in research studies. Importantly, approximately two-thirds of these results would have been classified as very reliable or reliable according to the revised definitions. The prevalence of poorly reliable results observed in our study is slightly lower than that of Boursier et al (19) (4.9% versus 9.1%). This likely reflects differences in the study populations, particularly the lower prevalence of advanced fibrosis in our study (median liver stiffness 6.3 kPa versus 8.1 kPa in Boursier et al [19]) because higher liver stiffness (≥7.1 kPa) is a criterion in the definition for reliability (see below). Moreover, liver stiffness was measured using the XL probe in 25% of our patients, whereas only the M probe was used in the French study. Because liver stiffness measured with the XL probe is consistently lower than with the M probe, a lower rate of poorly reliable results could also be anticipated in our study.

Because TE is increasingly being used in clinical decision making, it is important to understand factors that influence its reliability because poorly reliable results are less accurate than reliable examinations. Specifically, in the study by Boursier et al (19), poorly reliable results were only 70% accurate for the diagnosis of cirrhosis compared with 86% and 90% in patients with reliable and very reliable results, respectively. Corresponding AUROCs for cirrhosis were 0.82, 0.90 and 0.97, respectively. With these facts in mind, we examined several patient- and operator-related characteristics as potential predictors of unreliable examinations. As previously reported, older age was associated with an increased risk of unreliable LSM (18). The exact reasons for this finding have never been identified; however, we speculate that age-related alterations in the chest wall are involved. It is known that chest wall compliance decreases with age due to structural changes of the intercostal muscles, intercostal joints and rib-vertebral articulations. In addition, age-associated osteoporosis may increase kyphosis, resulting in changes in the geometry of the thorax (37). On a related note, we identified a 1.6-fold increase in the risk of poorly reliable results among patients with chronic lung disease, predominantly chronic obstructive pulmonary disease (data not shown). This novel finding may also relate to structural changes in the chest wall (eg, pulmonary hyperinflation) or technical difficulties with the FibroScan procedure due to deep respirations in these patients. Because an increased risk of LSM failure or unreliable results has not been reported in cohorts with cystic fibrosis (38), additional studies are necessary to confirm this finding and to elucidate potential mechanisms.

Although previous studies have reported that women have a higher rate of unreliable FibroScan examinations compared with men (18), we did not observe a significant impact of sex using the updated definition of reliability. As previously reported (18), obesity was associated with a nearly threefold risk of unreliable results in a subanalysis of patients with available BMI data. The importance of obesity as a predisposing factor for poorly reliable results is supported by the borderline effect of XL probe use (P=0.08), considered a surrogate marker for obesity in the absence of BMI data in all patients. Presumably, subcutaneous and prehepatic adipose tissue in obese patients interferes with transmission of the mechanical shear wave and/or the measurement of its propagation by the FibroScan device (7).

Previous studies by Lucidarme et al (39) and Myers et al (40) have demonstrated an impact of fibrosis stage on the rate of discordance between fibrosis estimated by LSM and liver biopsy; however, an impact on poorly reliable results has not been reported. In the current study, elevated liver stiffness was an independent predictor of poorly reliable LSM. Presumed cirrhosis was the most important risk factor, with fivefold higher odds of poorly reliable results in cirrhotic patients. This finding is not surprising because an LSM ≥7.1 kPa is one criterion in the definition of poor reliability (19). The other factor, IQR/M, also likely played a role because LSM variability tends to be greater in patients with cirrhosis (data not shown). The reason for this is unclear, but may relate to the broader range of potential LSMs in cirrhotic patients (ie, approximately 12.5 kPa to 75 kPa) compared with those who have lower liver stiffness (ie, 2.5 kPa to 12.4 kPa) (31). Interestingly, coagulopathy was associated with a twofold risk of poorly reliable results. Because there is no clear physical explanation for this finding, we suspect it reflects more severe liver disease and, therefore, higher liver stiffness in coagulopathic patients. The majority of these patients had diagnosis codes for thrombocytopenia as opposed to hereditary or acquired coagulation defects (data not shown). Because the effect of coagulopathy on poorly reliable results was independent of liver stiffness, it likely reflects the imperfect sensitivity of FibroScan for the diagnosis of cirrhosis.

A strength of our study was our analysis of the impact of specific liver conditions and comorbidities on FibroScan reliability using administrative data. In addition to uncovering a novel association between chronic lung disease and poorly reliable results, this approach revealed several other associations. First, patients with HBV had a lower likelihood of unreliable results. Because HBV-infected patients in our practice tend to be Asian and of smaller stature, this finding is not unexpected. In fact, we previously reported no FibroScan failures with the M probe in a study examining the value of the pediatric (S2) probe in this patient population (41). Second, hypertension and diabetes, components of the metabolic syndrome that have been associated with unreliable LSMs in previous studies (18), were significant in unadjusted, but not adjusted, analyses. Similarly, patients with congestive heart failure or arrhythmias had a twofold higher risk of poorly reliable LSM in univariate analyses. These findings may relate to hepatic congestion due to cardiac dysfunction, a well-described cause of liver stiffness overestimation (42). Because the power of our multivariate analysis may have been limited due to a small number of poorly reliable results (n=113), studies that use this novel definition of reliability in larger patient populations will be necessary to confirm or refute these findings.

In addition to patient-related predictors of FibroScan reliability, we examined the impact of procedural characteristics including the operator and operator experience. Castera et al (18) reported a lower risk of unreliable results among seven operators who had performed at least 500 examinations, challenging previous assertions that that a novice can consistently obtain reliable results after a short training period of only 50 examinations. In our study, however, there was no difference in the proportion of poorly reliable results between the first 500 and subsequent examinations by our two operators. On the contrary, OP1 was twice as likely to produce a poorly reliable LSM as OP2. This finding supports the importance of adequate operator training and ongoing quality control when using the FibroScan in clinical decision making. It is important to note, however, that these results were confounded by the availability of the FibroScan XL probe only during the final two years of the study. Therefore, OP1 – who was employed before OP2 – scanned many obese patients using the M probe during the early part of the study. This likely led to an overestimation of her true rate of unreliable results. In fact, OP1 was twice as likely to have FibroScan failure as OP2, presumably for the same reason.

Our study has several limitations that warrant discussion. First, we did not have histological data to confirm whether poorly reliable LSMs were less accurate for staging fibrosis than reliable examinations. Second, because this was a retrospective study, we did not prospectively collect data regarding BMI and other anthropometric measures (eg, waist circumference, thoracic perimeter, skin-capsular distance) that may have influenced FibroScan reliability. Similarly, we relied on administrative data to define patient comorbidities and hepatic diagnoses. Although many of these codes have been validated by medical record review (20,24-28), additional validation is necessary.

CONCLUSION

Poorly reliable FibroScan results are uncommon, occurring in approximately 5% of individuals. The most important determinants of poorly reliable LSM are older age, obesity, higher liver stiffness and the operator, the latter emphasizing the need for adequate training and quality control. A novel association between chronic pulmonary disease and poorly reliable results requires confirmation. Additional studies should be conducted to identify means of improving the reliability of FibroScan examinations so as to improve the accuracy of this valuable tool.

DISCLOSURES: Dr Myers was supported by a salary support award from the Canadian Institutes for Health Research (CIHR). Dr Kaplan is supported by salary support awards from the CIHR and Alberta Innovates-Health Solutions (AI-HS). Dr Swain is supported by the Cal Wenzel Family Foundation Chair in Hepatology. This study was supported, in part, by grants from AI-HS, CIHR (#84371) and the Canadian Liver Foundation. This study was based, in part, on data provided by Alberta Health. The interpretation and conclusions contained herein are those of the researchers and do not necessarily represent the views of the Government of Alberta. Neither the Government nor Alberta Health express any opinion in relation to this study. The authors have no financial disclosures or conflicts of interest to declare.

APPENDIX 1
Diagnosis codes used to define underlying liver disease etiologies

Hepatic diagnoses	Diagnosis code(s) (reference)	
	ICD-9-CM (32)	ICD-10 (33)
Hepatitis B	070.2, 070.3	B16, B18.0, B18.1, B19.1
Hepatitis C	070.41, 070.44, 070.51, 070.54, 070.7	B17.1, B18.2, B19.2
Nonalcoholic fatty liver disease	571.8	K75.81, K76.0
Alcoholic liver disease	571.0, 571.1, 571.2, 571.3	K70
Primary biliary cirrhosis	571.6	K74.3
Primary sclerosing cholangitis	576.1	K83.0
Autoimmune hepatitis	571.42	K75.4
Hemochromatosis	275.0	E83.1

ICD International Classification of Diseases

REFERENCES
1. Rockey DC, Caldwell SH, Goodman ZD, Nelson RC, Smith AD. Liver biopsy. Hepatology 2009;49:1017-44.
2. Regev A, Berho M, Jeffers LJ, et al. Sampling error and intraobserver variation in liver biopsy in patients with chronic HCV infection. Am J Gastroenterol 2002;97:2614-8.
3. Ratziu V, Charlotte F, Heurtier A, et al. Sampling variability of liver biopsy in nonalcoholic fatty liver disease. Gastroenterology 2005;128:1898-906.
4. Myers RP, Fong A, Shaheen AA. Utilization rates, complications and costs of percutaneous liver biopsy: A population-based study including 4275 biopsies. Liver Int 2008;28:705-12.
5. Sandrin L, Fourquet B, Hasquenoph JM, et al. Transient elastography: A new noninvasive method for assessment of hepatic fibrosis. Ultrasound Med Biol 2003;29:1705-13.
6. Myers RP, Elkashab M, Ma M, Crotty P, Pomier-Layrargues G. Transient elastography for the noninvasive assessment of liver fibrosis: A multicentre Canadian study. Can J Gastroenterol 2010;24:661-70.
7. Myers RP, Pomier-Layrargues G, Kirsch R, et al. Feasibility and diagnostic performance of the FibroScan XL probe for liver stiffness measurement in overweight and obese patients. Hepatology 2012;55:199-208.
8. Castera L, Forns X, Alberti A. Non-invasive evaluation of liver fibrosis using transient elastography. J Hepatol 2008;48:835-47.
9. Friedrich-Rust M, Ong MF, Martens S, et al. Performance of transient elastography for the staging of liver fibrosis: A meta-analysis. Gastroenterology 2008;134:960-74.
10. Steadman R, Myers RP, Leggett L, et al. A health technology assessment of transient elastography in adult liver disease. Can J Gastroenterol 2013;27:149-58.
11. Vergniol J, Foucher J, Terrebonne E, et al. Noninvasive tests for fibrosis and liver stiffness predict 5-year outcomes of patients with chronic hepatitis C. Gastroenterology 2011;140:1970-9.
12. Klibansky DA, Mehta SH, Curry M, Nasser I, Challies T, Afdhal NH. Transient elastography for predicting clinical outcomes in patients with chronic liver disease. J Viral Hepat 2012;19:e184-e193.
13. Merchante N, Rivero-Juarez A, Tellez F, et al. Liver stiffness predicts clinical outcome in human immunodeficiency virus/hepatitis C virus-coinfected patients with compensated liver cirrhosis. Hepatology 2012;56:228-38.
14. Robic MA, Procopet B, Metivier S, et al. Liver stiffness accurately predicts portal hypertension related complications in patients with chronic liver disease: A prospective study. J Hepatol 2011;55:1017-24.
15. Kim SU, Lee JH, Kim do Y, et al. Prediction of liver-related events using fibroscan in chronic hepatitis B patients showing advanced liver fibrosis. PLoS One 2012;7:e36676.
16. Masuzaki R, Tateishi R, Yoshida H, et al. Prospective risk assessment for hepatocellular carcinoma development in patients with chronic hepatitis C by transient elastography. Hepatology 2009;49:1954-61.
17. Jung KS, Kim SU, Ahn SH, et al. Risk assessment of hepatitis B virus-related hepatocellular carcinoma development using liver stiffness measurement (FibroScan). Hepatology 2011;53:885-94.
18. Castera L, Foucher J, Bernard PH, et al. Pitfalls of liver stiffness measurement: A 5-year prospective study of 13,369 examinations. Hepatology 2010;51:828-35.
19. Boursier J, Zarski JP, de Ledinghen V, et al. Determination of reliability criteria for liver stiffness evaluation by transient elastography. Hepatology 2013;57:1182-91.
20. Myers RP, Liu M, Shaheen AA. The burden of hepatitis C virus infection is growing: A Canadian population-based study of hospitalizations from 1994 to 2004. Can J Gastroenterol 2008;22:381-7.
21. Kaplan GG, Gregson DB, Laupland KB. Population-based study of the epidemiology of and the risk factors for pyogenic liver abscess. Clin Gastroenterol Hepatol 2004;2:1032-8.
22. Myers RP, Shaheen AA, Fong A, et al. Epidemiology and natural history of primary biliary cirrhosis in a Canadian health region: A population-based study. Hepatology 2009;50:1884-92.
23. Myers RP, Shaheen AA, Li B, Dean S, Quan H. Impact of liver disease, alcohol abuse, and unintentional ingestions on the outcomes of acetaminophen overdose. Clin Gastroenterol Hepatol 2008;6:918-25.
24. Myers RP, Leung Y, Shaheen AA, Li B. Validation of ICD-9-CM/ICD-10 coding algorithms for the identification of patients with acetaminophen overdose and hepatotoxicity using administrative data. BMC Health Serv Res 2007;7:159.
25. Quan H, Parsons GA, Ghali WA. Assessing accuracy of diagnosis-type indicators for flagging complications in administrative data. J Clin Epidemiol 2004;57:366-72.
26. Quan H, Parsons GA, Ghali WA. Validity of information on comorbidity derived from ICD-9-CCM administrative data. Med Care 2002;40:675-85.
27. Quan H, Parsons GA, Ghali WA. Validity of procedure codes in International Classification of Diseases, 9th revision, clinical modification administrative data. Med Care 2004;42:801-9.
28. Quan H, Sundararajan V, Halfon P, et al. Coding algorithms for defining comorbidities in ICD-9-CM and ICD-10 administrative data. Med Care 2005;43:1130-9.
29. Data Disclosure Handbook. In: Alberta Health and Wellness; 2003:1-15.

30. Williams JI, Young W. A summary of studies on the quality of health care administrative databases in Canada. In: Goel V, Williams JI, Anderson GM, Blackstein-Hirsch P, Fooks C, Naylor CD, eds. Patterns of Health Care in Ontario: The ICES Practice Atlas, 2nd edn. Ottawa: The Canadian Medical Association, 1996:339-345.

31. Castera L, Vergniol J, Foucher J, et al. Prospective comparison of transient elastography, Fibrotest, APRI, and liver biopsy for the assessment of fibrosis in chronic hepatitis C. Gastroenterology 2005;128:343-50.

32. International Classificiation of Diseases, 9th Revision, Clinical Modification (ICD-9-CM). Los Angeles: Practice Management Information Corporation, 2001.

33. WHO. International Statistical Classification of Diseases and Related Health Problems, Tenth Revision (ICD-10) Geneva: World Health Organization, 1992.

34. Elixhauser A, Steiner C, Harris DR, Coffey RM. Comorbidity measures for use with administrative data. Med Care 1998;36:8-27.

35. Myers RP, Quan H, Hubbard JN, Shaheen AA, Kaplan GG. Predicting in-hospital mortality in patients with cirrhosis: Results differ across risk adjustment methods. Hepatology 2009;49:568-77.

36. Li B, Evans D, Faris P, Dean S, Quan H. Risk adjustment performance of Charlson and Elixhauser comorbidities in ICD-9 and ICD-10 administrative databases. BMC Health Serv Res 2008;8:12.

37. Sprung J, Gajic O, Warner DO. Review article: Age related alterations in respiratory function – anesthetic considerations. Can J Anaesth 2006;53:1244-57.

38. Witters P, De Boeck K, Dupont L, et al. Non-invasive liver elastography (Fibroscan) for detection of cystic fibrosis-associated liver disease. J Cyst Fibros 2009;8:392-9.

39. Lucidarme D, Foucher J, Le Bail B, et al. Factors of accuracy of transient elastography (Fibroscan) for the diagnosis of liver fibrosis in chronic hepatitis C. Hepatology 2009;49:1083-9.

40. Myers RP, Crotty P, Pomier-Layrargues G, Ma M, Urbanski SJ, Elkashab M. Prevalence, risk factors and causes of discordance in fibrosis staging by transient elastography and liver biopsy. Liver Int 2010;30:1471-80.

41. Pradhan F, Ladak F, Tracey J, Crotty P, Myers RP. Feasibility and reliability of the FibroScan S2 (pediatric) probe compared with the M probe for liver stiffness measurement in small adults with chronic liver disease. Ann Hepatol 2013;12:100-7.

42. Millonig G, Friedrich S, Adolf S, et al. Liver stiffness is directly influenced by central venous pressure. J Hepatol 2010;52:206-10.

32

Caesarean section to prevent transmission of hepatitis B: A meta-analysis

Matthew S Chang MD[1], Sravanya Gavini MD[1], Priscila C Andrade PharmD[2], Julia McNabb-Baltar MD[1]

MS Chang, S Gavini, PC Andrade, J McNabb-Baltar. Caesarean section to prevent transmission of hepatitis B: A meta-analysis. Can J Gastroenterol Hepatol 2014;28(8):439-444.

BACKGROUND: Vertical transmission of hepatitis B virus (HBV) occurs in up to 10% to 20% of births.
OBJECTIVE: To assess whether Caesarean section, compared with vaginal delivery, prevents HBV transmission.
METHODS: A systematic review and meta-analysis was conducted. Two investigators independently searched PubMed, EMBASE and other databases for relevant studies published between 1988 and 2013. A manual search of relevant topics and major conferences for abstracts was also conducted. Randomized trials, cohort and case-control studies assessing the effect of delivery mode on vertical transmission of HBV were included. Studies assessing antiviral therapy and patients with coinfection were excluded. The primary outcome was HBV transmission rates according to delivery method.
RESULTS: Of the 430 studies identified, 10 were included. Caesarean section decreased the odds of HBV transmission by 38% compared with vaginal delivery (OR 0.62 [95% CI 0.40 to 0.98]; P=0.04) based on a random-effects model. Significant heterogeneity among studies was found (I^2=63%; P=0.003), which was largely explained by variation in hepatitis B immune globulin (HBIG) administration. Meta-regression showed a significant linear association between the percentage of infants receiving HBIG per study and the log OR (P=0.005), with the least benefit observed in studies with 100% HBIG administration. Subgroup analysis of hepatitis B e-antigen-positive women who underwent Caesarean section did not show a significant reduction in vertical transmission.
DISCUSSION: Caesarean section may protect against HBV transmission; however, convincing benefit could not be demonstrated due to significant study heterogeneity from variable HBIG administration, highlighting the importance of HBIG in HBV prevention.
CONCLUSION: More high-quality studies are needed before any recommendations can be made.

Key Words: *Hepatitis; Hepatitis B immune globulin; Prophylaxis; Vaccination*

La césarienne pour éviter la transmission de l'hépatite B : une méta-analyse

HISTORIQUE : Dans 10 % à 20 % des accouchements, le virus de l'hépatite B (VHB) est transmis verticalement au nouveau-né.
OBJECTIF : Évaluer si la césarienne permet mieux d'éviter la transmission du VHB que l'accouchement vaginal.
MÉTHODOLOGIE : Une analyse systématique et une méta-analyse ont été menées. Deux chercheurs ont fait des recherches indépendantes dans PubMed, EMBASE et d'autres bases de données pour en extraire les études pertinentes publiées entre 1988 et 2013. On a également procédé à une recherche manuelle des sujets pertinents et des grands congrès et colloques afin d'en dépouiller les résumés. Les essais aléatoires, les études de cohortes et les études cas-témoins évaluant l'effet du mode d'accouchement sur la transmission verticale du VHB ont été inclus, mais les études évaluant la thérapie antivirale et les patients co-infectés ont été exclues. Le résultat primaire était le taux de transmission du VHB en fonction du mode d'accouchement.
RÉSULTATS : Dix des 430 études repérées ont été incluses. D'après un modèle à effets aléatoires, la césarienne réduisait de 38 % le risque de transmission du VHB par rapport à l'accouchement vaginal (RC 0,62 [95 % IC 0,40 à 0,98]; P=0,04). L'importante hétérogénéité entre les études (I^2=63 %; P=0,003) s'expliquait en grande partie par la variation dans l'administration d'immunoglobuline de l'hépatite B (IgHB). La méta-régression a démontré une association linéaire significative entre le pourcentage de nourrissons recevant de l'IgHB dans chaque étude et le logarithme du rapport de cotes (P=0,005), le moins grand avantage étant observé dans des études où 100 % des sujets avaient reçu de l'IgHB. L'analyse de sous-groupe des femmes porteuses de l'antigène e du VHB qui avaient subi une césarienne a établi que la transmission verticale ne diminuait pas de manière significative.
DISCUSSION : La césarienne protège peut-être contre la transmission du VHB, mais il été impossible de dégager des avantages convaincants en raison de l'hétérogénéité importante des études, attribuable à la variabilité dans l'administration d'IgHB, ce qui en fait ressortir l'importance pour prévenir le VHB.
CONCLUSION : Il faudra mener plus d'études de haute qualité avant de proposer des recommandations.

Four hundred million individuals are infected with hepatitis B virus (HBV) worldwide (1), which can lead to chronic hepatitis, cirrhosis and hepatocellular carcinoma. Most chronic infections are acquired perinatally via vertical transmission from the mother (2). HBV transmission has declined dramatically with the advent of universal screening of pregnant women in conjunction with passive and active immunization using hepatitis B immune globulin (HBIG) and HBV vaccine in the neonatal period. However, transmission remains as high as 10% to 20% in cases for which the mother has high viral DNA or positive hepatitis B e antigen (HBeAg) levels (3,4).

With HIV, Caesarean section has been shown to be efficacious in reducing vertical transmission from highly contagious mothers to their infants (5). In contrast, the effect of delivery mode on HBV transmission remains controversial (6,7). Accordingly, we performed a systematic review and meta-analysis to determine whether Caesarean section, compared with vaginal delivery, prevented transmission of HBV from infected mother to infant.

METHODS

Data sources and searches

The Cochrane Collaboration methodology was applied to search PubMed, EMBASE, LILACS, BIOSIS and the Cochrane databases for articles in English, Portuguese, French or Spanish from 1988 to 2013. In addition, references of relevant articles and abstracts from major conferences were manually searched. The following search terms were used as both keywords and medical subject heading terms, where applicable, after consultation with a reference librarian (Paul Bain

[1]*Division of Gastroenterology, Hepatology, and Endoscopy, Brigham and Women's Hospital;* [2]*Laboratory of Neuromodulation & Center for Clinical Research Learning, Spaulding Rehabilitation Hospital, Harvard Medical School, Boston, Massachusetts, USA*
Correspondence: Dr Julia McNabb-Baltar, Division of Gastroenterology, Hepatology, and Endoscopy, Brigham and Women's Hospital, Harvard Medical School, 75 Francis Street, Boston, Massachusetts 02115 USA e-mail jmcnabb-baltar@partners.org

PhD, Harvard Medical School, Countway Library of Medicine, Boston, USA): Hepatitis B, Hepatitis B Virus, HBV, HBsAg, HBeAg, Caesarean Section, C section, "Mode of delivery", Pregnancy, Vertical Transmission, Perinatal Transmission, mother-to-child transmission, prevention. PubMed was searched for "Hepatitis B"[Mesh] OR "Hepatitis B virus"[Mesh] OR hepatitis b[tiab] OR HBV[tiab] OR HBsAg[tiab] OR HBeAg[tiab] AND (c section*[tiab] OR Caesarean*[tiab] OR "Caesarean Section"[Mesh] OR ECS[tiab]) and EMBASE was searched for 'hepatitis B'/exp OR 'hepatitis b':ti,ab OR HBV:ti,ab OR HBsAg:Ti,ab OR HBeAg:ti,ab, combined with 'Caesarean section'/exp OR caesarean*:ti,ab OR 'c section':ti,ab OR 'c sections':ti,ab OR ecs:ti,ab. Authors were contacted when data were ambiguous or missing.

Study selection

Inclusion criteria were determined a priori among the authors. Published and in-print randomized controlled trials, cohort studies and case-control studies were included. Overlapping studies, meta-analyses, systematic reviews, case reports/series, expert opinion, editorials, duplicates and animal studies were excluded. Eligible studies evaluated infants of pregnant mothers with chronic HBV infection, defined as positive hepatitis B surface antigen (8) who underwent Caesarean section or vaginal delivery. The intervention of interest was Caesarean section and the comparator was vaginal delivery. The outcome was vertical transmission of HBV. Studies in which the primary intervention was nucleos(t)ide therapy were excluded.

Data extraction and quality assessment

Two authors performed the database search independently and compared their search results; another independent author reviewed discrepancies. Two authors independently conducted the data extraction process and disagreements were resolved by discussion between the two review authors. When agreement could not be reached, a third author acted as an arbiter. Additional data from one abstract presented at the annual European Association for the Study of the Liver conference (9) was obtained from the authors via e-mail (personal communication, Dr Sheng-Nan Lu, Kaohsiung Chang Gung Memorial Hospital, Kaohsiung, Taiwan). Data extraction from articles was performed using a form that was designed a priori to include study design, source country, exclusion criteria, number of infants and rates of vertical HBV transmission stratified according to Caesarean section and vaginal delivery, percentage of mothers who were HBeAg positive (HBeAg+), percentage of mothers that had HBV DNA >10^6 copies/mL, percentage of infants who received HBIG and dose administered, and percentage of infants who received HBV vaccine and schedule. During the data extraction process, the following details were added to the a priori form: elective versus urgent Caesarean section and use of assist devices during vaginal delivery, such as forceps or vacuum suction. During data extraction, the meta-estimate was changed from risk ratios to ORs for all studies because one study was a case control. The final search was performed on August 11, 2013.

The methodological quality of each study was assessed using the Newcastle-Ottawa Quality Assessment Scale (NOS), which is a method for assessing the quality of nonrandomized studies in meta-analyses (10). The NOS allocates a maximum of nine stars to assess three domains: quality of study group selection, comparability of intervention and nonintervention groups, and ascertainment of the exposure and outcome.

Data synthesis and analysis

The outcome of interest was HBV transmission to the infant, defined as either hepatitis B surface antigen positive or detectable HBV DNA level. The ORs of developing HBV in infants were obtained from the studies and stratified analyses were performed according to maternal HBV DNA levels >10^6 copies/mL and HBeAg+ status, which are measures of high viral infectivity. Also performed was an additional subgroup analysis of elective versus urgent Caesarean section because this may modify HBV transmission through excess blood exposure.

The primary meta-estimate – the OR of HBV transmission in Caesarean section compared with vaginal delivery – was calculated for all studies including 95% CIs. Meta-analyses using both fixed-effects (11) and a random-effects models were conducted (12). It was anticipated that there would be high level of heterogeneity among the studies; results were reported using the random-effects model. Binary outcomes are presented as OR with 95% CI. Pooled ORs and 95% CI were determined using a Mantel-Haenszel random-effects model. An OR of <1 favoured Caesarean section as having a preventive effect on HBV transmission while an OR of >1 indicated that Caesarean section was harmful and increased HBV transmission. The point estimate of the OR was considered to be statistically significant at the P<0.05 level if the 95% CI did not include the value 1.

Statistical between-study heterogeneity was assessed using the I^2 test to measure the extent of inconsistency among the results and χ^2 test, with statistical significance set at P<0.05. Publication bias was assessed using funnel plot (13). An asymmetric funnel plot suggests publication bias or a systematic difference between smaller and larger studies ('small study effects') or the use of an inappropriate effect measure. Publication bias was also evaluated by the Duval and Tweedie trim-and-fill method (14). To evaluate the impact of each individual study, sensitivity analyses using a one-study-removed method were performed. Temporal trends and secular changes were assessed with the cumulative analysis approach.

Because HBV transmission rates are directly influenced by prophylaxis with HBIG and vaccination, subgroup analyses were performed in an attempt to explain possible sources of heterogeneity and used the test for interaction (χ^2 statistic) to estimate differences between groups. Unrestricted maximum likelihood random effects meta-regression was applied to percentage of HBIG administered as a continuous variable to evaluate for the impact of HBIG on HBV transmission rates. For all tests, a two-tailed P<0.05 was considered to be statistically significant. All analyses were performed in Comprehensive Meta Analysis Version 2.0 (Biostat, USA). The study is reported according to the Meta-analysis Of Observational Studies in Epidemiology (MOOSE) group reporting guidelines (15). All authors had access to the study data, and reviewed and approved the final manuscript.

RESULTS

Study selection

The search strategy identified 430 articles, of which 420 were excluded and 10 were included for analysis (Figure 1). Of the 10 studies included, eight were full-text articles (6,7,16-21) and two were major society meeting abstracts (9,22). One abstract (22) was found in EMBASE. The other abstract (9) was identified by searching the reference lists of the retrieved full-text articles.

Study characteristics are described in Table 1. Nine studies were retrospective cohort studies and one was a case-control study. The primary meta-estimate measured was the OR of HBV transmission from mothers to newborns among women who underwent Caesarean section (n=2352) compared with vaginal delivery (n=2739), yielding a total of 5091 newborns. The HBV transmission rate was 8% overall: 5% (116 of 2352) for mothers who underwent Caesarean section and 10% (283 of 2739) for those who underwent vaginal delivery. Three studies were conducted in HBeAg+ women exclusively, one study did not specify, and the remaining studies had mixed HBeAg+ and negative populations (range 25% to 55% HBeAg+). Prophylaxis rates with HBIG and HBV vaccination of infants varied across studies: three reported 100% prophylaxis with HBIG and vaccination, one did not mention prophylaxis rate, and the remaining studies reported a wide range (HBIG 51% to 76%, vaccination 1% to 100%). Four studies differentiated urgent from elective Caesarean section; only one study described whether instrumentation (forceps or suction) was used during delivery. Only four studies explicitly stated their exclusion criteria; all four excluded HIV, three excluded HCV coinfection and three excluded any form of recent HBV therapy (nucleos[t]ide analogues or

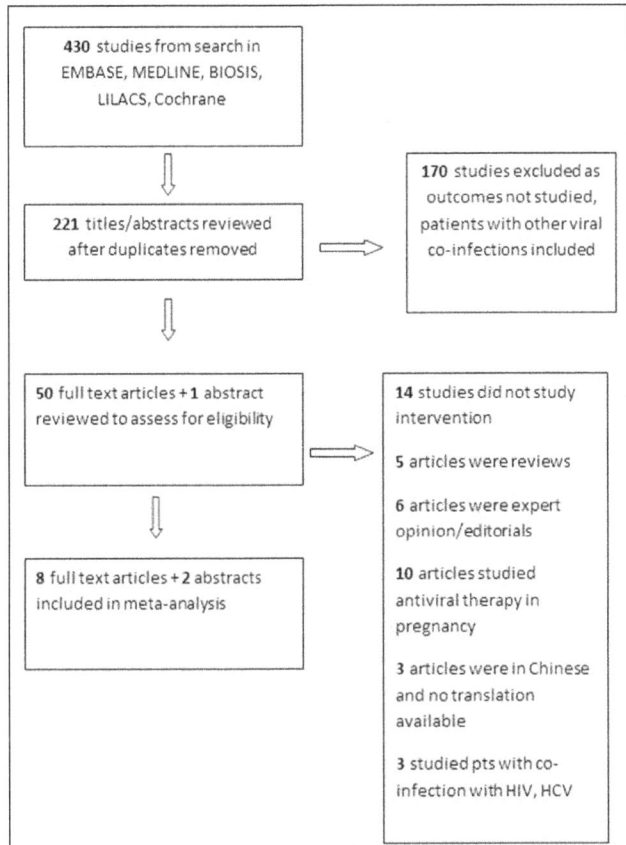

Figure 1) *Flow diagram of the study search and selection process. HCV Hepatitis C virus; pts Patients*

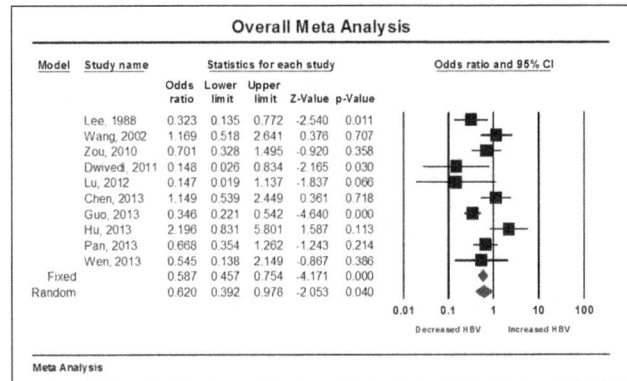

Figure 2) *Meta-analysis of hepatitis B virus transmission risk with Caesarean section versus vaginal delivery*

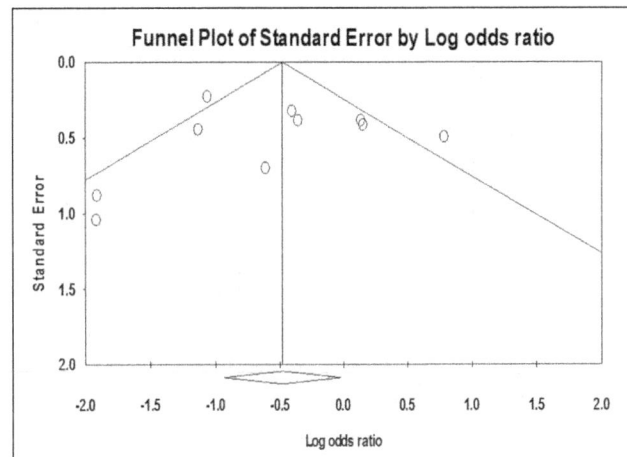

Figure 3) *Funnel plot of standard error according to hepatitis B virus transmission risk*

interferon). Seven studies were conducted in China, two in Taiwan and one in India. According to the NOS, nine studies were high quality (scores between 6 and 9) and one study was low quality (score 4); however, only three of the studies controlled for potential confounders.

Meta-analysis

Seven studies demonstrated decreased odds of HBV transmission, of which three were statistically significant, while three demonstrated increased odds of HBV transmission, but none were statistically significant (Figure 2). The overall meta-analysis demonstrated a statistically significant decrease in HBV vertical transmission with Caesarean section compared with vaginal delivery, with an OR of 0.62 (95% CI [0.40 to 0.978]; P=0.04). As expected, there was significant heterogeneity among the studies (Q test 25.58; P=0.003; I^2=63%).

A one-study-removed analysis was generally consistent with the overall finding that Caesarean section was associated with a reduction in HBV transmission, although this resulted in having the upper limit of the 95% CI cross 1 (null) in seven of 10 cases (Wang et al [20] [OR 0.57 [95% CI 0.35 to 0.93], Chen et al [16] [OR 0.57 [95% CI 0.35 to 0.92] and Hu et al [6] [OR 0.55 [95% CI 0.36 to 0.83], forest plot not shown). A cumulative analysis demonstrated a persistent trend toward a protective effect of Caesarean section on HBV transmission as studies were added to the model over time, but this did not consistently reach statistical significance (data not shown). This finding may have been due to the publication of five studies in the same year. When including only high-quality studies (NOS ≥6) and excluding Chen et al (16) (NOS 4), Caesarean section still reduced HBV transmission (OR 0.57 [95% CI 0.35 to 0.92]). However, this effect was no longer significant when limiting the analysis to cohort studies (excluded Guo et al [18], which was a case control study) (OR 0.70 [95% CI 0.44 to 1.11]) or when considering only high-quality cohort studies (excluding both Chen et al [16] and Guo et al [18]) (OR 0.635 [95% CI 0.38 to 1.07]) (forest plots not shown).

A funnel plot was only mildly asymmetric, suggesting that smaller studies at the right margin of the plot, favouring an increase in HBV transmission with Caesarean section, may be missing (Figure 3). The Duval and Tweedie trim-and-fill method (14) did not add any studies, indicating that publication bias was not a significant factor.

Of the studies with <100% of HBIG administration in infants, the study by Hu et al (6) collected HBV prophylaxis administration data primarily using surveys one to seven years after childbirth, rendering the study vulnerable to recall bias. Additionally, the HBV transmission rate in the vaginal delivery group was disproportionately lower than expected (2%). While this may, in part, be due to the low HBeAg+ prevalence of 25%, the HBV transmission rate was still lower than Wen et al (21), which had a similar HBeAg+ prevalence of 27%, but a much higher HBV transmission rate of 4% in the vaginal delivery group, suggesting that the population in Hu et al (6) study may be fundamentally different from the other study populations. To better account for this persistent heterogeneity, a meta-regression was performed to evaluate a potential linear relationship between the percentage of patients administered HBIG and the log OR of HBV transmission. While there was no association in the initial model (P=0.78 [model not shown]), a subsequent meta-regression excluding Hu et al (6) (Figure 4) revealed a significant linear relationship, such that the log OR increased by 0.02 times for each percentage point increase in HBIG administered (P=0.005) This confirmed the expected clinical finding that HBV transmission decreased as HBIG use approached 100%, accounting for the underlying heterogeneity among studies.

TABLE 1
Characteristics of eligible studies

Author (reference), year (country)	Study design	Quality score	Exclusion criteria	Newborns by Caesarean/vaginal, n/n	HBV+ newborns by Caesarean/vaginal, n/n	HBeAg+/>10^6 copies/mL, %	Given HBIG/vaccine, %	HBIG dosing	Vaccine schedule	Follow-up	Caesarean section, % Elective	Caesarean section, % Urgent	Forceps or vacuum, %
Lee et al (19), 1988 (China)	Retrospective cohort	6/9	Not reported	62/385	6/96	100/–	76/100	50 IU ≤9 h ± at 1 month	2 weeks, 1, 2 months, 1 year	6 months	Not reported	Not reported	Not reported
Wang et al (20), 2002 (China)	Retrospective cohort	7/9	Not reported	117/184	11/15	Not reported	All since 1997	100 IU	1, 2, 7 months	12 months	Not reported	Not reported	13
Zou et al (22), 2010 (China)	Retrospective cohort/abstract	7/9	Not reported	283/286	12/17	100/–	100/100	200 IU ≤12 h, 2 weeks	Delivery, 1, 6 months	12 months	33	17	Not reported
Dwivedi et al (17), 2011 (India)	Retrospective cohort	7/9	Not reported	11/25	2/15	41/–	Not reported	Not reported	Not reported	At delivery	11	19	Not reported
Lu et al (9), 2012 (Taiwan)	Retrospective cohort/abstract	8/9	Not reported	44/132	1/18	100	74/–	Not reported	Not reported	Not stated	Not reported	Not reported	Not reported
Chen et al (16), 2013 (China)	Retrospective cohort	4/9	HIV, HCV, TB, Ig, nuc	98/73	21/14	35/29	100/100	200 IU ≤24 h	≤24 h, 1, 6 months	At delivery	Not reported	Not reported	Not reported
Guo et al (18), 2013 (China)	Case control	7/9	Not reported	584/549	29/72	39/–	69/1	Not reported	Not reported	24 h	Not reported	Not reported	Not reported
Hu et al (6), 2013 (China)	Retrospective cohort	7/9	HIV, HCV, nuc, threatened abortion	285/261	14/6	25/–	51/100	No dose, ≤24 h	3 doses total	1–7 years	52	0	Not reported
Pan et al (7), 2013 (China)	Retrospective cohort	9/9	HIV, HCV, HDV, nuc/IFN within 6 months	736/673	17/23	55/48	100/100	200 IU ≤6 h	Delivery, 1, 6 months	7–12 months	35	17	Not reported
Wen et al (21), 2013 (Taiwan)	Retrospective cohort	8/9	HIV	132/171	3/7	27/–	75*/100	100 IU ≤24 h	Within 1 week, 1, 6 months	3 years	Not reported	Not reported	Not reported

*All hepatitis B e antigen-positive (HBeAg+) women received hepatitis B immune globulin (HBIG) and HBeAg-negative women were given the option to purchase HBIG. HCV Hepatitis C virus; Ig Immunoglobulin; HDV Hepatitis D virus; IFN Interferon; nuc Nucleos(t)ide analogue; TB Tuberculosis

A subgroup analysis stratified according to 100% HBV vaccination use found only a modest decrease in heterogeneity among studies that had 100% vaccination rates (Q test 9.86; P=0.08; I^2=49% [data not shown]). Further stratification within individual studies according to delivery type among women who received appropriate prophylaxis was not possible given the insufficient data. In three studies, data regarding rates of HBV transmission in HBeAg+ women, high risk for transmission, specified by delivery type were available. A separate analysis was performed that suggested a reduction in HBV transmission with Caesarean section but was not statistically significant (OR 0.71 [95% CI 0.47 to 1.08]; low heterogeneity, Q=0.18; P=0.92; I^2=0%).

DISCUSSION

Using a random-effects pooled meta-analysis, we detected a statistically significant decrease in the overall odds of HBV transmission in women who underwent Caesarean section compared with vaginal delivery. In contrast, a majority of the individual studies had point estimates favouring a reduction in HBV transmission with Caesarean section, but were inconclusive because the 95% CI crossed 1. Our findings are consistent with the findings of meta-analyses before 2012: one was inconclusive and another found a benefit with Caesarean section (23,24). We were able to include six additional studies (3738 newborns) that have been published since 2012, making our meta-analysis the largest and most robust to date.

There was significant heterogeneity among studies, which was largely explained by varying rates of HBIG prophylaxis. In the adjusted meta-regression model, as HBIG use approached 100%, the protective benefit of Caesarean section appeared to decrease, confirming the importance of HBIG in preventing vertical transmission.

Despite demonstrating a benefit in HBV transmission, our findings should be interpreted within the context of the study limitations, particularly given the high heterogeneity and deficits in primary study quality. Although NOS scores were generally high, several of the studies were missing key study details, as depicted in the evidence table (Table 1), and only two studies controlled for confounders such as high viral levels and nucleos(t)ide use. Most studies were conducted in China, with a varying HBeAg+ prevalence and, therefore, may be less generalizable to other countries. Two of the more recent studies (9,22) were only available in abstract form, which significantly limits in-depth analysis. Follow-up periods in several studies spanned decades when HBV prophylaxis was not yet standard of care and many infants may not have received it; this may have elevated the risk for transmission in these studies. HBV transmission also differs in cases of elective compared with urgent Caesarean section for which there is potential for more bleeding and, thus, a greater opportunity for viral transmission. However, this level of detail was not available in most of the studies.

Interpretation of our study findings in the clinical setting is challenging because Caesarean section carries its own complex set of risks. HBIG administration and HBV vaccination should be the first-line measure based on established guidelines (1). All women diagnosed with HBV should be referred to a provider experienced in the management of chronic liver disease (8). Our meta-analysis demonstrated that Caesarean section may offer additional protection against vertical transmission of HBV from the mother to the newborn, but the exact degree of benefit remains uncertain and is heavily influenced by HBIG administration rates. Any protective benefit from Caesarean section most likely occurs in higher-risk mothers, namely those who are HBeAg+ or have persistently elevated DNA levels despite nucleos(t)ide therapy before delivery, and should be studied further. It would be difficult to perform an adequately powered study, which would require 475 women with high viremia who failed nucleos(t)ide therapy, for each delivery method (vaginal versus Caesarean) to have 80% power to detect a decrease in HBV transmission rates from 10% to 5%. Additionally, differences in HBV transmission rates among women undergoing elective versus urgent Caesarean section are still unknown and also require further investigation. Based on fair evidence, we

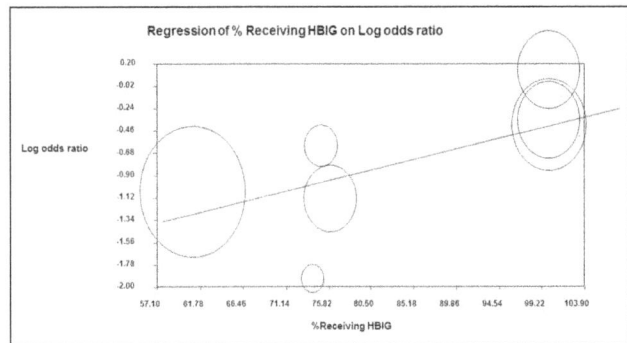

Figure 4) *Adjusted meta-regression of percent of women receiving hepatitis B immune globulin (HBIG) and log OR after removal of the study by Hu et al (6) (size of circles are proportional to study sample size)*

cannot make formal recommendations for or against the use of Caesarean section to prevent transmission of HBV (Grade C). Ultimately, more definitive studies, such as large population-based cohort studies or planned meta-analyses that include 100% HBIG and vaccination use, are needed to confirm our findings before Caesarean section can be adopted in clinical practice as a preventive measure against vertical transmission of HBV.

ACKNOWLEDGEMENTS: The authors thank Michael Stoto PhD and Deanna Alexis Carere MA MS CGC CCGC (Harvard School of Public Health) for their meta-analysis guidance.

DISCLOSURES: PCA is an employee of Johnson & Johnson Medical, Brazil. The remaining authors have no financial disclosures or conflicts of interest to declare. This study was not funded.

REFERENCES

1. Keeffe EB, Dieterich DT, Han SH, et al. A treatment algorithm for the management of chronic hepatitis B virus infection in the United States: 2008 update. Clin Gastroenterol Hepatol 2008;6:1315-41.
2. Pan CQ, Duan ZP, Bhamidimarri KR, et al. An algorithm for risk assessment and intervention of mother to child transmission of hepatitis B virus. Clin Gastroenterol Hepatol 2012;10:452-9.
3. Han GR, Cao MK, Zhao W, et al. A prospective and open-label study for the efficacy and safety of telbivudine in pregnancy for the prevention of perinatal transmission of hepatitis B virus infection. J Hepatol 2011;55:1215-21.
4. Pan CQ, Han GR, Jiang HX, et al. Telbivudine prevents vertical transmission from HBeAg-positive women with chronic hepatitis B. Clin Gastroenterol Hepatol 2012;10:520-6.
5. Read JS, Newell MK. Efficacy and safety of cesarean delivery for prevention of mother-to-child transmission of HIV-1. Cochrane Database Syst Rev 2005:CD005479.
6. Hu Y, Chen J, Wen J, et al. Effect of elective cesarean section on the risk of mother-to-child transmission of hepatitis B virus. BMC Pregnancy Childbirth 2013;13:119.
7. Pan CQ, Zou HB, Chen Y, et al. Cesarean section reduces perinatal transmission of hepatitis B virus infection from hepatitis B surface antigen-positive women to their infants. Clin Gastroenterol Hepatol 2013;11:1349-55.
8. Lok AS, McMahon BJ. Chronic hepatitis B: Update 2009. Hepatology 2009;50:661-2.
9. Lu SN, Wu CH, Ou CY, et al. Outcomes of combination of hepatitis B immunoglobuin and hepatitis B vaccination in high-risk newborns born to HBeAg-positive mothers. J Hepatol 2012;56:S31-2.
10. Wells G, Shea B, O'Connell D, et al. The New Castle-Ottawa Scale (NOS) for assessing the quality of non-randomized studies in meta-analysis. <www.ohri.ca/programs/clinical_epidemiology/oxford.asp> (Accessed August 16, 2013).
11. Demets DL. Methods for combining randomized clinical trials: Strengths and limitations. Stat Med 1987;6:341-50.

12. DerSimonian R, Laird N. Meta-analysis in clinical trials. Controlled Clin Trials 1986;7:177-88.
13. Egger M, Davey Smith G, Schneider M, et al. Bias in meta-analysis detected by a simple, graphical test. BMJ 1997;315:629-34.
14. Duval S, Tweedie R. Trim and fill: A simple funnel-plot-based method of testing and adjusting for publication bias in meta-analysis. Biometrics 2000;56:455-63.
15. Stroup DF, Berlin JA, Morton SC, et al. Meta-analysis of observational studies in epidemiology: A proposal for reporting. Meta-analysis Of Observational Studies in Epidemiology (MOOSE) group. JAMA 2000;283:2008-12.
16. Chen Y, Wang L, Xu Y, et al. Role of maternal viremia and placental infection in hepatitis B virus intrauterine transmission. Microbes Infect 2013;15:409-15.
17. Dwivedi M, Misra SP, Misra V, et al. Seroprevalence of hepatitis B infection during pregnancy and risk of perinatal transmission. Indian J Gastroenterol 2011;30:66-71.
18. Guo Z, Shi XH, Feng YL, et al. Risk factors of HBV intrauterine transmission among HBsAg-positive pregnant women. J Viral Hepatit 2013;20:317-21.
19. Lee SD, Lo KJ, Tsai YT, et al. Role of caesarean section in prevention of mother-infant transmission of hepatitis B virus. Lancet 1988;2:833-4.
20. Wang J, Zhu Q, Zhang X. Effect of delivery mode on maternal-infant transmission of hepatitis B virus by immunoprophylaxis. Chinese Med J 2002;115:1510-2.
21. Wen WH, Chang MH, Zhao LL, et al. Mother-to-infant transmission of hepatitis B virus infection: Significance of maternal viral load and strategies for intervention. J Hepatol 2013;59:24-30.
22. Zou H, Chen Y, Duan Z, et al. A retrospective study for clinical outcome of caesarean section on perinatal transmission of hepatitis B virus in infants born to HBeAg positive mothers with chronic hepatitis B (CHB). Hepatology 2010;(Suppl):235A. (Abst)
23. Wang HH, Wang ZP. [A Meta analysis: Mother to infant transmission of hepatitis B virus via different combined immunoprophylaxis delivery modes]. Zhonghua yu fang yi xue za zhi [Chinese journal of preventive medicine] 2010;44:221-3.
24. Yang J, Zeng XM, Men YL, et al. Elective caesarean section versus vaginal delivery for preventing mother to child transmission of hepatitis B virus – a systematic review. Virol J 2008;5:100.

33

Serrated adenoma prevalence in inflammatory bowel disease surveillance colonoscopy, and characteristics revealed by chromoendoscopy and virtual chromoendoscopy

Marietta Iacucci MD PhD[1], Cesare Hassan MD[1], Miriam Fort Gasia MD[1], Stefan Urbanski MD[2], Xianyong Gui MD[2], Bertus Eksteen MD[1], Gregory Eustace MD[1], Gilaad G Kaplan MD[1], Remo Panaccione MD[1]

M Iacucci, C Hassan, M Fort Gasia, et al. Serrated adenoma prevalence in inflammatory bowel disease surveillance colonoscopy, and characteristics revealed by chromoendoscopy and virtual chromoendoscopy. Can J Gastroenterol Hepatol 2014;28(11):589-594.

BACKGROUND: Sessile or nonpolypoid neoplastic lesions, including sessile serrated adenomas (SSAs), are difficult to detect in patients with inflammatory bowel disease (IBD).

OBJECTIVES: To assess the prevalence and endoscopic features of SSA in IBD patients undergoing surveillance colonoscopy using novel endoscopic techniques.

METHODS: Histology results of biopsies from a cohort of 87 patients (47 men; median age 51.4 years; median duration of disease 16.9 years; ulcerative colitis [n=40], Crohn disease [n=43], ischemic colitis [n=4]) with longstanding colonic IBD undergoing surveillance colonoscopy were reviewed. Lesions of dysplasia (adenoma-like mass, or dysplasia-associated lesion or mass), SSAs, adenoma-like polyps, hyperplastic polyps and inflammatory polyps were identified. Surveillance colonoscopy using high-definition alone, or with iScan (Pentax, USA) dye-sprayed or virtual chromoendoscopy was performed. Lesion characteristics were described before histological diagnosis.

RESULTS: Fourteen SSAs were detected in 87 (11%) IBD patients. The endoscopic characteristics of SSA lesions were: nonpolypoid appearance (86%), predominant localization in the proximal colon (79%), >6 mm in size (79%), cloudy cover (64%), Kudo pit pattern modified type IIO (86%) and irregular spiral vascular pattern (79%). Among the 44 SSAs and hyperplastic polyps found in the present study, the above characteristics of SSA at colonoscopy had a sensitivity of 92.86% (95% CI 66.06% to 98.8%) and specificity of 93.33% (95% CI 77.89% to 98.99%) in predicting a histological diagnosis of SSA (positive predictive value 86.67%, negative predictive value 96.55%).

CONCLUSION: SSAs are a common finding at surveillance colonoscopy in IBD and have several characteristic features. Further studies are needed to evaluate the natural history of these lesions in IBD patients.

Key Words: *High-definition iScan virtual and dye chromoendoscopy; Inflammatory bowel disease; Sessile serrated adenoma*

La prévalence d'adénome dentelé lors des coloscopies de surveillance de la maladie inflammatoire de l'intestin et les caractéristiques révélées par chromoendoscopie standard ou virtuelle

HISTORIQUE : Les lésions néoplasiques sessiles ou non polypoïdes, y compris les adénomes dentelés sessiles (ADS), sont difficiles à déceler chez les patients atteints d'une maladie inflammatoire de l'intestin (MII).

OBJECTIFS : Évaluer la prévalence et les caractéristiques endoscopiques de l'ADS chez les patients atteints d'une MII qui subissent une coloscopie de surveillance au moyen de nouvelles techniques endoscopiques.

MÉTHODOLOGIE : Des chercheurs ont analysé les résultats histologiques des biopsies d'une cohorte de 87 patients (47 hommes; âge médian de 51,4 ans; durée médiane de la maladie de 16,9 ans; colite ulcéreuse [n=40], maladie de Crohn [n=43], colite ischémique [n=4]) atteints d'une MII du côlon de longue date qui avaient subi une coloscopie de surveillance. Des lésions de dysplasie (masse adénomateuse ou lésion ou masse associée à la dysplasie), d'ADS, de polypes adénomateux, de polypes hyperplasiques et de polypes inflammatoires avaient été constatées. Une coloscopie de surveillance à haute définition, seule ou accompagnée d'une chromoendoscopie à coloration standard ou virtuelle iScan (Pentax, États-Unis), avait été effectuée. Les caractéristiques des lésions étaient décrites avant le diagnostic histologique.

RÉSULTATS: Quatorze ADS ont été décelés chez 87 patients atteints d'une MII (11 %). Les caractéristiques endoscopiques des lésions d'ADS étaient une apparence non polypoïde (86 %), un foyer prédominant dans le côlon proximal (79 %), une dimension de plus de 6 mm (79 %), une opacité (6 4 %), un motif ulcéreux de Kudo modifié de type IIO (86%) et des motifs vasculaires irréguliers en spirale (79 %). Sur les 44 ADS et polypes hyperplasiques relevés dans la présente étude, les caractéristiques précédentes d'ADS à la coloscopie avaient une sensibilité de 92,86 % (95 % IC 66,06 % à 98,8 %) et une spécificité de 93,33 % (95 % IC 77,89 % à 98,99 %) pour prédire un diagnostic histologique d'ADS (valeur prédictive positive de 86,67 %, valeur prédictive négative de 96,55 %).

CONCLUSION : Les ADS sont des observations courantes lors des coloscopies de surveillance des MII et possèdent plusieurs caractéristiques. D'autres études s'imposent pour en évaluer l'évolution naturelle chez les patients atteints d'une MII.

The risk of developing dysplasia and colorectal cancer in patients with longstanding inflammatory bowel disease (IBD) is well recognized (1-4). Random biopsies during white-light standard-definition colonoscopy (33 to 50 biopsies) with or without dye spraying chromoendoscopy (CE) has been the recommended strategy in North America to detect dysplastic lesions in patients with IBD (5). Several studies have shown that CE-guided targeted biopsies are more accurate in detecting dysplasia in patients with longstanding IBD (6-9) compared with white-light endoscopy (WLE). In fact, a recent consensus guideline (10) endorsed the use of CE as the standard surveillance colonoscopy in these patients.

The new generation of high-definition (HD) endoscopes with electronic filter technology provide minute details of colonic mucosal and vascular patterns, and may identify subtle flat, multifocal, polypoid, and pseudopolypoid neoplastic and non-neoplastic lesions (11-13). In addition, the newly developed iScan (Pentax, Japan) technology uses a digital contrast method to enhance mucosal and vascular patterns, and enhances endoscopic images. Advantages of electronic virtual CE over traditional CE include its convenience, lower cost and straightforward reversibility (14-17).

Emerging evidence has shown that serrated adenomas are also associated with longstanding IBD colitis, which may contribute to the

[1]*IBD Clinic, Division of Gastroenterology;* [2]*Department of Pathology, University of Calgary, Calgary, Alberta*
Correspondence: Dr Marietta Iacucci, Division of Gastroenterology, Department of Medicine, University of Calgary, 2500 University Drive Northwest, Calgary, Alberta T2N 1N4. e-mail miacucci@ucalgary.ca

development of colorectal cancer (18). Recently, the 'serrated neoplasia pathway' in IBD was defined according to morphological and molecular characteristics, and appears to be involved in IBD-related colorectal oncogenesis. The penultimate stage in the progression to carcinoma of this pathway are serrated polyps including hyperplastic polyps (HPs), traditional serrated adenomas and the more recently described sessile serrated adenomas (SSAs). Furthermore, some categories of serrated polyps previously classified as HPs are actually the precursors of serrated adenoma (19-21). However, these lesions may be overlooked during endoscopy due to their flat morphology, indefinite margins and cloudy pale colour, and they are often covered by mucus. Moreover, due to the morphological similarity with HPs, most detected SSAs are left in situ when they are misinterpreted by colonoscopists as clinically irrelevant HPs (22-26).

There is uncertainty regarding the real prevalence of SSA in IBD patients with known high risk for developing dysplasia. The endoscopic features of SSA in IBD are subtle and easily missed. Thus, in the present study, we aimed to assess the prevalence and characteristics of SSA detected in IBD patients undergoing surveillance endoscopies using novel digital endoscopic modalities.

METHODS

Study design

The present analysis was a retrospective cohort study performed at a single tertiary referral centre. All histology was reviewed by two gastrointestinal pathologists (XG and SU), and all colonoscopies were performed by a single experienced operator (MI) who was well trained in novel endoscopic techniques in IBD.

Patients

All patients diagnosed with inactive (Mayo subscore 0 to 1 and Harvey-Bradshaw <4) longstanding ulcerative colitis (UC) or Crohn disease (CD) (27,28) at the IBD clinic at the University of Calgary (Calgary, Alberta) from September 2011 to November 2013 were identified and enrolled in the study. All procedures were performed using HD iScan virtual CE or dye CE at the discretion of the endoscopist. During the study period, there was no clinical preference or specific recommendation for one of the two techniques. Exclusion criteria were: previous history of sporadic colon cancer; reported allergy to dye spray; liver cirrhosis; blood coagulation disorders; moderate to severe disease activity; inability to complete colonoscopy because of poor bowel preparation or patient intolerance; and pregnancy.

The extent of IBD was described according to the Montreal classification and clinical-endoscopic disease activity was determined using the Mayo score for UC, Harvey-Bradshaw and SES-CD for CD (27-30). Focal findings and abnormalities outside of markedly inflamed mucosa were classified according to the pit pattern classification of Kudo and Paris (31,32), and the routine practice of the endoscopist (MI) .

The Calgary Laboratory Services and the Conjoint Health Research Ethics Board of the University of Calgary approved the study.

Colonoscopic assessment

All colonoscopies were performed using an EPK-I (Pentax EC-3490Fi; Pentax, Japan) processor with HD alone, HD-iScan virtual CE using the three iScan settings in sequence from set 1 to set 3, devoting a mean time of 20 s for each single iScan setting or HD dye CE, in which methylene blue 0.2% was sprayed in a segmental fashion for the entire withdrawal procedure. The methylene blue dye was sprayed using a catheter through the working channel of the endoscope, according to routine practice.

iScan technology

The iScan is a new digital virtual CE system developed by Pentax, Japan. It is a postprocessing imaging technology that analyzes endoscopic images in real time, and consists of three types of algorithms: surface enhancement (SE), contrast enhancement and tone enhancement, each of

which can be selected by pressing a preassigned button on the handpiece of the endoscope. SE enhances light-dark contrast by obtaining luminance intensity data for each pixel. With SE, the difference in luminance intensity between the pixels of interest and the surrounding pixels is analyzed and the edge components are enhanced. Contrast enhancement digitally adds blue colour to relatively dark areas. The iScan system can provide detailed analysis based on vessel (iScan v), mucosal pattern (iScan p) or surface architecture (iScan SE), (16,29). The vascular pattern, surface architecture and mucosal pattern can characterize inflammation and colonic neoplastic lesions (13-15).

Biopsy protocol

Mucosal abnormalities were analyzed with regard to location (anatomy and distance from the anus [in cm]), morphology (polypoid, flat or depressed) and size using the Paris classification (31). The Paris classification divides lesions into three main categories: I – protruding lesions (Is sessile or Ip pedunculated); II – nonprotruding and nonexcavated lesions (IIa flat elevated, IIb completely flat and IIc slightly depressed); and III – excavated lesions (31).

For each lesion, mucosal pit pattern was characterized according to the Kudo classification (32). On withdrawal of the colonoscope from the cecum to the anus, sequential targeted biopsy specimens from targeted areas of suspected dysplasia (circumscribed lesions with irregular surface) were obtained. Any suspicious lesions detected during examination were sampled or immediately removed. This conforms to current guidelines for targeted biopsies of detected lesions.

Histological assessment

A comprehensive histological assessment was performed by two gastrointestinal histopathologists (XG and SU) who were blinded to the endoscopic findings. Pathology classification of inflammatory activity were graded using the Harpaz New York Mount Sinai score into no inflammation, mild to moderate inflammation, or severe inflammation. Neoplastic changes were classified according to the recently revised Vienna classification (33-35).

An SSA was defined as a serrated lesion with irregular dilated crypts, including dilation of the base of the crypts, which often have a boot, L or inverted T shape.

Statistical analysis

Interobserver agreement was calculated using the Fleiss kappa measurement. Interobsever and intraobserver agreement were expressed using the kappa coefficient: a kappa value <0.20 indicates poor agreement, 0.20 to 0.40 fair, 0.41 to 0.60 moderate, 0.61 to 0.80 good and 0.81 to 1.0 excellent. The study was observational and not powered to show superiority of any specific technique.

RESULTS

Patient demographic characteristics and procedure indications

A cohort of 87 consecutive IBD patients (47 [54%] male), median age 51.4 years (range 23 to 86 years), median duration of disease (UC [n=40], CD [n=43], ischemic colitis [n=4]) 16.9 years with longstanding (≥8 years) colonic IBD undergoing surveillance colonoscopy was included for study analysis. The demographic characteristics of the patients are summarized in Table 1.

At the discretion of the endoscopist (MI), a specialist in IBD colonoscopy, 24 (27.6%) patients underwent surveillance using HD colonoscopy alone, 35 (40.2%) using HD-iScan virtual CE and 28 (32.2%) using HD dye CE (Table 2).

Prevalence of SSA in the surveillance cohort

Fourteen SSAs were noted in 10 of 87 (11%) IBD patients, accounting for 19% of all lesions detected. None of the IBD patients with SSAs had a family history of colon cancer or personal history of polyps or dysplastic lesions.

TABLE 1
Demographic characteristics in each group of inflammatory bowel disease (IBD) patients

	Endoscopy		
Characteristic	HD alone (n=24)	HD + CE (n=35)	HD iScan* + DCE (n=28)
Male sex	15 (62.5)	15 (42.8)	17 (60.7)
Age, years, mean ± SD	47.62±14.46	51.94±11.07	54.11±14.48
Ulcerative colitis/Crohn disease/ischemic colitis, n/n/n	10/13/1	18/14/3	12/16/–
Pancolitis	7 (70)	10 (55.5)	8 (66.7)
Left-sided colitis	3 (30)	8 (44.4)	4 (33.3)
Duration of IBD, years, mean ± SD	15.58±7.88	18.31±8.94	13.75±8.5
Treatment with mesalazine	6 (25)	14 (40)	12 (42.9)
Treatment with immunosuppressants	5 (21)	4 (11.4)	5 (17.9)
Treatment with biological	4 (17)	5 (14.3)	5 (17.9)
Combination treatment	2 (8)	3 (8.5)	1 (3.5)
No treatment	7 (33.3)	8 (22.8)	4 (14.2)
Family history of colorectal cancer	3 (12.5)	2 (5.7)	1 (3.5)
Personal history of colorectal adenoma	7 (33.3)	5 (14.3)	9 (32.1)
Primary sclerosing cholangitis	5 (21)	3 (8.5)	1 (3.5)

*Data presented as n (%) unless otherwise indicated. *Pentax, Japan. CE Chromoendoscopy; DCE Dye sprayed CE; HD High definition*

TABLE 2
Baseline characteristics of colonic lesions in inflammatory bowel disease patients

	Endoscopy		
Characteristic	HD alone (n=24)	HD + CE (n=28)	HD + iScan* DCE (n=35)
Serrated adenoma	2 (8.3)	5 (17.8)	6 (17.1)
Hyperplastic polyps	13 (54.1)	7 (25.0)	10 (28.5)
Inflammatory polyps	7 (29.1)	8 (28.6)	3 (8.6)
Tubular adenoma	2 (8.3)	6 (21.4)	3 (8.6)
DALM/ALM	1 (4.1)	–	–
Intraepithelial neoplasia	–	–	–

*Data presented n (%) unless otherwise indicated. *Pentax, Japan. ALM Adenoma-like mass; CE Chromoendoscopy; DALM Dysplasia-associated lesion or mass; DCE Dye-sprayed CE; HD High definition*

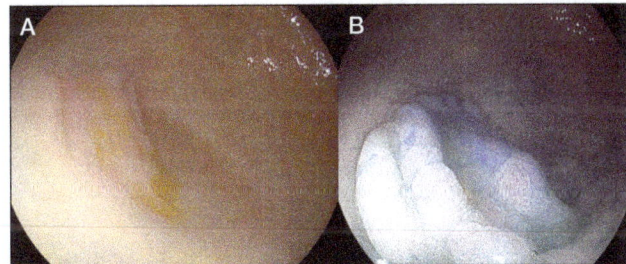

Figure 1) A *High-definition colonoscopy showing flat lesion covered with mucus with irregular indefinite margins at the base of the appendix.* **B** *High-definition + dye chromoendoscopy with 0.2% methylene blue characterize and enhance the Kudo pit pattern type IIO and the edge of the lesion*

Endoscopic features of SSA

Eleven (79%) of the SSA lesions were localized in the proximal colon (five in the ascending colon, three in the cecum, one in the appendix and two in the hepatic flexure). Most were nonpolypoid lesions type IIb (86%) and ≥6 mm in size (78%) with indefinite margins. The Kudo pit pattern was type IIO in 12 (86%) and the vascular pattern appeared as spiral and irregular in 11 (79%) (Table 3). The other two SSAs were localized in the sigmoid colon. They were sessile, <6 mm in size and with Kudo pit pattern type I. The interobserver agreement was calculated (kappa coefficient 0.86). The intraobserver agreement was also graded as excellent, with a kappa coefficient of 0.90.

The classical features of SSA on HD white-light colonoscopy were nonpolypoid, covered by mucus and cloudy-appearing lesions. However, on HD iScan virtual CE, additional features characterized SSA such as Kudo pit pattern type II or IIO with indefinite margins and spiral isolated vessels. Similarly, with HD dye CE, characteristic features of SSA as above were found (Figures 1 to 4). In the present study, among the 44 SSAs and HPs, the above characteristics of SSA at colonoscopy had a sensitivity of 92.86% (95% CI 66.06% to 98.8%) and specificity of 93.33% (95% CI 77.89% to 98.99%) in predicting a histological diagnosis of SSA. The positive predictive value of endoscopic features of SSA was 86.67% (95% CI 59.55% to 97.95%) and the negative predictive value was 96.55% (95% CI 82.17% to 99.42%).

Of the SSAs, detection according to technique were: two in the HD group (8%); six in the HD-iScan virtual CE group (17%); and six in the HD dye CE with methylene blue (21%).

Prevalence of other lesions at surveillance colonoscopy

Eleven adenomatous polyps were detected: two (8%) in the HD group, three (9%) in the HD iScan virtual CE group and six (21%) in the HD dye CE group. Thirty hyperplastic polyps were detected, 23 (77%) of which were localized in the left colon, mainly in the sigmoid colon. Only one patient had a dysplastic-associated lesion or mass (Table 2, Figure 4). This was a 44-year-old woman with longstanding Crohn's colitis and primary sclerosing cholangitis who underwent colectomy.

DISCUSSION

We report that SSAs may be detected in a significant proportion of IBD patients who undergo surveillance colonoscopy. Novel endoscopic techniques, such as iScan, virtual CE and dye-sprayed CE, may help in the detection of these lesions, although these findings require confirmation in a randomized controlled study.

In the present study, the prevalence of serrated sessile lesions located in IBD colitic mucosa was 16% in patients who underwent surveillance colonoscopy. The incidence of serrated sessile lesions was high in our population. However, this finding may not be generalizable to all gastroenterology practice because IBD patients were recruited from a tertiary care centre that specializes in dysplasia surveillance. The detection rates of SSA may vary according to centre, but is reported to be approximately 6% in average-risk patients undergoing screening colonoscopies for colorectal cancer detection (36). Thus, population-based studies are necessary to establish the incidence of SSA in IBD patients undergoing colonoscopy. A significant variable may be the experience of the colonoscopist in recognizing SSAs because they may otherwise be misintepreted as HPs.

TABLE 3
Baseline characteristics and endoscopic features of serrated adenoma in patients with inflammatory bowel disease

Female sex	Age, years, median	UC/CD/IC	Localization		Size		Paris classification		Kudo pit pattern	
			Right colon	Left colon	<6 mm	>6 mm	Is	IIb*	I	IIO
7	**50**	5/6/2	11	2	2	11	3	10	1	12

*Data presented as n. *Completely flat nonprotruding nonexcavating lesion. CD Crohn disease; IC Ischemic colitis; Is Sessile protruding lesion; UC Ulcerative colitis*

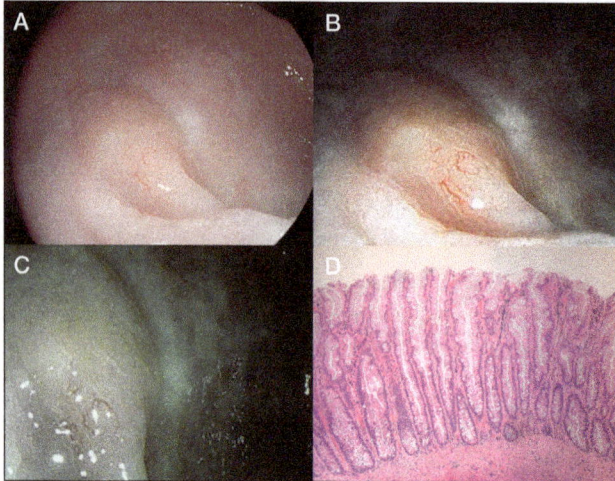

Figure 2) A to C *High-definition + iScan (Pentax, Japan) virtual chromoendoscopy showing flat lesion with indefinite margins and irregular spiral vessels.* D *Histological examination revealing serrated adenoma (hematoxylin and eosin stain, original magnification ×100)*

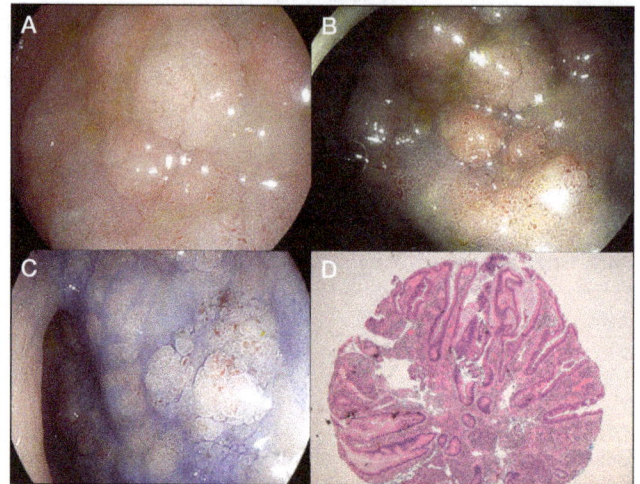

Figure 4) A *and* B *High-definition iScan (Pentax, Japan) virtual chromoendoscopy showing dysplasia-associated lesion or mass with mixture of Kudo pit pattern types IIIL-IV.* C *High-definition with dye chromoendoscopy with 0.2% methylene blue better characterize details in the edge of the lesions and pit pattern.* D *Histological examination showing low-grade intraepithelial neoplasia (hematoxylin and eosin stain, original magnification ×40)*

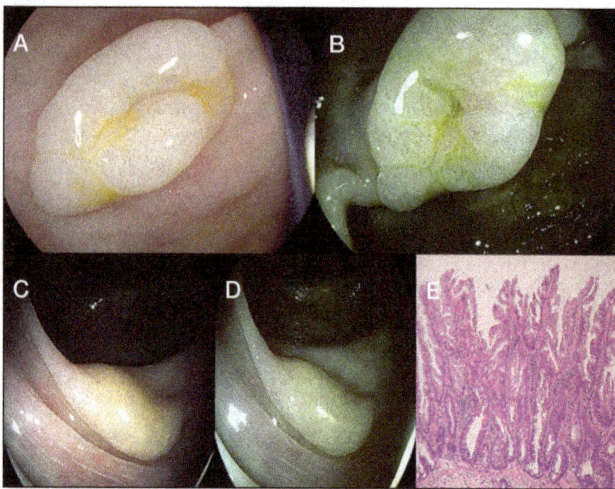

Figure 3) A to D *High-definition iScan (Pentax, Japan) virtual chromoendoscopy showing Kudo pit pattern type IIO.* E *Histological examination revealing serrated adenoma (hematoxylin and eosin stain, original magnification ×100)*

Serrated lesions exist in the inflammatory mucosa of IBD and are associated with a characteristic molecular profile. The appearance of the *BRAF* mutation is the early molecular change at the HP stage followed by microsatellite instability at the carcinoma stage (19,20). Rubio et al (18) assessed the histological phenotype of the dysplastic lesion juxtaposing colorectal carcinomas in 100 consecutive colectomy specimens from 50 patients with IBD and in 50 control (non-IBD) patients. They reported that 81.2% of the dysplastic lesions juxtaposing IBD carcinomas were villous or serrated adenoma, but only 55.1% in control cases. In particular, serrated adenoma accounted for nearly 29% of the noninvasive dysplastic lesions arising in IBD carcinomas but only 3% in control specimens.

In our case cohort study, the percentage of SSA detection was high. Recently, Johnson et al (37) retrospectively assessed serrated lesion detection rates in IBD and documented incidence of subsequent colorectal neoplasia in single-centre cohort study. They reported that serrated epithelial changes and sessile serrated polyps are uncommonly detected in IBD patients. An underestimation of detection of these lesions may be due, in part, to the use of WLE and random biopsies in performing surveillance colonoscopy in IBD patients, which could easily miss these lesions due to lack of recognition of characteristic features. In addition, because HPs have traditionally been considered to be nonprogressive lesions with no malignant potential (37), they are often ignored and not biopsied or removed by endoscopists. Most of the previous studies using novel filter-enhanced technologies, such as narrow-band imaging (NBI), were mostly based on the endoscopists' experience and, in most of the circumscribed sigmoid or rectal flat lesions with a regular mucosal pit pattern (Kudo types I and II) and with a weak vascular intensity on NBI, were considered to be HPs and often did not undergo biopsy (38-43). However, using novel endoscopic techniques, the endoscopic features of SSAs are very similar to HPs and require experience to differentiate.

More of our patients had SSA detected by HD-iScan virtual CE (17%) and by dye-sprayed CE (21%) than by HD endoscopy alone (8%). However, it cannot be concluded from the present study whether novel endoscopic techniques are better at detecting SSAs because the sample size was small and the study was not randomized. Unfortunately, these lesions are often subtle in appearance at endoscopy and pose challenges for endoscopic detection and removal, especially in IBD colitic mucosa, in which the mucosa often appears atrophic with scars and pseudopolyps.

The new generation of HD endoscopes with electronic filter technology have the potential to improve neoplasia detection and may contribute to reducing random biopsies by obtaining targeted biopsies for histological evaluation. HD endoscopy offers resolution superior to standard endoscopy and may significantly improve the detection and characterization of intraepithelial neoplasia in UC (11,12).

Conventional CE is the oldest and simplest method to improve the diagnosis of subtle epithelial changes and flat dysplastic lesions, and can improve characterization of margins that often can be difficult or impossible to detect using WLE. Several prospective randomized trials using methylene blue or indigo carmine for pan-CE in patients with longstanding UC have shown the unique benefit of CE in increasing the detection of intraepithelial neoplasia in IBD patients (5-9). HD-virtual CE, also known as dyeless CE, is a recently introduced image-enhancement technique.

There is controversy about the real role of NBI in dysplasia detection in UC patients. A recent study suggested that NBI offers no advantage over dye CE in IBD surveillance (38,41,43).

iScan remains a relatively unexplored technology in surveillance colonoscopy in IBD patients. However, it is a promising technique for differentiating neoplastic from non-neoplastic lesions of the colon. Hoffman et al (13) demonstrated that iScan was also able to predict neoplasia as precisely as dye CE, with an accuracy of 89% to 97%. Recently, in a prospective, randomized, back-to-back trial evaluating the utility of iScan in screening colonoscopy, Hong et al (15) demonstrated that iScan may fail to improve adenoma detection rates and the prevention of missed polyps; however, iScan appears to be effective for real-time histological prediction of polyp pathology compared with conventional HD white-light colonoscopy.

Finally, we have characterized and, for the first time, described the endoscopic findings of serrated adenoma in IBD patients using the iScan technique. SSAs tend to occur more often in the right colon compared with HPs; with a diameter exceeding 10 mm; with the type IIO pit pattern proposed by Kimura et al (23), which correspond to 'dilation of crypts'; and colouration may be yellowish due to mucin. They also have a cloud-like surface and indistinct borders that were predictive features on both HD-WLE and NBI, whereas dark spots and an irregular shape were predictive characteristics solely on NBI (24-26). However, these endoscopic vascular pattern findings (Figures 1 to 4) need to be validated.

The current study had several limitations. First, it was performed in a single referral tertiary academic centre and by one expert endoscopist. Additionally, the sample size of the study populations was not sufficiently large to detect subtle differences in dysplasia detection rates and to differentiate Crohn's colitis from UC. The study was observational and not powered to show superiority of any specific technique in diagnosing SSA in IBD. Thus, an appropriately randomized controlled trial comparing these dysplasia surveillance modalities is required to establish which is most effective.

Furthermore, a larger sample size is needed to better understand and characterize the morphology of the SSA in IBD patients compared with non-IBD patients. In the future, these data may aid endoscopists in recognizing and characterizing SSA in IBD patients, and facilitate real-time endoscopic therapeutic decisions.

CONCLUSION

Emerging evidence suggests that SSAs are common colonic lesions in IBD patients. It is possible that, as in non-IBD patients, these may be involved in the oncongenic pathway of colorectal cancer in IBD patients. SSAs are considered to be preneoplastic lesions, even if they do not show dysplasia at histology. Unfortunately, these lesions are often overlooked due to endoscopic features that are similar to HPs. Similar to dye CE, iScan CE has the potential to efficiently perform detailed characterization of the lesions and enable endoscopic targeting of biopsies or endoscopic therapeutic management.

DISCLOSURES: The authors have no financial disclosures or conflicts of interest to declare.

REFERENCES

1. Eaden JA, KR Abrams, JF Mayberry. The risk of colorectal cancer in ulcerative colitis: A meta-analysis. Gut 2001;48:526-35.
2. Beaugerie L, Svrcek M, Seksik P, et al. Risk of colorectal high-grade dysplasia and cancer in a prospective observational cohort of patients with inflammatory bowel disease. Gastroenterology 2013;145:166-75.
3. Jess T, Simonsen J, Jørgensen KT, et al. Decreasing risk of colorectal cancer in patients with inflammatory bowel disease over 30 years. Gastroenterology 2012;143:375-81
4. Lutgens MW, van Oijen MG, van der Heijden GJ, et al. Declining risk of colorectal cancer in inflammatory bowel disease: An updated meta-analysis of population-based cohort studies. Inflamm Bowel Dis 2013;19:789-99.
5. Francis A. Farraye, Robert D. Odze, Jayne Eaden, et al. AGA medical position statement on the diagnosis and management of colorectal neoplasia in inflammatory bowel disease. Gastroenterology 2010;138:738-45.
5. Rutter M, Bernstein C, Matsumoto T, et al. Endoscopic appearance of dysplasia in ulcerative colitis and the role of staining. Endoscopy 2004;36:1109-14.
6. Rutter MD, Saunders BP, Schofield G, et al. Pancolonic indigo carmine dye spraying for the detection of dysplasia in ulcerative colitis. Gut 2004;53:256-60.
7. Kiesslich, R Fritsch J, Holtmann M, et al. Methylene blue-aided chromoendoscopy for the detection of intraepithelial neoplasia and colon cancer in ulcerative colitis. Gastroenterology 2003;124:880-8.
8. Marion JF, Waye JD, Present DH, et al. Chromoendoscopy-targeted biopsies are superior to standard colonoscopic surveillance for detecting dysplasia in inflammatory bowel disease patients: A prospective endoscopic trial. Am J Gastroenterol 2008;103:2342-9.
9. Konijeti GG, Shrime MG, Ananthakrishnan AN, et al. Cost-effectiveness analysis of chromoendoscopy for colorectal cancer surveillance in patients with ulcerative colitis. Gastrointest Endosc 2013;S0016-5107.
10. Mowat C, Cole A, Windsor A, et al. Guidelines for the management of inflammatory bowel disease in adults. Gut 2011;60:571-607.

11. Subramanian V, Mannath J, Ragunath K, et al. Meta-analysis: The diagnostic yield of chromoendoscopy for detecting dysplasia in patients with colonic inflammatory bowel disease. Aliment Pharmacol Ther 2011;33:304-12.
12. Subramanian V, Ramappa V, Telakis E, et al. Comparison of high definition with standard white light endoscopy for detection of dysplastic lesions during surveillance colonoscopy in patients with colonic inflammatory bowel disease. Inflamm Bowel Dis 2013;19:350-5.
13. Kodashima S, Fujishiro M. Novel image-enhanced endoscopy with i-Scan technology. World J Gastroenterol 2010;16:1043-9.
14. Hoffman A, Kagel C, Goetz M, et al. Recognition and characterization of small colonic neoplasia with high-definition colonoscopy using i-Scan is as precise as chromoendoscopy. Dig Liver Dis 2010;42:45-50.
15. Hong S.N, Choe WH, Lee JH, et al. Prospective, randomized, back-to-back trial evaluating the usefulness of i-Scan in screening colonoscopy. Gastrointest Endosc 2012;75:1011-21.
16. Ignjatovic A, East JE, Subramanian V, et al. Narrow band imaging for detection of dysplasia in colitis: A randomized controlled trial. Am J Gastroenterol 2012;10:885-90.
17. Efthymiou M, Allen PB, Taylor AC, et al. Chromoendoscopy versus narrow band imaging for colonic surveillance in inflammatory bowel disease. Inflamm Bowel Dis 2013;19:2132-8.
18 Rubio CA, Befrits R, Jaramillo E, et al. Villous and serrated adenomatous growth bordering carcinomas in inflammatory bowel disease. Anticancer Res 2000;20:4761-4.
19. Bossard C, Denis MG, Bezieau S, et al. Involvement of the serrated neoplasia pathway in inflammatory bowel disease-related colorectal oncogenesis Oncol Rep 2007;18:1093-7.
20. O'Brien MJ, Yang S, Mack C, et al. Comparison of microsatellite instability, CpG island methylation phenotype, BRAF and KRAS status in serrated polyps and traditional adenomas indicates separate pathways to distinct colorectal carcinoma end-points. Am J Surg Pathol 2006;30:1491-501.

21. Chaubert P, Benhattar J, Saraga E, et al. K-ras mutations and p53 alterations in neoplastic and non-neoplastic lesions associated with longstanding ulcerative colitis. Am J Pathol 1994;144:767-75.

22. Ishigooka S, Nomoto M, Obinata N, et al. Evaluation of magnifying colonoscopy in the diagnosis of serrated polyps. World J Gastroenterol 2012;18:4308-16.

23. Kimura T, Yamamoto E, Yamano HO, et al. A novel pit pattern identifies the precursor of colorectal cancer derived from sessile serrated adenoma. Am J Gastroenterol 2012;107:460-9.

24. Kahi CJ, Li X, Eckert GJ, Rex DK. High colonoscopic prevalence of proximal colon serrated polyps in average-risk men and women. Gastrointest Endosc 2012;75:515-20.

25. Hazewinkel Y, López-Cerón M, East JE, et al. Endoscopic features of sessile serrated adenomas: Validation by international experts using high-resolution white-light endoscopy and narrow-band imaging Gastrointest Endosc 2013;7:916-24.

26. Iacucci M, Xianyong G, Love J, et al. Novel irregular vascular pattern features of serrated adenoma detected by high-definition iScan endoscopic technique. Gastrointest Endosc 2014;79:182-4.

27. Schroeder KW, Tremaine WJ, Ilstrup DM. Coated oral 5-aminosalicylic acid therapy for midly to moderately active ulcerative colitis: A randomized study. N Engl J Med 1987;317:1625-9.

28. D'Haens G, Sandborn WJ, Feagan BG, et al. A review of activity indices and efficacy endpoints for clinical trials of medical therapy in adults with ulcerative colitis. Gastroenterology 2007;132:763-86.

29. Montreal World Congress of Gastroenterology. Montreal classification. Can J Gastroenterol 2005;19:5-36.

30. Daperno M, D'Haens G, Van Assche G, et al. Development and validation of a new, simplified endoscopic activity score for Crohn's disease: The SES-CD. Gastrointest Endosc 2004;60:505-12.

31. Participants in the Paris Workshop. The Paris endoscopic classification of superficial neoplastic lesions: Esophagus, stomach, and colon. Gastrointest Endosc 2003;58:S3-43.

32. Kudo S, Tamura S, Nakajima T, et al. Diagnosis of colorectal tumorous lesions by magnifying endoscopy. Gastrointest Endosc 1996;44:8-14.

33. Itzkowitz SH, Harpaz N. Diagnosis and management of dysplasia in patients with inflammatory bowel diseases. Gastroenterology 2004;126:1634-48.

34. Riddell RH, Goldman H, Ransohoff DF, et al. Dysplasia in inflammatory bowel disease: Standardized classification with provisional clinical applications. Hum Pathol 1983;14:931-68.

35. Schlemper RJ, Riddell RH, Kato Y, et al. The Vienna classification of gastrointestinal epithelial neoplasia. Gut 2000;47:251-5.

36. Payne SR, Church TR, Wandell M, et al. Endoscopic detection of proximal serrated lesions and pathologic identification of sessile serrated adenomas/polyps very on the basis of center. Clin Gastroenterol Hepatol 2014;12:1119-26.

37. Johnson DH, Khanna S, Smyrk TC, et al. Detection rate and outcome of colonic serrated epithelial changes in patients with ulcerative colitis or Crohn's colitis. Aliment Pharmacol Ther 2014;39:1408-17.

38. Dekker E, van den Broek FJ, Reitsma JB, et al. Narrow-band imaging compared with conventional colonoscopy for the detection of dysplasia in patients with longstanding ulcerative colitis. Endoscopy 2007;39:216-21.

39. van den Broek FJ, Fockens P, van Eeden S, et al. Narrow-band imaging versus high-definition endoscopy for the diagnosis of neoplasia in ulcerative colitis. Endoscopy 2011;43:108-15.

40. Ignjatovic A, East JE, Subramanian V, et al. Narrow band imaging for detection of dysplasia in colitis: A randomized controlled trial. Am J Gastroenterol 2012;10:885-90.

41. Efthymiou M, Allen PB, Taylor AC, et al. Chromoendoscopy versus narrow band imaging for colonic surveillance in inflammatory bowel disease. Inflamm Bowel Dis 2013;19:2132-8.

42. Pellisé M, López-Cerón M, Rodríguez de Miguel C, et al. Narrow-band imaging as an alternative to chromoendoscopy for the detection of dysplasia in long-standing inflammatory bowel disease: A prospective, randomized, crossover study. Gastrointest Endosc 2011;74:840-84.

43. Pellisé M, Fernández-Esparrach G, Cárdenas A, et al. Clinical impact of wide-angle, high-resolution endoscopy in the diagnosis of colorectal neoplasia in a non-selected population: A prospective randomized controlled trial. Gastroenterology 2008;135:1062-8.

34

Comparing outcomes of donation after cardiac death versus donation after brain death in liver transplant recipients with hepatitis C:
A systematic review and meta-analysis

Malcolm Wells MD MSc[1], Kris Croome MD MS[2], Toni Janik MLIS AHIP[3],
Roberto Hernandez-Alejandro MD[2], Natasha Chandok MD MPH[1]

M Wells, K Croome, T Janik, R Hernandez-Alejandro, N Chandok.
Comparing outcomes of donation after cardiac death versus
donation after brain death in liver transplant recipients with
hepatitis C: A systematic review and meta-analysis. Can J
Gastroenterol Hepatol 2014;28(2):103-108.

BACKGROUND: Liver transplantation (LT) using organs donated
after cardiac death (DCD) is increasing due, in large part, to a shortage
of organs. The outcome of using DCD organs in recipients with hep-
atits C virus (HCV) infection remains unclear due to the limited
experience and number of publications addressing this issue.
OBJECTIVE: To evaluate the clinical outcomes of DCD versus donation after brain death (DBD) in HCV-positive patients undergoing LT.
METHODS: Studies comparing DCD versus DBD LT in HCV-positive
patients were identified based on systematic searches of seven electronic databases and multiple sources of gray literature.
RESULTS: The search identified 58 citations, including three studies,
with 324 patients meeting eligibility criteria. The use of DCD livers
was associated with a significantly higher risk of primary nonfunction
(RR 5.49 [95% CI 1.53 to 19.64]; P=0.009; I^2=0%), while not associated with a significantly different patient survival (RR 0.89 [95% CI
0.37 to 2.11]; P=0.79; I^2=51%), graft survival (RR 0.40 [95% CI 0.14 to
1.11]; P=0.08; I^2=34%), rate of recurrence of severe HCV infection
(RR 2.74 [95% CI 0.36 to 20.92]; P=0.33; I^2=84%), retransplantation
or liver disease-related death (RR 1.79 [95% CI 0.66 to 4.84]; P=0.25;
I^2=44%), and biliary complications.
CONCLUSIONS: While the literature and quality of studies assessing
DCD versus DBD grafts are limited, there was significantly more primary nonfunction and a trend toward decreased graft survival, but no
significant difference in biliary complications or recipient mortality
rates between DCD and DBD LT in patients with HCV infection.
There is insufficient literature on the topic to draw any definitive
conclusions.

Key Words: *Biliary complications; Donation after cardiac death; Hepatitis C;
Liver transplantation; Outcomes*

**Comparer les issues du don d'organe après un décès
cardiaque plutôt qu'après un décès cérébral chez
des greffés du foie atteints d'hépatite C : une
analyse systématique et une méta-analyse**

HISTORIQUE : La transplantation hépatique (TH) au moyen de
dons d'organes après un décès cardiaque (DDCa) augmente, en grande
partie à cause d'une pénurie d'organes. Les issues de l'utilisation
d'organes DDCa chez des greffés atteints d'une infection par le virus de
l'hépatite C (VHC) demeure nébuleux, en raison de l'expérience limitée et du peu de publications sur la question.
OBJECTIF : Évaluer les issues cliniques du DDCa par rapport au don
d'organe après un décès cérébral (DDCé) chez des patients positifs au
VHC qui ont subi une TH.
MÉTHODOLOGIE : Les chercheurs ont extrait les études comparant
la TH DDCa et la TH DDCé chez des patients positifs au VHC au
moyen de recherches systématiques menées dans sept bases de données
électroniques et de multiples sources de non publiées.
RÉSULTATS : La recherche a permis d'extraire 58 citations, dont trois
études comptant 324 patients qui respectaient les critères d'admissibilité.
Le recours à des foies DDCa s'associait à un risque significativement
plus élevé de non-fonction primaire (RR 5,49 [95 % IC 1,53 à 19,64];
P=0,009; I^2= 0 %), mais la différence n'était pas significative sur le
plan de la survie des patients (RR 0,89 [95 % IC 0,37 à 2,11]; P=0,79;
I^2=51 %), de la survie après la transplantation (RR 0,40 [95 % IC
0,14 à 1,11]; P=0,08; I^2=34 %), du taux de récurrence de grave infection par le VHC (RR 2,74 [95 % IC 0,36 à 20,92]; P=0,33; I^2=84 %),
des nouvelle transplantations ou des décès liés à l'insuffisance hépatique (RR 1,79 [95 % IC 0,66 à 4,84]; P=0,25; I^2=44 %) et des complications biliaires.
CONCLUSIONS : Les publications et la qualité des études évaluant
les TH DDCa par rapport aux TH DDCé sont limitées. Toutefois, on
observait une non-fonction primaire beaucoup plus importante et une
tendance vers une diminution de la survie après la transplantation,
mais aucune différence significative sur le plan des complications
biliaires ou des décès chez les greffés infectés par le VHC après un
DDCa ou un DDCé. Les publications sont insuffisantes pour qu'il soit
possible de tirer des conclusions définitives.

L iver transplantation (LT) is a life-saving modality for treating
well-selected patients with acute liver failure, end-stage liver disease, certain metabolic disorders and early hepatocellular carcinoma.
The current practice of LT is limited by the significant disparity
between organ availability and the number of patients awaiting transplantation. Donation after cardiac death (DCD) has become a significant source of transplantable organs in an attempt to expand the
donor pool and increase organ supply (1-4). While DCD allografts
have the potential to help address the disparity between organ availability and the number of patients awaiting LT, their use has been
associated with higher rates of graft failure and biliary complication,
particularly ischemic cholangiopathy, compared with donation after
brain death (DBD) allografts (5,6).

Hepatitis C virus (HCV) infection is currently a leading indication
for LT, constituting approximately 30% to 50% of all transplants
(7-10). Previous studies have suggested that HCV-positive recipients

[1]*Department of Medicine;* [2]*Department of Surgery, Schulich School of Medicine and Dentistry, Western University, London;* [3]*Hotel Dieu Grace Hospital,
Windsor, Ontario*
*Correspondence: Dr Natasha Chandok, Department of Medicine, Schulich School of Medicine and Dentistry, Western University, 339 Windermere Road,
PO Box 5339, London, Ontario N6A 5A5. e-mail nchandok@uwo.ca*

of DBD LT have worse outcomes than HCV-negative recipients, largely due to a more rapid and severe manner of recurrence of their HCV-related liver disease (9,11). Recurrence of HCV after LT is universal, with 20% to 40% of patients progressing to cirrhosis within five years of LT (12). Previous studies have shown that liver allografts from extended-criteria donors, such as those with advanced age, are at an increased risk of earlier and more severe HCV recurrence; this has deleterious impact on both patient and graft outcomes (13-16). It has also been suggested that organ cold/warm ischemia is a risk factor for increased severity of recurrence of HCV after LT. DCD organs experience warm ischemic injury not characteristic of DBD donors because of hypoperfusion and hypoxia during the agonal period of time of withdrawal of life support (11). It has, therefore, been theorized that HCV patients receiving DCD allografts may be at an increased risk for graft injury and accelerated HCV recurrence. Despite this theoretical risk, the literature investigating the outcomes of HCV-positive patients receiving DCD allografts is scant and conflicting reports have been published.

Tao et al (17) performed a retrospective matched control trial of 111 HCV-positive patients (37 receiving DCD LT and 74 matched controls receiving DBD LT). Although the two groups had similar donor and recipient characteristics, immunosuppression regimens, rates of acute cellular rejection and HCV profiles, the patients receiving DCD LT had a higher incidence of primary nonfunction (19% versus 3%; P=0.006) and significantly higher peak aspartate aminotransferase levels compared with DBD subjects. Although the survival rates were not significantly different, DCD LT recipients had lower one- and five-year survival rates (83% and 69% versus 84% and 78%, respectively; P=0.75) and graft survival rates (70% and 61% versus 82% and 74%, respectively; P=0.24). A total of 314 liver biopsies were performed; mixed modelling analysis showed that fibrosis progression rates were similar for the two groups (0.6 fibrosis units/year according to the Ishak modified staging system). The rates of severe HCV recurrence (retransplantation or death due to recurrent HCV and/or the development of stage 4/6 fibrosis or worse within two years) were not significantly different (three [8%] DCD patients versus 11 [15%] DBD patients; P=0.38). Cytomegalovirus infection (HR 7.9 [95% CI 2.1 to 28.9]; P=0.002) and acute cellular rejection (HR 6.2 [95% CI 2.0 to 19.7]; P=0.002) were the only independent risk factors for severe recurrence.

Taner et al (18) performed a retrospective analysis of 77 HCV-positive patients who received DCD liver grafts and 77 matched HCV-positive patients who received DBD liver grafts. There were no differences in one-, three- and five-year patient or graft survival rates among the groups. Multivariate analysis showed that the Model for End-Stage Liver Disease score (HR 1.037 [95% CI 1.006 to 1.069]; P=0.018]) and post-transplant cytomegalovirus infection (HR 3.367 [95% CI 1.493 to 7.593]; P=0.003) were significant factors for graft loss. A comparison of five-year protocol biopsy samples for fibrosis progression in HCV-positive patients post-transplant did not show a difference between DCD and DBD grafts. The authors concluded that DCD liver graft utilization does not cause untoward effects on disease progression or patient and graft survival compared with DBD liver grafts in HCV-positive patients.

Hernandez-Alejandro et al (19) performed a retrospective, matched-control trial evaluating 17 recipients with HCV who received a DCD graft and a matched group of 42 HCV recipients transplanted with a DBD graft. They found a statistically significant decrease in graft survival in HCV-positive patients undergoing DCD transplant (73%) compared with DBD transplant (93%) (P=0.01). There was a statistically significant increase in HCV recurrence at three months (76% versus 16%; P=0.005) and severe HCV recurrence within the first year (47% versus 10%) in the DCD group (P=0.004). The authors concluded that HCV recurrence is more severe and progresses more rapidly in HCV recipients who receive DCD grafts compared with those who receive DBD grafts. DCD LT in HCV recipients is associated with a higher rate of graft failure compared with those who receive DBD grafts.

The objective of the present study was to perform a systematic review and meta-analysis of studies comparing clinical outcomes of DCD versus DBD orthotopic LT in patients with HCV. The primary outcomes of interest were patient survival rates, graft survival rates, recurrence of severe HCV, primary nonfunction, acute cellular rejection, biliary strictures (diffuse or localized, anastomotic or nonanastomotic), biliary leaks and vascular complications (hepatic artery stenosis, hepatic artery thrombosis, portal vein thrombosis).

METHODS

Primary objectives
To compare one-year patient and graft survival rates in recipients transplanted for HCV with DCD versus DBD grafts; and to compare one-year patient and graft survival rates in recipients with versus without HCV undergoing DCD versus DBD LT.

Secondary objectives
To determine whether DCD LT compared with DBD LT in HCV-positive patients increases rates of primary nonfunction, acute cellular rejection, biliary strictures (diffuse or localized, anastomotic or nonanastomotic), biliary leaks or vascular complications (hepatic artery stenosis, hepatic artery thrombosis portal vein thrombosis).

Eligibility criteria
Inclusion criteria were studies that compared DCD versus DBD LT in patients with HCV, as well as DCD LT in patients with and without HCV; and studies that evaluated adult recipients (age ≥18 years) who underwent primary LT. To be included, studies had to include at least one of the prespecified outcomes. There was no limitation on randomized control trials and no restrictions on language. Results duplicated in multiple articles were included only once.

Information sources
A clinical librarian experienced in conducting systematic reviews in the health care field assisted with the literature search. The following electronic databases were searched to March 29, 2012: MEDLINE, Cochrane Database of Systematic Reviews (Cochrane Reviews); Database of Abstracts of Reviews of Effects (Other Reviews); Cochrane Central Register of Controlled Trials (Clinical Trials); Cochrane Methodology Register (Methods Studies); Health Technology Assessment Database (Technology Assessments); and the NHS Economic Evaluation Database (Economic Evaluations). Relevant articles from incompletely and nonpublished literature were identified by consulting with experts in the field. Searches were supplemented by reviewing the reference lists of all citations that met inclusion criteria by screening the first 50 citations in the 'See related articles' function on PubMed of the included studies, and by searching www.clinicaltrials.gov for relevant trials. Corresponding authors were e-mailed when additional information was needed.

Study selection
Two investigators (MW and NC) independently screened the title and abstract of the citations. If either investigator believed that a citation was relevant, it was marked for full-text retrieval. Two investigators independently evaluated the retrieved full-text articles for eligibility. Cohen's kappa statistic was used to quantify agreement between the investigators. Disagreements were resolved by discussion, and a third investigator (KC) was consulted in case of impasse.

Data collection
Two reviewers independently abstracted the data from included trials using a data collection form. Any disagreement in the abstracted data between the two reviewers was resolved by consensus. A third investigator resolved outstanding disagreements. In cases in which the data were incomplete or unclear, the study authors were contacted.

Data items

The following items were abstracted from the articles: demographic data of the study population and comparison group including age and sex; DCD versus DBD liver donations; features of the study design including allocation concealment, blinding, intention-to-treat analysis, number of patients lost to follow-up, rate of premature termination and funding source; the outcome measures of patient survival rate and graft survival rate; rates of primary nonfunction, acute cellular rejection, biliary strictures (diffuse or localized, anastomotic or nonanastomotic), biliary leaks, ischemic cholangiography, vascular complications (hepatic artery stenosis, hepatic artery thrombosis, portal vein thrombosis), HCV recurrence and retransplantation/liver-related death.

Risk of bias

The risk of bias on a study level was assessed by determining the adequacy of the method of randomization, allocation concealment, blinding of the trial participants, care providers and outcome assessors. Also assessed were whether the trial was terminated prematurely, whether the analysis was an intention-to-treat and the funding source.

The Grading of Recommendations, Assessment, Development and Evaluation approach (20) was used to characterize the risk of bias for each of the outcomes that had available data.

Statistical analysis

The meta-analysis was performed using the Cochrane Collaboration and the Quality of Reporting of Meta-analyses (QUORUM) guidelines. Statistical analyses were performed using Review Manager 5 (www.cochrane.org/). The RR was used as a summary measure of efficacy for dichotomous data and the mean difference between groups for continuous data to summarize the outcomes for patients treated with duct-to-duct versus Roux-en-Y loop anastomosis. For all RRs and mean differences, a 95% CI was reported. All analyses were conducted on an intention-to-treat basis.

Synthesis of results

Results were pooled using a Mantel-Haenszel random-effects model for dichotomous outcomes and mean difference for continuous outcomes. Statistical heterogeneity was evaluated using the I^2 statistic. An I^2 value of 0% to 25%, 25% to 50% and >50% were considered to be indicative of low, moderate and high heterogeneity, respectively.

Risk of publication bias

Funnel plots were used to assess the risk of publication bias across trials for all outcome measures.

RESULTS

Study selection

Fifty-eight citations were screened, of which 15 were selected for full-text retrieval. Of these, three articles (17-19) fulfilled eligibility criteria and were, thus, selected (Figure 1).

There was no disagreement regarding eligibility of full-text articles (Cohen's kappa = 1.00), and consensus was reached among all authors on inclusion and exclusion of all articles.

Twelve of the retrieved articles were excluded due to the absence of a comparison of DCD versus DBD liver donation in patients with HCV (n=10) (8,21-29) or the article was an editorial (n=1) (30).

Study characteristics

A total of 324 study participants in three trials comparing DCD versus DBD liver transplantation in HCV-positive patients. Study characteristics are included in Table 1.

Risk of bias within trials

The included trials had a high risk of bias. All three trials were retrospective analyses performed at single centres. There was no blinding and concealment.

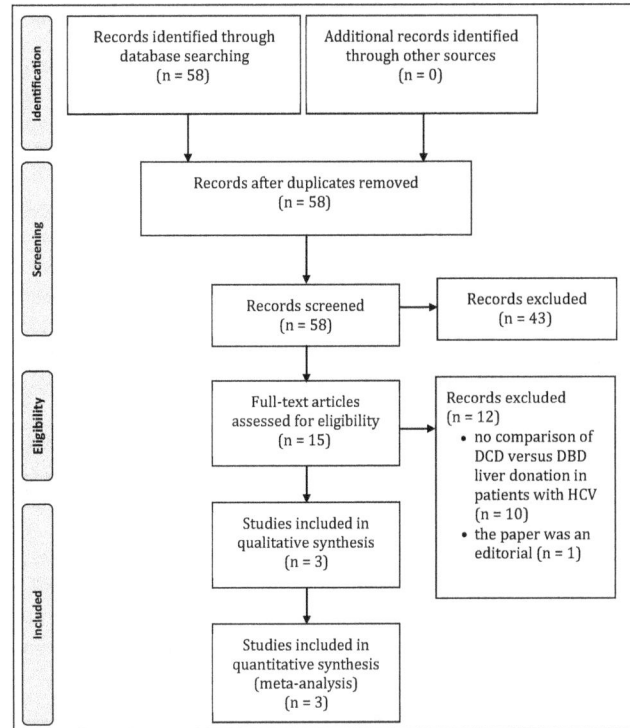

Figure 1) *Study selection. DBD Donation after brain death; DCD Donation after cardiac death; HCV Hepatitis C virus*

Risk of bias across trials

The funnel plots of the RR for all outcomes did not show evidence of publication bias.

Recipient survival

Compared with DBD, orthotopic LT with a DCD liver was not associated with a significantly decreased patient survival (three studies; risk ratio 0.89 [95% CI 0.37 to 2.11]; P=0.79; I^2=51%) (Figure 2). Heterogeneity was potentially explained by differences in length of follow-up. The overall quality of evidence was low (20).

Graft survival

DCD LT trended toward, but was not significantly associated with, a decrease in graft survival (n=2; RR 0.40 [95% CI 0.14 to 1.11]; P=0.08; I^2=34%) (Figure 3). Heterogeneity was potentially explained by differences in length of follow-up. The overall quality of evidence was low (20).

Biliary complications

The risk of biliary leaks was not statistically significantly higher (n=2; risk ratio 2.22 [95% CI 0.42 to 11.88]; P=0.35; I^2=35%) (Figure 4) in patients receiving a DCD versus a DBD LT. The level of heterogeneity was explained by length of follow-up, differences in the definition of biliary leak, and differences in postoperative imaging or investigations for leak. The overall quality of evidence was low (20).

Biliary strictures were not statistically different (n=2; RR 1.15 [95% CI 0.59 to 2.26]; P=0.68; I^2=0%) (Figure 4) in patients receiving a DCD versus a DBD LT. The quality of evidence was low (20).

Patients receiving LT from a DCD versus a DBD did not have a significantly increased risk of ischemic cholangiopathy (n=3; RR 6.67 [95% CI 0.84 to 52.66]; P=0.07; I^2=35%) (Figure 4). The quality of evidence was low (20).

Recurrence of HCV infection

Recurrence of HCV was not significantly different in patients receiving DCD versus DBD LT when patients from two studies were pooled, with a risk ratio of 2.74 (95% CI 0.36 to 20.92; P=0.33; I^2=84%) (Figure 5). The overall quality of evidence was low (20).

TABLE 1
Characteristics of included studies

	Hernandez-Alejandro et al (13), 2011		Taner et al (18), 2011		Tao et al (17), 2010	
	DCD	DBD	DCD	DBD	DCD	DBD
Study design	Retrospective cohort		Retrospective cohort		Retrospective cohort	
Transplantations, n	17	42	77	77	37	74
Donor characteristics						
Age, years, mean ± SD	44±13	46±9	37.7±13.5	37.6±13.2	37.9±16.4	38.1±16.2
Sex, male:female, n:n	N/A	N/A	N/A	N/A	27:10	45:31
Body mass index, kg/m², mean ± SD	N/A	N/A	N/A	N/A	26.6±5.3	28.3±9.6
Cold ischemic time, h, mean ± SD	5.32±1.4	5.9±0.8	5.9±1.4	6.3±1.3	11.2±2.4	11.3±2.7
Warm ischemic time, min, mean ± SD	29±16	N/A	32.0±11.3	33.9±10.4	N/A	N/A
Height, cm, mean ± SD	171.1±8.5	171.9±10	N/A	N/A	N/A	N/A
Donor COD (CVA/trauma/anoxia/other), n	10/5/2/0	28/6/6/2	19/37/18/3	37/22/18/0	N/A	N/A
Recipient characteristics						
Age, years, mean ± SD	54.2±5	48±10	54.5±5.9	53.4±6.0	51±6.7	51±6.2
Sex, male:female, n:n	15:2	30:12	59:18	55:22	31:6	58:16
Race (Caucasian/African American/other), n	17/0/0	41/0/1	69/7/1	73/4/0	N/A	N/A
Body mass index, kg/m²	N/A	N/A	28.6	29.8	29.2±4.9	28.7±5.0
MELD, mean ± SD	17.8±8.1	19.7±5.3	19.9±7.5	18.6±7.4	16.1±7.3	16.2±7.1
Hepatocellular carcinoma, n (%)	N/A	N/A	24 (31.2)	20 (26.0)	N/A	N/A
Hepatitis C genotype 1, n (%)	12 (70.6)	30 (71.4)	N/A	N/A	N/A	N/A

COD Cause of death; CVA Cerebral vascular accident; DBD Donation after brain death; DCD Donation after cardiac death; MELD Model for End-stage Liver Disease; N/A Not available

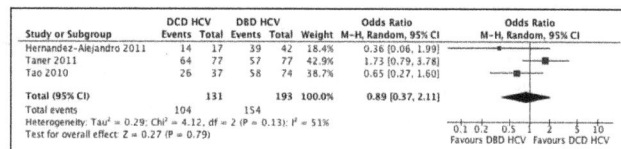

Figure 2) *Forest plot of recipient survival. DBD Donation after brain death; DCD Donation after cardiac death; HCV Hepatitis C virus*

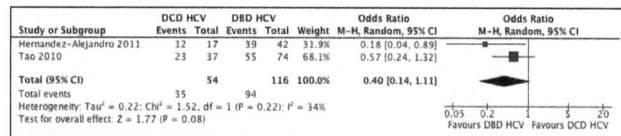

Figure 3) *Forest plot of graft survival. DBD Donation after brain death; DCD Donation after cardiac death; HCV Hepatitis C virus*

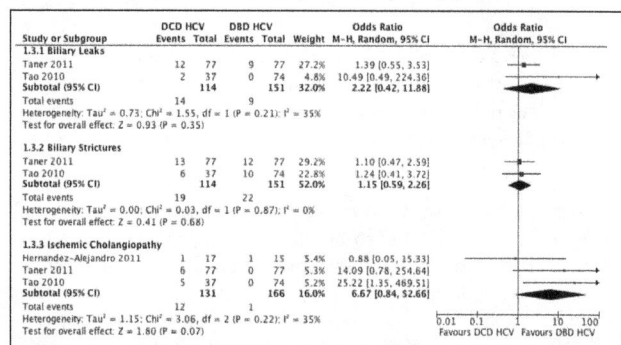

Figure 4) *Forest plot of biliary complications. DBD Donation after brain death; DCD Donation after cardiac death; HCV Hepatitis C virus*

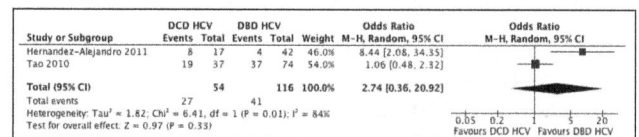

Figure 5) *Forest plot of recurrence of hepatitis C virus (HCV) infection. DBD Donation after brain death; DCD Donation after cardiac death*

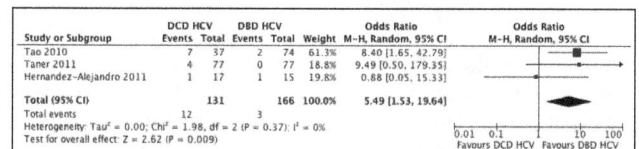

Figure 6) *Forest plot of primary nonfunction. DBD Donation after brain death; DCD Donation after cardiac death; HCV Hepatitis C virus*

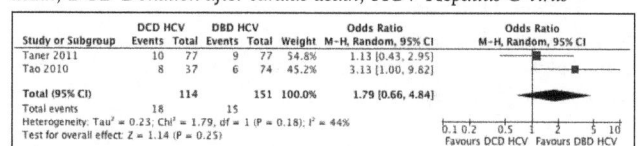

Figure 7) *Forest plot of retransplantation. DBD Donation after brain death; DCD Donation after cardiac death; HCV Hepatitis C virus*

DISCUSSION AND CONCLUSIONS

Summary of evidence

Three trials evaluated DCD versus DBD LT in recipients with HCV infection. The use of DCD livers in HCV-positive recipients was associated with a significant increase in primary nonfunction, but no significant difference in biliary complications, graft survival rates and recipient mortality rates (Table 1).

Limitations

The conclusions that can be drawn from the present systematic review were limited by the small numbers of patients and the retrospective nature of the trials included. Length of follow-up varied substantially among the studies. Techniques and experience also vary among institutions. In addition, there was a lack of histopathological correlation and generalizability of results, in addition to potential selection biases. There were significant differences in rates of HCV recurrence that could, at least partially, be explained by differences in rates of antiviral treatment within the first year post-LT.

Transplant liver primary nonfunction

Compared with DBD, LT with a DCD liver was associated with significantly increased primary liver nonfunction (three studies; risk ratio 5.49 [95% CI 1.53 to 19.64]; P=0.009; I²=0%) (Figure 6). The overall quality of evidence was low (20).

Retransplantation

DCD LT was not significantly associated with an increased risk of retransplantation (two studies; RR 1.79 [95% CI 0.66 to 4.84]; P=0.25; I²=44%) (Figure 7). The overall quality of evidence was low (20).

Despite these limitations, there is still value in the current meta-analysis because it is the first study of its kind and contributes to the knowledge base. Published experiences will likely never be prospective or randomized given the nature of transplantation, the complexities of organ allocation and important issues involving medical ethics. Therefore, high-grade evidence for this topic may never emerge.

Implications for clinical practice

Although significant for limitations, our meta-analysis indicates there is a substantial increase in primary nonfunction and a trend toward a decrease in graft survival, but no significant difference in other important clinical outcomes between DCD and DBD allografts in HCV-positive LT recipients.

Controversy remains in the use of DCD LT in HCV-positive patients. Individually, DCD LT and the presence of HCV have negative impact on patient and graft survival (11). It remains unclear whether the combination of DCD LT and HCV synergistically confers a worse outcome. The two studies that demonstrated no significant difference in patient outcomes with use of DCD LT in HCV-positive patients (17,18) included younger patients than the study that found a significant decrease in graft survival in HCV-positive patients undergoing DCD versus DBD LT (19).

DCD grafts are not contraindicated in well-selected HCV recipients and this is potentially an underutilized method to expand the donor pool. Over the past 10 years, approximately 700 to 800 patients have died awaiting LT (www.unos.org); DCD LT may be one of many solutions requiring further investigation.

Implications for research

DCD allografts have become a significant source of transplantable organs in an attempt to bridge the gap between supply and demand in LT. Our meta-analysis indicates an increased number of adverse events (namely primary nonfunction) with DCD allografts in HCV-positive patients and a trend toward decreased graft survival, but no significant decrease in patient survival.

Ideally, DBD allografts appear to be better suited to HCV-positive patients; however, organ availability necessitates the use of DCD allografts. The quality of evidence in the three included articles was low; a randomized control trial with protocolized liver biopsies would be ideal. However, this is not feasible because recipients could not be randomized because the process of listing recipients is complex and not amenable to a randomized control trial. In the absence of a trial, more observational, prospective and multicentre data are needed.

DISCLOSURES: All authors declare no support from any organization for the submitted work; no financial relationships with any organizations that may have an interest in the submitted work in the previous three years; and no other relationships or activities that could appear to have influenced the submitted work.

AUTHOR CONTRIBUTIONS: All authors contributed to the concept and design, and provided intellectual content of critical importance to this work. Dr Wells, Ms Janik and Dr Chandok performed the electronic literature search and manual search for potential articles. Dr Wells and Dr Chandok retrieved citations, reviewed full text papers and abstracted the data. All authors participated in the analysis and interpretation. All authors approved the final version of this article.

FUNDING: Supported by Western University Department of Medicine Program of Experimental Medicine (POEM) Research Award.

ACKNOWLEDGEMENTS: The authors acknowledge Valerie Kowalkovski of the University Hospital Library, London Health Sciences Centre for her help in retrieving the articles selected for full-text retrieval.

REFERENCES

1. de Vera ME, Lopez-Solis R, Dvorchik I, et al. Liver transplantation using donation after cardiac death donors: Long-term follow-up from a single center. Am J Transpl 2009;9:773-81.
2. Grewal HP, Willingham DL, Nguyen J, et al. Liver transplantation using controlled donation after cardiac death donors: An analysis of a large single-center experience. Liver Transpl 2009;15:1028-35.
3. Fujita S, Mizuno S, Fujikawa T, et al. Liver transplantation from donation after cardiac death: A single center experience. Transplantation 2007;84:46-9.
4. Pine JK, Aldouri A, Young AL, et al. Liver transplantation following donation after cardiac death: An analysis using matched pairs. Liver Transpl 2009;15:1072-82.
5. Foley DP, Fernandez LA, Leverson G, et al. Donation after cardiac death: The University of Wisconsin experience with liver transplantation. Ann Surg 2005;242:724-31.
6. Chan EY, Olson LC, Kisthard JA, et al. Ischemic cholangiopathy following liver transplantation from donation after cardiac death donors. Liver Transpl 2008;14:604-10.
7. Watt K, Veldt B, Charlton M. A practical guide to the management of HCV infection following liver transplantation. Am J Transpl 2009;9:1707-13.
8. Uemura T, Ramprasad V, Hollenbeak CS, Bezinover D, Kadry Z. Liver transplantation for hepatitis C from donation after cardiac death donors: An analysis of OPTN/UNOS data. Am J Transpl 2012;12:984-91.
9. Forman LM, Lewis JD, Berlin JA, Feldman HI, Lucey MR. The association between hepatitis C infection and survival after orthotopic liver transplantation. Gastroenterology 2002;122:889-96.
10. Berenguer M, Lopez-Labrador FX, Wright TL. Hepatitis C and liver transplantation. J Hepatol 2001;35:666-78.
11. Harring TR, Nguyen NT, Cotton RT, et al. Liver transplantation with donation after cardiac death donors: A comprehensive update. J Surg Res 2012;178:502-11.
12. Neumann UP, Berg T, Bahra M, et al. Long-term outcome of liver transplants for chronic hepatitis C: A 10-year follow-up. Transplantation 2004;77:226-31.
13. Hernadez-Alejandro R, Wall W, Jevnikar A, et al. Organ donation after cardiac death: Donor and recipient outcomes after the first three years of the Ontario experience. Can J Anaesthes 2011;58:599-605.
14. Furukawa H, Taniguchi M, Fujiyoshi M, Oota M. Experience using extended criteria donors in first 100 cases of deceased donor liver transplantation in Japan. Transpl Proc 2012;44:373-5.
15. Cameron A, Busuttil RW. AASLD/ILTS transplant course: Is there an extended donor suitable for everyone? Liver Transpl 2005(11 Suppl 2):S2-5.
16. Baccarani U, Adani GL, Toniutto P, et al. Liver transplantation from old donors into HCV and non-HCV recipients. Transpl Proc 2004;36:527-8.
17. Tao R, Ruppert K, Cruz RJ Jr, et al. Hepatitis C recurrence is not adversely affected by the use of donation after cardiac death liver allografts. Liver Transpl 2010;16:1288-95.
18. Taner CB, Bulatao IG, Keaveny AP, et al. Use of liver grafts from donation after cardiac death donors for recipients with hepatitis C virus. Liver Transpl 2011;17:641-9.
19. Hernandez-Alejandro R, Croome KP, Quan D, et al. Increased risk of severe recurrence of hepatitis C virus in liver transplant recipients of donation after cardiac death allografts. Transplantation 2011;92:686-9.
20. Guyatt GH, Oxman AD, Vist GE, et al. GRADE: An emerging consensus on rating quality of evidence and strength of recommendations. BMJ 2008;336:924-6.
21. Allam N, Al Saghier M, El Sheikh Y, et al. Clinical outcomes for Saudi and Egyptian patients receiving deceased donor liver transplantation in China. Am J Transpl 2010;10:1834-41.
22. Chen T, Jia H, Li J, Chen X, Zhou H, Tian H. New onset diabetes mellitus after liver transplantation and hepatitis C virus infection: Meta-analysis of clinical studies. Transpl Int 2009;22:408-15.
23. Feng S, Goodrich NP, Bragg-Gresham JL, et al. Characteristics associated with liver graft failure: The concept of a donor risk index. Am J Transpl 2006;6:783-90.

24. Grewal HP, Willingham DL, Nguyen J, et al. Liver transplantation using controlled donation after cardiac death donors: An analysis of a large single-center experience. Liver Transpl 2009;15:1028-35.

25. Hong JC, Yersiz H, Kositamongkol P, et al. Liver transplantation using organ donation after cardiac death: A clinical predictive index for graft failure-free survival. Arch Surg 2011;146:1017-23.

26. Mathur AK, Heimbach J, Steffick DE, Sonnenday CJ, Goodrich NP, Merion RM. Donation after cardiac death liver transplantation: Predictors of outcome. Am J Transpl 2010;10:2512-9.

27. Ortiz J, Feyssa EL, Parsikia A, et al. Severe hepatitis C virus recurrence is nearly universal after donation after cardiac death liver transplant. Exp Clin Transpl 2011;9:105-12.

28. Watt KD, Pedersen RA, Kremers WK, Heimbach JK, Charlton MR. Evolution of causes and risk factors for mortality post-liver transplant: Results of the NIDDK long-term follow-up study. Am J Transpl 2010;10:1420-7.

29. Xirouchakis E, Triantos C, Manousou P, et al. Pegylated-interferon and ribavirin in liver transplant candidates and recipients with HCV cirrhosis: Systematic review and meta-analysis of prospective controlled studies. J Viral Hepat 2008;15:699-709.

30. Garcia-Valdecasas JC. DCD donors: A unique source to significantly increase organ donation. J Hepatol 2011;55:745-6.

35

A survey of perceptions and practices of complementary alternative medicine among Canadian gastroenterologists

Zane Gallinger MD BSc(H)[1], Brian Bressler MD MS[2], Shane M Devlin MD[3], Sophie Plamondon MD[4], Geoffrey C Nguyen MD PhD[1]

Z Gallinger, B Bressler, SM Devlin, S Plamondon, GC Nguyen. A survey of perceptions and practices of complementary alternative medicine among Canadian gastroenterologists. Can J Gastroenterol Hepatol 2014;28(1):45-49.

BACKGROUND: Despite a high prevalence of complementary alternative medicine (CAM) use among inflammatory bowel disease (IBD) patients, there is a dearth of information about the attitudes and perceptions of CAM among the gastroenterologists who treat these patients.
OBJECTIVE: To characterize the beliefs, perceptions and practices of gastroenterologists toward CAM use in patients with IBD.
METHODS: A web-based survey was sent to member gastroenterologists of the Canadian Association of Gastroenterology. The survey included multiple-choice and Likert scale questions that queried physician knowledge and perceptions of CAM and their willingness to discuss CAM with patients.
RESULTS: Fifty-three per cent of respondents considered themselves to be IBD subspecialists. The majority (86%) of gastroenterologists reported that less than one-half of their patient population had mentioned the use of CAM. Only 8% of physicians reported initiating a conversation about CAM in the majority of their patient encounters. Approximately one-half (51%) of respondents were comfortable with discussing CAM with their patients, with lack of knowledge being cited as the most common reason for discomfort with the topic. Most gastroenterologists (79%) reported no formal education in CAM. While there was uncertainty as to whether CAM interfered with conventional medications, most gastroenterologists believed it could be effective as an adjunct treatment.
CONCLUSION: Our findings demonstrate that gastroenterologists were hesitant to initiate discussions about CAM with patients. Nearly one-half were uncomfortable or only somewhat comfortable with the topic, and most may benefit from CAM educational programs. Interestingly, most respondents appeared to be receptive to CAM as adjunct therapy alongside conventional IBD treatment.

Key Words: CAM; *Complementary alternative medicine; Crohn disease; IBD; Inflammatory bowel disease; Ulcerative colitis*

Un sondage des perceptions et des pratiques en médecine parallèle et complémentaire chez les gastroentérologues canadiens

HISTORIQUE : Malgré la forte prévalence de la médecine complémentaire et parallèle (MCP) chez les patients ayant une maladie inflammatoire de l'intestin (MII), il y a pénurie d'information sur les attitudes et perceptions de la MCP chez les gastroentérologues qui traitent ces patients.
OBJECTIF : Caractériser les croyances, les perceptions et les pratiques des gastroentérologues envers l'utilisation de la MCP chez les patients atteints d'une MII.
MÉTHODOLOGIE : Les gastroentérologues membres de l'Association canadienne de gastroentérologie ont reçu un sondage virtuel. Ce sondage contenait des questions à choix multiples et des questions sur l'échelle de Likert pour s'informer de leurs connaissances et perceptions de la MCP et de leur volonté à parler de MCP avec leurs patients.
RÉSULTATS : Cinquante-trois pour cent des répondants se considéraient comme des surspécialistes des MII. Selon la majorité (86 %) des gastroentérologues, moins de la moitié de leur population de patients indiquait utiliser la MCP. Seulement 8 % des médecins ont affirmé lancer une conversation sur la MCP lors de la majorité de leurs rencontres avec les patients. Environ la moitié (51 %) des répondants était à l'aise de discuter de MCP avec les patients, le manque de connaissances étant cité comme la principale raison d'être mal à l'aise d'aborder le sujet. La plupart des gastroentérologues (79 %) ont indiqué ne pas posséder de formation officielle sur la MCP. Même s'ils n'étaient pas certains de la possibilité d'interaction de la MCP avec les médicaments classiques, la plupart des gastroentérologues croyaient qu'elle pouvait être efficace comme traitement d'appoint.
CONCLUSION : Nos observations démontrent que les gastroentérologues hésitaient à lancer des discussions sur la MCP avec leurs patients. Près de la moitié n'était pas à l'aise ou plutôt mal à l'aise de parler de ce sujet, et la plupart pourraient profiter de programmes de formation sur la MCP. Fait intéressant, la plupart des répondants semblent réceptifs à la MCP comme traitement d'appoint à la thérapie classique des MII.

Patients with inflammatory bowel disease (IBD), including ulcerative colitis (UC) and Crohn disease, use complementary alternative medicine (CAM) more frequently than the general population (1,2). The popularity of CAM among IBD patients is due, in part, to the chronicity and severity of these diseases, resulting in patients seeking alternative treatments. Furthermore, patients with IBD comprise a well-educated population with a desire to gain control over their illness (3,4). CAM can serve as a coping mechanism through which patients can retain a sense of influence and independence in their treatment course. In addition, adverse effects experienced while taking some IBD medications may prompt patients to seek alternative treatments. Given the correlation between steroid use and CAM use among IBD patients, it is speculated that the adverse effects of these commonly used drugs drives the use of CAM (5,6). Due to the increasing use of information technology, along with a more informed and educated patient population, it can be expected that CAM will continue to play a prominent role in the holistic care of patients with IBD.

CAM may provide IBD patients with a greater sense of control over their disease treatment; however, its use remains controversial

[1]*Mount Sinai Hospital Centre for Inflammatory Bowel Disease, University of Toronto, Toronto, Ontario;* [2]*Division of Gastroenterology, University of British Columbia, Vancouver, British Columbia;* [3]*Inflammatory Bowel Disease Clinic, Division of Gastroenterology and Hepatology, University of Calgary, Calgary, Alberta;* [4]*Division of Gastroenterology, Centre Hospitalier Universitaire de Sherbrooke and Centre de Recherche Étienne-LeBel, Université de Sherbrooke, Sherbrooke, Québec*
Correspondence: Dr Geoffrey C Nguyen, Mount Sinai Hospital, 600 University Avenue, Suite 437, Toronto, Ontario M5G 1X5.
e-mail geoff.nguyen@utoronto.ca

TABLE 1
Practice characteristics of respondents

Years in practice, mean ± SD	13.5±9.0
Primary practice setting	
Academic	54 (62)
Community	29 (33)
Both	4 (5)
Scope of practice	
Limited to adult gastroenterology	60 (69)
Gastroenterology and internal medicine	16 (18)
Pediatric gastroenterology	11 (12)
Surgery	0 (0)
Other	0 (0)
Gastroenterology practice patients with IBD, %	
<10	16 (18)
10–25	36 (41)
25–50	20 (23)
>50	15 (17)
Subspecialist in IBD	
Yes	46 (53)
No	41 (47)

Data presented n (%) unless otherwise indicated. IBD Inflammatory bowel disease

among gastroenterologists (7,8). CAM has traditionally been difficult to study for multiple reasons including: a universally accepted definition of CAM does not exist; studies investigating CAM have significant limitations including a lack of randomized controlled trials, small sample sizes and selection biases; and an inability to study CAM methods without the use of concurrent conventional medications (3,9). There is also skepticism of CAM because of its potential to cause harm. Herbal therapies – the most common form of CAM used by IBD patients – have contributed to liver and renal failure (1,10,11). Other dangers include the addition of prescription medications in 'natural' products, along with the transmission of infectious diseases through contamination of needles and other sharps (4,12). Despite the inconsistencies and potential harm, CAM use continues to rise among the general population (5,13-16).

A survey suggested that 47% of Canadian patients with IBD used CAM to treat their IBD at some point in time (7). Studies from other countries have found similar rates of CAM use among IBD patients (17). Interestingly, most patients do not receive information about CAM from their gastroenterologists (18,19), which is concerning for several reasons. For example, adverse interactions between CAM therapies and conventional medications have been documented (20). As a result, patients who withhold information about their CAM use from their gastroenterologists may be putting themselves at risk. Interestingly, one study found that 50% of patients with IBD who use CAM do not believe there is scientific evidence to support their practices (19). This apparent contradiction may further represent a lack of meaningful communication between patients and their gastroenterologists.

While many studies have investigated the patterns of CAM use among IBD patients, limited data regarding gastroenterologist perceptions and beliefs regarding CAM (6,7,20) exist. To address this gap in knowledge, a survey study was directed toward Canadian gastroenterologists. The present article reports findings on how gastroenterologists communicate with patients regarding CAM; their reactions to patient CAM use; and potential ways in which CAM can be incorporated into the treatment of IBD.

METHODS

A questionnaire was developed to assess gastroenterologist attitudes and opinions regarding CAM. Situational questions involving CAM use by patients, as well as questions regarding specific CAM

modalities, were used. In the survey, CAM referred to 'complementary alternative medicine', which included but was not limited to meditation, acupuncture, traditional Chinese medicine, probiotics, massage and herbal diets. Multiple IBD specialists reviewed the survey and provided input to increase validity. Demographic data were solicited. The questionnaire was administered using an online survey engine (Novi-Survey).

The survey was sent to active members of the Canadian Association of Gastroenterology, who were medical doctors and not trainees, via their monthly e-mail invitation. Participants were encouraged to only complete the survey once. Surveys were sent in English only. After selecting the link to the survey site, participants were given an explanation of the study. Consent was implied if participants proceeded with the survey.

Before accessing the survey, participants were screened for suitability for the study. Participants were required to be practicing physicians, who in the past 12 months had participated in the care of patients with IBD, and had completed medical, specialty and/or subspecialty training. A combination of contingency, matrix and closed-ended questions were used in the questionnaire. All data were collected anonymously. Continuous variables are presented as means and SDs.

Some groups were collapsed for comparisons and analysis. IBD subspecialists and those with >50% of their practice including IBD patients were combined to categorize the comparison group 'IBD subspecialist'. In classifying comfort level with CAM, 'somewhat comfortable' and 'not comfortable' were combined into a single category of 'uncomfortable', while 'comfortable' and 'very comfortable' were combined into the category 'comfortable'. Certain categorical data of percentages were collapsed for comparison among groups. Comparisons of categorical variables between subgroups were performed using the χ^2 test or Fisher's exact test.

The study protocol was approved by the Research Ethics Board of Mount Sinai Hospital, Toronto, Ontario.

RESULTS

All active clinical, nontrainee members of the the Canadian Association of Gastroenterology were invited to participate in the survey via e-mail. There were 96 respondents to the survey, yielding a response rate of 22%. Among these, 87 met the inclusion criteria and completed the survey. The mean (± SD) length of time in practice was 13.5±9.0 years (Table 1). One-third of the respondents practiced primarily in a community setting, while the remaining two-thirds practiced in an academic setting or had an academic affiliation. The majority (69%) of respondents' clinical practices were limited to adult gastroenterology, while 18% practiced both internal medicine and gastroenterology; and 13% practiced only pediatric gastroenterology. Slightly more than one-half (53%) identified themselves as IBD subspecialists. However, a majority (60%) reported that fewer than one-quarter of their practice comprised IBD patients (Table 1).

The survey explored the nature of the patient-physician interaction with respect to CAM use. A vast majority (86%) of gastroenterologists reported that fewer than one-half of their patients mentioned the use of CAM in their discussion of IBD treatment. A minority (18%) of gastroenterologists reported that they initiated discussions about CAM in the majority of their patient encounters. IBD subspecialists were more inclined to do so than nonsubspecialists (28% versus 5%, respectively; P=0.02). However, academic gastroenterologists were not more likely to initiate discussions regarding CAM than their community counterparts (20% versus 14%; P=0.3). Only a minority (12%) of gastroenterologists believed that more than one-half of their patients used CAM without reporting it (Table 2). Physicians perceived the most common reason to not report CAM use was fear of physician disapproval (Figure 1).

Only one-half of respondents (51%) were comfortable or very comfortable discussing CAM with their patients (Figure 2A). There was no difference in comfort level between IBD subspecialists and nonsubspecialists (57% versus 43%, respectively; P=0.20) or between

TABLE 2
Gastroenterologist perceptions and practices regarding complementary alternative medicine (CAM)

	<10%	10% – 25%	>25% – 50%	>50%
What percentage of your patients has mentioned the use of CAM as a part of their treatment of inflammatory bowel disease?	18 (21)	36 (41)	21 (24)	12 (14)
How often do you initiate a discussion with your patients about their use of CAM?	34 (40)	24 (28)	11 (13)	15 (18)
How often does a patient with IBD initiate a discussion about their use of CAM?	20 (23)	34 (39)	26 (13)	7 (8)
What percentage of your patients do you think use CAM and do not tell you about it?	10 (12)	33 (38)	33 (38)	10 (12)

Data presented as n (%). IBD Inflammatory bowel disease

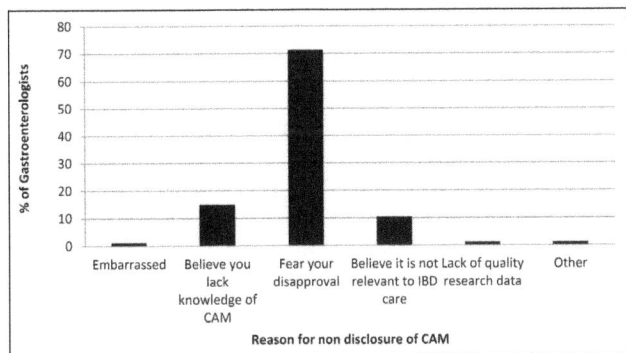

Figure 1) *Perceived reasons by gastroenterologists that patients do not disclose their use of complementary alternative medicine (CAM). IBD Inflammatory bowel disease*

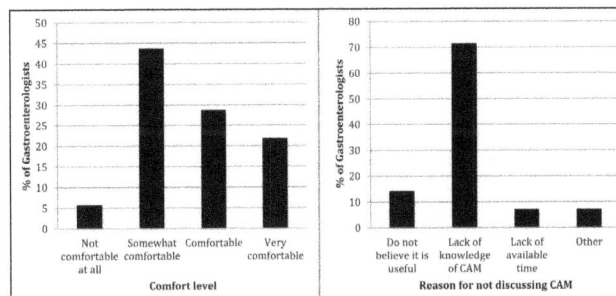

Figure 2) A *Comfort levels of gastroenterologists when discussing complementary alternative medicine (CAM) with their patients.* **B** *Reason that respondents were not comfortable or only somewhat comfortable discussing CAM with patients*

community and academic gastroenterologists (57% versus 38%, respectively; P=0.12). The most commonly cited reason for feeling uncomfortable or somewhat comfortable was a lack of knowledge on CAM (Figure 2B). Most gastroenterologists (79%) reported having never attended a formal education program on CAM, which included training in medical school, continuing medical education (CME) sessions, hospital workshops or structured independent learning. Among the minority that received formal training in CAM, 72% gained exposure through CME activities. IBD subspecialists were no more likely to have undergone formal training in CAM than nonsubspecialists (28% versus 13%; P=0.11). Community and academic gastroenterologists also reported similar exposure to formal CAM education (22% versus 17%; P=0.78).

Nearly one-half of physicians (47%) reported that they did not have a systematic or standardized approach to the discussion of CAM, and that their conversations with patients on the topic of CAM varied from individual to individual. Nearly one-third (32%) of gastroenterologists were willing to at least participate in an initial discussion regarding CAM, while a minority (15%) were doubtful that they would be able to add to such a discussion due to lack of knowledge on the topic. Only two gastroenterologists outright dismissed CAM, and two referred patients to an alternative practitioner, while one actively recommended its use.

Overall, gastroenterologists reported broad familiarity with the types of CAM. The majority (77%) of respondents had heard of and recommended probiotics (Figure 3). More than three-quarters of respondents had heard of each of the following CAM modalities: probiotics, prebiotics, herbal remedies, aloe vera, marijuana, fish oil and acupuncture. However, none of these modalities were recommended by more than 30% of gastroenterologists (Figure 3). The vast majority (90%) of gastroenterologists had, at some point, recommended at least one form of CAM listed on the survey. IBD subspecialists were no more likely to recommend CAM than non-IBD subspecialists (87% versus 93%; P=0.5). Similarly, the proportion of academic and community gastroenterologists who recommended at least one form of CAM did not significantly differ (91% versus 86%; P=0.47).

Table 3 summarizes gastroenterologists' beliefs and attitudes toward CAM. Most respondents believed that patients who respond poorly to conventional therapy exhibited more willingness to use CAM. A vast majority believed that their patients would still use CAM irrespective

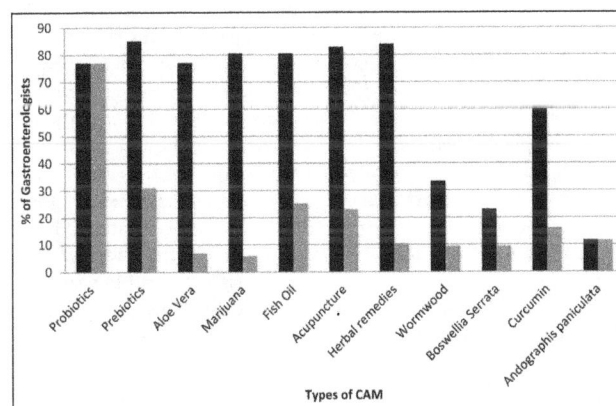

Figure 3) *Gastroenterologists' familiarity with and recommendation practices for specific modalities of complementary alternative medicine (CAM). Black bars represent the proportion of respondents who were familiar with a specific type of CAM and grey bars represent the proportion who recommended that specific modality*

of the physician's recommendations. Most respondents affirmed that CAM should be subjected to strict regulations by health agencies and that research in CAM efficacy should be a high priority. There was moderate uncertainty as to whether CAM would interfere with adherence to conventional medical management of IBD. However, the majority (57%) of respondents posited that CAM could serve as an effective adjunct to conventional therapy.

DISCUSSION

The present survey reports data regarding the current practices and attitudes of Canadian gastroenterologists toward patients who use CAM to treat IBD. Considering the widespread and increasing use of CAM, we believe it is necessary to gain an understanding of physician opinions and comfort levels with CAM, along with how these attitudes influence their interaction with patients. This information may help enhance the overall patient-physician encounter by fostering increased opportunities for communication. To our knowledge, the present study was the first to assess Canadian gastroenterologists' beliefs and practices related to CAM use.

TABLE 3
Perceptions of complementary alternative medicine (CAM) efficacy, user characteristics and utility in patients who use CAM to treat inflammatory bowel disease

	Strongly disagree	Disagree	Somewhat disagree	Undecided	Somewhat agree	Agree	Strongly agree
Patients that have poor response to conventional inflammatory bowel disease therapy tend to use more CAM	0 (0)	1 (1)	9 (11)	8 (10)	37 (44)	22 (26)	7 (8)
My patients will pursue CAM despite my recommendations for or against it	1 (1)	1 (1)	7 (8)	13 (16)	34 (45)	24 (29)	4 (5)
Women, high income and high education patients are more likely to use CAM	0 (0)	3 (4)	10 (12)	23 (28)	26 (31)	17 (21)	4 (5)
My patients would benefit from a wellness centre at my institution that could provide access to CAM providers	4 (5)	9 (11)	15 (18)	21 (25)	19 (23)	11 (13)	5 (6)
CAM can be an effective adjunct to the management of inflammatory bowel disease	2 (2)	7 (8)	11 (13)	16 (19)	32 (38)	13 (16)	3 (4)
CAM should be subject to strict regulations by governing health agencies	2 (2)	1 (1)	4 (5)	11 (13)	16 (19)	24 (29)	26 (31)
Research in the efficacy and safety of CAM should be a high priority	1 (1)	2 (2)	4 (5)	9 (11)	24 (29)	28 (34)	15 (19)
CAM interferes with the adherence to medical management of inflammatory bowel disease	1 (1)	13 (16)	25 (30)	19 (23)	21 (25)	5 (6.0)	0 (0)
When in doubt about potential drug-drug interactions of a CAM supplement, I call a pharmacist for clarification	3 (4)	18 (21)	11 (13)	10 (12)	19 (23)	14 (17)	9 (11)

Data presented as n (%)

Understanding the dynamics that surround the discussion of CAM can promote more open discussions between patients and their treating physicians. In our study, gastroenterologists perceived that patients most often instigate conversations regarding CAM. However, a majority of respondents believed that fewer than one-half of their patient population failed to disclose CAM use. Previous studies using patient self-report questionnaires have presented conflicting data regarding patient disclosure of CAM use. A survey sent to members of the Crohn's and Colitis Foundation found that 71% of IBD patients had discussed CAM with their doctors, while only 13% were uncomfortable doing so (7). Ganguli et al (1) found that 43% of IBD patients had discussed CAM with their gastroenterologist. However, another study of IBD patients found that only 34% had consulted with their gastroenterologist before using CAM (3). The variations in findings likely reflect inherent differences in study populations, design and tools, but underscore the underlying gravity of the problem. Physicians in our study speculated that fear of physician disapproval was a major contributing factor for the lack of disclosure, which mirror concerns expressed by Hilsden (7). Thus, physicians may need to initiate discussions about CAM with their patients to assure them that they will not be judged negatively for discussing alternative therapies. Regardless of the physician's initial beliefs regarding CAM, these conversations to ascertain whether a patient is using CAM for the treatment of IBD are important for assessing whether it is interfering with adherence to prescribed conventional therapies and the safety of the particular type of CAM being used. These discussions also provide an opportunity for physicians to disseminate accurate information, reliable sources of patient information and evidence-based recommendations regarding CAM.

Unfortunately, our study showed that fewer than one-quarter of physicians initiated discussions regarding CAM primarily because of discomfort with and lack of knowledge of the topic. Encouragingly, respondents appeared to be receptive to the role of CAM as adjunct therapy alongside conventional treatment. For more physicians to gain the confidence and comfort level to instigate conversations about CAM, more educational directives may be needed, either during training or CME programs, that address the topic. The vast majority of respondents had no formal education on CAM. Even guidance on a standardized approach to discussing CAM may facilitate these conversations because most physicians did not have one. One strategy is to routinely ask about CAM use during review of medications.

Given the high prevalence of CAM use, an increasingly important therapeutic consideration for gastroenterologists is the impact of alternative therapies on adherence to conventional IBD treatment; there was uncertainty among our respondents as to whether this was the case. A previous questionnaire-based study found that 24% of IBD patients agreed that CAM resulted in abandoning their use of conventional medicine (7). However, in a cross-sectional study conducted by Weizman et al (3), overall medication adherence did not significantly differ between CAM users and nonusers. A concerning finding from one survey on CAM use found that one in 12 patients reported being told by CAM practitioners to change their conventional medications prescribed by physicians (1). Similar data from the United Kingdom showed that CAM providers occasionally advised patients with celiac disease to adjust their prescribed medication dosage, without consulting the treating physicians (21).

Another reason gastroenterologists cited for not initiating discussions regarding CAM was lack of time. These concerns introduce the possible role of other health providers in educating patients about CAM – particularly pharmacists. In the current survey, there was also little consensus from gastroenterologists regarding the role of pharmacists in managing conventional medications and those prescribed by alternative practitioners. The role of the pharmacist in CAM has not been well elucidated in general. While pharmacists agree that they could serve an important role by performing medication reviews of patients who use CAM, they also report a need for additional formal and interprofessional training on CAM (13).

One unifying concern regarding CAM among gastroenterologists was the lack of evidence-based data. Numerous randomized controlled trials have tested the efficacy of certain CAM modalities on gastrointestinal symptoms and disease end points. However, design flaws and small sample sizes remain a reason for skepticism among gastroenterologists (14,16). The majority of gastroenterologists in the present survey agreed that research on the efficacy of CAM should remain a high priority. Herbal medications and probiotics are the most commonly used CAM for IBD (7,18,22). Results from our study showed that gastroenterologists frequently recommended probiotics for IBD, which may be attributable to evidence from clinical trials for pouchitis and UC (23). A meta-analysis from a Cochrane review (24) found limited evidence that probiotics added to standard therapy was modestly effective at inducing remission of disease activity in mild to moderate UC. A separate Cochrane review found insufficient evidence that probiotics were effective in the maintenance of remission of UC compared with placebo (25). Interestingly, most gastroenterologists surveyed did not recommend herbal remedies. Therefore, it is likely that the majority of IBD patients are being prescribed herbal supplements by nonphysicians.

There were several limitations to our survey, the first of which was the possiblity of response bias. Although the response rate (22%) was low, it is not unexpected for an e-mail-based survey that targeted all gastroenterologists throughout Canada. We could have increased the response rate by inviting only academic gastroenterologists, but we believed that it was also important to include representation from community gastroenterologists. We should note that our survey likely reflected under-representation from community gastroenterologists; however, there were no statistically significant different responses between academic and community gastroenterologists. An additional limitation was the lack of a unifying definition for CAM and, thus, the likelihood that the entire spectrum of CAM practices was not captured. The survey did provide an option to mention CAM modalities that we did not list. It does not appear that we omitted major forms of CAM because only eight gastroenterologists suggested additional forms of CAM.

CAM will continue to play a role in the physician-patient relationship. The use of CAM has risen steadily in the United Kingdom and Canada, and will likely continue to rise (5,15,26). As a result of the increasing use of CAM, the College of Physicians and Surgeons of Ontario recently revised a policy statement regarding how physicians should address patient use of CAM (27). Among other points, the policy recommends that "physicians inquire about patient use of CAM on a regular basis," and document this in the medical record (27). It is recommended that physicians read these policies to gain a better understanding of the most productive way to engage and advise their patients. In the present study, there was a lack of consensus among gastroenterologists on how CAM use may influence the patient-physician relationship. Additional educational opportunities, along with a unifying training and CME approach, possibly mandated from specific subspecialty organizations, may guide physicians in effectively counselling and guiding patients.

REFERENCES

1. Ganguli SC, Cawdron R, Irvine EJ. Alternative medicine use by Canadian ambulatory gastroenterology patients: Secular trend or epidemic? Am J Gastroenterol 2004;99:319-26.
2. Haas L, McClain C, Varilek G. Complementary and alternative medicine and gastrointestinal diseases. Curr Opin Gastroenterol 2000;16:188-96.
3. Weizman AV, Ahn E, Thanabalan R, et al. Characterisation of complementary and alternative medicine use and its impact on medication adherence in inflammatory bowel disease. Aliment Pharmacol Ther 2001;35:342-9.
4. Mooer G, Tillinger W, Sachs G, et al. Relationship between the use of unconventional therapies and disease-related concerns: A study of patients with inflammatory bowel disease. J Psychoso Res 1996;40:503-9.
5. Li FX, Verhoef MJ, Best A, Otley A, Hilsden RJ. Why patients with inflammatory bowel disease use or do not use complementary and alternative medicine: A Canadian national survey. Can J Gastroenterol 2005;19:567-73.
6. Langhorst J, Anthonisen IB, Steder-Neukamm U, et al. Amount of systemic steroid medication is a strong predictor for the use of complementary and alternative medicine in patients with inflammatory bowel disease: Results from a German national survey. Inflamm Bowel Dis 2005;11:287-95.
7. Hilsden R. Complementary and alternative medicine use by Canadian patients with inflammatory bowel disease: Results from a national survey. Am J Gastroenterol 2003;98:1563-8.
8. Hilsden RJ, Scott CM, Verhoef MJ. Complementary medicine use by patients with inflammatory bowel disease. Am J Gastroenterol 1998;93:697-701.
9. Bernstein CN. Complementary and alternative medicine use by patients with inflammatory bowel disease: Are Canadian physicians failing with conventional therapy, or not. Can J Gastroenterol 2004;18:47-8.
10. Barnes J. Pharmacovigilance of herbal medicines. Drug Safety 2003;26:829-51.
11. Langmead L, Rampton D. Review article: Complementary and alternative therapies for inflammatory bowel disease. Aliment Pharmacol Ther 2006;23:341-9.
12. Ernst E, Sherman KJ. Is acupuncture a risk factor for hepatitis? Systematic review of epidemiological studies. J Gastroenterol Hepatol 2003;18:1231-6.
13. Koh H-L, Teo H-H, Ng H-L. Pharmacists' patterns of use, knowledge, and attitudes toward complementary and alternative medicine. J Altern Complement Med 2003;9:51-63.
14. Koretz RL, Rotblatt M. Complementary and alternative medicine in gastroenterology: The good, the bad, and the ugly. Clin Gastroenterol Hepatol 2004;2:957-67.
15. Eisenberg DM, Davis RB, Ettner SL, et al. Trends in alternative medicine use in the United States, 1990-1997: Results of a follow-up national survey. JAMA 1998;280:1569-75.
16. Hilsden RJ, Verhoef MJ. Complementary and alternative medicine: Evaluating its effectiveness in inflammatory bowel disease. Inflamm Bowel Dis 1998;4:318-23.
17. Burgmann T, Rawsthorne P, Bernstein CN. Predictors of alternative and complementary medicine use in inflammatory bowel disease: Do measures of conventional health care utilization relate to use? Am J Gastroenterol 2004;99:889-93.
18. Limdi JK, Butcher RO. Complementary and alternative medicine use in inflammatory bowel disease. Inflamm Bowel Dis 2011;17:E86-8.
19. Gangl A. Alternative and complementary therapies for inflammatory bowel disease. Nat Clin Pract Gastroenterol Hepatol 2006;3:180-1.
20. Kong SC, Hurlstone DP, Pocock CY, et al. The incidence of self-prescribed oral complementary and alternative medicine use by patients with gastrointestinal diseases. J Clin Gastroenterol 2005;39:138-41.
21. Moody GA, Eaden JA, Bhakta P, Sher K, Mayberry JF. The role of complementary medicine in European and Asian patients with inflammatory bowel disease. Public Health 1998;112:269-71.
22. Tillisch K. Complementary and alternative medicine for gastrointestinal disorders. Clin Med 2007;7:224-7.
23. Holubar SD, Cima R, Sandborn WJ, et al. Treatment and prevention of pouchitis after ileal pouch-anal anastomosis for chronic ulcerative colitis. Cochrane Database Syst Rev 2010;(6):CD001176.
24. Naidoo, K, Gordon M, Fagbemi O, Thomas G, Akobeng A. Probiotics for maintenance of remission in ulcerative colitis. Cochrane Database Syst Rev 2011;(12):CD007443.
25. Mallon P, McKay D, Kirk S, Gardiner K. Probiotics for induction of remission in ulcerative colitis. Cochrane Database Syst Rev 2007;(4):CD005573.
26. Maha N, Shaw A. Academic doctors' views of complementary and alternative medicine (CAM) and its role within the NHS: An exploratory qualitative study. BMC Complement Altern Med 2007;7:17.
27. College of Physicians and Surgeons of Ontario Policy Statement #3-11. Dialogue. 2011:1;4.

36

Physician attitudes toward the use of fecal microbiota transplantation for the treatment of recurrent *Clostridium difficile* infection

Jonathan S Zipursky MD[1], Tivon I Sidorsky MD MBA[2], Carolyn A Freedman MD[3], Misha N Sidorsky AB[4], Kathryn B Kirkland MD[5]

JS Zipursky, TI Sidorsky, CA Freedman, MN Sidorsky, KB Kirkland. Physician attitudes toward the use of fecal microbiota transplantation for the treatment of recurrent *Clostridium difficile* infection. Can J Gastroenterol Hepatol 2014;28(6):319-324.

BACKGROUND: Fecal microbiota transplantation (FMT) is a safe and effective, yet infrequently used therapy for recurrent *Clostridium difficile* infection (CDI).

OBJECTIVE: To characterize barriers to FMT adoption by surveying physicians about their experiences and attitudes toward the use of FMT.

METHODS: An electronic survey was distributed to physicians to assess their experience with CDI and attitudes toward FMT.

RESULTS: A total of 139 surveys were sent and 135 were completed, yielding a response rate of 97%. Twenty-five (20%) physicians had treated a patient with FMT, 10 (8%) offered to treat with FMT, nine (7%) referred a patient to receive FMT, and 83 (65%) had neither offered nor referred a patient for FMT. Physicians who had experience with FMT (performed, offered or referred) were more likely to be male, an infectious diseases specialist, >40 years of age, fellowship trained and practicing in an urban setting. The most common reasons for not offering or referring a patient for FMT were: not having 'the right clinical situation' (33%); the belief that patients would find it too unappealing (24%); and institutional or logistical barriers (23%). Only 8% of physicians predicted that the majority of patients would opt for FMT if given the option. Physicians predicted that patients would find all aspects of the FMT process more unappealing than they would as providers.

CONCLUSIONS: Physicians have limited experience with FMT despite having treated patients with multiple recurrent CDIs. There is a clear discordance between physician beliefs about FMT and patient willingness to accept FMT as a treatment for recurrent CDI.

Key Words: Clostridium difficile *infection; Fecal microbiota transplantation; Fecal transplant; Physician attitudes; Shared decision making*

Les attitudes des médecins envers l'utilisation de la transplantation fécale pour le traitement de l'infection récurrente à *Clostridium difficile*

HISTORIQUE : La transplantation fécale (TF) est un traitement sécuritaire et efficace, mais peu utilisé pour soigner l'infection à *Clostridium difficile* (ICD) récurrente.

OBJECTIF : Caractériser les obstacles à l'adoption de la TF au moyen d'un sondage auprès des médecins sur leurs expériences et leurs attitudes envers l'utilisation de ce traitement.

MÉTHODOLOGIE : Un sondage électronique a été distribué aux médecins pour évaluer leur expérience de l'ICD et leurs attitudes envers la TF.

RÉSULTATS : Au total, 139 sondages ont été envoyés et 135 ont été remplis, pour un taux de réponse de 97 %. Vingt-cinq médecins (20 %) avaient traité un patient par TF, dix (8 %) avaient offert de le faire, neuf (7 %) avaient aiguillé un patient en vue d'une TF et 83 (65 %) n'avaient ni offert la TF ni aiguillé le patient pour qu'il la reçoive. Les médecins qui avaient l'expérience de la TF (effectuée, offerte ou aiguillée) étaient plus susceptibles d'être de sexe masculin, d'être spécialisés en infectiologie, d'avoir plus de 40 ans, de détenir un postdoctorat et d'exercer en milieu urbain. Les principales raisons de ne pas offrir une TF ou de ne pas aiguiller un patient pour qu'il la reçoive étaient de ne pas être dans « la bonne situation clinique » (33 %), de penser que les patients la trouveraient trop désagréable (24 %) et de se heurter à des obstacles logistiques ou posés par l'établissement (23 %). Seulement 8 % des médecins prédisaient que la majorité des patients opteraient pour la TF si on la leur offrait. Les médecins prédisaient que les patients trouveraient tous les aspects du processus de TF plus désagréable qu'eux-mêmes à titre de dispensateurs.

CONCLUSIONS : Les médecins avaient une expérience limitée de la TF, même s'ils avaient traité des patients ayant de multiples ICD récurrente. On constate une divergence claire entre les croyances des médecins au sujet de la TF et la volonté des patients à l'accepter comme traitement des ICD récurrentes.

Clostridium difficile infection (CDI) is an inflammatory diarrheal illness frequently associated with antibiotic use and characterized by disruptions in the normal intestinal microbiota (1). In recent years, CDIs have become more frequent, severe and refractory to therapy (2-9). It is estimated that 10% to 35% of patients treated with standard antibiotic therapy will progress to develop a recurrence (10-12). Up to 65% of patients treated with antibiotics for recurrent CDI will progress to develop a chronic, recurring form of the disease (13,14).

Fecal microbiota transplantation (FMT) has demonstrated significant value as a therapy for recurrent CDI. A systematic review found that 92% of patients treated with FMT for CDI or pseudomembranous colitis experienced rapid resolution of infection and symptoms (15). More recently, the first randomized controlled trial (RCT) of FMT was stopped early because of the treatment failure rate in the control groups; 94% of patients with recurrent CDI were cured with FMT, compared with 31% treated with vancomycin and 23% treated with vancomycin and sham FMT (gastric lavage) (16).

Despite increasing evidence supporting its safety and efficacy, FMT is infrequently used in medical practice. There is a widely held belief that FMT was seldom used because patients had a strong aversion to

[1]Faculty of Medicine, Geisel School of Medicine at Dartmouth, Hanover, New Hampshire; [2]Department of Dermatology, University of California, San Francisco, San Francisco, California, USA; [3]University of Toronto Faculty of Medicine, Toronto, Ontario; [4]Dartmouth College, Hanover; [5]Section of Infectious Diseases and International Health, Dartmouth-Hitchcock Medical Center, Lebanon, New Hampshire, USA
Correspondence: Dr Jonathan S Zipursky, Department of Medicine, University of Toronto, St Michael's Hospital, 30 Bond Street, Toronto, Ontario M5B 1W8.
e-mail jonathan.zipursky@mail.utoronto.ca

TABLE 1
Demographics of physician survey respondents (n=135)

Characteristic	
Sex	
Female	48 (37)
Male	82 (63)
Missing data	5 (4)
Age, years	
20–29	12 (9)
30–39	52 (40)
40–49	37 (28)
50–65	22 (17)
>65	8 (6)
Missing data	4 (3)
Level of training	
Currently in residency	20 (15)
Finished residency and did not enter fellowship	24 (18)
Finished residency and in a fellowship	10 (8)
Finished fellowship	77 (59)
Missing data	4 (3)
Type of specialty (either planning or currently practicing)	
Infectious diseases	45 (33)
General internal medicine	43 (32)
Gastroenterology	25 (19)
Other	18 (13)
Missing data	4 (3)
Practice setting	
Urban academic hospital	45 (34)
Urban community hospital	12 (9)
Urban private or group practice	7 (5)
Suburban academic hospital	2 (2)
Suburban community hospital	4 (3)
Suburban private or group practice	3 (2)
Rural academic hospital	52 (40)
Rural community hospital	2 (2)
Rural private or group practice	3 (2)
Government	1 (1)
Missing data	4 (3)

Data presented as n (%)

the procedure based on its unappealing nature (4,10,11,14,17,18). However, we recently published data suggesting that while patients find many aspects of FMT unappealing, these concerns do not interfere with their willingness to accept it in the setting of recurrent CDI (19). In fact, we found that up to 94% of patients would be willing to accept FMT as a treatment if it were recommended by their physician (19). These findings suggest that there are other significant barriers to FMT adoption. In the present study, we attempted to characterize these barriers by surveying physicians regarding their experiences with and attitudes toward the use of FMT for recurrent CDI.

METHODS

Survey development and validation
An electronic survey was developed using the online program Zoomerang. The survey was intended for physicians only and was distributed electronically between May 2011 and February 2012. It was comprised of five sections: physician experience with CDI; physician treatment patterns for CDI; physician experience with FMT; physician perceptions and attitudes toward FMT; and demographic data. A focus group including gastroenterologists in the Department of Gastroenterology at Dartmouth-Hitchcock Medical Center (DHMC, New Hampshire, USA) reviewed the survey for content and comprehension before distribution.

Physicians were first asked about their experience treating CDI and the volume of patients they currently treat for CDI. They were asked to describe their clinical experience treating both primary and recurrent CDI, and the treatment modalities they most commonly recommend for an initial episode, and for a first, second or third or greater recurrence.

Physicians were then asked about their knowledge of the published literature regarding FMT and their experience with FMT. Physicians were asked a series of questions about reasons for performing or recommending, or not performing or recommending FMT, and methods of performing FMT, if they have performed it.

After reading a summary of published data regarding the epidemiology and clinical outcomes of CDI and the efficacy of various treatment modalities compiled from Centers for Disease Control and Prevention (Georgia, USA) publications (20) and UpToDate (21), physicians rated the degree to which this information was consistent with their previous beliefs. They answered questions about what conditions would need to be met for them to offer FMT as a therapy both for nonfulminant and fulminant recurrent CDI. They then were asked to rate aspects of the FMT procedure on a five-point Likert scale, in which 1 represented "I don't find this unappealing at all"; 3 represented "Very unappealing, but not necessarily prohibitive"; and 5 represented "Definitely unappealing to the point of being prohibitive." Finally, using the same scale, physicians rated the degree to which they believed patients and donors would find aspects of the FMT procedure unappealing.

Study participants and recruitment
Participants were comprised of a convenience sample of primary care and subspecialty physicians, including those practicing internal medicine, family medicine, infectious diseases and gastroenterology. Surveys were distributed electronically to these physicians at DHMC and Baylor College of Medicine (Texas, USA). Physicians were also recruited through a posting by one of the authors (KBK) on the Emerging Infectious Diseases Network. Participation was voluntary, anonymous and uncompensated. All participants were provided with a general description of the survey before agreeing to participate. To help limit selection bias, the description did not reference FMT.

Ethical issues
The study protocol was reviewed and exempted by the Dartmouth College Committee for Protection of Human Subjects.

Analysis
Simple and stratified analyses of the data were performed using SPSS version 20 (IBM Corporation, USA). In some cases, Likert scales were collapsed into two categories for analysis: 'unappealing enough to interfere with acceptability' (scores 4 and 5) versus 'not unappealing enough to interfere with acceptability' (scores 1 to 3). The McNemar test was used to compare paired proportions and the χ^2 test was used to compare the relationship between categorical variables; $P<0.05$ was considered to be statistically significant.

RESULTS

A total of 139 surveys were sent and 135 were completed, yielding a response rate of 97%. Of the respondents reporting demographic information, 82 (63%) were male, 52 (40%) were between 30 and 39 years of age, and 77 (59%) had completed a clinical fellowship (Table 1). Of physicians providing medical specialty information (n=131), 43 (33%) were general internal medicine physicians, 45 (35%) were infectious disease specialists and 25 (19%) were gastroenterologists. Twenty (15%) respondents were completing residency training.

Among the participants, 100% had treated a patient with primary CDI and a first recurrence, 95% had treated a second recurrence of CDI and 77% had treated a third or greater recurrence. There were 127 (95%) physicians who were generally aware of FMT as a treatment modality, 71 (56%) indicated they were moderately informed about the FMT literature and 31 (24%) indicated they were very informed about FMT.

TABLE 2
Physician experience with *Clostridium difficile* infection (CDI)

Recommended treatment for CDI	Initial episode (n=135)	Recurrence		
		First (n=135)	Second (n=129)	Third (n=105)
PO metronidazole	116 (86)	76 (56)	6 (5)	3 (3)
PO vancomycin	28 (21)	77 (57)	85 (66)	34 (32)
IV metronidazole	13 (10)	6 (4)	9 (7)	7 (7)
Pulsed and tapered PO vancomycin	1 (1)	7 (5)	55 (43)	70 (67)
Probiotics	27 (20)	37 (27)	40 (31)	34 (32)
Rifaximin	0 (0)	0 (0)	11 (9)	23 (22)
Cholestyramine	0 (0)	1 (1)	1 (1)	8 (8)
IV immunoglobulins	0 (0)	1 (1)	1 (1)	8 (8)
Fecal biotherapy	0 (0)	0 (0)	3 (2)	20 (19)
Other	10 (7)	8 (6)	3 (2)	11 (11)
Has not treated	0 (0)	0 (0)	6 (4)	30 (22)

Data presented as n (%). IV Intravenous; PO Per oral

Physician experience with recurrent CDI and FMT

For an initial or first recurrent episode of CDI, most physicians recommended a course of oral metronidazole (86%) or oral vancomycin (21%). Physicians began recommending FMT for a second or greater recurrent CDI, and 19% of physicians would consider FMT as treatment for a third or greater recurrence of CDI (Table 2). Twenty-five (20%) of the physicians in the sample had treated a patient with FMT, 10 (8%) had offered to treat with FMT but the patient declined, nine (7%) had referred a patient to receive FMT, and 83 (65%) had neither offered FMT nor referred for FMT. Physicians who had experience with FMT (performed or offered) were more likely to be male, an infectious diseases specialist, >40 years of age, fellowship trained and practicing in an urban setting (Table 3). Among the 25 physicians who had performed FMT, 88% reported that, on average, the patients they treated with FMT had none or one recurrences of CDI after FMT.

Of the 44 (33%) physicians who had performed or offered FMT, or referred for FMT, the most common indication for recommending FMT was a third or greater recurrent CDI (96% who performed FMT, 90% who offered but not performed FMT, and 100% who referred). There were 83 (65%) physicians who had neither offered FMT nor referred for FMT. The three most frequent reasons for not offering FMT or referring for FMT were: not having what they considered to be 'the right clinical situation' (33%); the belief that patients would find FMT too unappealing (24%); and institutional or logistical barriers (23%) (Table 4).

Physician beliefs about FMT

Of 127 respondents, 27 (21%) indicated that the existing evidence was sufficient for them to recommend FMT routinely for nonfulminant, recurrent CDI; 74 (58%) and 16 (12%) indicated that an RCT or formal practice guidelines would be necessary, respectively, and 10 (8%) responded 'other'. For patients experiencing fulminant recurrent CDI, 48 respondents (38%) believed that the existing evidence was sufficient for them to recommend FMT, 46 (36%) indicated the need for an RCT in this population, 24 (19%) believed that practice guidelines were necessary, eight (6%) responded 'other' and one (1%) responded that under no circumstances would they offer FMT.

After reading a summary of information about CDI and the efficacy of different treatment modalities: 16 (12%) of 135 respondents indicated that the efficacy of antibiotics for recurrent CDI was much lower than they believed and 15 (11%) that deaths from CDI were much higher than they believed. Among 135 respondents, 31 (23%) indicated that the reported efficacy of FMT was higher than they believed, 23 (17%) were surprised that there were so few published reports on FMT, and 16 (12%) believed that RCTs for FMT had already been published.

TABLE 3
Physician characteristics associated with having treated with fecal microbiota transplantation (FMT), or offered or referred patients for FMT

Physician characteristic	Treated, offered to treat or referred for treatment with FMT, n (%)	P
Sex		0.02
Female (n=46)	10 (22)	
Male (n=78)	34 (44)	
Age, years		<0.001
<40 (n=61)	12 (20)	
≥40 (n=64)	32 (50)	
Specialty		<0.001
Infectious diseases (n=45)	30 (67)	
Non-Infectious diseases (n=80)	14 (18)	
Level of training		<0.001
Has not completed fellowship (n=50)	7 (14)	
Has completed fellowship (n=75)	37 (49)	
Setting of training		<0.001
Urban (n=61)	28 (46)	
Rural (n=54)	8 (15)	

TABLE 4
Reasons given by physicians for not offering fecal microbiota transplantation (FMT)* (n=83)

Reasons for not offering FMT	Physicians reporting this reason, n (%)
Have not had the right clinical situation[†]	27 (33)
Believe that patients will find the concept too unappealing	20 (24)
Institutional barriers (eg, IRB) make it difficult	19 (23)
I (physicians) find the concept too unappealing	15 (18)
Do not know enough about it[†]	10 (12)
Do not know whom to refer to[†]	6 (7)
Have concerns about the safety of the treatment	6 (7)
Do not believe it is effective based on data	3 (4)
Do not believe that I will receive reimbursement	1 (1)
Other	10 (12)

*Respondents were allowed to choose more than one option; [†]Options added based on free-text responses. IRB Institutional review board

When asked to consider a scenario in which a group of patients with recurrent CDI were fully informed of both the recurrence rates following antibiotic therapy and the reported efficacy and safety of FMT, and then given a choice of FMT or antimicrobial therapy alone, only 10 (8%) of 131 respondents predicted that the majority of informed patients would choose FMT. Fifty-six (43%) predicted that "a fair number" of patients would choose FMT, 63 (47%) that only a small number of patients would choose FMT, one (1%) predicted that all patients would choose FMT and one (1%) predicted that no patients would choose FMT.

Physicians' rating aspects of the FMT procedure

Physicians rated all aspects of FMT as at least somewhat unappealing (mean score >2) with the most negative scores associated with administering stool by nasogastric tube (3.2 of 5.0; with 44% of physicians rating at either a 4 or 5) and collecting, blending and straining the stool specimen (3.0 of 5.0; with 29% of physicians rating at either a 4 or 5). Among respondents, the least unappealing aspect of the treatment process was administering the stool by colonoscopy (2.0 of 5) (Table 5). While large percentages of providers found various aspects of FMT to

TABLE 5
Likert rating scale* of physician responses to questions regarding their own views about aspects of fecal microbiota transplatation (FMT) and their predictions about how patients would answer the same questions

	Physician responses			Physician predictions about patients			
Aspect of FMT	FMT unappealing, but would consider (rating 1, 2 or 3)	FMT too unappealing to consider (rating 4 or 5)	Missing, n	FMT unappealing, but would consider (rating 1, 2 or 3)	FMT too unappealing to consider (rating 4 or 5)	Missing, n	P
Collecting, blending and transferring stool specimen	80 (70.8)	33 (29.2)	22	53 (45.7)	63 (54.3)	19	<0.001
Cleaning all the required preparation and delivery equipment	82 (74.5)	28 (25.5)	25	52 (44.8)	64 (55.2)	19	< 0.001
Administering (receiving) the stool via enema	89 (79.5)	23 (20.5)	23	86 (74.8)	29 (25.2)	20	0.629
Administering (receiving) the stool via colonoscopy	86 (82.7)	18 (17.3)	31	82 (76.6)	25 (23.4)	28	0.549
Administering (receiving) the stool via NG tube	63 (55.8)	50 (44.2)	22	44 (38.9)	69 (61.1)	22	0.002
The smell and appearance of the stool throughout the process	82 (72.6)	31 (27.4)	22	57 (50.4)	56 (49.6)	22	<0.001
Finding a donor				76 (66.7)	38 (33.3)	21	

Data presented as n (%) unless otherwise indicated. *1 = Not unappealing at all; 3 = Very unappealing but could deal with it; 5 = Too unappealing to deal with. McNemar test was used to compare physician responses to their predictions about patients in the category 'FMT too unappealing to consider' (4,5). P<0.05 was considered to be statistically significant. NG Nasogastric

be unappealing to the point of being potentially prohibitive (rating of 4 or 5), no single aspect was deemed prohibitively unappealing by a majority of providers.

When asked to predict how patients and donors would rate potentially unappealing aspects of FMT, physicians predicted that patients and donors would rate all aspects of FMT as at least 'very unappealing, but not necessarily prohibitive' (mean score >3). Physicians predicted that the most negative scores would be associated with receiving FMT through an nasogastric tube (3.8 of 5.0; 61% rated either a 4 or 5). Physicians predicted that the least unappealing aspect of FMT for patients/donors would be receiving FMT by colonoscopy (2.8 of 5) or enema (3.0 of 5).

Physicians believed that four aspects of the FMT process would be more unappealing for patients and donors than for providers themselves, and that, in fact, the majority of patients would find them so unappealing that they would interfere with acceptability (ie, rated as 4 or 5). Physicians predicted that 54% of patients (versus 29% of physicians; P<0.001) would find collecting, blending and transferring the stool specimen unappealing enough to interfere with acceptability. They predicted 55% of patients (versus 26% of physicians; P<0.001) would find cleaning all of the required preparation and delivery equipment this unappealing. They predicted that 61% of patients (versus 44% of physicians; P=0.002) would find administering versus receiving the stool via nasogastric tube this unappealing. Finally physicians predicted 50% of patients (versus 29% of physicians; P<0.001) would find the smell and appearance of stool throughout the process unappealing enough to interfere with acceptability.

DISCUSSION

FMT is a safe, effective and seldom-used therapy for recurrent CDI. Editorialists have speculated on likely barriers to FMT adoption by physicians, suggesting that its aesthetically unappealing nature, logistical challenges and a previous lack of efficacy data from RCTs may be among the most common (22). The present study was the first to gather information regsarding barriers directly from physicians. Our study confirms that most physicians lack experience with FMT and offers several possible explanations for the fact that this treatment is still infrequently used, despite the growing CDI epidemic.

Our survey found that while 100% of the physicians reported treating patients with recurrent CDI, only 20% have treated a patient with FMT, and most (65%) have neither offered FMT nor referred for FMT.

Among the 65% of physicians, 80% indicated the following three most frequent reasons for not doing so. The most common reason (cited by 27 [33%] of 83 physicians) was not having encountered what they considered to be an appropriate clinical situation. Of note, all physicians had treated patients with recurrent CDI (100%, 95% and 77% had treated patients with one, two, or three or more recurrences, respectively) and most considered themselves to be familiar with FMT's efficacy and safety in recurrent CDI. Interestingly, of the 27 physicians who reported that they had not encountered an appropriate clinical situation, 25 (96%) had treated a second recurrent CDI and 15 (56%) had treated a third or greater recurrent CDI. One possible explanation for this apparent contradiction may be that many physicians are not entirely clear on what may justify an appropriate patient because many also stated that they would need formal practice guidelines to offer FMT to a patient with recurrent CDI. The second most common reason (cited by 24%) was the belief that patients would find the concept of FMT too unappealing. It appears possible that this belief may have also been ingrained within physicians' conceptualization of what constitutes an appropriate patient, helping to explain their having not encountered such a patient as the most common reason for having not offered FMT or referred for FMT, as discussed above. The third most common reason (cited by 23%) was institutional or logistical barriers including the need for institutional review board approval. Notably, 18% of physicians also cited their own aversion to FMT as a reason for not offering it to patients. Also of note, only one respondent cited concern about reimbursement (Table 4).

Physicians' responses regarding the efficacy and safety of FMT were somewhat inconsistent. Although a majority of physicians indicated that more evidence or practice guidelines would be needed before they would offer FMT to patients, a very small minority cited skepticism about the evidence supporting FMT's effectiveness (4%) or safety (7%) as reasons for not offering it. Furthermore, most respondents indicated familiarity with current efficacy and safety data supporting FMT, and few were surprised by the evidence presented. The incongruence of these responses make it difficult to predict what impact the recently published RCT (16) will have on FMT adoption. It may be a necessary, but insufficient, factor in changing practice; significantly increased adoption may require that the more commonly cited reasons for not recommending FMT are also addressed.

Our findings confirm the fact that physicians, similar to patients, find aspects of FMT unappealing. Physicians and patients tend to find the same aspects (administering and receiving FMT by nasogastric tube and the need to handle the stool [19]) most unappealing, but interestingly, physicians believe patients will find all aspects of FMT more unappealing than physicians do. Using a recently published survey on patient attitudes toward FMT for comparison (19), physician respondents dramatically overestimated both the intensity of patients' aversion and the degree to which the unappealing nature of FMT would act as a deterrent to patients' willingness to consider the treatment. Less than 10% of physicians believed that the majority of patients with recurrent CDI would consider FMT if informed about FMT's current safety and efficacy data. However, the patient survey found that up to 94% of patients would consider FMT, especially if it were recommended by their physician (19). This misperception about patients' receptivity to FMT may be an important and modifiable barrier keeping physicians from recommending this treatment.

Overcoming physician aversion to certain aspects of FMT may also lead to wider use of FMT. In fact, up to 29% of physicians categorized certain aspects of FMT (particularly those that involved handling and smelling fecal material) as unappealing enough to prevent them from offering the treatment. Creating protocols for reducing the need to contact stool (23) or shifting the handling of stool away from physicians (24) may remove this barrier. Moreover, innovations in preparation of fecal material or even synthetic stool (25) may improve the aesthetics of the procedure and, thus, its acceptance.

Our survey illustrates that logistical issues, including uncertainty about the need for institutional review board approval and the lack of a universally accepted protocol – although standardized protocols do exist (23) – certainly pose additional barriers to FMT. While planning to use enforcement discretion, the recent guidance by the Food and Drug Administration urging physicians to obtain investigational new drug approval before performing FMT (26) may also add some complexity. We are hopeful and optimistic that ongoing communication and collaboration between physician organizations and the Food and Drug Administration, in tandem with additional forthcoming RCT data (27), will soon lead to a reduction in the degree to which these perceived potential logistical complexities limit FMT adoption.

Although it provides the first systematically collected data on physician attitudes toward FMT, our study was limited in size and scope and may not be generalizable to all practicing physicians. We had relatively fewer female and gastroenterologist respondents. Thus, our stratified analysis of the data according to medical specialty was underpowered. Although the survey was performed before the publication of the first RCT for FMT, a strength of the study was its similarity to the survey used for our tandem patient study (19). In addition, the timing of the survey distribution enabled us to collect physician responses before the publication of our survey of patient attitudes and beliefs (19). Therefore, the physician respondents were not biased by previous knowledge of the patient responses.

The discordance revealed between patient attitudes and willingness to accept FMT and physicians' beliefs that patients will not accept FMT is the most important finding of the two surveys. It suggests that there is an opportunity for more dialogue between physicians and patients about the increasingly rigorous evidence supporting the use of FMT for recurrent CDI and shared decision making regarding whether the unappealing nature of the treatment is a barrier that can be overcome. Technological innovations that can reduce the need to handle stool and further efforts to systematize protocols and eliminate regulatory restrictions may significantly increase the adoption of FMT as well.

ACKNOWLEDGEMENTS: The authors thank the physicians in the Division of Gastroenterology at Dartmouth-Hitchcock Medical Center for their help in reviewing the survey and all of the physicians who voluntarily participated in the survey.

DISCLOSURES: Tivon and Misha Sidorsky have a pending patent related to the field of fecal microbiota transplantation. The other authors have no financial disclosures or conflicts of interest to declare.

FUNDING: This work was supported by a scholarship from the Infectious Disease Society of America (IDSA) 2011 Medical Scholars Program.

REFERENCES

1. Kachrimanidou M, Malisiovas N. *Clostridium difficile* infection: A comprehensive review. Crit. Rev. Microbiol 2011;37:178-87.
2. Bartlett J. Narrative Review: The new epidemic of *Clostridium difficile*-associated enteric disease. Ann Intern Med 2006;145:758-64.
3. McDonald LC, Owings M, Jernigan DB. *Clostridium difficile* infection in patients discharged from US short-stay hospitals, 1996-2003. Emerg Infect Dis 2006;12:409-15.
4. Kelly C, LaMont J. *Clostridium difficile* – more difficult than ever. N Engl J Med 2008;359:1932-40.
5. Gravel D, Miller M, Simor A, et al. Health care-associated *Clostridium difficile* infection in adults admitted to acute care hospitals in Canada: A Canadian Nosocomial Infection Surveillance Program Study. Clin Infect Dis 2009;48:568-76.
6. Pépin J, Valiquette L, Cossette B. Mortality attributable to nosocomial *Clostridium difficile*-associated disease during an epidemic caused by a hypervirulent strain in Quebec. CMAJ 2005;173:1037-42.
7. United Kingdom national statistics. Newport, United Kingdom: Office for National Statistics, UK Statistics Authority. <www.statistics.gov.uk> (Accessed September 26, 2012).
8. Pepin J, Alary M-E, Valiquette L, et al. Increasing risk of relapse after treatment of *Clostridium difficile* colitis in Quebec, Canada. Clin Infect Dis 2005;40:1591-7.
9. Cohen SH, Gerding DN, Johnson S, et al. Clinical practice guidelines for *Clostridium difficile* infection in adults: 2010 update by the Society for Healthcare Epidemiology of America (SHEA) and the Infectious Diseases Society of America (IDSA). Infect Control Hosp Epidemiol 2010;31:431-55.
10. Nood E Van, Speelman P, Kuijper E, et al. Struggling with recurrent *Clostridium difficile* infections: Is donor faeces the solution? Euro Surveill 2009;359:1-6.
11. Bakken JS. Fecal bacteriotherapy for recurrent *Clostridium difficile* infection. Anaerobe 2009;15:285-9.
12. Huebner ES, Surawicz CM. Treatment of recurrent *Clostridium difficile* diarrhea. Gastroenterol Hepatol 2006;2:203-8.
13. Pépin J, Routhier S, Gagnon S, et al. Management and outcomes of a first recurrence of *Clostridium difficile*-associated disease in Quebec, Canada. Clin Infect Dis 2006;42:758-64.
14. Borody TJ, Warren EF, Leis SM, et al. Bacteriotherapy using fecal flora: Toying with human motions. J Clin Gastroenterol 2004;38:475-83.
15. Gough E, Shaikh H, Manges AR. Systematic review of intestinal microbiota transplantation (fecal bacteriotherapy) for recurrent *Clostridium difficile* infection. Clin Infect Dis 2011;53:994-1002.
16. van Nood E, Vrieze A, Nieuwdorp M, et al. Duodenal infusion of donor feces for recurrent *Clostridium difficile*. N Engl J Med 2013;368:407-15.
17. Kahn SA, Gorawara-Bhat R, Rubin DT. Fecal bacteriotherapy for ulcerative colitis: Patients are ready, are we? Inflamm Bowel Dis 2012;18:676-84.
18. Borody TJ, Campbell J. Fecal microbiota transplantation: Current status and future directions. Expert Rev Gastroenterol Hepatol 2011;5:653-5.
19. Zipursky JS, Sidorsky TI, Freedman CA, et al. Patient attitudes toward the use of fecal microbiota transplantation in the treatment of recurrent *Clostridium difficile* infection. Clin Infect Dis 2012;55:1-7.
20. *Clostridium difficile* Infection. Centers Dis Control Prev Heal Infect <www.cdc.gov/hai/organisms/cdiff/cdiff_infect.html> (Accessed September 26, 2012).
21. Kelly CP, LaMont J. *Clostridium difficile* in adults: Treatment. UpToDate. <www.uptodate.com> (Accessed September 26, 2012).

22. Kelly CP. Fecal microbiota transplantation – an old therapy comes of age. N Engl J Med 2013;368:4745.
23. Bakken JS, Borody T, Brandt LJ, et al. Treating *Clostridium difficile* infection with fecal microbiota transplantation. Clin Gastroenterol Hepatol 2011;9:1044-9.
24. Silverman MS, Davis I, Pillai DR. Success of self-administered home fecal transplantation for chronic *Clostridium difficile* infection. Clin Gastroenterol Hepatol 2010;8:471-3.
25. Petrof EO, Gloor GB, Vanner SJ, et al. Stool substitute transplant therapy for the eradication of *Clostridium difficile* infection: "RePOOPulating" the gut. Microbiome 2013;1:3.
26. Guidance for Industry: Enforcement Policy Regarding Investigational New Drug Requirements for Use of Fecal Microbiota for Transplantation to Treat *Clostridium difficile* Infection Not Responsive to Standard Therapies. 2013. <GuidanceComplianceRegulatoryInformation/Guidances/Vaccines/ucm361379.htm> (Accessed June 26, 2013).
27. Kelly CR, Brandt LJ. Fecal Transplant for Relapsing C. *Difficile* Infection. ClinicalTrials.gov. <www.clinicaltrials.gov/ct2/show/NCT 01703494?term=fecal+transplant+brandt&rank=1> (Accessed June 26, 2013).

37

Safety and efficacy of Hemospray® in upper gastrointestinal bleeding

Alan Hoi Lun Yau MD[1], George Ou MD[1], Cherry Galorport MD[2], Jack Amar MD FRCPC[2], Brian Bressler MD MS FRCPC[2],

Fergal Donnellan MD FRCPC[2], Hin Hin Ko MD FRCPC[2], Eric Lam MD FRCPC[2], Robert Allan Enns MD FRCPC[2]

AHL Yau, G Ou, C Galorport, et al. Safety and efficacy of Hemospray® in upper gastrointestinal bleeding. Can J Gastroenterol Hepatol 2014;28(2):72-76.

BACKGROUND: Hemospray (Cook Medical, USA) has recently been approved in Canada for the management of nonvariceal upper gastrointestinal bleeding (UGIB).
OBJECTIVE: To review the authors' experience with the safety and efficacy of Hemospray for treating UGIB.
METHODS: A retrospective chart review was performed on patients who required endoscopic evaluation for suspected UGIB and were treated with Hemospray.
RESULTS: From February 2012 to July 2013, 19 patients (mean age 67.6 years) with UGIB were treated with Hemospray. A bleeding lesion was identified in the esophagus in one (5.3%) patient, the stomach in five (26.3%) and duodenum in 13 (68.4%). Bleeding was secondary to peptic ulcers in 12 (63.2%) patients, Dieulafoy lesions in two (10.5%), mucosal erosion in one (5.3%), angiodysplastic lesions in one (5.3%), ampullectomy in one (5.3%), polypectomy in one (5.3%) and an unidentified lesion in one (5.3%). The lesions showed spurting hemorrhage in four (21.1%) patients, oozing hemorrhage in 11 (57.9%) and no active bleeding in four (21.1%). Hemospray was administered as monotherapy in two (10.5%) patients, first-line modality in one (5.3%) and rescue modality in 16 (84.2%). Hemospray was applied prophylactically to nonbleeding lesions in four (21.1%) patients and therapeutically to bleeding lesions in 15 (78.9%). Acute hemostasis was achieved in 14 of 15 (93.3%) patients. Rebleeding within seven days occurred in seven of 18 (38.9%) patients. Potential adverse events occurred in two (10.5%) patients and included visceral perforation and splenic infarct. Mortality occurred in five (26.3%) patients but the cause of death was unrelated to gastrointestinal bleeding with the exception of one patient who developed hemoperitoneum.
CONCLUSIONS: The high rates of both acute hemostasis and recurrent bleeding suggest that Hemospray may be used in high-risk cases as a temporary measure or a bridge toward more definitive therapy.

Key Words: Efficacy; Hemospray; Safety; Upper gastrointestinal bleeding

La sécurité et l'efficacité de la poudre Hemospray[MC] **en cas de saignements œsogastroduodénaux**

HISTORIQUE : La poudre Hemospray (Cook Medical, États-Unis) a récemment été approuvée au Canada pour la prise en charge des saignements œsogastroduodénaux (SOGD) non variqueux.
OBJECTIFS : Examiner l'expérience des auteurs à l'égard de la sécurité et de l'efficacité de la poudre Hemospray pour traiter les SOGD.
MÉTHODOLOGIE : Les chercheurs ont effectué une analyse rétrospective des dossiers des patients qui avaient besoin d'une évaluation endoscopique en raison d'une présomption de SOGD et qui ont été traités à l'aide de poudre Hemospray.
RÉSULTATS : De février 2012 à juillet 2013, 19 patients (d'un âge moyen de 67,6 ans) ayant des SOGD ont été traités à l'aide de poudre Hemospray. Une lésion hémorragique a été décelée dans l'œsophage d'un patient (5,3 %), l'estomac de cinq patients (26,3 %) et le duodénum de 13 patients (68,4 %). Les saignements étaient secondaires à un ulcère gastroduodénal chez 12 patients (63,2 %) et à des ulcères de Dieulafoy chez deux patients (10,5 %). Chez cinq patients (5,3 % chacun), les saignements étaient respectivement causés pas une érosion muqueuse, une angiodysplasie, une ampullectomie, une polypectomie et une lésion non identifiée. Les lésions ont révélé une hémorragie pulsatile chez quatre patients (21,1 %), une hémorragie suintante chez 11 patients (57,9 %) et aucun saignement actif chez quatre patients (21,1 %). La poudre Hemospray a été administrée en monothérapie à deux patients (10,5 %), en première ligne à un patient (5,3 %) et en traitement de sauvetage à 16 patients (84,2 %). Elle a été appliquée en prophylaxie aux lésions non hémorragiques de quatre patients (21,1 %) et en traitement des lésions hémorragiques de 15 patients (78,9 %). Quatorze des 15 patients (93,3 %) sont parvenus à une hémostase aiguë. Sept des 18 patients (38,9 %) ont saigné de nouveau dans les sept jours. Deux patients (10,5 %) ont souffert d'effets indésirables potentiels, soit une perforation viscérale et un infarctus splénique. Cinq patients (26,3 %) sont décédés, mais la cause du décès n'était pas liée au saignement gastro-intestinal, à l'exception d'un patient qui a subi un hémopéritoine.
CONCLUSIONS : D'après les taux élevés d'hémostase aiguë et de saignements récurrents, dans les cas à haut risque, la poudre Hemospray peut être utilisée temporairement ou en attendant un traitement plus définitif.

Hemospray (TC-325) (Cook Medical, USA), a novel proprietary inorganic powder, has recently been approved in Canada for the management of nonvariceal upper gastrointestinal bleeding (UGIB) (1). It achieves hemostasis by adhering to the bleeding site, which leads to mechanical tamponade and, by concentrating and activating platelets and coagulation factors, promotes thrombus formation (2). Preliminary results on safety and efficacy appear to be promising for various types of gastrointestinal bleeding including those secondary to peptic ulcers (3-6), gastric varices (6-8), esophageal tear (5), gastric antral vascular ectasia (4), duodenal diverticula (6), colonic ulcer (9), radiation proctitis (10), Dieulafoy lesions (4,6,10), malignancy (4,6,11,12), sphincterotomy (5,12,13), ampullectomy (6,12), polypectomy (4,5,10) and endoscopic mucosal resection (4,12).

Endoscopic hemostasis has been widely accepted as first-line treatment for nonvariceal UGIB (3,14). Combined endoscopic therapy using injection, thermal and mechanical modalities is highly effective, with initial hemostasis achieved in 85% to 95% of cases (14,15); however, recurrent bleeding still occurs in 5% to 10% of cases (16). In addition, conventional endoscopic therapies may not be feasible in patients with active multifocal bleeding sites, particularly those with challenging anatomy and coagulopathy, in which contact coagulation efforts may be hampered by further tissue damage and induction of more bleeding (3). In contrast, Hemospray can quickly cover large areas and does not require en face view or direct contact with the bleeding lesion (10). However, the optimal indications and technical limitations of Hemospray are still being characterized (5). The present study provides additional experience with regard to the safety and efficacy of Hemospray in patients presenting with UGIB in a real-life setting outside of the clinical trial experience.

[1]Department of Medicine; [2]Division of Gastroenterology, University of British Columbia, Vancouver, British Columbia
Correspondence: Dr Robert Allan Enns, Division of Gastroenterology, St Paul's Hospital, 770-1190 Hornby Street, Vancouver, British Columbia V6Z 2K5. e-mail renns@interchange.ubc.ca

TABLE 1
Patient characteristics

Patient	Age, years	Sex	Hematemesis	Melena	Pre-syncope	Syncope	SBP	HR	Hgb, g/L (nadir)	PLT	INR	Antiplatelet	Anticoagulant
1	55	M	–	Yes	Yes	–	84	95	79	232	1.1	ASA (160 mg PO × 1)	–
2	74	M	–	Yes	Yes	–	55	122	42	168	1.5	ASA (325 mg PO × 1) Clopidogrel (600 mg PO × 1)	Heparin (therapeutic)
3	49	M	Yes	Yes	Yes	–	115	93	101	183	1.0	Ibuprofen (PO as needed)	–
4	61	M	–	Yes	–	–	98	86	90	180	1.0	ASA (81 mg PO daily) Clopidogrel (75 mg PO daily)	Heparin (therapeutic)
5	67	F	Yes	Yes	Yes	–	119	121	53	135	1.1	Diclofenac (50 mg PR twice per day)	–
6	88	F	–	Yes	–	–	82	135	70	86	2.0	ASA (81 mg PO daily)	Heparin (prophylactic) Warfarin (3 mg PO × 1)
7	71	M	–	Yes	–	–	132	129	72	362	1.9	–	Heparin (therapeutic) Warfarin (2.5 mg PO daily)
8	90	M	–	Yes	Yes	–	75	94	54	175	1.2	ASA (325 mg PO daily)	–
9	29	M	Yes	Yes	–	–	115	97	68	241	1.2	–	–
10	54	M	Yes	–	Yes	–	139	125	76	55	2.0	Ibuprofen (PO as needed)	Heparin (prophylactic)
11	94	F	Yes	Yes	–	–	101	82	85	210	1.2	ASA (81 mg PO daily) Clopidogrel (75 mg PO daily)	Heparin (prophylactic)
12	88	M	–	Yes	Yes	Yes	69	100	64	100	1.2	ASA (325 mg PO daily)	–
13	56	F	Yes	Yes	–	–	76	>100	64	43	2.4	–	Heparin (prophylactic)
14	40	M	–	Yes	–	–	80	113	74	384	1.5	ASA (81 mg PO daily)	Heparin (prophylactic)
15	72	M	–	Yes	–	–	98	110	71	17	1.2	–	–
16	86	M	–	Yes	–	–	142	68	107	144	1.1	–	–
17	72	M	–	Yes	–	–	78	120	87	122	–	–	–
18	53	F	Yes	Yes	–	–	60	98	41	118	1.8	–	Heparin (prophylactic)
19	85	M	Yes	–	Yes	–	112	86	76	206	1.0	–	Heparin (prophylactic)

ASA Acetylsalicylic acid; F Female; Hgb Hemoglobin (normal range 135 g/L to 170 g/L); HR Heart rate (beats/min); INR International normalized ratio (normal range 0.9 to 1.2); M Male; PLT Platelet count (normal 150×10^9/L to 440 ×10^9/L); PO Per oral; PR Per rectum; SBP Systolic blood pressure

METHODS

From February 2012 to July 2013, 19 patients who required endoscopic evaluation for suspected UGIB were treated with Hemospray. A retrospective chart review was performed collecting demographic data (age and sex); clinical data (symptoms, vital signs, medical history and medications); diagnostic data (complete blood count, renal function, coagulation study and endoscopic findings); and therapeutic data (resuscitative measures, hemostatic interventions and hemostatic outcomes). All patients provided written informed consent for study participation. The study was approved by the institutional review board.

Patients were resuscitated as needed to achieve hemodynamic stability before undergoing endoscopy. Hemospray was used as monotherapy (Hemospray only); first-line modality (Hemospray followed by conventional endoscopic therapy) or rescue modality (conventional endoscopic therapy followed by Hemospray) at the discretion of the endoscopist. Hemospray was delivered through a 10 Fr catheter that was inserted into the working channel of a therapeutic endoscope (Olympus, Japan). The bleeding site was observed for 5 min under endoscopy and, if recurrent bleeding occurred, Hemospray was reapplied as needed to a maximum of 20 g (one canister). Endoscopy was repeated and Hemospray was reapplied as needed in patients with clinical or laboratory evidence of recurrent bleeding.

The primary end point was acute hemostasis (defined as endoscopic observation of bleeding cessation for >5 min). The secondary end points were: recurrent bleeding at seven and 30 days (defined as clinical presentation of hematemesis or melena; hemoglobin level decrease >20 g/L within 48 h or direct visualization of active bleeding at the previously treated lesion at repeat endoscopy); mortality at seven and 30 days (related to gastrointestinal bleeding); and adverse events in hospital (related to Hemospray use). Hemospray failure was defined as the inability to achieve acute hemostasis after application

of 20 g of Hemospray or recurrent bleeding despite application of Hemospray on two separate occasions.

RESULTS

Patient characteristics (Table 1)

A total of 19 patients (mean age 67.6 years; range 29 to 94 years; five [26.3%] women) with UGIB were treated with Hemospray during the study period (February 2012 to July 2013).

Clinical presentation included hematemesis in eight (42.1%) patients, melena in 17 (89.5%), presyncope in eight (42.1%) and syncope in one (5.3%). Physical examination revealed hypotension (systolic blood pressure <90 mmHg) in nine (47.4%) patients and tachycardia (heart rate >100 beats/min) in 10 (52.6%). Laboratory investigations showed a mean hemoglobin nadir of 72.3 g/L (normal 135 g/L to 170 g/L), thrombocytopenia (platelets <150×10^9/L) in nine (47.4%) patients and coagulopathy (international normalized ratio >1.2) in seven (38.9%).

Medication review found the use of antiplatelet agents in 11 (57.9%) patients and anticoagulants in 10 (52.6%). Acetylsalicylic acid, clopidogrel and heparin (therapeutic dose) were administered to one patient who presented with unstable angina before cardiac catheterization (patient 4) and another who was admitted for transfemoral closure of severe mitral prosthetic paravalvular leak (patient 2). Warfarin and heparin (therapeutic dose) were given to one patient who had developed bilateral deep vein thrombosis in the lower extremities (patient 7).

Endoscopic findings (Table 2)

A bleeding lesion was identified in the esophagus in one (5.3%) patient, the stomach in five (26.3%) and duodenum in 13 (68.4%). Bleeding originated from peptic ulcers in 12 (63.2%) patients, Dieulafoy lesions in two (10.5%), mucosal erosion in one (5.3%), angiodysplastic lesions in one (5.3%), ampullectomy site in one (5.3%), polypectomy site in one (5.3%) and an unidentified lesion in

TABLE 2
Endoscopic findings

Patient	Location	Lesion	Stigmata
1	Gastric (prepylorus)	Ulcer	Oozing, clot
2	Gastric (cardia, fundus)	No discrete lesions	Adherent clots
3	Gastric (incisura)	Ulcers × 3 (5 mm)	Oozing
4	Gastric (fundus)	Angiodysplastic lesions × few	Oozing
5	Duodenal (D1/D2)	Ulcer	Multiple red spots, clean base
6	Duodenal (D2)	Ulcers × several	Spurting, visible vessel
7	Duodenal (D1/D2)	Ulcer (2 cm)	Oozing, large clot
8	Duodenal (D1/D2)	Dieulafoy lesion	Oozing
9	Duodenal (D1/D2)	Ulcer	Oozing, visible vessel
10	Esophageal (mid, 34 cm to 36 cm)	Ulcer with distal varices (3 cm)	Oozing, surrounding clot
11	Gastric (lesser curvature)	Dieulafoy lesions × 2	Oozing, clot
12	Duodenal (bulb)	Ulcer (hemicircumferential)	Spurting, visible vessel, adherent clots
13	Duodenal (D1/D2)	Ulcers × 2 (1.5 cm)	Spurting, visible vessel
14	Duodenal (D2)	Ulcers × 3 (hemicircumferential)	Adherent clots
15	Duodenal (D1/D2)	Erosion (linear)	Oozing
16	Duodenal (D1/D2)	Polypectomy site (3 cm, sessile)	Bleeding artery
17	Duodenal (major papilla)	Ulcer at ampullectomy site	Oozing, visible vessels × 4
18	Duodenal (D1/D2)	Ulcers × multiple (7 mm to 8 mm)	Spurting, visible vessel
19	Duodenal (bulb)	Ulcer	No active bleeding

D1 First part of the duodenum; D2 Second part of the duodenum

TABLE 3
Hemostatic interventions

Patient	Hemospray*	Injection (volume)	Thermal	Mechanical (frequency)	Transarterial embolization	Surgical oversewing
1	Rescue modality	Epinephrine (8 mL)	–	Clips (× 3)	–	–
2	Monotherapy	–	–	–	–	–
3	Monotherapy	–	–	–	–	–
4	Rescue modality	Epinephrine (4 mL)	–	–	–	–
5	Rescue modality	Epinephrine (8 mL)	BICAP cautery	Clips (× 2)	Yes	–
6	Rescue modality	Epinephrine (16 + 9 mL)	Cautery	Clips (× 5)	–	–
7	Rescue modality	Epinephrine (12 mL)	–	–	–	–
8	Rescue modality	Epinephrine (15 mL × 2)	Gold probe	–	–	–
9	Rescue modality	Epinephrine (6 mL)	BICAP cautery	–	–	–
10	Rescue modality	Epinephrine (2 + 6 mL) Tromboject sclerosant (2.5 mL)	–	Bands (× 5)	–	–
11	Rescue modality	Epinephrine (4 mL)	–	Clips (× 4)	–	–
12	Rescue modality	–	–	Clips (× 2)	Yes	–
13	Rescue modality	Epinephrine (8 mL)	Gold probe	Clips (× 6)	–	–
14	Rescue modality	Epinephrine x 2	BICAP cautery	Clips (× 3)	–	Yes
15	Rescue modality	Epinephrine (3 mL)	–	–	–	–
16	Rescue modality	Epinephrine (3 mL)	Hot biopsy forceps	Clips (× 2)	–	–
17	First modality	Epinephrine (4.5 mL)	Hot cautery forceps	–	–	–
18	Rescue modality	Epinephrine (10 mL)	BICAP cautery	–	–	–
19	Rescue modality	Epinephrine (3 mL)	Cautery	–	–	–

*BICAP Bipolar electrocoagulation; First modality (Hemospray [*Cook Medical, USA] followed by conventional endoscopic therapy); Monotherapy (Hemospray only); Rescue modality (Conventional endoscopic therapy followed by Hemospray)*

one (5.3%). The lesions demonstrated spurting hemorrhage in four patients (21.1%), oozing hemorrhage in 11 (57.9%) and no active bleeding in four (21.1%). Importantly, all four patients with spurting hemorrhage were found to have hemodynamic instability, thrombocytopenia and coagulopathy.

Hemostatic interventions (Table 3)
Hemospray was administered as monotherapy in two (10.5%) patients, first modality in one (5.3%) and rescue modality in 16 (84.2%). Other hemostatic modalities were injection methods in 16 (84.2%) patients, thermal methods in 10 (52.6%), mechanical methods in nine (47.4%), transarterial embolization in two (10.5%) and surgical oversewing in one (5.3%). Interestingly, in the latter three patients who ultimately required aggressive hemostatic interventions, all had received antiplatelets and demonstrated hemodynamic instability, but only one was found to have spurting hemorrhage on endoscopy.

Hemostatic outcomes (Table 4)
Hemospray was applied prophylactically to nonbleeding lesions in four (21.1%) patients and therapeutically to bleeding lesions in 15 (78.9%). Among patients with bleeding lesions, acute hemostasis was achieved in 14 of 15 (93.3%). The one patient who did not achieve acute hemostasis essentially had Hemospray failure and, ultimately, required transarterial embolization for spurting hemorrhage. Recurrent bleeding was found in seven of 18 (38.9%) patients and all developed within seven days of Hemospray application to lesions with spurting hemorrhage in two, oozing hemorrhage in three and no active bleeding in two. One of these patients required transarterial embolization and another required surgical oversewing. Repeat endoscopy was performed in seven (38.9%) patients and all occurred within seven days with the exception of one patient who received it at seven weeks. Four of these patients were found to have active bleeding of the previously treated lesion at repeat endoscopy, and Hemospray was reapplied to the one patient who only had minor oozing with acute hemostasis once again achieved.

Adverse events (Table 4)
Adverse events potentially related to Hemospray use were identified in two (10.5%) patients. One patient developed acute abdominal distension

TABLE 4
Hemostatic outcomes

Patient	Acute hemostasis	Recurrent bleeding	Repeat endoscopy	Repeat Hemospray	Hemospray failure	Adverse event	Mortality
1	Yes	No	No	N/A	No	–	–
2	N/A*	No	No	N/A	No	? Visceral perforation (day 0)	Hemoperitoneum, hypovolemic shock (day 0)
3	Yes	Yes (day 3)	Yes (day 4)	No	No	–	–
4	Yes	No	No	N/A	No	–	–
5	N/A*	Yes (day 2)	No	N/A	No	–	–
6	Yes	Yes (day 5)	Yes (day 6)†	No	No	–	Hospital-acquired pneumonia (day 13)
7	Yes	No	Yes (day 3)	No	No	–	–
8	Yes	Yes (day 1)	Yes (day 3)†	No	No	–	–
9	Yes	No	Yes (day 48)	No	No	–	–
10	Yes	No	Yes (day 3)‡	Yes	No	–	–
11	Yes	No	No	N/A	No	–	–
12	No	N/A	No	N/A	Yes	–	AV fistula blockage, hemodialysis withdrawal (day 21)
13	Yes	Yes (day 4)	No	N/A	No	–	Acute renal failure, newly diagnosed cryptogenic cirrhosis (day 12)
14	N/A*	Yes (day 7)	No	N/A	No	–	MSSA bacteremia, ventilator-acquired pneumonia (day 74)
15	Yes	No	No	N/A	No	–	–
16	Yes	No	No	N/A	No	–	–
17	Yes	Yes (day 1)	Yes (day 2)†	No	No	–	–
18	Yes	No	No	N/A	No	? Splenic infarct (day 29)	–
19	N/A*	No	No	N/A	No	–	–

*Hemospray (Cook Medical, USA) was applied prophylactically to nonbleeding lesions; †Active bleeding of the previously treated lesion; ‡Minor oozing of the previously treated lesion. AV Arteriovenous; MSSA Methicillin-sensitive Staphylococcus aureus; N/A Not applicable

with hemoperitoneum on diagnostic paracentesis in the hours following Hemospray application; however, a coroner's autopsy was not performed to determine whether visceral perforation had occurred. This patient was admitted with severe mitral prosthetic paravalvular leak requiring percutaneous transfemoral closure. He had a history of hypertension, coronary artery disease, atrial fibrillation, congestive heart failure and chronic kidney disease. Another patient developed radiological evidence of new-onset splenic infarct on abdominal computed tomography scan after Hemospray use. This patient was admitted for a compound fracture of the left proximal tibia requiring open reduction and internal fixation. She had a history of hepatic steatosis, cholelithiasis, end-stage renal disease, gout and osteoporosis.

Mortality (Table 4)

Mortality occurred in five (26.3%) patients; however, with the exception of the patient who had developed hemoperitoneum and hypovolemic shock on day 0, the cause of death in the other four patients was not directly related to gastrointestinal bleeding. These included hospital-acquired pneumonia on day 13; hemodialysis withdrawal secondary to arteriovenous fistula blockage on day 21; acute renal failure and newly diagnosed cryptogenic cirrhosis on day 12; and methicillin-susceptible bacteremia and ventilator-acquired pneumonia on day 74.

DISCUSSION

Our study examined the use of Hemospray in UGIB (n=19), which originated from peptic ulcers in 63.2% of patients. Hemospray was frequently administered as a rescue modality (84.2%), with an overall rate of acute hemostasis in 93.3% and rebleeding in 38.9% of patients. In the largest four case series performed by Sung et al (3 [n=20]), Smith et al (4 [n=82]), Holster et al (6 [n=16]) and Leblanc et al (12 [n=17]), Hemospray was used as monotherapy in 50% to 95%, first modality in 0% to 19% and rescue modality in 0% to 33% of patients, with an overall rate of acute hemostasis in 81% to 100%, and recurrent bleeding in 11% to 31%. The higher rates of recurrent bleeding and Hemospray use

as a rescue modality in our study could be due to selection bias in the tertiary care setting, with frequent encounters of thrombocytopenia (47.4%), coagulopathy (38.9%), antiplatelet use (57.9%), anticoagulant use (52.6%) and spurting hemorrhage (21.1%).

Our finding that spurting hemorrhage was present in the one patient in whom acute hemostasis was not achieved with Hemospray is consistent with the experience of Sung et al (3) and Holster et al (6); however, Leblanc et al (12) reported effective control of pulsatile bleeding with Hemospray. Recurrent bleeding may be expected to occur because the hemostatic powder does not directly induce healing of the underlying lesion and is sloughed off from the mucosal wall within two to three days, leaving behind a clean remnant (10,11). The high rates of both acute hemostasis and recurrent bleeding suggest that Hemospray is probably best used as a bridge toward more definitive therapy such as transjugular intrahepatic portosystemic shunt in variceal bleeding (8) and radiation therapy in malignancy-related bleeding (11).

One patient in our study developed hemoperitoneum on day 0 and another developed splenic infarct on day 29, although it remained unclear whether these were directly related to Hemospray use. Perforation appears unlikely because the pressure of carbon dioxide is only 12 mmHg when the catheter is placed at 1 cm to 2 cm from the target lesion (10). Embolization also appears unlikely based on the safety study performed in a porcine model by Giday et al (17) using a sevenfold greater dose of Hemospray than that used in most clinical cases; the authors found no histological evidence of powder embolization in systemic tissues including the spleen. In addition, case reports and series in humans have not reported the theoretical risks of Hemospray including thromboembolism, bowel perforation, bowel obstruction, coagulopathy, allergic reaction and powder inhalation (3-13). Transient biliary obstruction has been reported after Hemospray use in postsphincterotomy bleeding (13). However, this did not occur in our patient, who received Hemospray for bleeding from an ampullectomy site because a biliary stent had been previously inserted. Despite its apparent safety from limited data in short-term studies, Hemospray is contraindicated in variceal bleeding with low venous pressure and numerous collateral shunts due to the risk of thromboembolism (7), and in diverticular bleeding with thin mucosal wall and narrowed bowel lumen due to the risk of perforation and obstruction (10).

Conventional endoscopic therapies have been shown to be effective in decreasing the rates of recurrent bleeding, blood transfusion and surgical intervention in UGIB, but the mortality rate has remained at 7% to 10% in the past 30 years (18). It is, therefore, necessary to explore alternative methods of endoscopic hemostasis. Hemospray is a welcome addition to our current armamentarium given its many advantages. First, the ease of application without the need for advanced technical skills is desirable in emergency situations in which expert endoscopists are unavailable (12). Second, accurate localization and precise targeting are not necessary, making it useful in challenging anatomy compounded by endoscope angulation (10). Third, direct mucosal contact does not occur, reducing the risk of further tissue damage that could worsen bleeding and even result in perforation (11,12). Fourth, its ability to cover large areas with multiple bleeding points makes it a suitable choice for hemorrhagic gastritis, gastric antral vascular ectasia, radiation-induced mucosal injury and malignancy-related bleeding (3). Finally,

Hemospray can be used prophylactically or therapeutically and either alone or in combination with conventional endoscopic therapies depending on the risk of recurrent bleeding (19), with efficacy demonstrated in benign and malignant bleeding from the upper and lower gastrointestinal tract (3-13).

Limitations of our study included the small number of patients, the retrospective nature of data collection and the lack of documented information on the exact quantity of Hemospray applied. Future large-scale, prospective, randomized controlled trials should directly compare the relative efficacy of Hemospray with conventional endoscopic therapies, determine the exact duration of its hemostatic effect, establish its long-term safety in follow-up studies and characterize its optimal indications in mainstream endoscopy.

CONCLUSION

Hemospray appears to allow safe control of acute bleeding and may be used in high-risk cases as a temporary measure or a bridge toward more definitive therapy.

DISCLOSURES: The authors have no financial disclosures or conflicts of interest to declare.

REFERENCES

1. Giday SA. Preliminary data on the nanopowder hemostatic agent TC-325 to control gastrointestinal bleeding. Gastroenterol Hepatol 2011;7:620-2.
2. Aslanian HR, Laine L. Hemostatic powder spray for GI bleeding. Gastrointest Endosc 2013;77:508-10.
3. Sung JJY, Luo D, Wu JCY, et al. Early clinical experience of the safety and effectiveness of Hemospray in achieving hemostasis in patients with acute peptic ulcer bleeding. Endoscopy 2011;43:291-5.
4. Smith LA, Stanley A, Morris J. Hemospray for non-variceal upper gastrointestinal bleeding: Results of the SEAL dataset (survey to evaluate the application of hemospray in the luminal tract). Gut 2012;62:A61-A62.
5. Moosavi S, Barkun A. Case series: utility of Hemospray in management of benign upper and lower GI bleed of various etiologies: Preliminary experience. Can J Gastroenterol 2012;26:A081. (Abst)
6. Holster IL, Kuipers EJ, Tjwa ET. Hemospray in the treatment of upper gastrointestinal hemorrhage in patients on antithrombotic therapy. Endoscopy 2013;45:63-6.
7. Holster IL, Poley JW, Kuipers EJ, et al. Controlling gastric variceal bleeding with endoscopically applied hemostatic powder (Hemospray™). J Hepatol 2012;57:1391-402.
8. Stanley AJ, Smith LA, Morris AJ. Use of hemostatic powder (Hemospray) in the management of refractory gastric variceal hemorrhage. Endoscopy 2013;45:E86-E87.
9. Granata A, Curcio G, Azzopardi N, et al. Hemostatic powder as rescue therapy in a patient with H1N1 influenza with uncontrolled colon bleeding. Gastrointest Endosc 2013;78:451.
10. Soulellis C, Carpentier S, Chen YI, et al. Lower GI hemorrhage controlled with endoscopically applied TC-325 (with video). Gastrointest Endosc 2013;77:504-7.
11. Chen YI, Barkun AN, Soulellis C, et al. Use of the endoscopically applied hemostatic powder TC-325 in cancer-related upper GI hemorrhage: Preliminary experience (with video). Gastrointest Endosc 2012;75:1278-81.
12. Leblanc S, Vienne A, Dhooge M, et al. Early experience with a novel hemostatic powder used to treat upper GI bleeding related to malignancies or after therapeutic interventions (with videos). Gastrointest Endosc 2013;78:169-75.
13. Moosavi S, Chen YI, Barkun AN. TC-325 application leading to transient obstruction of a post-sphincterotomy biliary orifice. Endoscopy 2013;45:E130.
14. Barkun AN, Bardou M, Kuipers EJ, et al. International consensus recommendations on the management of patients with nonvariceal upper gastrointestinal bleeding. Ann Intern Med 2010;152:101-13.
15. Sung JJY, Tsoi KK, Lai LH, et al. Endoscopic clipping versus injection and thermo-coagulation in the treatment of non-variceal upper gastrointestinal bleeding: A meta-analysis. Gut 2007;45:1364-73.
16. Gralnek IM, Barkun AN, Bardou M. Management of acute bleeding from a peptic ulcer. N Engl J Med 2008;359:928-37.
17. Giday SA, Van Alstine W, Van Vleet J, et al. Safety analysis of a hemostatic powder in a porcine model of acute severe gastric bleeding. Dig Dis Sci 2013 (Epub ahead of print).
18. Giday SA, Kim Y, Krishnamurty DM, et al. Long-term randomized controlled trial of a novel nanopowder hemostatic agent (TC-325) for control of severe arterial upper gastrointestinal bleeding in a porcine model. Endoscopy 2011;43:296-9.
19. Barkun AN, Moosavi S, Martel M. Topical hemostatic agents: A systemic review with particular emphasis on endoscopic application in GI bleeding. Gastrointest Endosc 2013;77:692-700.

38

Rates of minor adverse events and health resource utilization postcolonoscopy

Vladimir Marquez Azalgara MDCM MSc[1], Maida J Sewitch PhD[2],
Lawrence Joseph PhD[3], Alan N Barkun MDCM FRCPC FACP FACG AGAF MSc[2]

V Marquez Azalgara, M Sewitch, L Joseph, AN Barkun. Rates of minor adverse events and health resource utilization post-colonoscopy. Can J Gastroenterol Hepatol 2014;28(11):595-599.

BACKGROUND: Little is known about minor adverse events (MAEs) following outpatient colonoscopies and associated health care resource utilization.

OBJECTIVE: To estimate the rates of incident MAE at two, 14 and 30 days postcolonoscopy, and associated health care resource utilization. A secondary aim was to identify factors associated with cumulative 30-day MAE incidence.

METHODS: A longitudinal cohort study was conducted among individuals undergoing an outpatient colonoscopy at the Montreal General Hospital (Montreal, Quebec). Before colonoscopy, consecutive individuals were enrolled and interviewed to obtain data regarding age, sex, comorbidities, use of antiplatelets/anticoagulants and previous symptoms. Endoscopy reports were reviewed for intracolonoscopy procedures (biopsy, polypectomy). Telephone or Internet follow-up was used to obtain data regarding MAEs (abdominal pain, bloating, diarrhea, constipation, nausea, vomiting, blood in the stools, rectal or anal pain, headaches, other) and health resource use (visits to emergency department, primary care doctor, gastroenterologist; consults with nurse, pharmacist or telephone hotline). Rates of incident MAEs and health resources utilization were estimated using Bayesian hierarchical modelling to account for patient clustering within physician practices.

RESULTS: Of the 705 individuals approached, 420 (59.6%) were enrolled. Incident MAE rates at the two-, 14- and 30-day follow-ups were 17.3% (95% credible interval [CrI] 8.1% to 30%), 10.5% (95% CrI 2.9% to 23.7%) and 3.2% (95% CrI 0.01% to 19.8%), respectively. The 30-day rate of health resources utilization was 1.7%, with 0.95% of participants seeking the services of a physician. No predictors of the cumulative 30-day incidence of MAEs were identified.

DISCUSSION: The incidence of MAEs was highest in the 48 h following colonoscopy and uncommon after two weeks, supporting the Canadian Association of Gastroenterology's recommendation for assessment of late complications at 14 days. Predictors of new onset of MAEs were not identified, but wide CrIs did not rule out possible associations. Although <1% of participants reported consulting a physician for MAEs, this figure may represent a substantial number of visits given the increasing number of colonoscopies performed annually.

CONCLUSION: Postcolonoscopy MAEs are common, occur mainly in the first two weeks postcolonoscopy and result in little use of health resources.

Key Words: *Colonoscopy; Health services utilization; Minor adverse events; Patient-centred care*

Le taux d'événements indésirables mineurs et d'utilisation des ressources de santé après une coloscopie

HISTORIQUE : On ne sait pas grand-chose des événements indésirables mineurs (ÉIM) qui suivent les coloscopies ambulatoires et de l'utilisation des ressources de santé qui s'y rattachent.

OBJECTIF : Évaluer le taux d'ÉIM deux, 14 et 30 jours après la coloscopie, de même que l'utilisation des ressources de santé s'y rapportant. L'objectif secondaire consistait à déterminer les facteurs associés à l'incidence d'ÉIM cumulatifs au bout de 30 jours.

MÉTHODOLOGIE : Les chercheurs ont mené une étude de cohorte auprès de personnes qui subissaient une coloscopie ambulatoire à l'Hôpital général de Montréal (HGM), au Québec. Avant la coloscopie, des personnes consécutives ont été enrôlées et interviewées. Elles ont donné de l'information sur leur âge, leur sexe, leurs comorbidités, leur utilisation d'antiplaquettaires et d'anticoagulants ainsi que leurs symptômes antérieurs. Les chercheurs ont examiné les rapports d'endoscopie pour connaître l'intervention privilégiée (biopsie, polypectomie). Lors du suivi par téléphone ou par Internet, les chercheurs ont obtenu les données relatives aux ÉIM (douleurs abdominales, gonflements, diarrhée, constipation, nausées, vomissements, sang dans les selles, douleurs rectales ou anales, céphalées, autre) et à l'utilisation des services de santé (visite à l'urgence, rendez-vous avec le médecin de première ligne ou le gastroentérologue, consultations avec une infirmière, un pharmacien ou une ligne téléphonique d'urgence). Ils ont évalué le taux d'ÉIM et d'utilisation des ressources de santé au moyen du modèle bayésien hiérarchique pour tenir compte du regroupement de patients au sein des pratiques des médecins.

RÉSULTATS : Sur les 705 personnes abordées, 420 (59,6 %) ont participé. Les taux d'ÉIM au suivi au bout de deux, 14 et 30 jours s'élevaient à 17,3 % (95 % intervalle de crédibilité [ICr] 8,1 % à 30 %), 10,5 % (95 % ICr 2,9 % à 23,7 %) et 3,2 % (95 % ICr 0,01 % à 19,8 %), respectivement. Le taux d'utilisation des ressources de santé au bout de 30 jours était de 1,7 %, puisque 0,95 % des participants avaient recouru aux services d'un médecin. Aucun prédicteur d'occurrence d'ÉIM n'a été déterminé.

EXPOSÉ : L'incidence d'ÉIM était plus élevée dans les 48 heures suivant la coloscopie et très basse au bout de deux semaines, ce qui appuie la recommandation d'évaluer les complications tardives au quatorzième jour, émise par l'Association canadienne de gastroentérologie. Les prédicteurs de nouveaux ÉIM n'ont pas été établis, mais les vastes ICr n'écartaient pas la possibilité d'associations. Même si moins de 1 % des participants déclaraient avoir consulté un médecin en raison d'ÉIM, ce résultat peut représenter un nombre substantiel de rendez-vous, car de plus en plus de coloscopies sont effectuées chaque année.

CONCLUSION : Les ÉIM sont courantes après la coloscopie, surtout dans les deux semaines suivant l'intervention, mais nécessitent peu de ressources de santé.

In Canada, colorectal cancer (CRC) is the second leading cause of cancer death and the fourth most common cancer diagnosed overall (1). It is possible to decrease the mortality related to CRC by screening, which is now recommended for all Canadians 50 through 75 years of age who are at average risk for developing CRC (ie, no personal or familiar risk factors other than age) (2). For most individuals, CRC screening begins with stool testing, followed by colonoscopy when the stool test is positive. Colonoscopy is the recommended modality for individuals at higher risk for CRC including those with a family history of CRC or personal history of polypectomy (3-5). While many Canadian provinces have implemented organized screening programs in the past three years, including quality assurance structures aimed at

[1]*Division of Gastroenterology, Vancouver General Hospital, Vancouver, British Columbia;* [2]*Department of Medicine;* [3]*Department of Epidemiology, Biostatistics and Occupational Health, McGill University, Montreal, Quebec*
Correspondence: Dr Maida J Sewitch, 687 Pine Avenue West, V Building, Room V2.15, Montreal, Quebec H3A 1A1. e-mail maida.sewitch@mcgill.ca

ensuring delivery of high standard care (6), most CRC screening in the province of Quebec is peformed opportunistically.

Extensive research and recommendations have been made to enhance the quality of all colonoscopies. The resulting quality indicators have focused primarily on physician performance (adenoma detection rate, cecal intubation rate and colonoscope withdrawal time) and safety (serious adverse events rate). As interest in the patient-centred care model shifts attention to patient satisfaction and comfort (7,8), information regarding the incidence of minor adverse events (MAEs), which do not result in hospitalization but cause significant discomfort, becomes important. To date, the few studies that have addressed MAEs after colonoscopy have reported rates that vary from 16.6% to 40.7% (9-15). These studies were heterogeneous in terms of the definitions of MAEs and the time points for their evaluation. Some studies failed to indicate the indication for colonoscopy (screening/nonscreening); calculate the MAE rates according to the endoscopic procedure (gastroscopy or colonoscopy); report the performance of intracolonoscopy procedures (polypectomy, biopsy) that could increase the risk of adverse events; and evaluate the presence of the discomfort before colonoscopy. In other studies, recall bias may have influenced the estimated rates, especially for lengthy follow-up intervals. Conducting a longitudinal study that includes short, medium and lengthy follow-up would not only provide better estimates of the rates and nature of MAEs, it would also yield information as to when these events occur.

Increasing our knowledge of the health resources used for post-colonoscopy MAEs would be helpful in decreasing unnecessary utilization. However, data are scant and substantial variability exists in the services assessed (12,13,16). Some studies included visits to the emergency department but did not include visits to primary care physicians, walk-in clinics or telephone consultations (16). In contrast, other studies considered visits to the emergency department as serious adverse events independent of the final discharge diagnosis (12,13), or relied on diagnosis and procedure codes (ie, *International Classification of Diseases, Ninth and 10th Revisions*) that would not capture MAEs.

Thus, the purpose of the present study was to estimate the rates and nature of incident MAEs at three assessment time points and 30-day cumulative incidence following outpatient colonoscopy, and the rate of health care resources use (visits to the emergency department, primary care doctor or gastroenterologist, and consultations with nurse(s), pharmacists or use of a telephone hotline) that resulted from MAEs. A secondary aim was to identify factors associated with the 30-day cumulative incidence of MAEs.

METHODS

Data collection

A longitudinal cohort study was conducted at the Montreal General Hospital (Montreal, Quebec). Eligible individuals were 40 to 76 years of age, scheduled for an outpatient colonoscopy, able to communicate in English or French, and provide informed consent. Individuals 40 to 50 years of age had to have a positive family history of CRC for whom the recommendation was to begin CRC screening at 40 years of age with colonoscopy (3,5).

Individuals were excluded if they were scheduled for a sigmoidoscopy, proctoscopy or same-day gastroscopy, had an active history of CRC, or were under investigation for a possible flare of known inflammatory bowel disease. Ethics approval was obtained from the McGill University Faculty of Medicine Institutional Review Board (Montreal, Quebec) before study inception, and all participants provided written informed consent.

Five trained research assistants were responsible for recruitment, administration of the baseline questionnaire, review of endoscopy reports and telephone follow-up. The baseline questionnaire collected data regarding medical history (diabetes, heart conditions, pulmonary diseases, kidney disease, liver disease, neurological conditions, inflammatory bowel disease), use of high-risk medications for colonoscopy outcomes (acetylsalicylic acid, clopidogrel [Plavix, sanofi, USA],

dabigatran, warfarin (Coumadin, Bristol-Myers Squibb, USA) ticagrelor, prasugrel and nonsteroidal anti-inflammatory drugs), presence of symptoms in the 30 days before the colonoscopy (abdominal pain, bloating, diarrhea, constipation, nausea or vomiting, blood in the stools, rectal or anal pain, headaches or migraine, other symptoms) and demographics (age, sex, ethnicity, smoking status, level of education). The endoscopy report provided data on the physician performing the colonoscopy, trainee participation during the index colonoscopy (yes/no), colonoscopy indication (screening/not screening), doses of midazolam (mg) and fentanyl (μg) used, physician's evaluation of bowel preparation quality (excellent, good, fair/poor), performance of biopsy or polypectomy (yes/no), method of colon insufflation (air/carbon dioxide) and duration of the colonoscopy (min).

For the purpose of the present study, screening colonoscopy was defined as a procedure performed in asymptomatic individuals 50 to 76 years of age (2). The presence/absence of symptoms was derived from the baseline questionnaire and the endoscopy report. Nonscreening colonoscopy was defined as one performed for investigation of gastrointestinal symptoms, dysplasia detection in inflammatory bowel disease, iron deficiency anemia; follow-up to resolution of an episode of acute diverticulitis, past polypectomy, surgically removed CRC, positive nonendoscopy CRC screening test (eg, fecal immunochemical test, fecal occult blood test, virtual colonoscopy, double-contrast barium enema); or family history of CRC.

Follow-up occurred by telephone interview, or e-mail and Internet-based survey at three time points: two, 14 and 30 days after the colonoscopy. The questions were exactly the same for the two modes of data collection. When participants were not reached, they were telephoned daily for the next three consecutive days (one attempt per day). When participants were not reached on the same day but within the next three consecutive days, the MAE was recorded as having occurred at that assessment time point. If the participant remained unreachable, the research assistants waited until the next scheduled follow-up to contact them again. Similarly, e-mails were sent for follow-ups, and a reminder e-mail daily for the next three consecutive days for non-response. The surveys were created using the Survey Monkey Internet service (www.surveymonkey.net).

MAE was defined as any discomfort the patient experienced after discharge home from the endoscopy unit that did not require any of the following: an overnight stay in the emergency room; hospitalization, blood product transfusion, prescription of antibiotics, surgical or endoscopic intervention or caused death, and that was not present in the 30 days before the colonoscopy as reported in the baseline questionnaire. Data regarding the nature of the discomfort (abdominal pain, bloating, diarrhea, constipation, nausea or vomiting, blood in the stools, rectal or anal pain, headaches or migraine or other symptoms) were obtained. The participant was asked about consulting a health professional/service for the discomfort, the type of professional/service consulted (*Info-Santé* Help Line, emergency room physician, family doctor, gastroenterologist, nurse, pharmacist or other professional), and whether the patient was hospitalized or received a blood transfusion. Predictors of MAEs were determined a priori based on previous studies, and included age (9,12), sex (12,13), presence of comorbidities (10), performance of a polypectomy (13,14), colonoscopy duration (13), trainee participation (10,12) and modality of colon insufflation (17). Information regarding the independent variables was obtained from the baseline questionnaire and the endoscopist report.

Statistical analysis

Description of the study population at entry included means and SDs for continuous data and frequency distributions for categorical data. The descriptive analyses were performed using STATA/SE version 11.2 (StataCorp, USA). Bayesian binomial hierarchical modelling was used to estimate the MAE rates in the cohort to account for patient clustering within physicians (18). Incident MAE rates at each assessment time point were calculated as the sum of individuals who reported at least one MAE at that time point. The 30-day cumulative incidence

MAE rate was calculated as the sum of all individuals who reported at least one MAE at any follow-up. Normal noninformative priors for all parameters were used. Univariate and multivariate logistic regression were used to identify factors associated with the 30-day cumulative incidence MAE rate. Missing data for independent variables were handled using multiple imputation. Bayesian analyses were performed using WinBUGS version 1.4.3 (MRC Biostatistics Unit, United Kingdom).

Sample size

The sample size calculation was based on the estimate of MAEs at seven days according to Ko et al (13). The proportion of patients with at least one MAE at two days was expected to be 34%, the aim was to estimate this proportion to an accuracy of ±5% using a 95% CI. This criterion suggested that 345 participants needed to be recruited. An 20% attrition rate was expected based on the completion rate observed in similar studies (10,13,14). Thus, a total of 414 participants was needed to attain the desired level of accuracy.

RESULTS

Recruitment

Of the 705 consecutive patients approached for participation, 451 (64%) eligible individuals accepted. After excluding 31 individuals (protocol violations, improper consent, age <40 or >76 years, concomitant gastroscopy, scheduled for a sigmoidoscopy, scheduled for an endoscopic ultrasound), the final sample size was 420. Response rates for the day 2, 14 and 30 follow-ups were 342 (81.4%), 335 (79.8%) and 310 (73.8%), respectively. In total, 268 (63.8%) participants responded to all follow-ups and 378 (90.0%) responded to at least one follow-up.

Participant and endoscopy characteristics

Table 1 summarizes participant and endoscopy characteristics. Participants were a mean (± SD) 58.7±8.3 years of age and 192 (45.7%) were female. Ninety-five (22.6%) participants reported at least one comorbidity (diabetes 7.1%, cardiac disease 5.2%, pulmonary disease 4.8%, inflammatory bowel disease 3.8%, kidney disease 2.6%, liver disease 1.4% and neurological disease 1.9%), and 89 (21.2%) reported regular use of at least one high-risk medication (acetylsalicylic acid 16.2%, nonsteroidal anti-inflammatory drugs 4.1%, clopidogrel 0.7%, warfarin [Coumadin, Bristol-Myers Squibb]/dabigatran 0.7%). Of all colonoscopies, 302 (71.9%) were performed by eight gastroenterologists and 118 (28.1%) by five general surgeons. Trainees participated in 30 (7.2%) colonoscopies. The 13 endoscopists performed between four and 80 (median 26) colonoscopies, and 10 reported carbon dioxide as the method of bowel insufflation. The endoscopy report was available for 418 (99.2%) participants. The cecal intubation rate was 96±0.2% and the polypectomy rate was 34±0.47%.

MAE rates

The day 2 follow-up occurred 2.6±0.99 days after the index colonoscopy. Of the 342 respondents, 59 reported at least one MAE, corresponding to an incident MAE rate of 17.3% (95% credible interval [CrI] 8.1% to 30%). The day 14 follow-up occurred 14.7±0.99 days after the index colonoscopy. Of the 335 respondents, 33 reported at least one MAE, yielding an incident MAE rate of 10.5% (95% CrI 2.9% to 23.7%). The 30-day follow-up occurred 30.7±1.07 days after the index colonoscopy. Of the 310 respondents, six reported at least one MAE, yielding an incident MAE rate of 3.2 % (95% CrI 0.01% to 19.8%). Of the 378 (90%) individuals who responded to at least one follow-up, 88 reported at least one MAE, corresponding to a 30-day cumulative incidence MAE rate of 23.3% (95% CrI 19.1% to 27.6%). Eight (1.9%) respondents reported a different symptom at a different assessment time point, and contributed only to the MAE rate for the earlier assessment time point. Table 2 summarizes the discomfort experienced at all three assessment time points. Abdominal pain and bloating were the most commonly reported symptoms at day 2 and day 14, while abdominal pain and constipation were the most commonly reported symptoms at day 30.

TABLE 1
Baseline patient and colonoscopy characteristics of the study population (n=420)

Patient characteristic	
Age, years mean ± SD	58.7±8.3
Female sex	192 (45.7)
Preferred contact method	
E-mail	267 (63.6)
Telephone	153 (36.4)
Comorbidities	95 (22.6)
High-risk medications	89 (21.2)
Symptoms in the 30 days before colonoscopy (n=418)	
Any symptom	237 (56.4)
Abdominal pain	73 (17.4)
Bloating	107 (25.5)
Diarrhea	56 (13.3)
Constipation	81 (19.3)
Nausea/vomiting	32 (7.6)
Blood in stools	39 (9.3)
Rectal pain	40 (9.5)
Headache/migraine	77 (18.3)
Other	57 (13.6)
Ethnic background	
White	367 (87.4)
Nonwhite	53 (12.6)
Endoscopy characteristics	
Colonoscopy indication	
Screening	200 (47.6)
Not screening	220 (52.4)
Fentanyl dose, μg, mean ± SD	83.6±35.9
Midazolam* dose, mg, mean ± SD	3.1±1.3
Endoscopy duration, min, mean ± SD	21.7±7.8
Trainee participation	30 (7.2)
Method of colon insufflation	
Air	100 (24)
Carbon dioxide	320 (76)
Cecal intubation, %, mean ± SD	96±0.2
Preparation quality	
Excellent or good	372 (88.6)
Poor or fair	44 (10.5)

*Data presented as n (%) unless otherwise indicated. *Versed (Roche, USA)*

Table 3 presents the results of the univariate and multivariate logistic regression models used to estimate the effect of participant and endoscopy characteristics on the 30-day incidence of MAE. No associations were found, although wide CrIs throughout preclude definitive conclusions.

Health resource utilization

Table 4 presents the health resources used in the 30 days following colonoscopy. Seven (1.7%) participants reported consulting a health professional for an MAE, four of whom consulted a physician. In addition, two participants reported experiencing a serious adverse event; each had visited the emergency department and required hospitalization for syncope and hemothorax (day 2 follow-up) and for post-polypectomy bleeding (day 30 follow-up).

DISCUSSION

The present longitudinal cohort study reports on the incidence, nature and predictors of outpatient postcolonoscopy MAEs. The incidence of MAEs was highest in the first 48 h following colonoscopy and

TABLE 2
Frequency of incident* minor adverse events reported at days 2, 14 and 30 postcolonoscopy

Minor adverse event	Assessment time point		
	Day 2 (n=342)	Day 14 (n=335)	Day 30 (n=310)
Abdominal pain	30 (8.6)	14 (4.1)	3 (0.9)
Bloating	22 (6.3)	17 (5.0)	0 (0)
Diarrhea	9 (2.6)	6 (1.8)	1 (0.3)
Constipation	9 (2.6)	7 (2.1)	3 (0.9)
Nausea/vomiting	6 (1.7)	2 (0.6)	0 (0)
Blood in the stools	2 (0.6)	2 (0.6)	0 (0)
Rectal/anal pain	9 (2.6)	1 (0.3)	2 (0.6)
Headache	13 (3.7)	2 (0.3)	0 (0)
Other	20 (5.8)†	7 (2.1)‡	1 (0.3)
Any	59 (17)	33 (9.7)	6 (1.9)

Data presented as n (%). *Defined as no report in the 30 days before colonoscopy; †Includes fatigue, dizziness, fever, shivers, nasal irritation, pain at venopuncture site, dehydration, back pain and anxiety; ‡Includes disorientation, fatigue, itchiness, fever and dehydration; 'reaction to anesthesia' does not total to 100 because more than one symptom could be reported

TABLE 3
Univariate and multivariate results for predictors of 30-day cumulative incidence of minor adverse events

Variable	Univariate	Multivariate
	OR (95% CI)	OR (95% CI)
Age	1.01 (0.97–1.03)	0.99 (0.97–1.02)
Sex		
Female	Reference	Reference
Male	0.81 (0.49–1.29)	0.81 (0.49–1.27)
Medical problem		
No	Reference	Reference
Yes	1.60 (0.89–2.66)	1.60 (0.87–2.68)
Trainee participation		
No	Reference	Reference
Yes	0.57 (0.14–1.41)	0.53 (0.15–1.27)
Duration, min	1.01 (0.99–1.03)	1.01 (0.99–1.04)
Polypectomy		
No	Reference	Reference
Yes	1.16 (0.68–1.85)	1.13 (0.64–1.85)
Insufflation with		
Air	Reference	Reference
Carbon dioxide	0.88 (0.41–1.58)	0.84 (0.41–1.50)

TABLE 4
Number of individuals who used health resources for minor adverse events according to assessment time point

Health resource	Day 2 (n=342)	Day 14 (n=335)	Day 30 (n=310)
Family physician	2	0	1
Gastroenterologist	0	1	0
Emergency department*	0	0	0
Pharmacist	0	1	0
Nurse	1	0	0
Info-Santé Help Line	0	0	0
Other	1†	0	0
Any use	4	2	1

Data presented as n. *Two individuals visited the emergency department for serious adverse events and they are not counted in the minor adverse events; †Acupuncture

showed a rate of 29%. Our 30-day incident MAE rate is lower than the sum of MAE rates at each assessment time point because patients who reported more than one MAE or at more than one assessment time point were counted only once in determining this rate.

We did not identify any predictors of new-onset MAEs, but wide CrIs meant that associations could not be ruled out. It is possible that the impact of polypectomy was diluted because we did not specify the method of polyp removal (eg, forceps or electrocautery-assisted); electrocautery has been associated with increased odds for MAEs (13). Contrary to a recent meta-analysis, the method of insufflation (air versus carbon dioxide) was not a predictor of postcolonoscopy discomfort in our study, possibly due to the lack of statistical power (17).

The evaluation of health care resources utilization for MAEs revealed that seven (1.7%) participants had contacted a health professional, a finding that supports the belief that MAEs are generally mild and short lived. Our follow-up relied on direct contact with patients to learn about the consultations to physicians and other health professionals, which represent real-world health care resources use. Four (0.95%) participants reported medical consultations; although this was a small percentage of our sample in the context of the large number of colonoscopies performed annually, it may represent a significant number of physician visits for MAEs. Some of these consultations may be avoided with a 24 h telephone follow-up because they were not avoided with the detailed discharge information that patients routinely received in the studied endoscopy unit.

Our findings showed that the majority of MAEs occur within 48 h after the colonoscopy and almost all occur within the first two weeks, supporting the Canadian Association of Gastroenterology's recommendation that late complications should be assessed at 14 days (19). Nevertheless, the timing for contacting the patient for colonoscopy follow-up is debatable and depends on the purpose of the assessment. If the purpose is to inquire about the patient's condition, satisfaction with the colonoscopy experience or to reinforce postdischarge instructions, then early follow-up (within two days) may be preferred. However, if the purpose is to monitor serious adverse events, then a longer time interval may be preferred. A population-based study by Rabeneck et al (20) found that a 14-day interval would capture the majority of bleeds requiring hospital admission. Similarly, we found that the majority of MAEs occurred within the first 14 days after colonoscopy. Our findings that polypectomy and/or comorbidities increase the risk for MAEs mirror those of others; these variables could be used to identify patients targeted for colonoscopy aftercare.

Our observational study had several limitations. Selection bias may have occurred if respondents were different from nonrespondents with regard to MAE occurrence. The endoscopic report software uses 'screening' as the default indication for colonoscopy, and this may have resulted in misclassification. However, we reviewed the patient's clinical history as summarized in the endoscopy report to classify the colonoscopy indication according to our definition. Limited generalizability

uncommon after 14 days. Abdominal pain and bloating were consistently the two most frequently MAEs reported at days 2 and 14, while abdominal pain and constipation were the most frequently reported at day 30. No predictors of the 30-day cumulative incidence rate of MAE were identified. Less than 1% of respondents sought the services of a physician for an MAE.

Our 30-day incident MAE rate was similar to rates found in some studies (9-11), but substantially different from others (12-15). Zubarik et al (14,15) conducted two studies. In one (14), the MAE rate at 30 days (16.6%) may have been underestimated due to recall bias and, in the other (15), the rate (36.6%) included symptoms that occurred in the endoscopy unit recovery area before discharge as well as those that occurred up to 30 days postcolonoscopy. The 34% MAE rate at seven days reported by Ko et al (13) did not account for previous symptoms and is likely an overestimate of incident MAEs. Finally, de Jonge et al (12) reported an MAE rate of 40.7% at 30 days; however, the subanalysis that restricted MAEs to those definitely related to the colonoscopy

of our findings is possible because the study was conducted in a large academic centre, where physicians had performed several thousand endoscopies. Finally, the small sample size produced very wide CrIs for predictors of MAEs precluding definitive conclusions.

CONCLUSIONS

Our study presents the first prospective estimates of incident MAE rates after outpatient colonoscopies. Our single-institution longitudinal findings provide empirical evidence on the timing and nature of MAE occurrence. Replication of our findings may be informative as to the type of after-care that could be implemented to avoid unnecessary physician consults.

FUNDING: This research was funded by the *Fonds de recherche du Québec – Santé* through an operating grant awarded to Maida Sewitch. Vladimir Azalgara MD, MSc was funded by the Research Institute of the McGill University Health Centre (RI-MUHC) through a RI-MUHC Master of Science studentship.

REFERENCES

1. Canadian Cancer Society. Canadian cancer statistics 2012. Toronto: Canadian Cancer Society, 2012.
2. Leddin DJ, Enns R, Hilsden R, et al. Canadian Association of Gastroenterology position statement on screening individuals at average risk for developing colorectal cancer: 2010. Can J Gastroenterol 2010;24:705-14.
3. Levin B, Lieberman DA, McFarland B, et al. Screening and surveillance for the early detection of colorectal cancer and adenomatous polyps, 2008: A joint guideline from the American Cancer Society, the US Multi-Society Task Force on Colorectal Cancer, and the American College of Radiology. Gastroenterology 2008;134:1570-95.
4. Lieberman DA, Rex DK, Winawer SJ, et al. Guidelines for colonoscopy surveillance after screening and polypectomy: A consensus update by the US Multi-Society Task Force on Colorectal Cancer. Gastroenterology 2012;143:844-57.
5. Rex DK, Johnson DA, Anderson JC, et al. American College of Gastroenterology guidelines for colorectal cancer screening 2009 [corrected]. Am J Gastroenterol 2009;104:739-50.
6. Zarychanski R, Chen Y, Bernstein CN, et al. Frequency of colorectal cancer screening and the impact of family physicians on screening behaviour. CMAJ 2007;177:593-7.
7. Sewitch MJ, Dube C, Brien S, et al. Patient-identified quality indicators for colonoscopy services. Can J Gastroenterol 2013;27:25-32.
8. Sewitch MJ, Gong S, Dube C, et al. A literature review of quality in lower gastrointestinal endoscopy from the patient perspective. Can J Gastroenterol 2011;25:681-5.
9. Baudet JS, Diaz-Bethencourt D, Aviles J, et al. Minor adverse events of colonoscopy on ambulatory patients: The impact of moderate sedation. Eur J Gastroenterol Hepatol 2009;21:656-61.
10. Bini EJ, Firoozi B, Choung RJ, et al. Systematic evaluation of complications related to endoscopy in a training setting: A prospective 30-day outcomes study. Gastrointest Endosc 2003;57:8-16.
11. Chen YK, Godil A, Thompson SA, et al. Telephone callback is unnecessary after outpatient endoscopy. J Clin Gastroenterol 1998;26:342-3.
12. de Jonge V, Sint Nicolaas J, van Baalen O, et al. The incidence of 30-day adverse events after colonoscopy among outpatients in the Netherlands. Am J Gastroenterol 2012;107:878-84.
13. Ko CW, Riffle S, Shapiro JA, et al. Incidence of minor complications and time lost from normal activities after screening or surveillance colonoscopy. Gastrointest Endosc 2007;65:648-56.
14. Zubarik R, Fleischer DE, Mastropietro C, et al. Prospective analysis of complications 30 days after outpatient colonoscopy. Gastrointest Endosc 1999;50:322-8.
15. Zubarik R, Ganguly E, Benway D, et al. Procedure-related abdominal discomfort in patients undergoing colorectal cancer screening: A comparison of colonoscopy and flexible sigmoidoscopy. Am J Gastroenterol 2002;97:3056-61.
16. Leffler DA, Kheraj R, Garud S, et al. The incidence and cost of unexpected hospital use after scheduled outpatient endoscopy. Arch Intern Med 2010;170:1752-7.
17. Wong WL, Wu ZII, Sun Q, et al. Meta-analysis: The use of carbon dioxide insufflation vs. room air insufflation for gastrointestinal endoscopy. Aliment Pharmacol Ther 2012;35:1145-54.
18. Gelman A, Carlin J, Stern H, Rubin D. Bayesian Data Analysis, 2nd edn. Boca Raton: Chapman and Hall, 2003.
19. Armstrong D, Barkun A, Bridges R, et al. Canadian Association of Gastroenterology consensus guidelines on safety and quality indicators in endoscopy. Can J Gastroenterol 2012;26:17-31.
20. Rabeneck L, Saskin R, Paszat LF. Onset and clinical course of bleeding and perforation after outpatient colonoscopy: A population-based study. Gastrointest Endosc 2011;73:520-3.

39

Physicians' practices for diagnosing liver fibrosis in chronic liver diseases: A nationwide, Canadian survey

Giada Sebastiani MD[1], Peter Ghali MD FRCPC MSc[1], Philip Wong MD FRCPC MSc[1],

Marina B Klein MD MSc[2], Marc Deschenes MD[1], Robert P Myers MD FRCPC [3]

G Sebastiani, P Ghali, P Wong, MB Klein, M Deschenes, RP Myers. Physicians' practices for diagnosing liver fibrosis in chronic liver diseases: A nationwide, Canadian survey. Can J Gastroenterol Hepatol 2014;28(1):23-30.

OBJECTIVE: To determine practices among physicians in Canada for the assessment of liver fibrosis in patients with chronic liver diseases.
METHODS: Hepatologists, gastroenterologists, infectious diseases specialists, members of the Canadian Gastroenterology Association and/or the Canadian HIV Trials Network who manage patients with liver diseases were invited to participate in a web-based, national survey.
RESULTS: Of the 237 physicians invited, 104 (43.9%) completed the survey. Routine assessment of liver fibrosis was requested by the surveyed physicians mostly for chronic hepatitis C (76.5%), followed by autoimmune/cholestatic liver disease (59.6%) and chronic hepatitis B (52.9%). Liver biopsy was the main diagnostic tool for 46.2% of the respondents, Fibroscan (Echosens, France) for 39.4% and Fibrotest (LabCorp, USA) for 7.7%. Etiology-specific differences were observed: noninvasive methods were mostly used for hepatitis C (63% versus 37% liver biopsy) and hepatitis B (62.9% versus 37.1% liver biopsy). For 42.7% of respondents, the use of noninvasive methods reduced the need for liver biopsy by >50%. Physicians' characteristics associated with higher use of noninvasive methods were older age and being based at a university hospital or in private practice versus community hospital. Physicians' main concerns regarding noninvasive fibrosis assessment methods were access/availability (42.3%), lack of guidelines for clinical use (26.9%) and cost/lack of reimbursement (14.4%).
CONCLUSIONS: Physicians who manage patients with chronic liver diseases in Canada require routine assessment of liver fibrosis stage. Although biopsy remains the primary diagnostic tool for almost one-half of respondents, noninvasive methods, particularly Fibroscan, have significantly reduced the need for liver biopsy in Canada. Limitations in access to and availability of the noninvasive methods represent a significant barrier. Finally, there is a need for clinical guidelines and a better reimbursement policy to implement noninvasive tools to assess liver fibrosis.

Key Words: *Canadian physicians; Chronic liver diseases; Liver biopsy; Liver fibrosis; Noninvasive fibrosis methods*

Les pratiques des médecins pour diagnostiquer la fibrose hépatique en cas de la maladie hépatique chronique : un sondage pancanadien

OBJECTIF : Déterminer les pratiques des médecins du Canada en matière d'évaluation de la fibrose hépatique chez des patients atteints d'une maladie hépatique chronique.
MÉTHODOLOGIE : Les hépatologistes, les gastroentérologues, les infectiologues, les membres de l'Association canadienne de gastroentérologie et ceux du Réseau pour les essais VIH qui prenaient en charge des patients ayant une maladie hépatique ont été invités à participer à un sondage virtuel national.
RÉSULTATS : Sur les 237 médecins invités, 104 (43,9 %) ont rempli le sondage. Les médecins demandaient une évaluation systématique de la fibrose hépatique surtout en cas d'hépatite C chronique (76,5 %), de maladie hépatique auto-immune ou de maladie cholestatique du foie (59,6 %) et d'hépatite B chronique (52,9 %). La biopsie hépatique était le principal outil diagnostique pour 46,2 % des répondants, le Fibroscan (Echosens, France), pour 39,4 % d'entre eux, et le Fibrotest (LabCorp, États-Unis), pour 7,7 % d'entre eux. Les chercheurs ont observé des différences propres à l'étiologie : les méthodes non effractives étaient surtout utilisées en cas d'hépatite C (63 % par rapport à 37 % de biopsie hépatique) et d'hépatite B (62,9 % par rapport à 37,1 % de biopsie hépatique). Chez 42,7 % des répondants, le recours à une méthode non effractive réduisait de plus de 50 % la nécessité de biopsie hépatique. Les caractéristiques des médecins associées à une plus forte utilisation de méthodes non effractives étaient le fait d'être plus âgés et de travailler dans un hôpital universitaire ou en pratique privée plutôt que dans un hôpital général. Les principales inquiétudes des médecins à l'égard de l'évaluation non effractive de la fibrose étaient l'accès ou la disponibilité (42,3 %), l'absence de directives cliniques (26,9 %) et le coût ou l'absence de remboursement (14,4 %).
CONCLUSIONS : Les médecins qui prennent en charge les patients ayant une maladie hépatique chronique au Canada demandent une évaluation systématique du stade de fibrose hépatique. Même si la biopsie demeure le principal outil diagnostique pour près de la moitié des répondants, les méthodes non effractives, notamment le Fibroscan, ont considérablement réduit la nécessité d'utiliser la biopsie hépatique au Canada. Les limites d'accès et de disponibilité des méthodes non effractives représentent un obstacle important. Enfin, il faudrait produire des directives cliniques et prévoir une meilleure politique de remboursement pour qu'on puisse adopter les outils non effractifs dans l'évaluation de la fibrose hépatique.

Chronic liver diseases (CLDs) are a major cause of morbidity and mortality worldwide, affecting 360 per 100,000 persons and ranking as the 12th leading cause of overall mortality (1,2). In Canada, 2748 deaths were attributed to CLDs and liver cirrhosis (11th leading cause of death) in 2008 (3). The main etiologies of CLDs are chronic infections with hepatitis C and B viruses (HCV and HBV, respectively), alcoholic liver disease (ALD) and nonalcoholic fatty liver disease (NAFLD). Chronic infections with HCV and HBV impose a significant medical and economic burden in Canada, affecting nearly 1% and 2% of the population, respectively (4,5). NAFLD is the most common liver disease in Canada, afflicting as much as 30% of the population (6). The consumption of alcohol is increasing in Canada and, as a result, the incidence of ALD is also increasing (7).

Independent of etiology, the progression of all CLDs occurs via a common histopathological pathway characterized by the formation of fibrosis leading to a progressive distortion of the hepatic architecture, the hallmark of evolution to cirrhosis. The accumulation of fibrosis in the liver is the event with the greatest impact on the prognosis of CLDs. Natural history studies indicate that approximately 20% to 40% of patients with CLDs will develop significant liver fibrosis (stage F2 according to METAVIR histological classification [8]), 10% will progress to cirrhosis and 1% to 5% will develop hepatocellular carcinoma

[1]*Division of Gastroenterology, Royal Victoria Hospital, McGill University Health Centre; [2]Department of Medicine, Division of Infectious Diseases/ Chronic Viral Illness Service, McGill University Health Centre, Montreal, Quebec; [3]Liver Unit, Division of Gastroenterology and Hepatology, Department of Medicine, University of Calgary, Alberta*
Correspondence: Dr Giada Sebastiani, Department of Medicine, Division of Gastroenterology, McGill University Health Centre, Royal Victoria Hospital, 687 Avenue Pine West, Montreal, Quebec H3A 1A1 e-mail giada.sebastiani@mcgill.ca

(HCC) within two to three decades (9,10). Cirrhosis requires specific follow-up including screening for esophageal varices and HCC with periodic gastroscopy and ultrasound (11,12).

The diagnosis of liver fibrosis stage is also critical for reinforcing behavioural interventions in patients with NAFLD and ALD, and for a definitive indication for antiviral therapy in individuals with chronic viral hepatitis.

For HCV, although guidelines from the Canadian Association for the Study of the Liver (CASL) state that there is no absolute fibrosis threshold to preclude antiviral therapy, prompt initiation of treatment should be considered in patients with advanced liver fibrosis (F3 or F4 according to METAVIR classification, corresponding to bridging fibrosis or cirrhosis [8]), who are at risk for end-stage hepatic complications (4). The landscape of antiviral therapy is rapidly changing in chronic hepatitis C. Until recently, the standard of care was dual therapy with pegylated interferon and ribavirin. Recently, the direct antiviral agents boceprevir and telaprevir have offered substantial improvements in response rates for patients infected with HCV genotype 1 (4). The future looks even brighter, considering the new compounds that will soon lead to interferon-free regimens (13). In this dynamic landscape, the assessment of liver fibrosis stage will remain of paramount importance for determining prognosis and guide HCV treatment. The CASL guidelines include liver fibrosis stage in the decisional algorithm for the treatment of hepatitis B (5). As such, an assessment for liver fibrosis stage is recommended for all patients infected with HBV and HCV (4,5).

In NAFLD, the recent guidelines from the American Association for the Study of Liver Diseases (AASLD) recommend histological assessment in individuals at risk for nonalcoholic steatohepatitis (NASH), such as individuals with the metabolic syndrome (14,15). Liver fibrosis assessment also has a prognostic and diagnostic role in ALD and autoimmune/cholestatic liver diseases (16-18).

Liver biopsy has long been the gold standard to stage liver fibrosis. This procedure, however, is invasive, costly, impractical as a screening tool and prone to sampling error (11,19). In recent years, noninvasive tools for liver fibrosis have been proposed. Fibrosis can be measured noninvasively based on a biological approach (serum biomarkers) or on a physical approach (liver stiffness). The most validated serum biomarkers include Fibrotest (LabCorp, USA, combining gamma-glutamyl transpeptidase, total bilirubin, α-2-macroglobulin, apolipoprotein A1, haptoglobin, age and sex) and aspartate aminotransferase-to-platelet ratio index (APRI) (20-22). Transient elastography (Fibroscan; Echosens, France) is an ultrasound-based device that measures liver stiffness as a surrogate of liver fibrosis (23). Other methods include magnetic resonance elastography and acoustic radiation force impulse elastography (24,25). Noninvasive methods for liver fibrosis diagnosis are gaining more credibility across guidelines and experts' recommendations, particularly in chronic HCV and HBV infections (4,5,21,26). However, there are no data regarding the adherence of Canadian physicians to guidelines with regard to routine assessment of liver fibrosis. Moreover, information regarding implementation of noninvasive methods instead of liver biopsy among Canadian physicians who manage CLD patients are lacking.

We conducted a web-based survey aimed at investigating practices of liver fibrosis assessment among physicians who manage CLD patients across Canada.

METHODS

The present study was a cross-sectional survey of Canadian specialists who manage patients with CLDs. The survey was developed by the first author (GS) and first distributed among the coauthors to assess satisfaction and face validity. Modifications were made based on feedback and comments. The final version consisted of six pages and 21 items divided into two sections: clinician profile; and practice profile and liver fibrosis assessment (Online Appendixes A to F [go to www.pulsus.com]).

The first section included questions about age, sex, primary specialty, years of practice, time dedicated to patient care, practice location and province of practice. The second section included questions regarding CLDs followed in practice, etiologies of CLDs for which assessment of liver fibrosis stage was requested, the main tool used to diagnose liver fibrosis, opinion on the best noninvasive tool to diagnose liver fibrosis, impact of noninvasive tools on the number of liver biopsies performed, impact of noninvasive methods for liver fibrosis on the number of HCV- and HBV-infected patients treated, and concerns regarding noninvasive tools for liver fibrosis. A link to the web-based survey was sent by e-mail between August 2012 and January 2013 to members of the Canadian Association of Gastroenterology (CAG) and Canadian HIV Trial Network who manage patients with CLDs. Confidentiality was preserved by the fact that e-mails were sent through the CAG National Office. All responses were anonymous and the investigators received no information that would identify the respondent or their site of practice. Ethics approval was sought from the McGill University Health Centre Research Ethics Office (Montreal, Quebec); an official research ethics board approval was not required.

Requested answers were either oriented (different items to choose from), based on a grading scale (ranking from 0 to 6 scale) or a matrix of choices with multiple answers per row. Standard descriptive statistics were used to describe response frequency. The χ^2 test was used to compare categorical variables; a two-sided P<0.05 was considered to be statistically significant.

RESULTS

Of 237 invited physicians, 104 (43.9%) completed the survey. Of these, 83 (79.8%) were members of the CAG and 21 (20.2%) were members of the Canadian HIV Trial Network. Table 1 summarizes the demographics of the surveyed physicians. Overall, most respondents were male (78.8%), had gastroenterology as their primary specialty (64.4%), were based at a university hospital (51%) and dedicated >75% of their time to patient care activities (71.1%). The majority of respondents were from Ontario (40.4%) and Quebec (36.6%).

Etiology of CLDs and practices of responding physicians

The etiologies of CLDs seen by the respondents were as follows: 87 (83.7%) physicians managed NAFLD patients; 84 (80.8%) saw patients with autoimmune/cholestatic liver disease; 83 (79.8%) saw ALD cases; 81 (77.9%) physicians managed patients with HCV; 70 (67.3%) managed HBV patients; and 33 (31.7%) saw HIV patients coinfected with HBV and/or HCV. The primary specialty impacted the etiology of CLDs managed by the responding physician (Table 2). As such, respondents with gastroenterology as their primary specialty managed fewer HBV patients compared with hepatologists (P=0.02). Similarly, gastroenterologists saw fewer HIV-coinfected patients than hepatologists or infectious diseases specialists (P<0.0001). Conversely, infectious diseases specialists were less likely to manage NAFLD patients compared with hepatologists (P=0.0004) and gastroenterologists (P<0.0001). Infectious diseases specialists saw fewer ALD cases compared with hepatologists (P=0.0002) and gastroenterologists (P<0.0001). Interestingly, hepatologists saw significantly fewer NAFLD (P=0.04) and ALD patients (P=0.05) than gastroenterologists. Finally, infectious diseases specialists managed fewer patients with autoimmune/cholestatic liver disease compared with hepatologists and gastroenterologists (P<0.0001).

The remainder of the surveyed physicians (9.6%) had family medicine or internal medicine as their primary specialty. They managed fewer HBV patients compared with gastroenterologists (20% versus 67.2%; P=0.004), hepatologists (20% versus 94.1%; P<0.0001) and infectious diseases specialists (20% versus 80%; P=0.007) (data not shown). When compared with gastroenterologists and hepatologists, they also managed fewer patients with NAFLD (20% versus 100% and 94.1%, respectively; P<0.0001) and ALD (40% versus 95.5%; P<0.0001; and versus 82.4%, respectively; P=0.02). Conversely, they saw more HIV-coinfected patients than gastroenterologists (60% versus 13.4%; P=0.0005), and managed fewer patients with autoimmune/cholestatic

TABLE 1
Characteristics of the surveyed physicians (n=104)

Age group, years	
<40	30 (28.8)
40–50	33 (31.7)
50–60	27 (26)
>60	14 (13.5)
Sex	
Male	82 (78.8)
Female	22 (21.2)
Primary specialty	
Gastroenterology	67 (64.4)
Hepatology	17 (16.4)
Infectious disease	10 (9.6)
Other (family medicine, internal medicine)	10 (9.6)
Years of practice	
<5	14 (13.5)
5–10	20 (19.2)
10–20	30 (28.8)
>20	40 (38.5)
Practice location	
University-based hospital	53 (51)
Community hospital	29 (27.9)
Private practice	22 (21.1)
Time dedicated to patients' care	
<50	11 (10.6)
50–75	19 (18.3)
>75	74 (71.1)
Province of practice	
Ontario	42 (40.4)
Quebec	38 (36.6)
British Columbia	10 (9.6)
Alberta	7 (6.7)
Rest of Canada	7 (6.7)

Data presented as n (%)

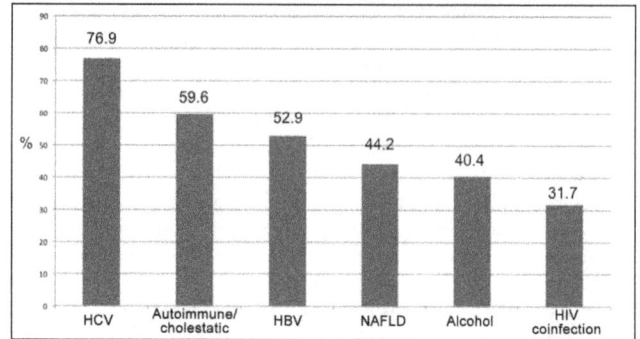

Figure 1) *Rate of surveyed physicians requiring routine assessment of liver fibrosis stage according to etiology of chronic liver diseases. HBV Hepatitis B virus; HCV Hepatitis C virus; NAFLD Nonalcoholic fatty liver disease*

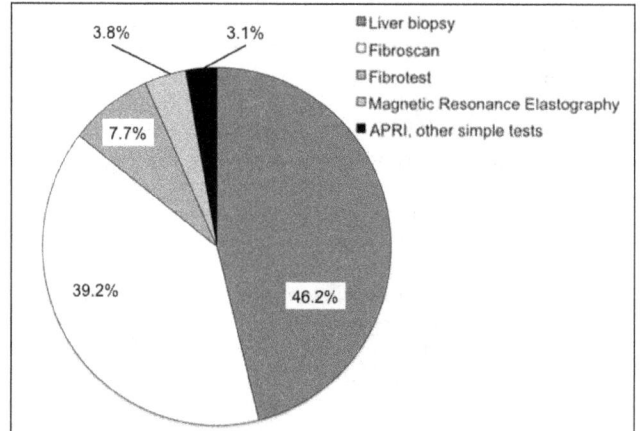

Figure 2) *Primary method used by the responding physicians for the assessment of liver fibrosis. APRI Aspartate aminotransferase-to-platelet ratio index; Fibroscan (Echosens, France); Fibrotest (LabCorp, USA)*

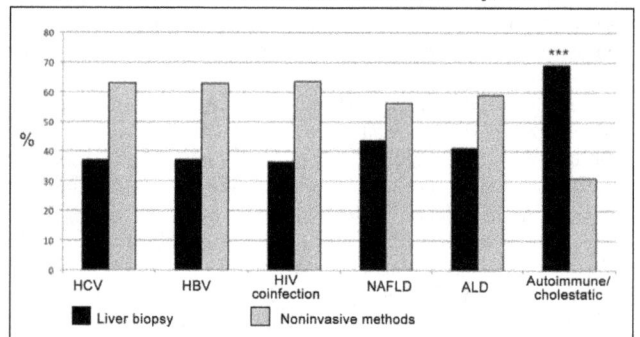

Figure 3) *Use of noninvasive methods for assessing liver fibrosis versus liver biopsy according to etiology of chronic liver diseaes. ***P<0.0001 compared with all other etiologies of chronic liver diseases. ALD Alcoholic liver disease; HBV Hepatitis B virus; HCV Hepatitis C virus; NAFLD Nonalcoholic fatty liver disease*

liver disease compared with gastroenterologists and hepatologists (20% versus 94% and 94.1%, respectively; P<0.0001).

The effect of CLD etiology and practice characteristics on diagnosing liver fibrosis

Figure 1 depicts the rate of physicians requiring routine assessment of liver fibrosis stage according to the etiology of CLD. Chronic HCV was the most common etiology (76.9%), followed by autoimmune/cholestatic liver disease (59.6%) and chronic HBV (52.9%). Figure 2 shows the primary method used by respondents for the assessment of liver fibrosis. Liver biopsy was the primary diagnostic tool for 46.2% of the physicians, followed by Fibroscan (39.4%) and Fibrotest (7.7%). When asked which tool was used as the secondary test, 35.6% answered liver biopsy, 32.7% Fibroscan, 13.5% none, 9.6% APRI and other simple biomarkers, 2.9% Fibrotest and 5.7% other (magnetic resonance, computed tomography scan, comparative radiological examinations).

Figure 3 depicts the use of liver biopsy versus noninvasive methods according to etiology of CLDs. Overall, in chronic viral hepatitis, including HCV, HBV and HIV-coinfected patients, there was a tendency for a higher use of noninvasive methods for liver fibrosis staging. Autoimmune/cholestatic liver disease was the only disease in which liver biopsy was significantly more used than noninvasive tools (69% versus 31%; P<0.0001 compared with the other etiologies of CLDs). Table 3 shows the detailed distribution of methods for liver fibrosis diagnosis according to etiology of CLDs. Fibroscan was the most used noninvasive method in all etiologies of CLDs. Interestingly, the use of Fibroscan was significantly higher in HCV versus ALD and autoimmune/cholestatic liver disease (53.1% versus 33.7% and 19%, respectively;

P=0.02 and P<0.0001). Simple serum biomarkers were more frequently used in ALD than HCV (16.9% versus 2.5%; P=0.0006). Figure 4 illustrates the impact of noninvasive methods in terms of reduction of liver biopsies performed in a physician's practice. Overall, for 42.7% of respondents, the use of noninvasive methods reduced the need for liver biopsy by >50%. Table 4 summarizes the etiology-specific decrease in the need for liver biopsy. The highest reduction in liver biopsies was observed in HCV, given that a ≥50% decrease was observed in 62.9% of respondents. This figure was significantly higher than that in NAFLD (43.7%; P=0.01), ALD (39%; P=0.04) and autoimmune/cholestatic liver disease (27.8%; P<0.0001).

The effect of physicians' demographics and characteristics on practices of liver fibrosis diagnosis is shown in Table 5. Older physicians used more noninvasive methods for liver fibrosis than younger respondents

TABLE 2
Etiology of chronic liver disease managed by surveyed physicians according to their primary specialty

Chronic liver disease	Primary specialty			P*		
	Gastroenterology	Hepatology	Infectious diseases			
Hepatitis C	53 (79.1)	16 (94.1)	9 (90)	0.14	0.41	0.69
Hepatitis B	45 (67.2)	16 (94.1)	8 (80)	**0.02**	0.41	0.25
HIV coinfection	9 (13.4)	12 (70.6)	8 (80)	**<0.0001**	**<0.0001**	0.58
Nonalcoholic fatty liver disease	67 (100)	16 (94.1)	3 (30)	**0.04**	**<0.0001**	**0.0004**
Alcoholic liver disease	64 (95.5)	14 (82.4)	1 (10)	**0.05**	**<0.0001**	**0.0002**
Autoimmune/cholestatic liver disease	63 (94)	16 (94.1)	2 (20)	0.98	**<0.0001**	**<0.0001**

*Data presented as n (%). Bolded values indicate statistical significance. *χ^2 test between Gastroenterology and Hepatology in the first column; between Gastroenterology and Infectious diseases in the second column; and between Hepatology and Infectious diseases in the third column*

TABLE 3
Primary method for assessment of liver fibrosis according to etiology of chronic liver disease

Chronic liver disease	Liver biopsy	Fibroscan*	Fibrotest†	APRI, other simple biomarkers	Magnetic resonance elastography
Hepatitis C	30 (37)	43 (53.1)	6 (7.4)	2 (2.5)	0 (0)
Hepatitis B	26 (37.1)	32 (45.7)	6 (8.6)	6 (8.6)	0 (0)
HIV coinfection	12 (36.4)	15 (45.4)	3 (9.1)	3 (9.1)	0 (0)
Nonalcoholic fatty liver disease	38 (43.7)	33 (37.9)	5 (4.6)	9 (1.1)	2 (2.3)
Alcoholic liver disease	34 (41)	28 (33.7)	4 (4.8)	14 (16.9)	3 (3.6)
Autoimmune/cholestatic liver disease	58 (69)	16 (19)	2 (2.4)	6 (7.2)	2 (2.4)

*Data presented as n (%). *Echosens, France; †LabCorp, USA. APRI Aspartate aminotransferase-to-platelet ratio index*

TABLE 4
Etiology-specific impact of noninvasive methods in terms of reductions of liver biopsies performed

Chronic liver disease	Liver biopsy no longer performed	Reduction, %		
		>50	25 to 50	<25
Hepatitis C	15 (18.5)	36 (44.4)	17 (21)	13 (16.1)
Hepatitis B	11 (15.7)	26 (37.1)	17 (24.3)	16 (22.9)
HIV coinfection	4 (12.1)	14 (42.4)	10 (30.3)	5 (15.2)
Nonalcoholic fatty liver disease	10 (11.5)	28 (32.2)	20 (23)	29 (33.3)
Alcoholic liver disease	10 (12)	29 (35)	14 (16.9)	30 (36.1)
Autoimmune/cholestatic liver disease	10 (11.9)	15 (17.9)	18 (21.4)	41 (48.8)

Data presented as n (%)

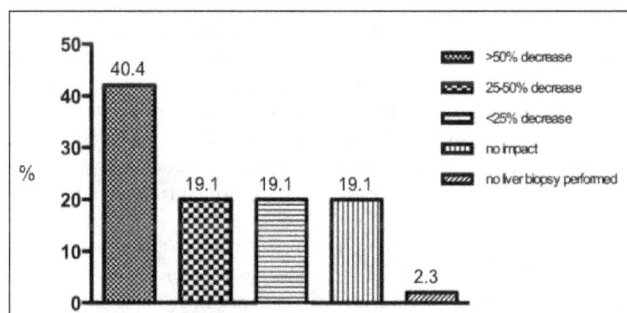

Figure 4) *Impact of noninvasive methods on the number of liver biopsies performed by the surveyed physicians*

(P=0.02). Hepatologists and infectious diseases specialists used more noninvasive methods for liver fibrosis (particularly Fibroscan) than gastroenterologists, although this difference was not statistically significant. Respondents practicing their primary specialty for longer tended to use more noninvasive methods for liver fibrosis assessment than those practicing for shorter durations. Interestingly, physicians based at a university hospital or in private practice used more non-invasive methods than those based at a community hospital (P=0.05). Although the province of practice did not impact the use of

noninvasive methods versus biopsy, a trend for regional variation in the use of noninvasive methods was observed (Table 6). In Ontario, Fibrotest was the primary noninvasive tool for fibrosis diagnosis for 30.5% of the surveyed physicians, and this figure was significantly higher than the other provinces (P=0.004).

Satisfaction with and concerns about noninvasive methods for liver fibrosis

When asked whether noninvasive methods for liver fibrosis provide an accurate assessment, 86 (82.6%) of respondents agreed, nine (8.7%) disagreed and nine (8.7%) neither agreed nor disagreed. For 91 (87.5%) of the participants, Fibroscan was ranked as the best noninvasive method for staging liver fibrosis. For 35 (33.7%) of the surveyed physicians, the implementation of noninvasive methods for liver fibrosis resulted in more patients treated with antiviral therapy, while there was no change in the remaining 69 (66.3%). The major concern regarding noninvasive methods for liver fibrosis was access/availability for 44 (42.3%) of respondents, lack of guidelines for use in clinical practice for 28 (26.9%), cost/lack of reimbursement for 15 (14.4%), unsatisfactory accuracy for eight (7.7%), poor reproducibility for six (5.8%) and delayed results for three (2.9%). Overall, 62 (59.6%) of the responding physicians did not have a Fibroscan in their clinics, and 38 (61.3%) physicians in this group reported no convenient access to the device. All responding phys-icians who did not have a Fibroscan nor convenient access to it would increase the use of noninvasive methods for liver fibrosis if access/availability was improved.

TABLE 5
Effect of physicians' demographics and practice characteristics on methods used to diagnose liver fibrosis

	Noninvasive methods	Liver biopsy	P
Age, years			**0.02**
<40	15 (26.8)	15 (31.3)	
40–50	13 (23.2)	20 (41.7)	
50–60	16 (28.6)	11 (22.9)	
>60	12 (21.4)	2 (4.1)	
Sex			0.22
Male	47 (83.9)	35 (72.9)	
Female	9 (16.1)	13 (27.1)	
Primary specialty			0.15
Gastroenterology	31 (55.4)	36 (75)	
Hepatology	11 (19.6)	6 (12.5)	
Infectious diseases	6 (10.7)	4 (8.3)	
Other	8 (14.3)	2 (4.2)	
Years of practice			0.09
<5	4 (7.1)	10 (20.8)	
5–10	12 (21.4)	8 (16.7)	
10–20	14 (25)	16 (33.3)	
>20	26 (46.5)	14 (29.2)	
Practice location			**0.05**
University-based hospital	32 (57.1)	21 (44)	
Community hospital	10 (17.9)	19 (40)	
Private practice	14 (25)	8 (17)	
Time dedicated to patients' care			0.90
<50	6 (10.7)	5 (10.4)	
50–75	9 (16.1)	10 (20.8)	
>75	41 (73.2)	33 (68.8)	
Province			0.62
Ontario	23 (41.1)	19 (39.6)	
Quebec	21 (37.6)	17 (35.4)	
British Columbia	5 (8.9)	5 (10.4)	
Alberta	6 (10.7)	1 (2.1)	
Rest of Canada	1 (1.7)	6 (12.5)	

Data presented as n (%). Bolded values indicate statistical significance

TABLE 6
Distribution of noninvasive methods to diagnose liver fibrosis according to province of practice of surveyed physicians

Province	Fibroscan*	Fibrotest[†]	APRI, other simple biomarkers	MRE
Ontario	14 (60.9)	7 (30.5)	1 (4.3)	1 (4.3)
Quebec	18 (85.7)	0 (0)	1 (4.8)	2 (9.5)
British Columbia	4 (80)	0 (0)	0 (0)	1 (20)
Alberta	5 (83.3)	1 (16.7)	0 (0)	0 (0)
Rest of Canada	0 (0)	0 (0)	1 (100)	0 (0)

*Data presented as n (%). *Echosens, France; [†]LabCorp, USA. APRI Aspartate aminotransferase-to-platelet ratio index; MRE Magnetic resonance elastography*

DISCUSSION

The present study was the first to evaluate practice patterns for diagnosing and staging liver fibrosis among Canadian physicians who manage patients with CLDs. Most surveyed physicians require a systematic assessment of liver fibrosis; thus, they adhere to current guidelines that recommend assessment of liver fibrosis in patients with CLDs (4,5). However, although a number of noninvasive diagnostic methods have been developed, almost one-half of Canadian physicians still use liver biopsy as their primary diagnostic tool. Importantly, most of the surveyed physicians believe that noninvasive methods, particularly Fibroscan, provide an accurate staging of liver fibrosis in CLDs. Nevertheless, limitations in access/availability represent a significant barrier. Our results highlight the importance of improving access to noninvasive methods for liver fibrosis diagnosis. Canadian physicians have also identified the emerging need for guidelines in clinical practice and an improved reimbursement policy.

In Canada, CLDs, mainly due to HCV, HBV, NAFLD and ALD, represent the 11th leading cause of death (3). Liver fibrosis stage is the single most important factor impacting the prognosis of patients with CLDs and it has a major role in management decisions, such as initiation of antiviral therapy and implementation of interventions including alcohol abstinence and control of dysmetabolisms (4,5,10,16,26). Once cirrhosis is established, it may lead to end-stage complications including decompensation, HCC and death. Identification of patients with cirrhosis is critical to begin appropriate surveillance measures such as endoscopy for esophageal varices or ultrasound for HCC screening. However, in 20% of patients with CLDs, the diagnosis is made on presentation of the first episode of hepatic decompensation due to cirrhosis (27). Thus, implementation of liver fibrosis staging and surveillance for cirrhosis at a preclinical stage will facilitate long-term planning for these patients. Similarly, the longitudinal assessment of fibrosis in a safe, noninvasive manner is desirable. Our study highlights that most Canadian physicians who follow patients with CLDs require routine assessment of liver fibrosis stage, thus recognizing its importance for decision making. Chronic hepatitis C is the etiology for which assessment of liver fibrosis is required by most physicians, followed by autoimmune/cholestatic liver disease, chronic hepatitis B, NAFLD and ALD. This is consistent with national and international guidelines. In fact, an assessment of liver fibrosis is recommended in chronic HBV and HCV infections; however, in some conditions, such as ALD and autoimmune/cholestatic liver disease, liver biopsy still has a diagnostic role in assessing severity or ruling out other forms of liver disease (4,5,14,16-18,26,28,29). Importantly, although patients with HIV and HCV and/or HBV coinfection experience higher rates of evolution toward cirrhosis than monoinfected individuals, routine assessment of liver fibrosis was requested by only 31.7% of respondents. This may be due to the fear of performing liver biopsy in HIV-positive patients given a possible higher chance of bleeding associated with clotting abnormalities (30,31).

In our experience, the primary specialty of the respondents impacted the etiology of CLDs seen. Gastroenterologists are more likely to manage NAFLD and ALD patients than hepatologists and infectious diseases specialists, and they manage fewer patients with HBV and HIV coinfection. Conversely, infectious diseases specialists manage fewer patients with autoimmune/cholestatic disease. This practice profile reflects a subspecialty in the management of CLDs that has been already observed in other Canadian studies (32,33).

For almost one-half of the surveyed physicians, liver biopsy remains the primary tool used to diagnose liver fibrosis. This procedure, however, is invasive and accompanied by several drawbacks including pain and risk of fibrosis underestimation (19,34). Cost is also a major issue. A cost-benefit analysis (35) showed that in the United States, the cost of a liver biopsy is USD$1,032 and could rise to USD$2,745 when complications occur. In Canada, the mean cost of a complicated liver biopsy requiring hospitalization is $4,579 (36). During the past two decades, scientific interest has been focused on implementing noninvasive approaches to diagnose liver fibrosis in

CLDs. The most validated among them include Fibroscan and serum biomarkers that are computed from readily available parameters, such as APRI and Fibrotest. Liver biopsy use increased by 41% between 1994 and 2002 in Canada, highlighting the increasing importance of liver fibrosis staging for clinicians managing CLD patients (36). On the other hand, at that time, noninvasive measures of fibrosis had not yet affected the utilization of liver biopsy in our health region, probably owing to their limited availability before 2003. Our data demonstrate that the introduction of noninvasive methods to assess liver fibrosis has impacted Canadian physicians' practices considering that 42.6% of respondents have reduced the number of liver biopsies performed by >50%.

Significant differences exist according to the etiology of liver disease. As such, liver biopsy is used significantly more in autoimmune/cholestatic patients compared with other types of CLDs. This most likely reflects the fact that liver biopsy remains important to diagnose the cause of liver disease in these patients, while for HBV and HCV the diagnosis is established by clinical information and serological tests. Although liver biopsy remains a major diagnostic tool to differentiate NASH from simple steatosis, liver biopsy is not used significantly more in NAFLD by Canadian physicians.

The most widely used noninvasive tool in Canada is Fibroscan, followed by Fibrotest. This finding is consistent with the most recommended noninvasive methods (4,21). Several surveyed physicians use magnetic resonance elastography as the primary tool for liver fibrosis assessment. This noninvasive method has recently shown excellent accuracy to diagnose liver fibrosis (24). However, it is costly, time consuming and has limited availability. Surprisingly, simple biomarkers, such as APRI, were used by only a minority of respondents. This can be explained by the fact that, although readily available and inexpensive, these biomarkers have significant lower diagnostic accuracy and higher rates of unclassified cases compared with sophisticated methods such as Fibroscan and Fibrotest (11,21). Interestingly, there is higher use of simple biomarkers in ALD versus HCV, in which Fibroscan is the predominant noninvasive method. This likely reflects the fact that the aspartate aminotransferase to alanine aminotranferase ratio, a simple and inexpensive biomarker, has long been known as a potential indicator of ALD (37,38).

Demographics and practice characteristics of surveyed physicians impact the diagnostic methods adopted. Older physicians use more noninvasive methods than younger respondents. Similarly, and contrary to our presurvey expectations, liver biopsy was used more often by the junior (years of practice) respondents versus senior physicians, who preferred noninvasive techniques, although this difference was not statistically significant. This may be due to a greater familiarity with the noninvasive methods and the ability to use them in clinical practice. Physicians based at a university hospital or practicing in private used more noninvasive tools than respondents based at a community hospital, likely reflecting easier access and availability of the noninvasive tools in these settings. Interestingly, surveyed physicians practicing in Ontario used Fibrotest more than any other Canadian province.

Most of the surveyed physicians demonstrate satisfaction with the accuracy of the currently available noninvasive methods for staging liver fibrosis. The implementation of noninvasive tools for liver fibrosis resulted in more patients treated with antiviral therapy for one-third of respondents. We speculate that access to and availability of noninvasive methods, which were the major concern for the surveyed physicians, represent a significant barrier to increasing the number of treated patients, given the critical role of liver fibrosis stage in guiding antiviral therapy in HCV and HBV patients. An additional barrier includes a lack of guidelines for use in clinical practice. The Asian Pacific Association for the Study of the Liver produced the only consensus recommendations on liver fibrosis in 2009 (39). At that time, the consensus statement read that clinical utility of noninvasive techniques would be proven by further studies in large numbers of patients. More recent guidelines on management of specific CLDs provide a

different perspective. As such, the European Association for the Study of the Liver (EASL) guidelines for HCV management state that, although liver biopsy remains the gold standard of reference, noninvasive methods can also be used (26). Similarly, the CASL guidelines state that acceptable methods to stage liver fibrosis include liver biopsy, Fibroscan and serum biomarkers (4). The EASL guidelines for HBV management state that a liver biopsy is often recommended to facilitate treatment decision (28). According to the CASL guidelines on HBV, clinicians should have access to transient elastography testing (5). In NAFLD, the AASLD guidelines recommend the use of a simple biomarker, the NAFLD fibrosis score, to direct patients at high risk for advanced fibrosis or NASH toward liver biopsy (14).

The variation in the strength of recommendation of noninvasive methods according to the etiology of CLDs and across different guidelines reflects the quality and number of validating studies and the local availability and reimbursement policy. Chronic hepatitis C is the etiology for which most studies have been conducted, and the abundance of data is reflected by the recommendation of implementing noninvasive tools.

Finally, reimbursement policy was a major concern for 14.4% of the respondents. While in France, *la Haute Autorité de Santé* has approved reimbursement for Fibroscan and Fibrotest since 2007, Fibroscan is currently reimbursed only in Quebec. However, work is in progress in British Columbia, Alberta, Ontario and Nova Scotia. Fibrotest is currently not reimbursed by any Canadian province.

Few studies have investigated physicians' practices regarding liver biopsy use and fibrosis assessment before our study. A French survey that interviewed 1177 general practitioners concluded that liver biopsy may be refused by up to 59% of patients with hepatitis C, and 22% of the physicians share the same concern due to the invasiveness of the procedure (40). Another survey performed at an American centre (41) showed that among 112 clinicians, 29.5% did not perform liver biopsy for the following reasons: concern about risks (72.7%); low reimbursement (66.7%); and logistical issues with space and recovery time (45.4%). Interestingly, in France, where noninvasive methods of liver fibrosis were first marketed and reimbursement policies have been implemented since 2007, a nationwide survey regarding assessment of liver fibrosis in hepatitis C among French hepatologists showed that liver biopsy is still systematically performed by only 4% of respondents (42). In agreement with our findings, this French study showed that updated guidelines for the use of noninvasive methods in clinical practice were required by 95% of respondents. Also, a survey by Ratziu et al (43) investigating diagnostic practices for NAFLD showed that in France, liver biopsy is rarely performed as a first-line diagnostic procedure and that the large majority use serum biomarkers or Fibroscan (43). The high rate of use of noninvasive methods in France reflects the high dissemination of knowledge and the presence of key opinion leaders in this area, which likely contributed to the implementation of these methods.

A limitation of our study was the relatively low response rate of 43.9%. This is similar to previous analogue surveys (43) but could bias the results because nonresponders may hold divergent views on some aspects of liver fibrosis practices and accuracy of noninvasive methods or have lower levels of overall interest in it. However, all responding and nonresponding physicians were active members of a scientific hepatogastroenterological or HIV society, thus forming a rather homogenous group in terms of training and medical interest. Also, the majority of respondents came from two provinces. The opinions and practices of physicians from the rest of Canada may, therefore, be under-represented. Nonetheless, the salient issues regarding fibrosis assessment faced by practitioners across the country are similar. Finally, we did not solicit responses from wider groups of physicians, including family medicine, infectious diseases and internal medicine specialists; therefore, there may be over- or underestimation of the use of noninvasive tests in these groups.

CONCLUSION

The present nationwide survey showed that most Canadian physicians who manage patients with CLDs adhere to current guidelines regarding the routine assessment of liver fibrosis. Although biopsy was the primary tool for fibrosis assessment for 50% of the surveyed physicians, noninvasive tools, particularly Fibroscan, have significantly reduced the need for liver biopsy in Canada. Limitations in access to/availability of the noninvasive tools represent a significant barrier. Finally, the present study emphasizes the need for 'ad hoc' clinical guidelines of use and an improved reimbursement policy to implement noninvasive methods to diagnose and stage fibrosis that will ultimately minimize costs and the use of liver biopsy in the Canadian health care system.

ACKNOWLEDGEMENTS: This work was supported by start-up operating funds from the Department of Medicine of McGill University and from the Research Institute of the McGill University Health Centre. GS holds a Chercheur-Boursier career award from the *Fonds de la Recherche en Santé du Quebéc* (FRSQ). MBK is supported by a *Chercheurs Nationaux* career award from the FRSQ. The authors are grateful to Ms Kathleen Rollet for the scientific contribution to the statistical analysis of the data.

CONTRIBUTIONS: GS contributed to the conception, study design, data, interpretation of the data and first draft of the article. PG, PW, MBK and MD contributed with data and interpretation of the data. RPM contributed to the conception, study design, data and interpretation of the data.

DISCLOSURES: GS has acted as speaker for Merck, Vertex, Gilead, served as an advisory board member for Boheringer Ingelheim and Novartis and has received research funding from Vertex. PG has acted as speaker for Merck, Vertex and Gilead and received research funding from Merck. PW has served as speaker and consultant for Bristol Myers Squibb, Gilead, Merck, Novartis, Roche, and as investigator for Merck, Novartis, Roche and Vertex. MBK has received honoraria and acted as a consultant for viiv, Gilead, Janssen and Merck and received research funding from Merck. MD has served as an advisory board member for Roche, Merck, Janssen, Vertex and Gilead. RPM has received consulting fees from Merck Canada Inc, Roche Canada, Genentech Inc, Johnson and Johnson, Norgine Ltd, GE Healthcare and Vertex, has served as speaker for Merck Canada Inc, Roche Canada, Vertex and KNS Canada, and has received research support from the Canadian Institutes for Health Research, Alberta Heritage Foundation for Medical Research (now Alberta Innovates-Health Solutions) and Echosens.

REFERENCES

1. Fleming KM, Aithal GP, Solaymani-Dodaran M, Card TR, West J. Incidence and prevalence of cirrhosis in the United Kingdom, 1992-2001: A general population-based study. J Hepatol 2008;49:732-8.
2. Kim WR, Brown RS Jr, Terrault NA, El-Serag H. Burden of liver disease in the United States: Summary of a workshop. Hepatology 2002;36:227-42.
3. Sanabria AJ, Dion R, Lucar E, Soto JC. Evolution of the determinants of chronic liver disease in Quebec. Chronic Dis Inj Can 2013;33:137-45.
4. Myers RP, Ramji A, Bilodeau M, Wong S, Feld JJ. An update on the management of hepatitis C: Consensus guidelines from the Canadian Association for the Study of the Liver. Can J Gastroenterol 2012;26:359-75.
5. Coffin CS, Fung SK, Ma MM; Canadian Association for the Study of the Liver. Management of chronic hepatitis B: Canadian Association for the Study of the Liver consensus guidelines. Can J Gastroenterol 2012;26:917-38.
6. Beaton MD. Current treatment options for nonalcoholic fatty liver disease and nonalcoholic steatohepatitis. Can J Gastroenterol 2012;26:353-7.
7. Kendall PRW. Public Health approach to alcohol policy: An updated report from the provincial health officer. National Library of Canada Cataloging in Publication Data, 2008.
8. Bedossa P, Dargere D, Paradis V. Sampling variability of liver fibrosis in chronic hepatitis C. Hepatology 2003;38:1449-57.
9. Friedman SL. Mechanisms of hepatic fibrogenesis. Gastroenterology 2008;134:1655-69.
10. Yano M, Kumada H, Kage M, et al. The long-term pathological evolution of chronic hepatitis C. Hepatology 1996;23:1334-40.
11. Sebastiani G, Alberti A. How far is noninvasive assessment of liver fibrosis from replacing liver biopsy in hepatitis C? J Viral Hepat 2012;19(Suppl 1):18-32.
12. de Franchis R. Revising consensus in portal hypertension: Report of the Baveno V consensus workshop on methodology of diagnosis and therapy in portal hypertension. J Hepatol 2010;53:762-8.
13. Pawlotsky JM. NS5A inhibitors in the treatment of hepatitis C. J Hepatol 2013;59:375-82.
14. Chalasani N, Younossi Z, Lavine JE, et al. The diagnosis and management of non-alcoholic fatty liver disease: Practice Guideline by the American Association for the Study of Liver Diseases, American College of Gastroenterology, and the American Gastroenterological Association. Hepatology 2012;55:2005-23.
15. Ratziu V, Bellentani S, Cortez-Pinto H, Day C, Marchesini G. A position statement on NAFLD/NASH based on the EASL 2009 special conference. J Hepatol 2010;53:372-84.
16. O'Shea RS, Dasarathy S, McCullough AJ. Alcoholic liver disease. Hepatology 2010;51:307-28.
17. EASL Clinical Practice Guidelines: Management of cholestatic liver diseases. J Hepatol 2009;51:237-67.
18. Manns MP, Czaja AJ, Gorham JD, et al. Diagnosis and management of autoimmune hepatitis. Hepatology 2010;51:2193-213.
19. Rockey DC, Caldwell SH, Goodman ZD, Nelson RC, Smith AD. Liver biopsy. Hepatology 2009;49:1017-44.
20. Wai CT, Greenson JK, Fontana RJ, et al. A simple noninvasive index can predict both significant fibrosis and cirrhosis in patients with chronic hepatitis C. Hepatology 2003;38:518-26.
21. Castera L. Noninvasive methods to assess liver disease in patients with hepatitis B or C. Gastroenterology 2012;142:1293-302; e1294.
22. Imbert-Bismut F, Ratziu V, Pieroni L, Charlotte F, Benhamou Y, Poynard T. Biochemical markers of liver fibrosis in patients with hepatitis C virus infection: A prospective study. Lancet 2001;357:1069-75.
23. Sandrin L, Fourquet B, Hasquenoph JM, et al. Transient elastography: A new noninvasive method for assessment of hepatic fibrosis. Ultrasound Med Biol 2003;29:1705-13.
24. Wang QB, Zhu H, Liu HL, Zhang B. Performance of magnetic resonance elastography and diffusion-weighted imaging for the staging of hepatic fibrosis: A meta-analysis. Hepatology 2012;56:239-47.
25. Cassinotto C, Lapuyade B, Ait-Ali A, et al. Liver fibrosis: Noninvasive assessment with acoustic radiation force impulse elastography – comparison with FibroScan M and XL probes and FibroTest in patients with chronic liver disease. Radiology 2013;269:283-92.
26. Craxi A. EASL Clinical practice guidelines: Management of hepatitis C virus infection. J Hepatol 2011;55:245-64.
27. Garcia-Tsao G, Friedman S, Iredale J, Pinzani M. Now there are many (stages) where before there was one: In search of a pathophysiological classification of cirrhosis. Hepatology 2010;51:1445-9.
28. EASL clinical practice guidelines: Management of chronic hepatitis B virus infection. J Hepatol 2012;57:167-85.
29. EASL clinical practical guidelines: Management of alcoholic liver disease. J Hepatol 2012;57:399-420.
30. Rosenthal E, Poiree M, Pradier C, et al. Mortality due to hepatitis C-related liver disease in HIV-infected patients in France (Mortavic 2001 study). AIDS 2003;17:1803-9.
31. Garcia-Ordonez MA, Colmenero JD, Jimenez-Onate F, Martos F, Martinez J, Juarez C. Diagnostic usefulness of percutaneous liver biopsy in HIV-infected patients with fever of unknown origin. J Infect 1999;38:94-98.
32. Myles A, Mugford GJ, Zhao J, Krahn M, Wang PP. Physicians' attitudes and practice toward treating injection drug users with hepatitis C: Results from a national specialist survey in Canada. Can J Gastroenterol 2011;25:135-9.
33. Bain VG, Wong WW, Greig PD, Yoshida EM. Hepatology and the Canadian gastroenterologist: Interest, attitudes and patterns of practice: Results of a national survey from the Canadian Association of Gastroenterology. Can J Gastroenterol 2003;17:25-9.

34. Colloredo G, Guido M, Sonzogni A, Leandro G. Impact of liver biopsy size on histological evaluation of chronic viral hepatitis: The smaller the sample, the milder the disease. J Hepatol 2003;39:239-44.

35. Wong JB, Koff RS. Watchful waiting with periodic liver biopsy versus immediate empirical therapy for histologically mild chronic hepatitis C. A cost-effectiveness analysis. Ann Intern Med 2000;133:665-75.

36. Myers RP, Fong A, Shaheen AA. Utilization rates, complications and costs of percutaneous liver biopsy: A population-based study including 4275 biopsies. Liver Int 2008;28:705-12.

37. Cohen JA, Kaplan MM. The SGOT/SGPT ratio – an indicator of alcoholic liver disease. Dig Dis Sci 1979;24:835-8.

38. Sorbi D, Boynton J, Lindor KD. The ratio of aspartate aminotransferase to alanine aminotransferase: Potential value in differentiating nonalcoholic steatohepatitis from alcoholic liver disease. Am J Gastroenterol 1999;94:1018-22.

39. Shiha G, Sarin SK, Ibrahim AE, et al. Liver fibrosis: Consensus recommendations of the Asian Pacific Association for the Study of the Liver (APASL). Hepatol Int 2009;3:323-33.

40. Bonny C, Rayssiguier R, Ughetto S, et al. [Medical practices and expectations of general practitioners in relation to hepatitis C virus infection in the Auvergne region]. Gastroenterol Clin Biol 2003;27:1021-5.

41. Muir AJ, Trotter JF. A survey of current liver biopsy practice patterns. J Clin Gastroenterol 2002;35:86-8.

42. Castera L, Denis J, Babany G, Roudot-Thoraval F. Evolving practices of non-invasive markers of liver fibrosis in patients with chronic hepatitis C in France: Time for new guidelines? J Hepatol 2007;46:528-529; author reply 529-530.

43. Ratziu V, Cadranel JF, Serfaty L, et al. A survey of patterns of practice and perception of NAFLD in a large sample of practicing gastroenterologists in France. J Hepatol 2012;57:376-83.

40

Practice and documentation of performance of colonoscopy in a central Canadian health region

Harminder Singh MD MPH[1,2,3,4,5], Lisa Kaita RN BN[3], Gerry Taylor MSc[3],
Zoann Nugent PhD[6], Charles Bernstein MD[1,2,3]

H Singh, L Kaita, G Taylor, Z Nugent, C Bernstein. Practice and documentation of performance of colonoscopy in a central Canadian health region. Can J Gastroenterol Hepatol 2014;28(4):185-190.

OBJECTIVE: To evaluate the reporting and performance of colonoscopy in a large urban centre.
METHODS: Colonoscopies performed between January and April 2008 in community hospitals and academic centres in the Winnipeg Regional Health Authority (Manitoba) were identified from hospital discharge databases and retrospective review of a random sample of identified charts. Information regarding reporting of colonoscopies (including bowel preparation, photodocumentation of cecum/ileum, size, site, characteristics and method of polyp removal), colonoscopy completion rates and follow-up recommendations was extracted. Colonoscopy completion rates were compared among different groups of physicians.
RESULTS: A total of 797 colonoscopies were evaluated. Several deficiencies in reporting were identified. For example, bowel preparation quality was reported in only 20%, the agent used for bowel preparation was recorded in 50%, photodocumentation of colonoscopy completion in 6% and polyp appearance (ie, pedunculated or not) in 34%, and polyp size in 66%. Although the overall colonoscopy completion rate was 92%, there was a significant difference among physicians with varying medical specialty training and volume of procedures performed. Recommendations for follow-up procedures (barium enema, computed tomography colonography or repeat colonoscopy) were recorded for a minority of individuals with reported poor bowel preparation or incomplete colonoscopy.
CONCLUSIONS: The present study found many deficiencies in reporting of colonoscopy in typical, city-wide clinical practices. Colonoscopy completion rates varied among different physician specialties. There is an urgent need to adopt standardized colonoscopy reporting systems in everyday practice and to provide feedback to physicians regarding deficiencies so they can be rectified.

Key Words: *Colonoscopy; Colonoscopy completion; Documentation*

L'exercice et la consignation de la coloscopie dans une région sanitaire du centre du Canada

OBJECTIF : Évaluer la consignation et l'exécution de la coloscopie dans un grand centre urbain.
MÉTHODOLOGIE : Les chercheurs ont extrait les coloscopies exécutées entre janvier et avril 2008 dans des centres hospitaliers communautaires et universitaires de l'Office régional de santé de Winnipeg, au Manitoba, contenues dans les bases de données des congés hospitaliers et l'analyse rétrospective d'un échantillon aléatoire de dossiers sélectionnés. Ils en ont tiré l'information relative à la consignation des coloscopies (y compris la préparation intestinale, la documentation photo du cæcum et de l'iléon, ainsi que la dimension, les caractéristiques et la méthode d'ablation des polypes), le taux d'achèvement des coloscopies et les recommandations de suivi. Ils ont comparé le taux d'achèvement des coloscopies entre les divers groupes de médecins.
RÉSULTATS : Au total, les chercheurs ont évalué 797 coloscopies, et ils ont repéré plusieurs lacunes de consignation. Par exemple, la qualité de la préparation intestinale était précisée dans 20 % des cas seulement, l'agent utilisé pour la préparation intestinale, dans 50 % des cas, la documentation photo de l'achèvement de la coloscopie, dans 6 % des cas, l'apparence des polypes (pédonculée ou non), dans 34 % des cas, et la dimension des polypes, dans 66 % des cas. Même si le taux global d'achèvement des coloscopies s'élevait à 92 %, il y avait des différences significatives entre médecins selon la spécialité et le volume d'interventions exécutées. Les recommandations sur les interventions de suivi (lavement baryté, coloscopie par tomodensitométrie ou reprise de la coloscopie) étaient consignées pour une minorité de patients dont la préparation était mauvaise ou la coloscopie, incomplète.
CONCLUSIONS : La présente étude a démontré plusieurs lacunes dans la consignation de la coloscopie au sein des pratiques cliniques urbaines ordinaires. Le taux d'achèvement des coloscopies variait selon les spécialités. Il est urgent d'adopter des systèmes standardisés de consignation des coloscopies dans la pratique quotidienne, de même que de souligner aux médecins les lacunes qui peuvent être rectifiées.

Colonoscopy has become the most commonly performed endoscopic procedure (1). The annual number of colonoscopies performed for both diagnostic and screening indications has increased rapidly as the population has grown older; the procedure has become preferred over radiology contrast imaging, and with increasing uptake of colorectal cancer (CRC) screening and surveillance (2). Irrespective of the initial test used for CRC screening, colonoscopy remains the essential final step in the screening and diagnosis of most CRCs and colon polyps.

Several studies, however, have reported that colonoscopy is much less effective in detecting proximal colon (ie, right-sided) CRCs than distal (ie, left-sided) CRCs (3-5). Several studies have also suggested that colonoscopy, as performed in usual clinical practice, is less effective in reducing CRC incidence and mortality due to proximal colon CRC than to distal colon CRC (4,6). However, other studies have reported a large reduction in subsequent incidence and mortality due to proximal colon CRC postcolonoscopy (7-9). The differences in the performance of colonoscopy by different health care providers may be responsible for these apparently inconsistent findings from different studies. While the biology of proximal and distal CRCs may be different, colonoscopy technique is considered to be an important cause of missed proximal colon lesions. This may be because of incomplete colonoscopies (not examining the entire proximal colon), lack of

[1]*Internal Medicine, University of Manitoba;* [2]*University of Manitoba IBD Clinical and Research Centre;* [3]*Winnipeg Regional Health Authority;*
[4]*CancerCare Manitoba, Department of Hematology and Oncology;* [5]*Community Health Sciences, University of Manitoba;* [6]*CancerCare Manitoba, Department of Epidemiology and Cancer Registry, Winnipeg, Manitoba*
Correspondence: Dr Harminder Singh, Section of Gastroenterology, University of Manitoba, 805-715 McDermot Avenue, Winnipeg, Manitoba R3E 3P4. e-mail singh@cc.umanitoba.ca

recognition of subtle lesions and/or poor bowel preparation. Hence, over the past decade, there has been an increasing emphasis on assessment and enhancement of colonoscopy performance (1,10).

We performed a retrospective review of reports of the colonoscopies performed in our large health care region to assess the performance and recording of colonoscopies in our region.

METHODS

Manitoba is a central Canadian province with a population of 1.25 million. Approximately two-thirds of the colonoscopies in the province are performed in the capital city of Winnipeg. The majority (85%) of the colonoscopies performed in the city are through the six hospitals and their affiliated endoscopy units, all of which are administered by a single regional health authority, the Winnipeg Regional Health Authority (WRHA). The current study was performed as a quality assessment and improvement project. The study was a practice audit performed for the WRHA's Medicine Standards Committee and was, therefore, exempt from ethics board review. Identifying information accessed by the WRHA Standards Committees and the audit teams are protected by law from disclosure to anyone, including WRHA management and administration.

All hospitals in Manitoba abstract admission and discharge information on outpatient (day surgery) endoscopies performed in hospitals, in addition to all inpatients. Hospital discharge abstracts are reported to Manitoba Health (MH), which reports to the Canadian Institute for Health Information. MH is the provincial agency with overall responsibility for health care in the entire province. In addition to submitting to MH, all hospitals in Winnipeg also submit hospital discharge abstracts to the WRHA, which maintains a decision support system to aid in the planning of the services in the city.

An electronic search of WRHA decision support system was performed to identify all individuals ≥16 years of age who underwent a lower gastrointestinal endoscopy at one of the six hospitals in Winnipeg between January 1 and March 31, 2008. The Canadian Classification of Interventions codes 1.NM.??.BA*, 2.NM.??.BA*, 1.NP.13.BA* and 2NK.??.BA.I were used to identify the lower gastrointestinal endoscopies. A random sample of 25% of the procedures performed in this time period was reviewed. Individuals identified in the chart review to have undergone previous colorectal surgery or flexible sigmoidoscopies instead of colonoscopies on the index date were excluded. However, the procedures reported as flexible sigmoidoscopy were included when the intent of the examination (determined from the review of the preprocedure information) was colonoscopy, but the procedure was stopped in the distal colon. For the individuals who underwent multiple colonoscopies, only the first colonoscopy performed in the study time period was included.

A trained, experienced nurse auditor abstracted information from the charts including patient demographics, comorbidities, indication for the procedures, laxative agent(s) used for bowel preparation, sedative agent and dose used, duration of the procedure, extent of the colon examined (as reported by the endoscopists), documentation of quality of bowel preparation on colonoscopy, documentation of colonic polyps, method of colonic polyp removal and follow-up recommendations, including that for those with incomplete colonoscopies, those with poor bowel preparation and polyps.

Statistical analysis

Results were tabulated using standard descriptive analyses. Fisher's exact test was used to compare differences in proportions. A priori, it was planned to compare colonoscopy reporting and completion rate between different groups of endoscopists (physician medical speciality, volume of procedures performed) and site of the procedure. Multivariate logistic regression analysis was performed to determine the association of physician medical speciality, volume of procedures performed or hospital site of the procedure with incomplete colonoscopies, with adjustment for patient age, sex, inpatient versus outpatient status and indication for the procedure (CRC screening/surveillance versus

diagnostic). There were correlations between volume of procedures performed, physician medical speciality and hospital site of endoscopy and, hence, to avoid multicolinearity, effect of physician medical speciality, volume of procedures performed and hospital site were assessed in separate models.

Because the number of colonoscopies performed by general practitioners was small, they were not included in the comparison between physician medical specialities. In addition, six cases, for which the end point reached during colonoscopy was not recorded, were excluded from the analysis of colonoscopy completion rate. In the primary analysis, the colonoscopy was considered to be complete when the end point reached was recorded to be the cecum, ileum or the ileocecal valve. Because visualization of the cecal pole is important to complete a colonoscopy and is not feasible in some cases, in sensitivity analyses, those with the recorded end point of ileocecal valve were considered to be incomplete colonoscopies. Overall colonoscopy completion rate and adjusted colonoscopy completion rate (excluding cases with mass lesions, strictures, and severe colitis from both the numerator and the denominator) were calculated.

RESULTS

A total of 797 patients (44% men; median age 59 years [interquartile range (IQR) 49 to 69 years]; 78% residents of Winnipeg) and their colonoscopies were included in the study. There were 65 (8%) inpatients and 239 (30%) were performed in one of the two teaching hospitals. Gastroenterologists performed 339 (43%) of the procedures, general surgeons 415 (52%) and general practitioners 43 (5%). Snare polypectomy was performed during 20% of the colonoscopies and biopsies during an additional 28%. A slightly higher proportion of colonoscopies performed for individuals >50 years of age were accompanied by snare polypectomy (24%).

The most common recorded comorbidities included hypertension (26%), diabetes (14%), obesity (9 %), previous diagnosis of any cancer (8%), coronary artery disease (6%) and asthma (6%).

Indications for the procedures

Of the 732 colonoscopies performed on outpatients, 25% (n=183) were performed for CRC screening and/or surveillance, but only 2% were recorded to be performed for primary, average-risk CRC screening. Other CRC screening/surveillance indications included family history of CRC (17%), a personal history of colon polyps (12%), positive fecal occult blood test (5%) and family history of colon polyps (1%). The most common symptoms for outpatient colonoscopy included rectal bleeding (20%), abdominal pain (11%), anemia (9%), diarrhea (7%), inflammatory bowel disease (4%) and change in bowel habits (4%).

The most common indications for colonoscopies for hospitalized inpatients included rectal bleeding (42%), diarrhea (21%), anemia (18%) and abdominal pain (15%).

Of the 74 colonoscopies performed for diarrhea, one-third (n=25) did not have a biopsy performed.

Agents used for bowel preparation before the colonoscopy

Five hospitalized patients underwent colonoscopy for rectal bleeding without bowel preparation. For another nine (1% [all outpatients]), there was no documentation as to whether bowel preparation was used. Of the remaining 783 procedures, the specific agent used was recorded for only 388 (49.6%). Sodium picosulfate was the most common agent used (67%), followed by polyethylene glycol 3350 with electrolytes oral solution (20%) and, for the remainder of cases, varying combinations of oral phospho soda, magnesium citrate, enemas and bisacodyl (oral or rectal) were used.

Quality of bowel preparation during colonoscopy

A vast majority (80%) of cases did not have documentation regarding the quality of the bowel preparation in the report, with wide variation among the six hospitals, but not between gastroenterologists and general surgeons or according to volume of procedures performed (Table 1).

The documentation was not limited to cases with poor bowel preparation because two-thirds of the cases in which quality of bowel preparation was recorded were rated to have adequate, good or excellent preparation.

The colonoscopy completion rate was 89% for the cases with recorded quality of bowel preparation during colonoscopy: 71% for those with poor preparation and 100% for those with excellent preparation. Of cases with poor preparation and complete colonoscopy, 36% were reported to have colonic polyps.

Sedation

A majority (99%) of the procedures were performed using midazolam and/or fentanyl (97% both drugs). Only four procedures were performed without sedation and another four received propofol. Most individuals (68%) received between 3 mg and 5 mg of midazolam and 50 µg to 100 µg of fentanyl (referred to as the 'usual dose' in the present study), with a median dose of 5 mg for midazolam and 100 µg for fentanyl.

Although there was no difference between the gastroenterologists and general surgeons with regard to the use of more than the usual dose of sedation, a higher proportion of procedures performed by gastroenterologist involved lower-than-usual doses (4% versus 12% for general surgeons; P<0.001). A higher proportion of incomplete colonoscopies received lower than the usual dose (23% versus 5%; P<0.001).

Colonoscopy completion rate

Photographic documentation of the cecum and/or ileum was recorded in 6% of cases and ileal biopsy was obtained in an additional 5%. For the remainder of the cases, the authors had to rely on self-reported end points. Of note, equipment for photodocumentation was available at all sites during the time period the colonoscopies in the study were performed.

The most common reasons listed for the 65 incomplete colonoscopies were: poor bowel preparation (22%); inability to advance because of patient discomfort (14%); patient safety (11%); and/or looping of the colonoscope (8%).

The overall colonoscopy completion rate was 92% (726 of 791 cases) and the adjusted colonoscopy completion rate was 94% (722 of 772 cases). After excluding cases with documented poor bowel preparation, the adjusted colonoscopy completion rate was 95% (686 of 723 cases). Considering the cases in which the recorded end point reached was the ileocecal valve as incomplete colonoscopies, the overall colonoscopy completion rate was 89% (703 of 791) and adjusted colonoscopy completion rate was 91% (700 of 772 cases).

The inpatients had a lower colonoscopy completion rate, as did the procedures performed by general surgeons (Table 2). There was no significant difference with regard to age, sex or indication of the procedure (CRC screening/surveillance versus diagnostic). There was a significant difference in colonoscopy completion rates among the different hospitals, with a higher proportion of the procedures performed by general surgeons at the hospitals with a lower completion rate. When the cases with the reported end point of ileocecal valve were included among the incomplete colonoscopies, the difference between gastroenterologists and general surgeons was larger (overall colonoscopy completion rate: general surgeons 84%, gastroenterologists 94%; adjusted colonoscopy completion rate: general surgeons 86%, gastroenterologists 97%; P<0.001 for both comparisons). The colonoscopy completion rate was higher for the group of endoscopists with higher procedure volume (Table 2). Of the 42 endoscopy physicians included in the present study, 10 with the lowest completion rate (eight general surgeons) performed 55% of the incomplete colonoscopies; the colonoscopy completion rate among these physicians ranged between 76% and 86%. In the multivariate analysis, the difference among hospitals, physician medical specialities and according to procedure volume persisted (Table 3).

TABLE 1
Documentation of quality of bowel preparation during colonoscopy performed in Winnipeg (Manitoba) hospitals between January 1 and March 31, 2008

	Proportion of cases with no documentation of quality of bowel preparation during colonoscopy, %	P
Hospital site		<0.001
A	94	
B	76	
C	70	
D	58	
E	83	
F	85	
Physician medical speciality		1.00
General surgery	80	
Gastroenterology	79	
Volume of procedures performed*		0.43
Quartile 1 (<16 procedures)	79	
Quartile 2 (17–21 procedures)	84	
Quartile 3 (22–25 procedures)	82	
Quartile 4 (>25 procedures)	78	

*Quartiles were defined by number of physicians, which were 11, 11, 10 and 10 in the four groups, respectively. The volume of procedures was based on the colonoscopies included in the study, which would translate to annualized procedure volume quartiles of <256, 272 to 336, 352 to 400, and >400 per year

Duration of procedure

The median duration of colonoscopy (without biopsy or polypectomy) was 14 min (IQR 10 min to 20 min) and for incomplete colonoscopies was 21 min (IQR 12 min to 26 min). The withdrawal time was not documented for any cases.

The median duration of patient stay at the hospitals from admission to discharge for outpatients was 2.9 h (IQR 2.5 h to 3.4 h).

Polyp findings

Thirty-one percent (n=250) of the cases were documented to have colonic polyps and 3.3% (n=26) had suspected CRC. Of the 401 polyps reported in the study, 66% (n=263) had comments regarding their size; among the 250 patients with polyps, size was mentioned for 72% (n=180). There was no mention of colonic site for 2% of the polyps and, for another 6%, the polyp site was mentioned as a distance from the anal verge. There was no mention as to how 10% of the polyps were managed; 41% were removed with a snare, 33% with biopsy, 11% with hot biopsy and 5% were cauterized. For only 34% of the polyps, there was mention as to whether the polyps were sessile, flat or pedunculated.

Complications

A reversal agent for sedation was used in a single case and two patients experienced vasovagal episodes.

Follow-up recommendations

Of the 52 cases with documented poor bowel preparation, recommendations for follow-up procedures (barium enema, computed tomography colonography or repeat colonoscopy) were recorded for 21% (n=11). Similarly, of the 50 cases with incomplete colonoscopy and no structural lesions, 50% (n=25) had recommendations for follow-up procedures recorded.

Of the 250 cases with polyps, no follow-up recommendations were recorded for 28% (n=69). Follow-up was considered to include scheduling an office visit to discuss pathology, follow-up colonoscopy or simply a mention that follow-up would be decided based on the pathology results. Of the 53 cases with one or two low-risk polyps (<1 cm in size

TABLE 2
Overall and adjusted colonoscopy completion rates, stratified according to type of procedure, indication of procedure, patient characteristics and site of the procedure for colonoscopies performed in Winnipeg (Manitoba) hospitals between January 1 and March 31, 2008

| | Colonoscopy | | | | |
Variable	Total number	Overall completion rate, %	P	Adjusted colonoscopy completion rate, %	P
Colonoscopy with or without additional procedures			0.08		0.01
Colonoscopy alone	416	90		91	
Colonoscopy with biopsy	219	95		97	
Colonoscopy with polypectomy	156	92		95	
Outpatient versus inpatient			<0.01		0.02
Outpatient	729	93		94	
Inpatient	62	76		85	
Patient age, years			0.24		0.87
<50	211	94		94	
≥50	580	91		93	
Patient sex			0.70		0.66
Male	352	92		94	
Female	439	91		93	
Sex and age, years			0.55		0.84
Male <50	91	96		96	
Female <50	120	93		92	
Male ≥50	261	91		93	
Female ≥50	319	91		93	
Procedure indication			0.17		0.39
Colorectal cancer screening/surveillance	182	95		95	
Diagnostic	609	91		93	
Hospital site			0.03		0.02
A	124	87		89	
B	99	87		88	
C	124	94		97	
D	115	92		93	
E	114	92		94	
F	215	96		97	
Physician medical speciality			<0.01		<0.01
Gastroenterology	337	96		97	
General surgery	411	89		91	
Volume of procedures performed*			<0.01		<0.01
Quartile 1 (<16 procedures)	73	89		89	
Quartile 2 (17–21 procedures)	156	87		89	
Quartile 3 (22–25 procedures)	180	90		92	
Quartile 4 (>25 procedures)	382	95		96	

*Quartiles were defined by number of physicians, which were 11, 11, 10 and 10 in the four groups, respectively. The volume of procedures is based on the colonoscopies included in the study, which would translate to annualized procedure volume quartiles of <256, 272 to 336, 352 to 400, and >400 per year

and no villous features or high-grade dysplasia on the subsequent pathology report) and a recommendation for follow-up colonoscopy, colonoscopy was recommended within five years for 58% (n=31).

DISCUSSION

The present study suggests that overall, the colonoscopy completion rate in the WRHA was within the recommended range in 2008, albeit at the lower limit and less than that reported in other major centres (11). However, completion rates are only one aspect of measuring the adequacy of colonoscopy. There were considerable differences between different groups of physicians performing the colonoscopy. There were several deficiencies in reporting, including quality of the bowel preparation, photodocumentation, polyp characteristics and follow-up recommendations. Many individuals with small colonic polyps were recommended surveillance colonoscopies at short intervals.

The recommended overall colonoscopy completion rate is at least 90% (10,11). In our study, the gastroenterologists, as a group, had an overall colonoscopy completion rate of 96%. Several other series involving expert endoscopists have also reported higher completion rates (11). Our study results from a large city wide practice suggest that overall colonoscopy completion rates >95% are achievable in usual clinical practice. Therefore, based on our study results and those of previous studies, and to ensure that most patients receive high-quality care, we believe the minimum acceptable overall colonoscopy completion rate should be immediately increased to >95%.

The wide variation in colonoscopy performance, including colonoscopy completion rates among different gastroenterologists versus surgical endsocopists, is potentially contributing to the variation in CRC incidence and mortality after performance of colonoscopy. This includes differences between proximal and distal colonic CRC cancer protection afforded by colonoscopy as well as in terms of interval cancers, all of which have been reported by us for colonoscopies performed in Manitoba (3,6,12).

Although the 31% polyp detection rate in our study was greater than the recommended adenoma detection rate of 25% for men and

15% for women (10) (and similar to the equivalent polyp detection rate of 40% and 30%, respectively, among men and women [13]), the poor recording of polyp characteristics is surprising. The follow-up for polyps is dependent on their size, which must be dependent on the assessment during colonoscopy for polyps resected piecemeal. In addition, the management of polyps found to be malignant on pathology assessments is different for pedunculated polyps (colonoscopic polypectomy is considered to be adequate and full treatment, if the histology is favourable) and nonpedunculated polyps (surgery must be considered for most).

The follow-up recommendations recorded in our study suggest many individuals may not be obtaining appropriate follow-up (no follow-up for incomplete colonoscopy or colonoscopy with poor bowel preparation) or surveillance colonoscopy at short intervals for those with low-risk polyps.

Our study highlights the need for standardized training, and clinical practice and colonoscopy reporting templates. Endoscopists should be provided with report cards detailing their colonoscopy completion rates and adequacy of procedure documentation. If one completes a colonoscopy to the cecum, but the bowel preparation was very poor, it has very different implications for outcomes and future plans. An electronic endoscopy reporting system with mandatory data entry fields would facilitate better recording of findings on colonoscopy, follow-up recommendations and generation of report cards for individual physicians. Regular provision of report cards to endoscopists has been associated with improved colonoscopy quality indicators (14) including colonoscopy completion rates (15). Alternatively, especially when electronic endoscopy reporting systems are not financially feasible, endoscopists could be mandated to participate in practice audit programs such as those offered by the Canadian Association of Gastroenterology, which provide feedback to individual endoscopists. However, such practice audit programs do not provide individual endoscopist-level data to the directors of endoscopy units and, therefore, do not allow for discussion among individual endoscopists and their unit directors, as may be necessary when feedback does not lead to practice change.

In the absence of independent verification of colonoscopy preparation quality, a report of 'poor prep' may be justification for – rather than the cause of – an incomplete colonoscopy. Therefore, the proportion of colonoscopies with reported poor colonoscopy preparation should be monitored as one of the colonoscopy quality measures. In addition, because of the possibility of attempts to 'game' the system by reporting 'poor prep' when the colonoscopy cannot be completed, we believe when colonoscopy quality measures are regularly recorded and reported, it is preferable to report on overall colonoscopy completion rates.

In 2008, an endoscopy redesign initiative was introduced by the WRHA internal medicine and surgery programs to streamline and standardize the delivery of the endoscopy services in Winnipeg. Our study results have provided background information on the practice patterns for the proposals submitted and currently pending with the provincial government for improving delivery and documentation of endoscopy services in the city, and for facilitating individual physician feedback as a nonthreatening learning and information tool.

Our results should be interpreted in the context of study strengths and limitations. The present study was an evaluation of a city-wide practice of a large number of endoscopists (n=42). Because the analysis was performed retrospectively, there was no incentive for the physicians to modify their usual clinical practices in response to observations (Hawthorne effect, which may skew actual practice). This was a chart review rather than an analysis of administrative claims data, in which the reporting of colonoscopy completion may be altered if the reimbursements are linked to the reported colonoscopy completion. We were able to incorporate intent of the procedures and, hence, the colonoscopies that were reported as flexible sigmoidoscopies were considered to be incomplete. However, because several potential predictors of interest (physician medical specialty, place of practice and procedure volumes) correlated with one another (general surgeons

TABLE 3
Multivariate logistic regression analysis for overall incomplete colonoscopies performed in Winnipeg (Manitoba) hospitals between January 1 and March 31, 2008

Variable*	Adjusted OR† (95% CI)
Physician medical specialty	
General surgery	3.19 (1.68–6.07)
Gastroenterology	Reference
Hospital site	
A	3.20 (1.35–7.59)
B	3.27 (1.33–8.04)
C	1.41 (0.52–3.96)
D	2.29 (0.89–5.91)
E	1.61 (0.60–4.30)
F	Reference
Volume of procedures performed‡	
Quartile 1 (<16 procedures)	2.91 (1.19–7.12)
Quartile 2 (17–21 procedures)	3.37 (1.71–6.62)
Quartile 3 (22–25 procedures)	2.30 (1.15–4.60)
Quartile 4 (>25 procedures)	Reference

Separate models were developed for physician medical specialty, hospital site and volume of procedures performed; †Adjusted for patient age, sex, inpatient versus outpatient status and indication of the procedure (colorectal cancer screening/surveillance versus diagnostic); ‡Quartiles were defined by number of physicians, which were 11, 11, 10 and 10 in the four groups, respectively. The volume of procedures is based on the colonoscopies included in the study, which would translate to annualized procedure volume quartiles of <256, 272 to 336, 352 to 400, and >400 per year

performed lower volume of procedures at certain hospitals), we were unable to determine the independent effect of some of these factors. Nevertheless, this does not limit the most important interpretation of our results in that there are significant differences among physicians with regard to reporting of colonoscopy and colonoscopy completion rates. Further improvement and education efforts should focus on individual physicians rather than groups of physicians because there is likely a difference, even within the different groups. We did not have a sufficient number of procedures per endoscopist to be able to provide stable individual estimates, which will be feasible only when data are collected electronically. Our colonoscopy completion rate calculations were based on individual physician reporting rather than photodocumentation. Our estimate of the effect of procedure volume was based on the colonoscopies randomly included in the study, which, however, does correlate with the annual volume of endoscopic procedures performed (data not shown). We have reported on colonoscopies performed several years ago and it is possible that practice patterns have changed regarding endoscopy in Winnipeg; however, considering that reporting methods have not changed across the entire region and our personal practice review of contemporary reports suggests they are still lacking, we do not believe the passage of five years would have markedly altered the data.

CONCLUSION

The present study demonstrated that, while recommended colonoscopy completion rates were being achieved by most physicians (of various backgrounds) in usual clinical practice in 2008, there were significant variations among different groups of physicians and some individual physicians may have much lower colonoscopy completion rates. Poor colonoscopy reporting is extremely common in usual clinical practice. There is an urgent need for adoption of standardized mandatory reporting systems.

DISCLOSURES: There are no conflicts of interest for any of the authors. HS, LK and GT were involved in the study concept and design; acquisition of data; analysis and interpretation of data and critical revision of the manuscript for important intellectual content. ZN was involved in data analysis. CB was involved in interpretation of data and critical revision of the manuscript. All authors read and approved the final manuscript. The results and conclusions are those of the authors, and no official endorsement by WRHA is intended or should be inferred.

REFERENCES

1. Lieberman D. How good is your dentist? How good is your endoscopist? The quality imperative. Gastroenterology 2012;142:194-6.
2. Singh H, Demers AA, Xue L, et al. Time trends in colon cancer incidence and distribution and lower gastrointestinal endoscopy utilization in Manitoba. Am J Gastroenterol 2008;103:1249-56.
3. Singh H, Nugent Z, Demers AA, et al. Rate and predictors of early/missed colorectal cancers after colonoscopy in Manitoba: A population-based study. Am J Gastroenterol 2010;105:2588-96.
4. Baxter NN, Goldwasser MA, Paszat LF, et al. Association of colonoscopy and death from colorectal cancer. Ann Intern Med 2009;150:1-8.
5. Baxter NN, Sutradhar R, Forbes SS, et al. Analysis of administrative data finds endoscopist quality measures associated with postcolonoscopy colorectal cancer. Gastroenterology 2011;140:65-72.
6. Singh H, Nugent Z, Mahmud SM, et al. Predictors of colorectal cancer after negative colonoscopy: A population-based study. Am J Gastroenterol 2010;105:663-73.
7. Brenner H, Chang-Claude J, Seiler CM, et al. Protection from colorectal cancer after colonoscopy: A population-based, case-control study. Ann Intern Med 2011;154:22-30.
8. Baxter NN, Warren JL, Barrett MJ, et al. Association between colonoscopy and colorectal cancer mortality in a US cohort according to site of cancer and colonoscopist specialty. J Clin Oncol 2012;30:2664-9.
9. Nishihara R, Wu K, Lochhead P, et al. Long-term colorectal-cancer incidence and mortality after lower endoscopy. N Engl J Med 2013;369:1095-105.
10. Rex DK, Petrini JL, Baron TH, et al. Quality indicators for colonoscopy. Am J Gastroenterol 2006;101:873-85.
11. Rabeneck L, Rumble RB, Axler J, et al. Cancer Care Ontario colonoscopy standards: Standards and evidentiary base. Can J Gastroenterol 2007;21(Suppl D):5D-24D.
12. Singh H, Nugent Z, Demers AA, et al. The reduction in colorectal cancer mortality after colonoscopy varies by site of the cancer. Gastroenterology 2010;139:1128-37.
13. Fayad NF, Kahi CJ. Quality measures for colonoscopy: A critical evaluation. Clin Gastroenterol Hepatol 2013 pii:S1542-3565(13)01465-1 (Epub ahead of print).
14. Lin OS, Kozarek RA, Arai A, et al. The effect of periodic monitoring and feedback on screening colonoscopy withdrawal times, polyp detection rates, and patient satisfaction scores. Gastrointest Endosc 2010;71:1253-9.
15. Kahi CJ, Ballard D, Shah AS, et al. Impact of a quarterly report card on colonoscopy quality measures. Gastrointest Endosc 2013;77:925-31.

41

E-mail communication in the management of gastroenterology patients: A review

Ian Plener MD[1], Andrew Hayward MD[1], Fred Saibil MD[1,2]

I Plener, A Hayward, F Saibil. E-mail communication in the management of gastroenterology patients: A review. Can J Gastroenterol Hepatol 2014;28(3):161-165.

E-mail correspondence between physicians and patients can be a useful tool to improve communication efficiency, provide economic and ecological benefits, improve therapeutic interventions and adherence, and enhance self-management. The model of self-management in chronic disease has become an integral component of North American and British medicine. From a practical standpoint, the use of e-mail between physicians and patients can complement the self-management model.

E-mail communication has many benefits from both patient and physician perspectives. E-mail contact reduces the inefficiencies associated with telecommunications. Physicians are able to better document out-of-office patient encounters and provide access to specialist care for patients in remote locations. This use of e-mail has the potential to increase patient safety through physician approval of self-manager actions, including earlier initiation of needed treatments. Fewer clinic visits afford additional time for new consultations and sicker patients, reducing the overall burden on referral and wait times.

The present article reviews some of the literature regarding physician-patient e-mail communication in the general ambulatory setting, in the context of chronic disease and with a specific focus on inflammatory bowel disease (IBD). The authors provide a framework for the use of e-mail communication in the IBD population, with emphasis on the concept of e-mail use. Also illustrated are the benefits and disadvantages, and examples of the e-mail contract as proposed by the Canadian Medical Protective Association. Examples of specific e-mail communication topics are provided for several IBD scenarios. Potential negative consequences of this mode of communication are also discussed.

Key Words: *Electronic mail; E-mail; Inflammatory bowel disease; Patient-physician communication; Self-management*

Les communications par courriel dans la prise en charge des patients en gastroentérologie

Les correspondances par courriel entre médecins et patients peuvent être utiles pour améliorer l'efficacité des communications, présenter des avantages d'ordre économique et écologique, accroître les interventions et l'observance thérapeutiques et améliorer l'autogestion. Le modèle d'autogestion des maladies chroniques fait désormais partie intégrante de la médecine nord-américaine et britannique. Sur le plan pratique, les courriels entre médecins et patients peuvent compléter ce modèle.

Les communications par courriel comportent de nombreux avantages pour les patients et les médecins. Ainsi, elles réduisent les inefficacités associées aux télécommunications. Les médecins sont mieux en mesure de répertorier les conseils aux patients hors du cabinet et d'offrir des soins spécialisés aux patients des régions éloignées. Cette utilisation des courriels peut accroître la sécurité des patients, car les médecins peuvent approuver leurs mesures d'autogestion, y compris l'amorce plus rapide de traitements nécessaires. La diminution du nombre de rendez-vous en cliniques dégage du temps pour les nouvelles consultations et les patients plus malades et réduit le fardeau global des aiguillages et des temps d'attente.

Le présent article présente une analyse bibliographique partielle des communications par courriel entre médecins et patients en milieu ambulatoire en cas de maladies chroniques, notamment les maladies inflammatoires de l'intestin (MII). Les auteurs présentent un cadre d'utilisation des communications par courriel au sein de la population atteinte de MII et s'attardent sur le concept d'utilisation des courriels. Ils en exposent également les avantages et les inconvénients et donnent des exemples du contrat d'utilisation des courriels proposé par l'Association canadienne de protection médicale. Ils proposent aussi des exemples de sujets de communications par courriel dans quelques scénarios liés aux MII. Ils abordent enfin le potentiel de conséquences négatives de ce mode de communication.

E-mail correspondence is a universal mode of communication; however, its implementation in medical practice is not widespread. According to Statistics Canada data from 2010, 80% of individuals >16 years of age used the Internet for personal use, from home, work or elsewhere (1). Of those, 64% conducted online searches for medical or health-related information (1). Increasingly, patients now use the Internet to access health web sites and physician web pages (2,3). Internet statistics in the United States indicate that e-mail has become the main form of communication for >90% of users (4). According to a Harris Online poll conducted in 2005, 70% of online adults in the United States wanted to be able to e-mail their doctors and, of those, 37% were willing to pay out-of-pocket to compensate physicians for this service (5,6). Additionally, there has been a significant increase in patient demand for e-mail contact with their physicians (7,8). E-mail has been evaluated as an avenue for communication between physicians and patients/caregivers for its potential benefits in improving service efficiency, cost savings, improvements to patient outcomes, ecological benefits and enhancement of self-management programs in chronic disease. As far back as 1994, the majority of patients from two studies in family practice and internal medicine regarded e-mail communication as a means to improved efficiency, access to medical care, and convenient for employees and students (9). Couchman et al (9) reported that 90% of surveyed patients in the ambulatory setting were interested in using e-mail for prescription refills, 78% in scheduling appointments, 87% in booking nonurgent consultations and 84% in obtaining diagnostic test results. However, the health care industry has been cautious in accepting this medium. In 1998, only 7% of American physicians e-mailed their patients (10). In a review of health care provided to university students in Finland, the volume of e-mail correspondence averaged 7.7 e-mails per patient per month (3,11). In this population, similar to many primary care scenarios, e-mail communication was used for nonurgent matters. More recently, however, American studies demonstrate that e-mail communication use among physicians has increased to 16% in primary

[1]*Department of Medicine, University of Toronto;* [2]*Division of Gastroenterology, Sunnybrook Health Sciences Centre, Toronto, Ontario*
Correspondence and reprints: Dr Fred Saibil, Sunnybrook Health Sciences Centre, 2075 Bayview Avenue, Room H-52, Toronto, Ontario M4N 3M5.
e-mail fred.saibil@utoronto.ca

```
┌─────────────────────────────────────────────┐
│          BOX 1: E-mail management*          │
│         Advantages to e-mail management     │
├─────────────────────────────────────────────┤
```

BOX 1: E-mail management*

Advantages to e-mail management

Enhanced convenience of communication outside of traditional office hours (30).

Improved documentation, correspondence audits and confirmation with read receipts.

Valuable written reference for the patient, improving information recall and providing evidence of the communication (6,32).

Improves physician accessibility for nonurgent communications (14).

Reliable communication modality for patients with disabilities.

Effective communication with patients who are temporarily traveling abroad, away for study or in remote communities.

Efficient and potentially minimizes cost of information delivery to patients (26).

Adjunct to self-management paradigm to free up clinic resources for sicker patients.

Disadvantages to e-mail management

Patient and physician concerns about privacy, confidentiality and potential misuse of information (7).

Physicians' concern regarding possibly increased, nonremunerated workload (32).

Patients' expectations regarding timely replies may be problematic (9,12).

Impersonal nature of email communication (16).

Potential misuse of email for urgent clinical matters (9).

Economics of implementing secure, encrypted web-based servers.

Medico-legal issues, including informed consent (33).

Technological glitches (eg, redirect back to sender, unintended recipients) (31).

Successful Implementation

Integrate a secure, encrypted, confidential web messaging system.

Discussions with patients regarding appropriate use of e-mail and legal implications (obtain informed consent).

Standardized e-mail contract in accordance with CMPA (25).

Select patients suitable for email communication and establish expectations (34).

Monitor level of usage – prescription renewals, appointment bookings, management dialogue

Establish mechanism for tracking and following up on e-mail misuse.

Numbers in parentheses refer to references

BOX 2: Sample e-mail dialogues for inflammatory bowel disease patients

Patient: colitis flaring; doubled my 5-ASA.

Gastroenterologist: good; report in 5-7 days; if no recent antibiotics/travel, and not getting better, start pred 40 mg daily – if you go on pred, tell us and my secretary will give you an apptmt (CC email to secretary)

Patient: think I've got another blockage, bloated, cramps, no BMs

Gastroenterologist: clear fluids only x 36 h, then try to progress diet; report in 48 h to 72 h

Patient: on azathioprine; had blood test yesterday

Gastroenterologist: test fine; repeat 3 mths

Patient: do you have my colonoscopy results?

Gastroenterologist: all biopsies fine; repeat in 2 yrs, but see you in 1 yr

ASA Aminosalicylic acid; BMs Bowel movements; mths Months; yr Year(s)

care, and as much as 72% in large outpatient settings (5). As with any form of new communication, transformation takes time. While telephone contact was initially met with some resistance, physicians now regularly use telephones, pagers and faxes.

E-MAIL USE IN PRIMARY CARE

E-mail communication between patients and health care professionals can take several forms as an adjunct to in-person consultation. Primary care physicians and their patients have demonstrated a preference for e-mail over telephone consultations for nonurgent matters such as uncomplicated urinary tract infections, chronic back pain, sore throats, hypercholesterolemia and Pap smear results (12-16). Patients and physicians managing primary care issues have endorsed e-mail use for many years (16). E-mail has also been used to optimize adherence and compliance to treatment, through communicating reminders to patients, as well as inquiries regarding medication side effects and treatment duration (17). Furthermore, e-mail use in the form of patient follow-ups (eg, after an initial appointment), when clarification or additional information may be required or before an office visit for medical updates may be beneficial (14,15,18). Physician-patient e-mail may also be used to notify patients of instructions in preparation for tests or to acquire screening information using a questionnaire.

E-MAIL USE IN CHRONIC DISEASE MANAGEMENT

E-mail can play a valuable role in enhancing the management of chronic diseases by improving continuity of care while allowing health care professionals flexibility in responding to nonurgent issues, with the side benefit of affording consultation time for sicker patients

(12,18). The model of self-management in chronic disease has become an integral component of North American and British medicine (7). Successful self-managers are now commonplace in the setting of reactive airway disease, type II diabetes mellitus, congestive heart failure, recurrent urinary tract infections, chronic obstructive pulmonary disease and long-term anticoagulation (19,20). Patients with inflammatory bowel disease (IBD) have also been successfully managed using this paradigm (21). E-mail correspondence between physicians and patients improves communication efficiency, leads to more rapid therapeutic interventions, improves compliance and adherence to therapeutic regimens, provides economic and ecological benefits, and enhances the self-management model.

Innovative physician-patient communication methods, such as e-mail, can help confront the issue of increasing wait times, provide patients in remote communities with easy access to specialist care and reduce office inefficiencies. We believe that the use of e-mail between physicians and patients provides a useful adjunct to the self-management model in chronic disease (Box 1).

E-MAIL USE IN GASTROENTEROLOGY

Little has been published related to the use of e-mail in the field of gastroenterology. With respect to patients with irritable bowel syndrome, patients' expectations regarding the quality and quantity of communication with their physician is paramount (5). E-mail communication may serve as a useful adjunct to provide patients with additional educational content, detailed explanations of their condition, serve to answer follow-up questions and enhance appointment scheduling (5). In an overwhelming majority of patients, the above are essential qualities that contribute to overall patient experience and their opinion of their gastroenterologist (5). To our knowledge, e-mail communication has not been studied in other areas of gastroenterology.

E-MAIL USE IN IBD

There is a paucity of literature regarding e-mail communication in the management of IBD. Specifically related to IBD, Cross and Finklestein (22) advanced the self-management paradigm with a study focusing on the feasibility of home telemanagement for patients. Telemanagement may be helpful in selected patients; however, e-mail requires only a computer and Internet access. For the past seven years, the senior author of the present article (FS) has been using e-mail to support self-managers. The integration of e-mail into the self-management paradigm has clear benefits in Canadian health care and should be applicable to all health care models (21) (Box 2).

IBD self-managers may also benefit from reassurance, via e-mail, when experiencing minor flares. A randomized controlled trial conducted by Kennedy et al (23) assessed quality of life, health service resource use and patient satisfaction in 700 patients after 12 months of implementing a self-management approach. Self-managers had fewer hospital visits without increases in primary care visits, an improvement in quality of life and reduction in anxiety (23). Based on a

---

BOX 3: Sample e-mail history form, with replies for new patient in italics

Have you ever been hospitalized overnight for anything? Any operations? Why? *Yes, in 1978 for bladder reflux surgery.*

Describe your problem – **if** you are having any gastro-intestinal symptoms, or say "none". *Cramping in lower abdomen, alternating between diarrhea and constipation, red blood in stool, gassy and bloated abdomen. Sore to touch and fatigue.*

Do you smoke? How much and for how many years? Quit? For how many per year? *Yes, quit approximately 2 months ago. Smoked since a teenager.*

Do you drink alcohol? How many beers/glasses of wine/drinks of liquor a day or a week or a month? Please reply for each type of beverage. *I do not consume alcohol. Never have.*

How's your appetite? Have you lost any weight recently? How much? On purpose? Still losing? *Appetite varies. Hunger to nausea. No significant weight loss or gain.*

Any trouble swallowing? Nausea? Vomiting? Heartburn or indigestion? If yes to any of these, how long is problem present, and how many times a day or a week or a month does it occur? *N/A*

Any pains in your abdomen? Please describe – where in your abdomen, constant or intermittent, duration of each episode if intermittent, severity, anything that makes it worse, anything that makes it better? *Yes, pain in lower abdomen. Radiates from centre to both sides. Somewhat constant over last two weeks.*

How often do you have a bowel movement (BM)? Daily? Every 2nd day? Solid or loose? Any bleeding? Do you get up from sleep to have bowel movements? Any urgency? If urgent, mild, moderate, or severe? *Bowel movement can range from daily to every few days. Intermittent blood in stool. Always suffered from irregularity. Do not get up during sleep.*

List **ALL** medications, doses and reasons for being on them, whether prescribed or not. *Not currently on any medications.*

Are you allergic to any drugs? If yes, describe reaction. *No*

Please tell me about your family history; anyone with colon cancer or colon polyps; any other kind of cancer in the family; any diseases that "run" in the family? *Diabetes on mother's side, paternal grandfather died of stomach cancer, mother has polyps.*

Do you have heart disease? Lung disease? Kidney disease? High blood pressure? Any other disease? *No diseases.*

Do you have sleep apnea? *No*

What do you do for a living? *Mental Health Community Crisis Worker.*

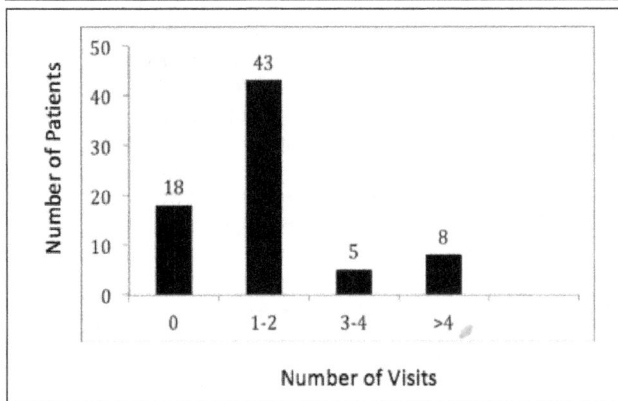

Figure 1) *Number of clinic visits by patients over a six-month period*

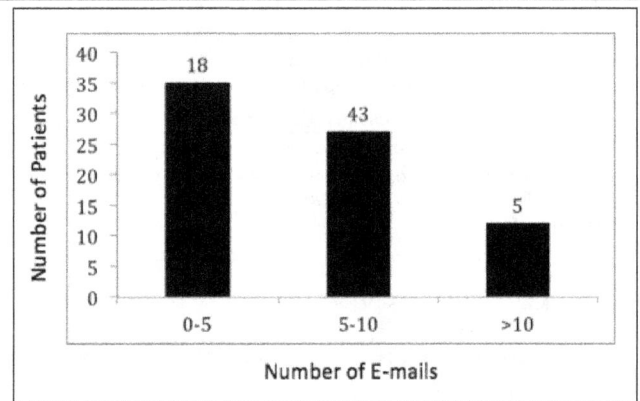

Figure 2) *Number of e-mail exchanges between patients and their specialist over a six-month period*

patient's report of a disclosed symptom set, the experienced physician can assess whether a patient needs to be seen in the same way that is currently achieved with telephone calls (21). In the senior author's (FS) practice, e-mail is being used frequently, especially for IBD patients living and working at a distance from the clinic. Although many of these communications pertain to blood test results, other common uses include advice regarding steroid dosing and fine-tuning of management regimens. Patients undergoing pharmacotherapy, such as immunosuppressants, frequently require regular blood work monitoring and assessment of adverse effects. Patients can easily inform physicians when they have gone for a blood test and then can receive a response indicating normal or abnormal values. Abnormal values would prompt some form of follow-up (which may be in the form of additional e-mail), whereas normal values would merely be noted by an e-mail indicating the time for the next routine test. By adding e-mail as a means of triaging self-managers, additional clinic time with shorter wait times can be made available for new consultations and sicker patients requiring in-person assessment.

AUTHORS' EXPERIENCE

In a pilot study conducted by the senior author and clinical trainees at Sunnybrook Health Sciences Centre (Toronto, Ontario) evaluating e-mail management in patients with IBD, e-mail communication appeared to have many benefits from both patient and physician perspectives (24). A patient questionnaire was administered via e-mail to 137 consenting IBD patients with a minimum six months of e-mail communication. Seventy-four (54%) patients responded to the survey.

The five main question categories included: e-mail usage, economic impact, number of clinic visits, convenience and demographics. Main outcomes measured included: e-mails sent, hours lost from work, distance travelled, specialist clinic visits, hours taken per appointment, anxiety scale and patient preference (Box 3).

Reviewing six months of e-mail communication, 76% of e-mail-managed IBD patients estimated that they made at least one to two fewer visits to the clinic (Figure 1). To attend the clinic, 65% of participants commuted >3.1 miles (5 km) to 6.2 miles (10 km) from home, and 73% >3.1 miles (5 km) to 6.2 miles (10 km) from their place of employment. More than 50% travelled for longer than 30 min. Fifty-three percent of participating patients exchanged e-mail with their specialist on more than five to 10 occasions during the six-month period (Figure 2). Additionally, 77% of patients reported a reduction in their stress level regarding their IBD management. When given a choice between traditional health care delivery (clinic visits only) and clinic visits combined with e-mail access, 90% of patients preferred the combined model. Further evaluation with a rigorous protocol is planned to better evaluate the short-term and long-term benefits of e-mail management in patients with IBD.

QUALITY, SAFETY AND LEGAL IMPLICATIONS

It is clear that e-mail consultations are not always suitable. Individuals with urgent questions and/or issues must be made aware that they should either telephone the doctor's office or go to an emergency department, particularly with symptoms such as neurological deficits, dyspnea, chest pain or severe pain in any other location (16).

Similarly, for intimate issues, such as mental health or substance abuse, a more direct interaction is generally preferable (14,17). In some circumstances, patients may require a follow-up by the physician through a telephone call or in-person consultation due to incomplete or vague details via e-mail (18). The potential for e-mail use will vary from patient to patient (13). In addition, if either a physician or patient would prefer to discuss an issue in the office setting, an in-person consultation should be arranged.

Many physicians have expressed concerns regarding the use of e-mail communication, with emphasis on potential legal and security implications. However, it should be noted that the danger of personal information being directed to unintended recipients is equally as plausible as most current methods of communication including fax machines, voice mail and regular mail. As with any proposed intervention, it is the primary responsibility of the physician to discuss the legal risks, ensure confidentiality, maintain optimal standards of practice and require informed consent. It is also advisable to conduct e-mail communication using high-security servers and single-user computers to avoid potential breaches in security. With many of these legal implications in mind, the Canadian Medical Protective Association developed a formal arrangement between physician and patient by means of an e-mail contract in 2005 with a revised version in June 2013 (25). This contract outlines the risks associated with this type of interaction and clarifies the appropriate situations when e-mail is an acceptable choice. The senior author of the present article (FS) uses a personalized version of this contract.

The main quality and safety issues surrounding e-mail consultation include: patient confidentiality; identifying appropriate clinical situations for e-mail use; transcription errors and liability; e-mail integration into clinical models; and practice economics (3,7,8,26). Secure, encrypted, web-based electronic messaging systems can address issues regarding security and liability that are associated with conventional e-mail communication (12). However, not all institutions have the available infrastructure and instead rely on standard e-mail communication (26). The responsibility for minimizing legal risks would fall on physicians who would be expected to adhere to the same rigid data protection rules expected of business and industry settings. E-mail encryption and safe data storage would also be required in addition to informed consent by the patient (26). It is important to select patients capable of using e-mail communication effectively (27). A subgroup of patients may be excluded from e-mail use for reasons including those with questionable reliability, the inability to understand appropriate use of e-mail and the technologically unskilled, among others. However, increased patient satisfaction has been noted in several studies of e-mail consultation, with patients preferring this method as a more convenient communication modality. In 2002, a United Kingdom-based survey by Potts and Wyatt (28) demonstrated that newly certified physicians have greater familiarity and comfort in using the Internet. This is not surprising given the expansion of technology into modern clinical practice and training. This illustrates a potential generational effect on Internet and e-mail consultation use.

FINANCIAL AND WORKLOAD IMPLICATIONS

When considering the use of e-mail in clinical practice, one needs to consider the time investment physicians require communicating with their patients. While time must be found for e-mailing, time will be freed up as a result of fewer telephone calls. Telephone calls require that both physician and patient be available at the same time within relatively few hours. On the other hand, e-mail enables patients to send messages at a time of convenience for them, and allows physicians to reply in the same fashion. In the senior authors' (FS) practice, patients are informed that e-mail is primarily for brief, nonurgent exchanges and that the physician may not reply for 24 h to 48 h. In addition, as stated above, if the physician or patient would prefer to discuss an issue in the office setting, that request should be granted.

In the United States, e-mail management has been a billable activity for several years. While no Canadian fee schedule compensates physicians for e-mail at this time, the Ontario government, in conjunction with the Ontario Medical Association, has recently agreed to incorporate 'e-consultations' into health care delivery (29). Given the obvious benefits, it is anticipated that a fee structure will be developed.

CONCLUSIONS

From a practical standpoint, e-mail communication reduces the inefficiencies present with telecommunications. Physicians are able to document out-of-office patient encounters, reach patients efficiently and provide access to specialist care for patients in remote locations. This type of access has the potential to increase patient safety through physician approval of self-manager actions and earlier initiation of needed treatments. Fewer clinic visits affords additional time for new consultations and sicker patients, reducing the overall burden on referral and wait times. From the patient perspective, e-mail communication has reduced the need for primary care, and specialist and emergency visits. This has direct impact in reducing time required off work, with elimination of travel and significant reduction of the ecological footprint from fuel emissions.

While e-mail communication has clear benefits, the legal implications must be considered. Canadian Medical Protective Association e-mail contract provides an effective way of documenting informed consent and outlining the situations for which e-mail is appropriate. Akin to the voice mail of a physician's office instructing patients how to proceed in the event of an emergency, the e-mail contract acts to direct patients on how to appropriately use this form of communication, as well as its limitations. The incorporation of e-mail into the self-management of chronic diseases, such as IBD, has the potential to enhance patient care and safety.

ACKNOWLEDGEMENTS: Dr Ian Plener was the 2010 Ilona Diener Clinical Summer Student in Inflammatory Bowel Disease. Dr Andrew Hayward was the 2005 Ilona Diener Clinical Summer Student in Inflammatory Bowel Disease.

REFERENCES

1. Statistic Canada. Individual Internet Use and E-commerce. <www.statcan.gc.ca/daily-quotidien/111012/dq111012a-eng.htm> (Accessed July 10, 2012)
2. Brooks R, Menachemi N. Physicians' use of email with patients: Factors influencing electronic communication and adherence to best practices. J Med Internet Res 2006;8:e2.
3. Gaster B, Knight C, DeWitt D, Sheffield J, Assefi NP, Buchwald D. Physicians' use of and attitudes toward electronic mail for patient communication. J Gen Intern Med. 2003;18:385-9.
4. Minitwatts Marketing Group. Internet World Stats. <www.internetworldstats.com/stats.htm> (Accessed June 30, 2012).
5. Halpert A, Dalton C, Palsson O, et al. Irritable bowel syndrome patient's ideal expectations and recent experiences with healthcare providers: A national survery. Dig Dis Sci 2010; 55:375-83.
6. Gullo K. Many nationwide believe in the potential benefits of electronic medical records and are interested in online communication with physicians. The Wall Street Journal Online Health Care Poll Newsletter, March 2005.
7. Kleiner K, Akers R, Burke B, Werner E. Parent and physician attitudes regarding electronic communication in pediatric practices. Pediatr 2002;109:740-4.
8. Moyer C, Stern D, Katz S, Fendrick AM. "We got mail": Electronic communication between physicians and patients. Am J Manag C 1999;5:1513-22.
9. Couchman G, Forjuoh S, Rascoe T. E-mail communications in family practice: What do patients expect? J Fam Pract 2001;50:414-8.
10. Lacher D, Nelson E, Bylsma W, Spena R. Computer use and needs of internists: A survey of members of the American College of Physicians-American Society of Internal Medicine. Proc AMIA Symp 2000:453-56.

11. Castren J, Niemi M, Virjo I. Use of email for patient communication in student health care: A cross-sectional study. Med Inf. 2005;5:2.

12. Liederman E, Morefield CS. Web messaging: A new tool for patient-physician communication. JAMA 2003;10:260-70.

13. Kassirer J. Patients, physicians, and the Internet. Health Aff 2000;19:115-23.

14. Katz S, Moyer C, Cox D, Stern D. Effect of a triage-based e-mail system on clinic resource use and patient and physician satisfaction in primary care: A randomized controlled trial. J Gen Intern Med 2003;18:736-44.

15. White C, Moyer C, Stern D, Katz S. A content analysis of e-mail communication between patients and their providers: Patients get the message. JAMA 2004;11:260-7.

16. Car J, Sheikh A. Email consultations in health care: 1 – scope and effectiveness. Br Med J 2004;329:435-8.

17. Dunbar P, Madigan D, Grohskopf L, et al. A two-way messaging system to enhance antiretroviral adherence. JAMA 2003;10:11-5.

18. Patt M, Houston T, Jenckes M, Sands D, Ford DE. Doctors who are using e-mail with their patients: A qualitative exploration. J Med Internet Res 2003;5:e9.

19. Deakin T, McShane C, Cade J, Williams R. Group based training for self-management strategies in people with type 2 diabetes mellitus. Cochrane Database Syst Rev 2005.

20. Bourbeau J, Julien M, Maltais F, et al. Reduction of hospital utilization in patients with chronic obstructive pulmonary disease: A disease-specific self-management intervention. Arch Intern Med 2003;163:585-91.

21. Saibil F, Lai E, Hayward A, Yip J, Gilbert C. Self-management for people with inflammatory bowel disease. Can J Gastroenterol 2008;22:281-7.

22. Cross R, Finkelstein J. Feasibility and acceptance of a home telemanagement system in patients with inflammatory bowel disease: A 6-month pilot study. Dig Dis Sci 2007;52:357-64.

23. Kennedy AP, Nelson E, Reeves D, et al. A randomised controlled trial to assess the effectiveness and cost of a patient orientated self-management approach to chronic inflammatory bowel disease. Gut 2004;53:1639-45.

24. AAFP. Making a case for online physician-patient communication. It can improve communications, practice efficiency and maybe even the bottom line. Fam Pract Manag 2008;15:A3-A6.

25. Canadian Medical Protective Association (CMPA). Use of email with your patients, legal risk. <www.cmpa-acpm.ca/cmpapd04/docs/resource_files/infosheets/2005/com_is0586-e.cfm> (Accessed July 5, 2012)

26. Car J, Sheikh A. Email consultations in health care: 2. Acceptability and safe application. BMJ 2004;329:439-42.

27. Medem Inc. eRisk Working Group for Healthcare's Guidelines for Online Communication. <www.medem.com/phy/phy_eriskguidelines.cfm 2007> (Accessed July 12, 2012)

28. Potts H, Wyatt J. Survey of doctors' experience of patients using the Internet. J Med Internet Res 2002;4:e5.

29. Ontario Government and Ontario Medical Association. McGuinty Government and OMA Protecting Gains in Health Care. <http://news.ontario.ca/mohltc/en/2012/11/ontario-and-oma-reach-agreement.html> (Accessed July 15, 2012).

30. Leong S, Gingrich D, Lewis P, Mauger D, George J. Enhancing doctor-patient communication using email: A pilot study. J Am Board Fam Pract 2005;18:180-8.

31. Virji A, Yarnall K, Krause K, et al. Use of email in a family practice setting: opportunities and challenges in patient- and physician-initiated communication. BMC Med 2006;4:18

32. Pondichetty V, Penn D. The progressive roles of electronic medicine: Benefits, concerns, and costs. Am J Med Sci 2004;328:94-9.

33. Ceresia P, Crolla D. Physician-patient email communication: Legal risks. The Canadian Medical Protective Association Information Sheet. December 2005.

34. Katz S, Moyer, C. The emerging role of online communication between patients and their providers. J Gen Intern Med 2004;19:978-83.

42

Association between proton pump inhibitor use and spontaneous bacterial peritonitis in cirrhotic patients with ascites

Mélissa Ratelle B Pharm MSc[1], Sylvie Perreault B Pharm PhD[2],
Jean-Pierre Villeneuve MD[3], Lydjie Tremblay B Pharm MSc[1,2]

M Ratelle, S Perreault, J-P Villeneuve, L Tremblay. Association between proton pump inhibitor use and spontaneous bacterial peritonitis in cirrhotic patients with ascites. Can J Gastroenterol Hepatol 2014;28(6):330-334.

BACKGROUND: There are data suggesting a link between proton pump inhibitor (PPI) use and the development of spontaneous bacterial peritonitis (SBP) in cirrhotic patients with ascites; however, these data are controversial.

OBJECTIVE: To assess whether the use of PPIs in cirrhotic patients with ascites is associated with an increased risk for SBP.

METHODS: A retrospective case-control study (June 2004 to June 2010) was conducted at the *Centre Hospitalier de l'Université de Montréal* in Montreal, Quebec. Fifty-one cirrhotic patients admitted with paracentesis-proven SBP ($\geq$250 neutrophils/mm^3), occurring within seven days of hospital admission, met the inclusion criteria. These patients were matched 1:2 (for age, Child-Pugh class and year of admission) with 102 comparable cirrhotic patients with ascites who were admitted for conditions other than SBP.

RESULTS: Patients with SBP had a significantly higher rate of prehospital PPI use (60.8%) compared with cirrhotic patients without SBP (42.2%; P=0.03). On multivariate analysis, PPI use was the only factor independently associated with SBP (OR 2.09 [95% CI 1.04 to 4.23]; P=0.04). Thirty-five (35%) patients in both groups had no documented indication for PPI use in their charts. Forty-five percent of the remaining cirrhotic patients with SBP had an inappropriate indication, as defined in the protocol, for PPI use compared with 25% of controls.

CONCLUSIONS: Cirrhotic patients with SBP were twice as likely to have taken PPIs than patients without SBP. These findings reinforce the association between PPI use and SBP observed in other studies. A high percentage of cirrhotic patients were taking a PPI without any documented indication.

Key Words: *Ascites; Cirrhosis; Proton pump inhibitor; Spontaneous bacterial peritonitis*

L'association entre l'utilisation d'inhibiteurs de la pompe à protons et la péritonite bactérienne spontanée chez des patients cirrhotiques souffrant d'ascite

HISTORIQUE : Selon certaines données, il y aurait un lien entre l'utilisation d'inhibiteurs de la pompe à protons (IPP) et l'apparition d'une péritonite bactérienne spontanée (PBS) chez les patients cirrhotiques souffrant d'ascite. Ces données sont toutefois controversées.

OBJECTIF : Évaluer si l'utilisation d'IPP chez des patients cirrhotiques souffrant d'ascite s'associe à une augmentation du risque de PBS.

MÉTHODOLOGIE : Les chercheurs ont mené une étude rétrospective cas-témoins (juin 2004 à juin 2010) au Centre hospitalier de l'Université de Montréal, au Québec. Cinquante et un patients cirrhotiques admis à cause d'une PBS démontrée par paracentèse ($\geq$250 neutrophiles/mm^3), s'étant manifesté dans les sept jours précédant l'hospitalisation, respectaient les critères d'inclusion. Ces patients ont été jumelés selon un ratio de 1:2 (pour l'âge, le score de Child-Pugh et l'année d'admission) à 102 patients cirrhotiques souffrant d'ascite comparables, qui avaient été admis pour d'autres problèmes qu'une PBS.

RÉSULTATS : Les patients ayant une PBS présentaient un taux considérablement plus élevé d'utilisation d'IPP avant l'hospitalisation (60,8 %) que les patients cirrhotiques sans PBS (42,2 %; P=0,03). À l'analyse multivariée, l'utilisation d'IPP était le seul facteur qui s'associait de manière indépendante à la PBS (RR 2,09 [95 % IC 1,04 à 4,23]; P=0,04). Dans les deux groupes, 35 patients (35 %) ne présentaient pas d'indication d'utilisation d'IPP au dossier. Quarante-cinq pour cent des autres patients cirrhotiques ayant une PBS présentaient une indication inappropriée d'utilisation d'IPP selon la définition du protocole, par rapport à 25 % des sujets-témoins.

CONCLUSIONS : Les patients cirrhotiques ayant une PBS étaient deux fois plus susceptibles d'avoir pris des IPP que les patients sans PBS. Ces résultats étayent l'association entre l'utilisation d'IPP et la PBS observée dans d'autres études. Un fort pourcentage de patients cirrhotiques prenaient des IPP sans qu'il y ait d'indication au dossier.

Spontaneous bacterial peritonitis (SBP) is a common and severe complication in patients with cirrhosis (1), and is associated with significant mortality (2). The initial step in the pathogenesis of SBP is bacterial translocation from the gut flora to mesenteric lymph nodes (1). Increased gut permeability and small intestinal bacterial overgrowth are apparent in liver cirrhosis and both can facilitate bacterial translocation (1,3-5). Cirrhotic patients are more susceptible to infections through different mechanisms including impaired immunity caused by decreased reticuloendothelial system phagocytic activity, complement deficiency and neutrophil dysfunction (6-8).

Gastric acid is a defense mechanism against ingested microorganisms; reduction of gastric acidity increases bacterial proliferation in the stomach and small intestine. This predisposes to enteric infections (9-11). Proton pump inhibitors (PPIs) are potent gastric acid inhibitors and their use has been associated with an increased susceptibility to enteric infections caused by various enteropathogens including *Salmonella, Campylobacter* and *Clostridium difficile* (12,13). Furthermore, some data suggest a link between PPI use and the development of SBP in cirrhotic patients with ascites; however, these data are controversial (14-18).

Different mechanisms have been postulated to explain the increased rate of enteric infections associated with PPI therapy. Among these are: increase in small intestinal overgrowth; alteration of the microbial flora; impairment of neutrophil function (in vitro); and delayed gastric emptying (13). Another factor that may influence the infectious risk related to PPI use in advanced cirrhosis is the fact that PPI metabolism may be significantly impaired (with the exception of rabeprazole). This can result in higher exposure to PPIs (19,20).

[1]Department of Pharmacy, Centre Hospitalier de l'Université de Montréal; [2]Université de Montréal; [3]Division of Hepatology, Department of Medicine, Hôpital St-Luc, Centre Hospitalier de l'Université de Montréal, Montréal, Québec

Correspondence: Ms Mélissa Ratelle, Department of Pharmacy, Centre Hospitalier de l'Université de Montréal, 3840 St-Urbain, Montréal, Québec H2W 1T8 e-mail melissa.ratelle.chum@ssss.gouv.qc.ca

PPIs are highly effective and well tolerated. They are extensively used and, potentially, overused in many acid-related disorders (21-23). PPI overuse in cirrhotic patients is documented in the literature (24,25).

The primary outcome of our study was to evaluate whether the use of PPIs is associated with the development of SBP in cirrhotic patients with ascites. The secondary outcome was to evaluate whether the indications for PPI use in our study population were appropriate.

METHODS

Study population and identification of cases and controls

A retrospective review of all consecutive patients admitted between June 2004 and June 2010 with the diagnosis of cirrhosis with ascites according to *International Classification of Diseases, Ninth Revision* codes was performed at the *Centre Hospitalier de l'Université de Montréal*, a tertiary care hospital located in Montreal, Quebec. After identification of these patients, the charts were reviewed for the presence or absence of SBP. SBP cases were defined as paracentesis yielding ≥250 polymorpho-nuclear white blood cells (PMNs) per cubic millilitre with or without a positive culture of ascitic fluid within seven days of admission. Also used was a computerized list of patients with a neutrophil count in their ascitic fluid to ensure that all potential patients were identified. The non-SBP patient group (controls) were cirrhotic patients who underwent diagnostic paracentesis but were negative for SBP (PMN count <250 cells/mm^3 and a negative ascitic culture). Patients who had an unreliable medication list on hospital admission, antibiotic use with the exception of metronidazole for treatment of hepatic encephalopathy, immunosuppressant use, gastrointestinal bleeding (within 14 days before hospital admission), HIV infection or previous episode of SBP were excluded. All identified cases were community-acquired SBP. Each SBP patient was then matched according to age, year of admission and Child-Pugh-Turcotte (CPT) class, with two cirrhotic patients with ascites admitted for reasons other than SBP (1:2 ratio).

Recorded information

Information regarding demographics, reason for hospital admission, cirrhosis etiology, history of variceal bleeding or hepatic encephalopathy, diabetes, CPT classification, Model for End-stage Liver Disease (MELD) score, history of PPI use before admission (indication, dose and duration) and 30-day survival rate was collected. The laboratory blood tests included total bilirubin, albumin, creatinine and sodium levels, and international normalized ratio on admission. Ascitic fluid data included polymorphonuclear neutrophils, protein levels (when available) and bacteriological confirmation of SBP (when available).

PPI use and indication definitions

Patients were defined as PPI users if they had taken a PPI daily for at least two weeks before hospital admission. Information regarding PPI exposure was retrieved from both physician admission/emergency notes and outpatient medication lists provided by retail pharmacies and/or pharmacist drug history. To assess the duration of and indication for PPI therapy, previous hospitalization medical records were reviewed in addition to outpatient follow-up medical notes because the majority of the authors' patients were already followed by hepatologists at their centre. Appropriate PPI indication was defined as gastroesophageal reflux disease, peptic ulcer disease, Barrett's esophagus, dyspepsia, alcoholic gastritis, *Helicobacter pylori* infection, and postesophageal variceal sclerotherapy or banding (EVL). Peptic ulcer disease treatment and post-EVL were considered to be inappropriate indications if the treatment duration exceeded three months or two months, respectively.

Statistical analysis

Non-normally distributed continuous variables are presented as median (quartile 1 to quartile 3). The Wilcoxon Mann-Whitney test was used to compare the two groups. Proportions were used for categorical variables and the Pearson χ^2 test (or the Fisher's exact test) was used to the compare the two groups. The relationship between SBP and exposure to PPIs was evaluated using conditional logistic regression (univariate and multivariate) to calculate the ORs. Multivariate analysis was used to measure the potential effect of confounders. The covariates included in the model were sex, diabetes, serum sodium level and MELD score. With regard to the secondary outcome, the percentage of patients receiving a PPI for an appropriate indication was calculated. In all analyses, P<0.05 was considered to be statistically significant. MELD scores were calculated according to the method used by the United Network for Organ Sharing (www.mayoclinic.org).

RESULTS

A total of 1083 charts from patients with cirrhosis and ascites were reviewed. Paracentesis-proven SBP was confirmed in 242 cases. In all cases, antibiotics were started after the diagnostic paracentesis. From these 242 cases, 72 were excluded because the infection was diagnosed >7 days after admission (nosocomial SBP), 19 because they experienced a previous SBP episode, 71 because they were receiving immunosuppressant medication, 22 because of antibiotic use and 14 because of bleeding within 14 days before hospitalization. The remaining 51 cases with community-acquired SBP were then matched according to age, CPT class and year of admission with 102 cirrhotic patients with ascites without SBP. The main reasons for hospital admission in patients without SBP were ascites (32%), hepatic encephalopathy (13%), pre-transplant evaluation (11%), alcoholic hepatitis (10%), acute-on-chronic liver failure (7%) and transjugular intrahepatic portosystemic shunt (5%).

The clinical characteristics of the two groups are summarized in Table 1. There were no significant differences in baseline demographics and clinical parameters. The median age was 60 years and the majority of patients were men. The percentage of patients with CPT class C (78%) and class B (22%) were similar in the two groups. There was no significant difference in ascitic fluid protein concentration in patients with SBP compared with those without SBP, but data were available from only 67% and 57% of patients, respectively.

Among the patients with SBP, the proportion taking PPIs before admission was 61% compared with 42% in those without SBP; the difference was significant (P=0.03) (Table 1). Details of PPI use in the two groups are shown in Table 2. No significant differences were observed for PPI dosage (standard versus double dosing) and overall indications between the two groups. Among documented indications, inappropriate indications for PPI use were found in 45% of SBP patients (nine of 20 cases) compared with 25% of patients without SBP (seven of 28 controls) (P=0.147). No documented indication for PPI use was found in 36% (11 of 31) of SBP patients compared with 35% of patients (15 of 43) without SBP.

On multivariate analysis, PPI use was the only factor independently associated with the occurrence of SBP (OR 2.09 [95% CI 1.04 to 4.23]; P=0.04) (Table 3).

Bacteriological confirmation was available in 26 of 51 (51%) cases. Gram-positive organisms were found in nine (18%) patients and Gram-negative organisms were found in 17 (33%) patients (Table 4). There was no statistical difference in Gram species between PPI users and nonusers. The mortality rate at 30 days was 20% among patients with SBP and 9% among patients without SBP, mostly from hepatic failure (P=0.057).

DISCUSSION

The results of the current study support an association between PPI use and the development of SBP in cirrhotic patients with ascites. At the time we initiated our study, there were only two published studies that evaluated the relationship between PPI use and SBP in cirrhotic patients as a primary end point but their results were contradictory (16,18).

TABLE 1
Demographic, clinical and laboratory data from patients with spontaneous bacterial peritonitis (SBP) and controls

	SBP		
	Yes (n=51)	No (n=102)	P*
Age, years	60.2 (55.5-69.7)	61.1 (52.0-68.1)	0.72
Male sex	41 (80)	73 (72)	0.238
Race			0.334
Caucasian	48 (94)	100 (98)	
Other	3 (6)	2 (2)	
History of hepatic encephalopathy	23 (45)	44 (43)	0.818
History of esophageal varices	35 (69)	62 (61)	0.342
Serum bilirubin at admission, μmol/L	66 (47-196)	72 (49-115)	0.595
Serum creatinine at admission, μmol/L	98 (70-133)	100 (66-124)	0.392
Serum sodium at admission, mmol/L	133 (129-136) n=34	134 (129-136) n=58	0.668
Ascites protein, g/L	12 (5-20)	8.5 (5-14)	0.238
Etiology of cirrhosis			0.491
Alcohol	25 (49)	44 (43)	
HCV/HBV	14 (28)	27 (27)	
NASH/cryptogenic	8 (16)	26 (26)	
Other	4 (8)	5 (5)	
Diabetes mellitus	16 (31)	33 (32)	0.903
Child-Pugh score	11 (10-12)	10 (10-11)	0.352
MELD score	21 (17-27)	20 (16-23)	0.112
PPI use	31 (61)	43 (42)	0.03

*Data presented as median (quartile 1-quartile 3) or n (%) unless otherwise indicated. *P<0.05 considered to be statistically significant. HBV Hepatitis B virus; HCV Hepatitis C virus; MELD Model for End-stage Liver Disease; NASH Nonalcoholic steatohepatitis; PPI Proton pump inhibitor*

TABLE 2
Details of proton pump inhibitor (PPI) use

	Spontaneous bacterial peritonitis		
	Yes (n=51)	No (n=102)	P
Double daily PPI dosing	6 (19); n=31	14 (33); n=43	0.207
PPI-appropriate indications	11 (55); n=20	21 (75); n=28	0.147
Indications	n=31	n=43	0.746
Postesophageal variceal banding	6 (19)	7 (16)	
Peptic ulcer disease	7 (23)	3 (7)	
Dyspepsia	2 (7)	6 (14)	
GERD	1 (3)	3 (7)	
Alcoholic gastritis	1 (3)	2 (5)	
Helicobacter pylori	1 (3)	2 (5)	
Gastroprotection	1 (3)	3 (7)	
Other	1 (3)	2 (5)	
No documentation	11 (36)	15 (35)	

Data presented as n (%) unless otherwise indicated. All patients were taking PPIs (daily versus twice daily) for at least 30 days. Inappropriate use was considered if peptic ulcer disease treatment >3 months, postesophageal variceal banding prophylaxis >2 months, portal hypertension gastritis and ulcer prophylaxis without proper indication. GERD Gastroesophageal reflux disease

First, Campbell et al (16) did not find an association between PPI use and SPB in a retrospective case-control study involving 116 consecutive cirrhotic patients with ascites (OR 1.22 [95% CI 0.52 to 2.87]; P=0.64). However, limitations of their study included the small number of patients with SBP (32 of 116) and the fact that the MELD score was significantly higher in the SBP group (P=0.002).

TABLE 3
Risk factors for spontaneous bacterial peritonitis

	OR (95% CI)	P
Univariate analysis		
Proton pump inhibitor use	2.12 (1.07–4.19)	0.032
Multivariate analysis		
Proton pump inhibitor use	2.14 (1.07–4.14)	0.04
Male sex	1.56 (0.67–3.67)	0.304
Diabetes mellitus	0.93 (0.44–1.97)	0.844
Serum sodium level	0.98 (0.92–1.05)	0.518
Model for End-stage Liver Disease score	1.05 (0.99–1.11)	0.055

TABLE 4
Bacteriological confirmation in patients with spontaneous bacterial peritonitis (n=26)

	n
Gram positive	
Staphyloccocus species	6
Streptoccocus species	3
Gram negative	
Escherichia coli	7
Klebsiella species	4
Enterobacter species	2
Haemophilus influenza	1
Campylobacter fetus	1
Pseudomonas aeruginosa	1
Bacteroides fragilis	1

Then, in 2009, Bajaj et al (18) performed a retrospective case-control study involving 70 patients with SBP matched 1:1 for age and CPT class with 70 comparable patients with cirrhosis and ascites. There was no significant difference in the CPT score and the MELD score between the two groups. On multivariate analysis, PPI use was independently associated with SBP (OR 4.31 [95% CI 1.34 to 11.7]; P=0.003) and ascitic fluid protein concentration was protective.

Since then, three other retrospective case-control studies involving cirrhotic patients with ascites have been published with the same primary end point (14,15,26). Choi et al (15) compared 83 patients with SBP with 93 controls who did not have SBP. On multivariate analysis, CPT class C, high MELD score and PPI use (OR 3.44 [95% CI 1.164 to 10.188]; P=0.025) were independent risk factors for SBP. H$_2$ receptor antagonist use was not associated with SBP. Goel et al (14) compared 65 cirrhotic patients with SBP with 65 patients without SBP. The CPT score was significantly higher in the SBP group (P=0.046). In the multivariate analysis, after adjusting for CPT score, patients who did not use PPI in the previous 90 days were 71% less likely to develop SBP than those who used PPI in the previous seven days (OR 0.29 [95% CI 0.13 to 0.68]; P=0.004). In this study, patients who received previous antibiotics were not excluded because it was performed in the previously described studies, but the authors believed that it did not influence their results. Finally, de Vos et al (26) compared 51 unmatched cirrhotic patients with SBP with 51 cirrhotic patients without SBP. The study showed that cirrhotic patients with SBP received PPIs twice as often as noninfected cirrhotic patients with ascites; however, in the multivariate analysis, PPI use was not associated with SBP (P=0.1). The only parameter significantly associated with SBP was international normalized ratio (P=0.007).

A recent meta-analysis including eight studies (n=3815) (27) showed that cirrhotic patients receiving a PPI had approximately three times the risk of developing SBP compared with patients not receiving PPIs (OR 3.15 [95% CI 2.09 to 4.74]). The five studies discussed above were included in the meta-analysis plus two retrospective cohort studies available as abstracts (28,29) and one prospective cohort study (30).

The methodology used in our study was very similar to the study by Bajaj et al (18). We matched cases and controls for age and CPT class, the latter factor being very important because the severity of the disease is associated with a greater risk for developing SBP. We also considered the potential bias of time on PPI prescribing habits by matching cases and controls according to year of admission. We hypothesized that if there was a change in PPI prescribing habits over the years, both groups would be affected equally. Confounding factors, such as previous gastrointestinal bleeding, SBP episode(s), or antibiotic or immunosuppressant use, were excluded. Due to our stringent inclusion and exclusion criteria, we were not able to recruit more than 51 cases, but we found two controls per SBP case. Because paracentesis is not performed routinely on admission in cirrhotic patients with ascites at our centre, it was difficult to recruit more than two controls for every case of SBP.

On multivariate analysis, PPI use was the only factor independently associated with SBP (OR 2.09 [95% CI 1.04 to 4.23]; P=0.04). MELD score was found to have a nonsignificant effect (OR 1.05 [95% CI 0.99 to 1.11]; P=0.06). It would have been interesting to know whether ascitic fluid protein concentration was protective against SBP but no conclusion can be drawn because data were missing for nearly 40% of the patients in both groups. These missing data could be explained by the fact that radiologists frequently perform parencentesis in our centre and they do not request ascitic fluid concentration routinely.

The secondary outcome of our study was to evaluate whether the indications for PPI use in the study population were appropriate. The results show, as in previous observations, an overuse of PPI in cirrhotic patients (24,25). The fact that 35% of patients with SBP and 36% of patients without SBP received a PPI without any documented indication is concerning. In addition, only 55% and 75% of SBP cases and controls, respectively, received a PPI for an appropriate indication as defined in our study.

It is a common practice to prescribe a PPIs after esophageal variceal sclerotherapy or banding to prevent or heal postprocedure ulcerations. Some data from uncontrolled nonrandomized studies showed that PPIs may have a role in the prevention and healing of ulcerations postesophageal sclerotherapy (31). In a double-blinded randomized placebo-controlled trial, the short-term use of pantoprazole (10 days) after elective band ligation was associated with a significant reduction of the size of ulcers but had no effect on the overall number of ulcers or in symptoms related to the procedure (32). In our study, PPI use post-EVL was considered to be appropriate if used for ≤2 months postvariceal ligation. Even with this broad definition, we observed that PPI use was pursued for longer periods post-EVL without medical or pharmacological reason.

One of the strengths of our study was the fact that we used two reliable sources to document PPI use. The medication list documented by physician notes and a complete medication list copy provided by retail pharmacies or hospital pharmacist drug history were considered to be trustworthy. Because PPIs are not available over the counter in Canada, it was easier to evaluate the duration of use. In our opinion, all patients taking PPIs for at least 30 days before admisson better reflects PPI use than the minimum of 14 days that was initially defined in our protocol.

CONCLUSION

Our study has shown that PPI use in cirrhotic patients with ascites is an independent risk factor for developing SBP. Our data reinforce the previous positive link between PPI use and SBP observed in other retrospective case-control studies. Ideally, a prospective randomized study should be conducted; however, such a study would be difficult to perform and ethically questionable. In the meantime, PPI indications in cirrhotic patients should be frequently re-evaluated with particular attention devoted to duration of use, especially following EVL. The minimal effective PPI dose should be used in advanced cirrhosis because it is known that PPI exposure is increased in these patients because of an altered pharmacokinetic profile. The double-standard dose should also be avoided whenever possible.

DISCLOSURES: The authors have no financial disclosures or conflicts of interest to declare.

REFERENCES

1. Gines P, Arroyo V, Rodes J. Pathophysiology, complications, and treatment of ascites. Clin Liver Dis 1997;1:129-55.
2. Pinzello G, Simonetti RG, Craxi A, Di Piazza S, Spano C, Pagliaro L. Spontaneous bacterial peritonitis: A prospective investigation in predominantly nonalcoholic cirrhotic patients. Hepatology 1983;34:545-9.
3. Scarpellini E, Valenza V, Gabrielli M, et al. Intestinal permeability in cirrhotic patients with and without spontaneous bacterial peritonitis: Is the ring closed? Am J Gastroenterol 2010;105:323-7.
4. Jun DW, Kim KT, Lee OY, et al. Association between small intestinal bacterial overgrowth and peripheral bacterial DNA in cirrhotic patients. Dig Dis Sci 2010;55:1465-71.
5. Chang CS, Chen CH, Lien HC, Yeh HZ. Small intestine dysmotility and bacterial overgrowth in cirrhotic patients with spontaneous bacterial peritonitis. Hepatology 1998;28:1187-90.
6. Such J, Guarner C, Enriquez J, Rodriguez JL, Seres I, Vilardell F. Low C3 in cirrhotic ascites predisposes to spontaneous bacterial peritonitis. J Hepatol 1988;6:80-4.
7. Rimola A, Soto R, Bory F, Arroyo V, Piera C, Rodes J. Reticuloendothelial system phagocytic activity in cirrhosis and its relation to bacterial infections and prognosis. Hepatology 1984;4:53-8.
8. Fiuza C, Salcedo M, Clemente G, Tellado J. In vivo neutrophil dysfunction in cirrhotic patients with advanced liver disease. J Infect Dis 2000;182:526-33.
9. Martinsen TC, Bergh K, Waldum HL. Gastric juice: A barrier against infectious diseases. Basic Clin Pharmacol Toxicol 2005;96:94-102.
10. Hunt RH. The protective role of gastric acid. Scand J Gastroenterol (Suppl) 1988;146:34-9.
11. Giannella RA, Broitman SA, Zamcheck N. Gastric acid barrier to ingested microorganisms in man: Studies in vivo and in vitro. Gut 1972;13:251-6.
12. Leonard J, Marshall JK, Moayyedi P. Systematic review of the risk of enteric infection in patients taking acid suppression. Am J Gastroenterol 2007;102:2047-56.
13. Bavishi C, Dupont HL. Systematic review: The use of proton pump inhibitors and increased susceptibility to enteric infection. Aliment Pharmacol Ther 2011;34:1269-81.
14. Goel GA, Deshpande A, Lopez R, Hall GS, van Duin D, Carey WD. Increased rate of spontaneous bacterial peritonitis among cirrhotic patients receiving pharmacologic acid suppression. Clin Gastroenterol Hepatol 2012;10:422-7.
15. Choi EJ, Lee HJ, Kim KO, et al. Association between acid suppressive therapy and spontaneous bacterial peritonitis in cirrhotic patients with ascites. Scand J Gastroenterol 2011;46:616-20.
16. Campbell MS, Obstein K, Reddy KR, Yang YX. Association between proton pump inhibitor use and spontaneous bacterial peritonitis. Dig Dis Sci 2008;53:394-8.
17. Bauer TM, Steinbruckner B, Brinkmann F, et al. Small intestinal bacterial overgrowth in patients with cirrhosis: Prevalence and relation with spontaneous bacterial peritonitis. Am J Gastroenterol 2001;96:2962-7.
18. Bajaj JS, Zadvornova Y, Heuman DM, et al. Association of proton pump inhibitor therapy with spontaneous bacterial peritonitis in cirrhotic patients with ascites. Am J Gastroenterol 2009;104:1130-4.
19. Robinson M, Horn J. Clinical pharmacology of proton pump inhibitors: What the practising physician needs to know. Drugs 2003;63:2739-54.
20. Branch RA. Drugs in liver disease. Clin Pharmacol Ther 1998;64:462-5.

21. Naunton M, Peterson GM, Bleasel MD. Overuse of proton pump inhibitors. J Clin Pharm Ther 2000;25:333-40.

22. Heidelbaugh JJ, Kim AH, Crang R, Walker PC. Overutilization of proton-pump inhibitors: What the clinician needs to know. Ther Adv Gastroenterol 2012;5:219-32.

23. Heidelbaugh JJ, Goldberg KL, Inadomi JM. Overutilization of proton pump inhibitors: A review of cost-effectiveness and risk in PPI. Am J Gastroenterol 2009;104:S27-32.

24. Kalaitzakis E, Bjornsson E. Inadequate use of proton-pump inhibitors in patients with liver cirrhosis. Eur J Gastroenterol Hepatol 2008;20:512-8.

25. Chavez-Tapia NC, Tellez-Avila FI, Garcia-Leiva J, Valdovinos MA. Use and overuse of proton pump inhibitors in cirrhotic patients. Med Sci Monit 2008;14:468-72.

26. de Vos M, De Vroey B, Garcia Garcia B, et al. Role of proton pump inhibitors in the occurrence and the prognosis of spontaneous bacterial peritonitis in cirrhotic patients with ascites. Liver Int 2013;33:1316-23.

27. Deshpande A, Pasupuleti V, Thota P. Acid-suppressive therapy is associated with spontaneous bacterial peritonitis in cirrhotic patients: A meta-analysis. J Gastroenterol Hepatol 2013;28:235-42.

28. Northup PG, Argo CL, Berg CL. Chronic proton pump inhibitor use is strongly associated with hepatorenal syndrome and spontaneous bacterial peritonitis in cirrhosis patients. Hepatology 2008;48:325A.

29. Bulsiewicz W, Scherer JR, Feinglass JM, Howden CW, Flam SL. Proton pump inhibitor (PPI) use is independently associated with spontaneous bacterial peritonitis (SBP) in cirrhotics with ascites. Gastroenterology 2009;136:A-11. (Abst)

30. van Vlerken LG, Huisman EJ, van Hoek B, et al. Bacterial infections in cirrhosis: Role of proton pump inhibitors and intestinal permeability. Eur J Clin Invest 2012;42:760-7.

31. Lodato F, Azzaroli F, Di Girolamo M, et al. Proton pump inhibitors in cirrhosis: Tradition or evidence based practice? World J Gastroenterol 2008;14:2980-5.

32. Shaheen NJ, Stuart E, Schmitz SM, et al. Pantoprazole reduces the size of postbanding ulcers after variceal band ligation: A randomized, controlled trial. Hepatology 2005;41:588-94.

43

Predictors of mortality among patients undergoing colectomy for ischemic colitis: A population-based, United States study

Matthew D Sadler MD[1], Nikila C Ravindran MD[1], James Hubbard MSc[1], Robert P Myers MD MSc[1], Subrata Ghosh MD[1], Paul L Beck MD PhD[1], Elijah Dixon MD MSc[3], Chad Ball MD[3], Chris Prusinkiewicz MD[4], Steven J Heitman MD MSc[1], Gilaad G Kaplan MD MPH[1,2]

MD Sadler, NC Ravindran, J Hubbard, et al. Predictors of mortality among patients undergoing colectomy for ischemic colitis: A population-based, United States study. Can J Gastroenterol Hepatol 2014;28(11):600-604.

BACKGROUND: Ischemic colitis is a potentially life-threatening condition that can require colectomy for management.

OBJECTIVE: To assess independent predictors of mortality following colectomy for ischemic colitis using a nationally representative sample of hospitals in the United States.

METHODS: The Nationwide Inpatient Sample was used to identify all patients with a primary diagnosis of acute vascular insufficiency of the colon (*International Classification of Diseases, Ninth Revision* codes 557.0 and 557.9) who underwent a colectomy between 1993 and 2008. Incidence and mortality are described; multivariate logistic regression analysis was performed to determine predictors of mortality.

RESULTS: The incidence of colectomy for ischemic colitis was 1.43 cases (95% CI 1.40 cases to 1.47 cases) per 100,000. The incidence of colectomy for ischemic colitis increased by 3.1% per year (95% CI 2.3% to 3.9%) from 1993 to 2003, and stabilized thereafter. The postoperative mortality rate was 21.0% (95% CI 20.2% to 21.8%). After 1997, the mortality rate significantly decreased at an estimated annual rate of 4.5% (95% CI −6.3% to −2.7%). Mortality was associated with older age, 65 to 84 years (OR 5.45 [95% CI 2.91 to 10.22]) versus 18 to 34 years; health insurance, Medicaid (OR 1.69 [95% CI 1.29 to 2.21]) and Medicare (OR 1.33 [95% CI 1.12 to 1.58]) versus private health insurance; and comorbidities such as liver disease (OR 3.54 [95% CI 2.79 to 4.50]). Patients who underwent colonoscopy or sigmoidoscopy (OR 0.78 [95% CI 0.65 to 0.93]) had lower mortality.

CONCLUSIONS: Colectomy for ischemic colitis was associated with considerable mortality. The explanation for the stable incidence and decreasing mortality rates observed in the latter part of the present study should be explored in future studies.

Key Words: *Colectomy; Incidence; Ischemic colitis; Mortality; Temporal trends*

Les prédicteurs de mortalité chez les patients qui subissent une colectomie secondaire à une colite ischémique : une étude en population menée aux États-Unis

HISTORIQUE : La colite ischémique est une maladie au potentiel mortel dont la prise en charge peut exiger une colectomie.

OBJECTIF : Évaluer les prédicteurs indépendants de mortalité après une colectomie secondaire à une colite ischémique au moyen d'un échantillon national représentatif d'hôpitaux des États-Unis.

MÉTHODOLOGIE : Pour repérer tous les patients ayant un diagnostic primaire d'insuffisance vasculaire aiguë du côlon (*Classification internationale des maladies, Neuvième révision*, codes 557.0 et 557.9), les chercheurs ont utilisé l'échantillon national de patients hospitalisé qui ont subi une colectomie entre 1993 et 2008. Ils en décrivent l'incidence et la mortalité et ont utilisé l'analyse par régression logistique pour déterminer les prédicteurs de mortalité.

RÉSULTATS : L'incidence de colectomie secondaire à la colite ischémique s'élevait à 1,43 cas (95 % IC 1,40 à 1,47 cas) sur 100 000 habitants. L'incidence de colectomie secondaire à la colite ischémique a augmenté de 3,1 % par année (95 % IC 2,3 % à 3,9 %) entre 1993 et 2003 et s'est stabilisée par la suite. Le taux de mortalité postopératoire était de 21,0 % (95 % IC 20,2 % à 21,8 %). Après 1997, le taux de mortalité a considérablement diminué, à un taux annuel estimatif de 4,5 % (95 % IC −6,3 % à −2,7 %). La mortalité s'associait à un âge plus avancé, de 65 à 84 ans (RC 5,45 [95 % IC 2,91 à 10,22]) par rapport à 18 à 34 ans; à l'assurance-maladie comme Medicaid (RC 1,69 [95 % IC 1,29 à 2,21]) et Medicare (RC 1,33 [95 % IC 1,12 à 1,58]) plutôt qu'à l'assurance-maladie privée, et à des comorbidités comme les hépatopathies (RC 3,54 [95 % IC 2,79 à 4,50]). Les patients qui avaient subi une coloscopie ou une sigmoïdoscopie (RC 0,78 [95 % IC 0,65 à 0,93]) présentaient une mortalité moins élevée.

CONCLUSIONS : La colectomie secondaire à la colite ischémique s'associait à une mortalité considérable. Dans le cadre de prochaines études, il faudrait chercher à expliquer la stabilisation de l'incidence et la diminution du taux de mortalité observées dans la dernière partie de la présente étude.

Ischemic colitis is a common disorder in elderly patients that is associated with significant morbidity, mortality and health care expenditures (1-3). Population-based studies reporting the incidence, morbidity and mortality of acute vascular insufficiency of the colon are lacking. A systematic review (4) reported that the incidence of ischemic colitis ranged from 4.4 to 44 cases per 100,000 person-years. Furthermore, three of every 1000 hospital admissions at one tertiary care centre in the United States (US) were for ischemic colitis (2); the same centre also reported that 1% of all colonoscopies and flexible sigmoidoscopies showed evidence of ischemic colitis (5).

The prognosis for ischemic colitis is variable, with many patients experiencing mild events that do not require hospitalization. However, others require admission to hospital for physiological support and risk stratification. Patients with severe presentations may require a segmental or total colectomy to manage complications of ischemic colitis. Mortality among patients with ischemic colitis who require colectomy is high. However, predictors for risk stratification for mortality are lacking in the literature.

We assessed in-hospital mortality following colectomy for ischemic colitis and determined independent predictors of mortality

[1]*Departments of Medicine;* [2]*Community Health Sciences;* [3]*Surgery;* [4]*Anesthesia, University of Calgary, Calgary, Alberta*
Correspondence: Dr Gilaad Kaplan, Teaching Research and Wellness Centre, 3280 Hospital Drive Northwest, 6D56, Calgary, Alberta T2N 4N1.
e-mail ggkaplan@ucalgary.ca

following colonic resection using a nationally representative sample of hospitals in the US.

METHODS

Data source

Data were extracted from the Healthcare Cost and Utilization Project Nationwide Inpatient Sample (NIS) database for the years 1993 to 2008. The NIS database contains hospital discharge abstracts from approximately 20% of nonfederal acute care hospitals in the US. Stratified random sampling was performed to ensure that the database was representative of the US population, and accounts for approximately 90% of all hospitalizations, including community and academic centres, but not long-term care facilities. The NIS contains information on demographic characteristics, up to 15 diagnostic and procedure codes based on the *International Classification of Diseases, Ninth Revision*, Clinical Modification (ICD-9-CM), outcomes and hospital characteristics. Because each record is for a single hospitalization – not a person – multiple records are possible for an individual with recurrent hospitalizations. NIS data compare favourably with the National Hospital Discharge Survey, supporting the validity of this database (6). Quality control and validation of the NIS are performed by the Agency for Healthcare Research and Quality in Rockville, Maryland (USA) (7). The NIS database has been used extensively to study nationwide outcomes for incidence, health service utilization and in-hospital mortality (8-11).

Study sample

ICD-9-CM diagnosis codes were used to identify 10,111 discharges of patients with a primary diagnosis of acute vascular insufficiency of the intestine (codes 557.0 and 557.9) who were admitted emergently from 1993 to 2008, and underwent a segmental or total colectomy (codes 45.7 or 45.8). Individuals with a co-existing ICD-9-CM procedural code for a small bowel resection (codes 45.50, 45.51, 45.6 and 45.72) were excluded to remove patients with ischemic small bowel. Patients with a secondary diagnosis of acute vascular insufficiency were excluded to avoid patients who experienced vascular insufficiency as a complication of their primary admission. Patients who were admitted electively were also excluded. The cohort was limited to adults 18 to 84 years of age.

Study variables

The primary outcome of interest was in-hospital mortality following colectomy for ischemic colitis. Demographic variables evaluated included: age at diagnosis, categorized as 18 to 34, 35 to 49, 50 to 64 and 65 to 84 years; sex; race and ethnicity, classified as Caucasian, African American, Hispanic, Asian or other/unknown; and health care insurance status, categorized as private, Medicare, Medicaid, self-pay or other/unknown. The following Charlson index comorbidities were assessed: myocardial infarction, congestive heart failure, peripheral vascular disease, cerebrovascular disease, dementia, chronic pulmonary disease, rheumatic disease, peptic ulcer disease, mild liver disease, moderate or severe liver disease, diabetes without chronic complications, diabetes with chronic complications, hemiplegia or paraplegia, renal disease, cancer, metastatic solid tumour and AIDS/HIV (12). Hospital characteristics evaluated included hospital location, classified as rural, urban teaching or urban nonteaching, and hospital region, categorized as Midwest, South, West or Northeast.

Statistical analysis

Calculation of percentages and logistic regression analyses were performed using SAS-callable SUDAAN release 11.0.0 (Research Triangle Institute, USA) to adjust for the complex sampling design of the NIS. Joinpoint Regression Program version 4.0.1 (Statistical Research and Applications Branch, National Cancer Institute, USA) was used to detect inflection points across time, and temporal analyses were performed using SAS version 9.3 (SAS Institute Inc, USA) Figures were created using Stata Statistical Software release 11.2 (StataCorp LP, USA).

Discharge-level weights were used to produce 95% CIs for point estimates and to reflect nationwide data during the study period. The annual incidence and mortality for patients who underwent colectomy for ischemic colitis in the US population were determined. The annual incidence and mortality rates were calculated by dividing the weighted estimate for all annual admissions/deaths in US hospitals by the annual civilian population size for the US using estimates from census data. For each annual incidence and mortality rate, 95% CIs were calculated. Temporal changes in the incidence and mortality rates were calculated using generalized linear regression models that assumed a Poisson distribution and adjusted for overdispersion. Additionally, Joinpoint models were used to assess for statistical inflection points in the temporal trends; models with zero, one or two inflection points were tested to determine whether the trend would be best modelled by zero, one or two regression segments.

Multivariable logistic regression using generalized estimating equations to account for clustering of discharges within hospitals was performed to evaluate factors that predicted in-hospital mortality in patients who underwent colectomy for ischemic colitis. Covariates assessed in the model included demographics, Charlson index comorbidities and procedures implemented in the management of acute vascular insufficiency of the colon (eg, colonoscopy). Point estimates were represented as adjusted ORs with 95% CIs. Two-sided P values were reported with a significance level of 0.05.

RESULTS

Between 1993 and 2008, the NIS database sampled 10,111 discharges for ischemic colitis patients who underwent colectomy. The characteristics of ischemic colitis patients requiring colectomy are summarized in Table 1.

Incidence

The overall incidence for colectomy for ischemic colitis was 1.43 cases per 100,000 person-years (95% CI 1.40 cases to 1.47 cases). Between 1993 and 2008, the incidence rate for colectomies in patients with ischemic colitis significantly increased (P=0.0004) (Figure 1). Over the 16-year study period, the estimated annual percent change (APC) in incidence rates was 1.4% (95% CI 0.6% to 2.3%; P=0.0004). A statistically significant inflection point was observed in 2003. Between 1993 and 2003, the incidence rate increased significantly at an annual rate of 3.1% (95% CI 2.3% to 3.9%), whereas the incidence rate between 2003 and 2008 was stable (APC −2.1% [95% CI −4.7% to 0.6%]).

Mortality

Among patients who were emergently admitted to hospital for ischemic colitis and underwent colectomy, 21.0% (95% CI 20.2% to 21.8%) died in hospital. The overall mortality rate in the US was 0.30 per 100,000 population (95% CI 0.29 to 0.31). A statistically significant inflection point for mortality was observed in 1997. Between 1993 and 1997, the mortality rate of colectomy for ischemic colitis increased significantly at an annual mean rate of 10.1% (95% CI 4.5% to 16.0%). After 1997, the mortality rate decreased significantly (APC −4.5% [95% CI −6.3% to −2.7%]) (Figure 2).

In multivariate logistic regression analysis, several factors were found to predict mortality following colectomy for ischemic colitis (Table 1). Patients 65 to 84 years of age were more likely to die (OR 5.45 [95% CI 2.91 to 10.22]) compared with the age group 18 to 34 years; and patients with Medicaid insurance (OR 1.69 [95% CI 1.29 to 2.21]) and Medicare insurance (OR 1.33 [95% CI 1.12 to 1.58]) were more likely to die compared with those with private insurance. Comorbidities such as liver disease (OR 3.54 [95% CI 2.79 to 4.50]) were associated with increased risk for mortality, whereas other comorbidities such as diabetes (OR 0.57 [95% CI 0.42 to 0.77]) were negatively associated with death (Table 1). Patients who underwent colonoscopy or sigmoidoscopy had a lower risk for death (OR 0.78 [95% CI 0.65 to 0.93]) (Table 1).

TABLE 1
Predictors of in-hospital mortality in patients who underwent colectomy for ischemic colitis between 1993 and 2008

Variable	% (95% CI) (n=10,111)	Mortality, % (95% CI) (n=2112)	Adjusted OR (95% CI)
Age, years			
18–34	2.1 (1.8–2.4)	5.2 (2.9–9.2)	1.00
35–49	6.6 (6.2–7.1)	10.4 (8.3–12.9)	1.84 (0.95–3.57)
50–64	22.5 (21.6–23.3)	15.4 (13.9–16.9)	3.17 (1.71–5.89)
65–84	68.8 (67.8–69.7)	24.3 (23.3–25.4)	5.45 (2.91–10.22)
Sex			
Male	38.7 (37.7–39.6)	21.6 (20.3–22.9)	1.00
Female	61.3 (60.4–62.3)	20.6 (19.6–21.6)	0.94 (0.85–1.04)
Race			
Caucasian	63.7 (62.3–65.1)	21.2 (20.2–22.2)	1.00
African American	6.3 (5.8–6.9)	21.6 (18.4–25.1)	0.93 (0.75–1.16)
Hispanic	3.0 (2.7–3.4)	20.6 (16.4–25.5)	0.94 (0.69–1.28)
Asian	0.5 (0.3–0.6)	15.3 (7.6–28.6)	0.66 (0.28–1.52)
Other/unknown	26.5 (25.1–27.9)	20.5 (18.9–22.1)	1.03 (0.91–1.18)
Health Insurance			
Private	21.2 (20.4–22.1)	12.9 (11.5–14.4)	1.00
Medicare	69.8 (68.8–70.7)	23.8 (22.8–24.9)	1.33 (1.12–1.58)
Medicaid	5.0 (4.5–5.4)	19.2 (16.0–22.8)	1.69 (1.29–2.21)
Self-pay	2.0 (1.8–2.3)	13.9 (9.7–19.6)	1.30 (0.84–2.03)
Other/unknown	2.0 (1.7–2.3)	18.3 (13.6–24.1)	1.41 (0.97–2.06)
Hospital location			
Rural	14.4 (13.5–15.3)	19.0 (16.8–21.3)	1.00
Urban, nonteaching	44.2 (42.9–45.5)	20.7 (19.5–21.9)	1.12 (0.95–1.33)
Urban, teaching	41.4 (40.1–42.7)	22.0 (20.7–23.4)	1.24 (1.05–1.47)
Hospital region, United States			
Northeast	22.1 (21.0–23.3)	22.6 (20.8–24.6)	1.00
Midwest	26.0 (24.9–27.1)	19.8 (18.2–21.4)	0.84 (0.71–0.98)
South	41.7 (40.5–43.0)	22.1 (20.8–23.4)	0.97 (0.85–1.12)
West	10.2 (9.3–11.1)	16.0 (13.8–18.4)	0.71 (0.57–0.88)
Myocardial infarction			
No	91.5 (90.9–92.0)	20.7 (19.9–21.6)	1.00
Yes	8.5 (8.0–9.1)	23.7 (20.9–26.6)	1.09 (0.91–1.30)
Congestive heart failure			
No	77.9 (77.1–78.7)	19.2 (18.3–20.1)	1.00
Yes	22.1 (21.3–22.9)	27.2 (25.4–29.2)	1.33 (1.18–1.50)
Peripheral vascular disease			
No	91.1 (90.5–91.7)	21.2 (20.3–22.0)	1.00
Yes	8.9 (8.3–9.5)	19.1 (16.7–21.8)	0.81 (0.68–0.98)
Cerebrovascular disease			
No	95.7 (95.3–96.1)	20.6 (19.8–21.5)	1.00
Yes	4.3 (3.9–4.7)	28.4 (24.2–33.0)	1.46 (1.15–1.86)
Dementia			
No	98.8 (98.6–99.0)	21.0 (20.2–21.8)	1.00
Yes	1.2 (1.0–1.4)	19.6 (12.9–28.7)	0.85 (0.50–1.44)
Chronic pulmonary disease			
No	71.8 (70.9–72.7)	20.4 (19.4–21.4)	1.00
Yes	28.2 (27.3–29.1)	22.5 (21.0–24.1)	1.04 (0.93–1.16)
Rheumatic disease			
No	96.9 (96.5–97.2)	20.9 (20.1–21.8)	1.00
Yes	3.1 (2.8–3.5)	22.6 (18.3–27.6)	1.22 (0.92–1.61)
Peptic ulcer disease			
No	97.9 (97.6–98.1)	20.8 (20.0–21.6)	1.00
Yes	2.1 (1.9–2.4)	29.3 (23.5–35.7)	1.50 (1.10–2.04)

Continued in next column

TABLE 1 – CONTINUED
Predictors of in-hospital mortality in patients who underwent colectomy for ischemic colitis between 1993 and 2008

Variable	% (95% CI) (n=10,111)	Mortality, % (95% CI) (n=2112)	Adjusted OR (95% CI)
Mild liver disease			
No	96.3 (95.9–96.7)	20.1 (19.3–20.9)	1.00
Yes	3.7 (3.3–4.1)	44.6 (39.6–49.8)	3.54 (2.79–4.50)
Diabetes without chronic complication			
No	84.7 (84.0–85.4)	21.6 (20.7–22.5)	1.00
Yes	15.3 (14.6–16.0)	17.5 (15.6–19.5)	0.71 (0.61–0.83)
Diabetes with chronic complication			
No	96.5 (96.1–96.9)	21.1 (20.3–22.0)	1.00
Yes	3.5 (3.1–3.9)	17.3 (13.7–21.6)	0.57 (0.42–0.77)
Hemiplegia or paraplegia			
No	99.1 (98.9–99.3)	21.0 (20.2–21.8)	1.00
Yes	0.9 (0.7–1.1)	19.8 (12.5–30.1)	0.98 (0.53–1.79)
Renal disease			
No	87.2 (86.5–87.9)	19.1 (18.3–20.0)	1.00
Yes	12.8 (12.1–13.5)	33.5 (30.9–36.3)	2.23 (1.92–2.58)
Cancer			
No	96.0 (95.6–96.4)	20.6 (19.7–21.4)	1.00
Yes	4.0 (3.6–4.4)	31.0 (26.8–35.6)	1.72 (1.35–2.18)
Moderate or severe liver disease			
No	99.5 (99.3–99.6)	20.8 (20.0–21.7)	1.00
Yes	0.5 (0.4–0.7)	47.4 (34.7–60.5)	2.17 (1.17–4.04)
Metastatic solid tumour			
No	98.5 (98.3–98.8)	20.8 (20.0–21.7)	1.00
Yes	1.5 (1.2–1.7)	30.2 (23.3–38.2)	1.41 (0.92–2.17)
AIDS/HIV			
No	99.86 (99.77–99.92)	21.0 (20.1–21.8)	1.00
Yes	0.14 (0.08–0.23)	34.2 (14.9–60.6)	2.43 (0.66–8.92)
Colonoscopy or sigmoidoscopy			
No	90.6 (90.0–91.2)	21.3 (20.4–22.2)	1.00
Yes	9.4 (8.8–10.0)	17.9 (15.6–20.5)	0.78 (0.65–0.93)

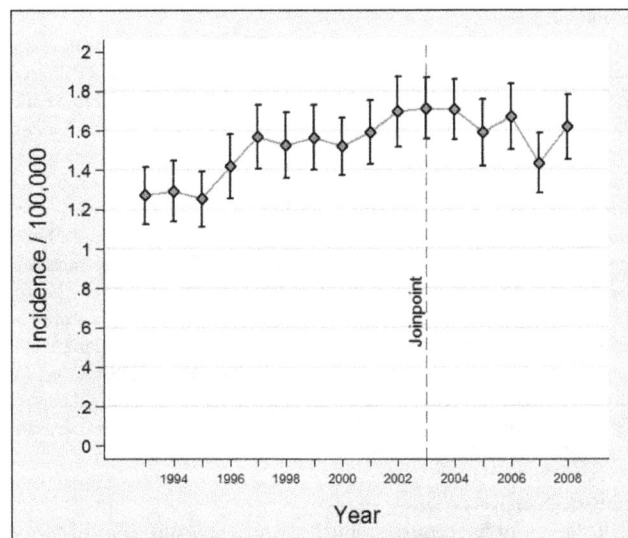

Figure 1) *Annual incidence rates of ischemic colitis for patients requiring colectomy in the United States between 1993 and 2008*

DISCUSSION

The present population-based study evaluated the incidence of and mortality from colectomy for ischemic colitis in the US using a nationally representative sample. As the North American population ages, we will likely observe an increasing number of admissions to hospital for ischemic colitis. Reassuringly, the annual incidence of colectomy for ischemic colitis has stabilized since 2003. This is important because colectomy for ischemic colitis was associated with significant mortality. Nearly one in five patients who were emergently admitted to hospital with ischemic colitis and required a colectomy subsequently died in hospital.

Our sample specifically assessed hospitalized patients with ischemic colitis who required colectomy. The present study was not designed to analyze patients with ischemic colitis not requiring hospital admission, or who were admitted to hospital but did not require colectomy. Furthermore, patients with ischemic colitis who died in hospital before colectomy were not evaluated. Additionally, acute vascular insufficiency of the colon occurring as an in-hospital complication (eg, postsurgery) was not included in the present study. Nonetheless, the high mortality associated with this condition necessitates prospective studies to evaluate modifiable factors that may prevent the occurrence of ischemic colitis or mitigate mortality among patients with ischemic colitis who require colectomy.

While the incidence of colectomy for ischemic colitis has not decreased, mortality rates have decreased significantly since 1997. These results suggest that clinical detection and management may be improving across time. Cardiovascular risk factor modification strategies (eg, smoking cessation, improved diabetes management, etc) have improved during our study period (13), and may have indirectly reduced the burden of disease. Further advances in surgical management and postoperative management, including intensive care management, may have improved mortality outcomes. Additional studies will be needed to explain potential causes of the decline in mortality rates observed after 1997.

Several important risk factors for mortality and surgery were identified. Our study demonstrated that colonic resection increased the risk for death. Brandt et al (14) also showed that mortality was higher (37%) in patients needing surgery compared with those managed medically (5.6%). However, surgical resection may simply act as a surrogate for patients with increased disease severity. Also, patients without private insurance were at increased risk for mortality and colonic resection. Such patients may have been disenfranchised with increased barriers to early access to health care, contributing to worse disease states and outcome (15). Furthermore, these patients may have had lower socioeconomic status and may have been more likely to have cardiovascular risk factors (eg, smoking).

Other predictors of mortality identified in our study included advancing age and specific comorbidities including liver disease, renal disease and congestive heart failure. Other studies have reported that hyperthyroidism, stroke, cancer, hepatitis C and renal dysfunction increase mortality (2,13,14,16-19). Thus, clinicians should cautiously monitor patients with these comorbidities who are admitted with ischemic colitis. Future studies are necessary to evaluate whether a prediction rule for mortality can be generated from at-risk comorbidities.

Patients who underwent colonoscopy or sigmoidoscopy were less likely to die. Patients who undergo these procedures present with more classic symptoms, such as hematochezia, which warrants earlier diagnostic intervention and medical management. Patients who undergo endoscopic evaluation may also represent those receiving additional expert management by a gastroenterologist or surgeon. Alternatively, gastroenterologists are less likely to endoscopically evaluate ill patients at risk for perforation or unable to tolerate sedation. Consequently, the reduced mortality associated with endoscopic evaluation may have been biased by confounding by indication.

Our results should be interpreted in the context of the limitations associated with the use of administrative databases (20,21). First, our study population was based on the ICD-9 code for vascular insufficiency of the intestine, which does not have the specificity to differentiate ischemic colitis from small bowel infarction. However, all of our patients underwent a partial or total colectomy, and we excluded all patients who underwent a concurrent small bowel resection. Also, a

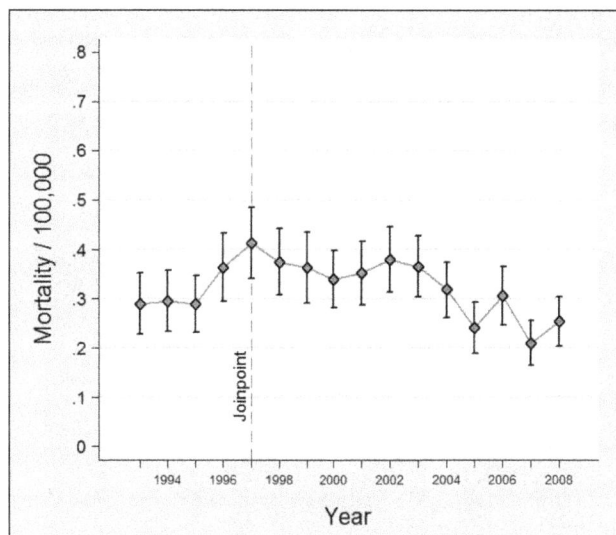

Figure 2) *Annual mortality rates for ischemic colitis patients requiring colectomy in the United States between 1993 and 2008*

study that validated ICD-9 coding demonstrated that the majority of cases represented ischemic colitis (22). Second, the NIS database extracts data from discharge abstracts, which prevents investigators from following patient outcomes postdischarge. Third, the NIS database does not provide data on preadmission or in-hospital medications and, thus, we could not directly study the effects of medication use that have been examined in other studies (23,24). Fourth, although the sampling frame of the NIS has been shown to represent >90% of all hospitalizations, Veteran Affairs hospitals were not included in the NIS database. Thus, the annual civilian population size for the US was used as the denominator for incidence and mortality calculations.

CONCLUSION
Our population-based study evaluated the incidence of colectomy for ischemic colitis in the US using a nationally representative sample. In the latter years of our study, the incidence of colectomy for ischemic colitis stabilized and mortality rates decreased. This was an important finding because 20% of patients died postoperatively. Additional prospective studies in this area will elucidate clinical and medication-related parameters for treatment, early detection, natural disease history, and risk factor modification to decrease adverse outcomes and overall burden of this important disease.

DISCLOSURES: The authors have no financial disclosures or conflicts of interest to declare.

ACKNOWLEDGEMENTS: Dr Gilaad Kaplan is supported by a New Investigator Award from the Canadian Institutes of Health Research and a Population Health Investigator Award from Alberta-Innovates Health Solutions.

AUTHOR CONTRIBUTIONS: Matthew D Sadler – participated in conceiving the study idea, developing the study design, interpreting results and writing of the manuscript. Nikila C Ravindran – participated in conceiving the study idea, developing the study design, interpreting results and editing the manuscript. James Hubbard – participated in developing the study design, analyzing the results and editing the manuscript. Robert P Myers – participated in developing the study design, interpreting results and editing the manuscript. Subrata Ghosh – participated in developing the study design, interpreting results and editing the manuscript. Paul L Beck – participated in developing the study design, interpreting results and editing the manuscript. Elijah Dixon – participated in developing the study design, interpreting results and editing the manuscript. Chad Ball – participated in developing the study design, interpreting results and editing the manuscript.

Chris Prusinkiewicz – participated in developing the study design, interpreting results and editing the manuscript. Steven J Heitman – participated in developing the study design, interpreting results and editing the manuscript. Gilaad G Kaplan – participated in conceiving the study idea, developing the study design, preparing the data, supervising the analysis, interpreting

results and writing the manuscript. Dr Kaplan confirms that he has had full access to all of the data in the study and had final responsibility for the decision to submit for publication. All authors reviewed and approved the final version of the manuscript.

REFERENCES

1. Huguier M, Barrier A, Boelle PY, Houry S, Lacaine F. Ischemic colitis. Am J Surg 2006;192:679-84.
2. Sotiriadis J, Brandt LJ, Behin DS, Southern WN. Ischemic colitis has a worse prognosis when isolated to the right side of the colon. Am J Gastroenterol 2007;102:2247-52.
3. Arnott ID, Ghosh S, Ferguson A. The spectrum of ischaemic colitis. Eur J Gastroenterol Hepatol 1999;11:295-303.
4. Higgins PD, Davis KJ, Laine L. Systematic review: The epidemiology of ischaemic colitis. Aliment Pharmacol Ther 2004;19:729-38.
5. Brandt LJ. Bloody diarrhea in an elderly patient. Gastroenterology 2005;128:157-63.
6. Whalen D EA. HCUP Nationwide Inpatient Sample (NIS) Comparison Report: U.S. Agency for Healthcare Research and Quality; 2004.
7. Gorham ED, Garland CF, Garland FC. Acid haze air pollution and breast and colon cancer mortality in 20 Canadian cities. Can J Public Health 1989;80:96-100.
8. Kaplan GG, Hubbard J, Panaccione R, et al. Risk of comorbidities on postoperative outcomes in patients with inflammatory bowel disease. Arch Surg 2011;146:959-64.
9. Kaplan GG, McCarthy EP, Ayanian JZ, Korzenik J, Hodin R, Sands BE. Impact of hospital volume on postoperative morbidity and mortality following a colectomy for ulcerative colitis. Gastroenterology 2008;134:680-7.
10. Meddings L, Myers RP, Hubbard J, et al. A population-based study of pyogenic liver abscesses in the United States: Incidence, mortality, and temporal trends. Am J Gastroenterol 2010;105:117-24.
11. Kaplan GG, Panaccione R, Hubbard JN, et al. Inflammatory bowel disease patients who leave hospital against medical advice: Predictors and temporal trends. Inflamm Bowel Dis 2009;15:845-51.
12. Deyo RA, Cherkin DC, Ciol MA. Adapting a clinical comorbidity index for use with ICD-9-CM administrative databases. J Clin Epidemiol 1992;45:613-9.
13. Lee TC, Wang HP, Chiu HM, et al. Male gender and renal dysfunction are predictors of adverse outcome in nonpostoperative ischemic colitis patients. J Clin Gastroenterol 2010;44:e96-100.
14. Brandt LJ, Feuerstadt P, Blaszka MC. Anatomic patterns, patient characteristics, and clinical outcomes in ischemic colitis: A study of 313 cases supported by histology. Am J Gastroenterol 2010;105:2245-52.
15. Nguyen GC, Bayless TM, Powe NR, Laveist TA, Brant SR. Race and health insurance are predictors of hospitalized Crohn's disease patients undergoing bowel resection. Inflamm Bowel Dis 2007;13:1408-16.
16. Montoro MA, Brandt LJ, Santolaria S, et al. Clinical patterns and outcomes of ischaemic colitis: results of the Working Group for the Study of Ischaemic Colitis in Spain (CIE study). Scand J Gastroenterol 2011;46:236-46.
17. Flobert C, Cellier C, Berger A, et al. Right colonic involvement is associated with severe forms of ischemic colitis and occurs frequently in patients with chronic renal failure requiring hemodialysis. Am J Gastroenterol 2000;95:195-8.
18. Paterno F, McGillicuddy EA, Schuster KM, Longo WE. Ischemic colitis: Risk factors for eventual surgery. Am J Surg 2010;200:646-50.
19. Mosele M, Cardin F, Inelmen EM, et al. Ischemic colitis in the elderly: Predictors of the disease and prognostic factors to negative outcome. Scand J Gastroenterol 2010;45:428-33.
20. Ma C, Crespin M, Proulx MC, et al. Postoperative complications following colectomy for ulcerative colitis: A validation study. BMC Gastroenterol 2012;12:39.
21. Molodecky NA, Panaccione R, Ghosh S, Barkema HW, Kaplan GG. Challenges associated with identifying the environmental determinants of the inflammatory bowel diseases. Inflamm Bowel Dis 2011;17:1792-9.
22. Sands BE, Duh MS, Cali C, et al. Algorithms to identify colonic ischemia, complications of constipation and irritable bowel syndrome in medical claims data: Development and validation. Pharmacoepidemiol Drug Saf 2006;15:47-56.
23. Walker AM, Bohn RL, Cali C, Cook SF, Ajene AN, Sands BE. Risk factors for colon ischemia. Am J Gastroenterol 2004;99:1333-7.
24. Cole JA, Cook SF, Sands BE, Ajene AN, Miller DP, Walker AM. Occurrence of colon ischemia in relation to irritable bowel syndrome. Am J Gastroenterol 2004;99:486-91.

Permissions

List of Contributors

Daniel J Smyth MD FRCPC, Duncan Webster MD FRCPC, Mark MacMillan MD FRCPC, Lisa McKnight MD FRCPC, Frank Schweiger MD FRCPC
Horizon Health Network, New Brunswick
Dalhousie University, Halifax, Nova Scotia

Lisa Barrett MD PhD FRCPC
Capital Health
Dalhousie University, Halifax, Nova Scotia

Robert P Myers MD MSc
Liver Unit, Division of Gastroenterology and Hepatology, Department of Medicine, University of Calgary, Calgary, Alberta

Mel Krajden MD
BC Centre for Disease Control, Vancouver, British Columbia

Marc Bilodeau MD
University of Montreal, Montreal, Quebec

Kelly Kaita MD
University of Manitoba, Winnipeg, Manitoba

Paul Marotta MD
Western University, London, Ontario

Kevork Peltekian MD
Dalhousie University, Halifax, Nova Scotia

Alnoor Ramji MD
University of British Columbia, Vancouver, British Columbia

Chris Estes MPH and Homie Razavi PhD
Center for Disease Analysis, Louisville, Colorado, USA

Morris Sherman MD
University of Toronto, Toronto, Ontario

Mamatha Bhat MD FRCPC, Marc Deschênes MD FRCPC and Peter Ghali MD FRCPC
Division of Gastroenterology and Hepatology, Department of Medicine, McGill University Health Centre, Montreal, Canada

Said A Al-Busafi MD FRCPC
Division of Gastroenterology and Hepatology, Department of Medicine, McGill University Health Centre, Montreal, Canada
Division of Gastroenterology, Sultan Qaboos University, Oman

Yidan Lu MD and Myriam Martel BSc
Divisions of Gastroenterology

Alan N Barkun MD MSc
Divisions of Gastroenterology
Epidemiology Biostatistics and Occupational Health, McGill University Health Centre, McGill University, Montreal, Quebec

Stephen Ip MD
Department of Medicine

AbdulRazaq AH Sokoro PhD
Department of Medicine
Department of Pathology, University of Manitoba
Diagnostic Services of Manitoba

Lisa Kaita BN, Claudia Ruiz BA and Elaine McIntyre RN
4Winnipeg Regional Health Authority;

Harminder Singh MD MPH
Department of Medicine
Department of Community Health Sciences, University of Manitoba
Department of Hematology and Oncology, CancerCare Manitoba
University of Manitoba IBD Clinical and Research Centre, Winnipeg, Manitoba

Alexander F Hagel MD, Martin Raithel MD, Wolfgang H Hagel MD, Heinz Albrecht MD, Thomas M de Rossi MD and Markus F Neurath MD
Department of Gastroenterology, University of Erlangen

Erwin Gäbele MD
Department of Gastroenterology, Asklepios Clinic Burglengenfeld, Burglengenfeld

Christine Singer MD
Institute of Employment Research, Nuremberg

Thomas Schneider MD and Michael J Farnbacher MD
Department of Gastroenterology, Clinical Centre Fuerth, Teaching Hospital of the University of Erlangen, Erlangen, Germany

Yingming Amy Chen MD, Anish Kirpalani MD, Paraskevi A Vlachou MD and Errol Colak MD
Department of Medical Imaging, St Michael's Hospital, Toronto

Patrick Cervini MD
Department of Diagnostic Imaging, Windsor Regional Hospital – Ouellette Campus, Windsor

Samir C Grover MD MEd
Division of Gastroenterology, St Michael's Hospital, Toronto, Ontario

Melissa Kelley MD, Nikhil Joshi MD, Yagang Xie MD and Mark Borgaonkar MD MSc
Faculty of Medicine, Memorial University, St John's, Newfoundland and Labrador

Sonya A MacParland PhD, Frank Bialystok PhD Eve Roberts MD and Jordan J Feld MD
University of Toronto, Toronto, Ontario

Marc Bilodeau MD and Norma Choucha
Liver Unit, Department of Medicine, Université de Montréal, Montréal, Québec

Jason Grebely PhD
The Kirby Institute, UNSW Australia, Sydney, Australia

Julie Bruneau MD
Department of Family Medicine, Université de Montréal, Montréal, Québec

Curtis Cooper MD and Louise Balfour PhD
Division of Infectious Diseases, University of Ottawa, Ottawa, Ontario

Marina Klein MD
Division of Infectious Diseases

Selena M Sagan PhD
Department of Microbiology & Immunology, McGill University, Montreal, Quebec

Mel Krajden MD
British Columbia Centre for Disease Control
University of British Columbia, Vancouver, British Columbia

Jennifer Raven PhD
Canadian Institutes of Health Research – Institute of Infection and Immunity, Ottawa, Ontario

Rodney Russell PhD
Division of Biomedical Sciences, Memorial University of Newfoundland, St John's, Newfoundland & Labrador

Michael Houghton PhD and D Lorne Tyrrell MD PhD
Li Ka Shing Institute of Virology, University of Alberta, Edmonton, Alberta

Muhammad Ali Khan MD, Abdur Rahman Khan MD, Tariq Hammad MD and Sehrish Kamal MD
Department of Internal Medicine

Aijaz Ahmed Sofi MD, Usman Ahmad MD, Osama Alaradi MD, Jennifer Pratt RN, Thomas Sodeman MD, William Sodeman MD and Ali Nawras MD
Department of Internal Medicine, Division of Gastroenterology, University of Toledo Medical Center, Toledo, Ohio, USA

Jennifer Chaulk MD, Michelle Carbonneau NP MN RN, Hina Qamar MD, Adam Keough BSc, Hsiu-Ju Chang MSc, Mang Ma MD FRCPC and Puneeta Tandon MD MSc FRCPC
Division of Gastroenterology, Department of Medicine

Deepali Kumar MD MSc FRCPC
Division of Infectious Diseases, Department of Medicine, University of Alberta, Edmonton, Alberta

James W Keck MD MPH
Epidemic Intelligence Service, Office of Surveillance, Epidemiology, and Laboratory Services, Centers for Disease Control and Prevention, Atlanta, Georgia
Arctic Investigations Program, Centers for Disease Control and Prevention

Karen M Miernyk BS and Brian J McMahon MD
Arctic Investigations Program, Centers for Disease Control and Prevention
Alaska Native Tribal Health Consortium

Lisa R Bulkow MS, Thomas W Hennessy MD MPH and Michael G Bruce MD MPH
Arctic Investigations Program, Centers for Disease Control and Prevention

Janet J Kelly MS MPH
Alaska Native Tribal Health Consortium

Frank Sacco MD
Department of Surgery, Alaska Native Medical Center, Anchorage, Alaska, USA

Sang Hyoung Park MD, Suk-Kyun Yang MD, Soo-Kyung Park MD, Dong-Hoon Yang MD, Kee Wook Jung MD, Kyung-Jo Kim MD, Byong Duk Ye MD, Jeong-Sik Byeon MD, Seung-Jae Myung MD and Jin-Ho Kim MD
Department of Gastroenterology, University of Ulsan College of Medicine, Asan Medical Center, Seoul

Jong Wook Kim MD
Division of Gastroenterology, Department of Internal Medicine, Inje University Ilsan Paik Hospital, Ilsanseo-gu, Goyang-si, Gyeonggi-do, Korea

Wael El-Matary MBBCh MD MSc FRCPCH FRCPC
Section of Pediatric Gastroenterology, Department of Pediatrics, and Manitoba Institute of Child Health, Faculty of Medicine, University of Manitoba, Winnipeg, Manitoba. Dr El-Matary is also affiliated with the University of Alexandria, Egypt

Jensen Tan MD MSc FRCSC and Jennifer Muir MD
Department of General Surgery, University of Toronto

Natalie Coburn MD MPH FRCSC FACS
Department of General Surgery, University of Toronto
Odette Cancer Centre, Sunnybrook Health Sciences Centre

Simron Singh MD MPH FRCPC
Odette Cancer Centre, Sunnybrook Health Sciences Centre

David Hodgson MD MPH FRCPC
Institute for Clinical and Evaluative Sciences
University Health Network

Refik Saskin MSc
Institute for Clinical and Evaluative Sciences

Alex Kiss PhD
Institute for Clinical and Evaluative Sciences
Sunnybrook Research Institute, Sunnybrook Health Sciences Centre, Toronto, Ontario

Lawrence Paszat MD MSc FRCPC and Craig Earle MD MSc FRCPC
Odette Cancer Centre, Sunnybrook Health Sciences Centre
Institute for Clinical and Evaluative Sciences

Abraham El-Sedfy MD MSc
Odette Cancer Centre, Sunnybrook Health Sciences Centre
Department of Surgery, Saint Barnabas Medical Center, Livingston, New Jersey, USA

Eva Grunfeld MD DPhil FCFP
Institute for Clinical and Evaluative Sciences
Department of Family and Community Medicine, University of Toronto, Toronto, Ontario

Calvin Law MD MPH FRCSC
Department of General Surgery, University of Toronto
Odette Cancer Centre, Sunnybrook Health Sciences Centre
Institute for Clinical and Evaluative Sciences
Sunnybrook Research Institute, Sunnybrook Health Sciences Centre, Toronto, Ontario

Jennifer G Stretton NP MN BScN
Division of Gastroenterology, St Joseph's Healthcare Hamilton, Hamilton, Ontario

Barbara K Currie NP MN BNRN
Division of Gastroenterology, QEII Health Sciences Centre, Halifax, Nova Scotia

Usha K Chauhan NP MN BScN
Division of Gastroenterology, Hamilton Health Sciences, Hamilton, Ontario

Sara El Ouali MD, Myriam Martel BSc and Davide Maggio MD
Divisions of Gastroenterology

Alan N Barkun MD MSc
Divisions of Gastroenterology
Clinical Epidemiology, McGill University, Montreal, Quebec

Curtis Cooper MD
University of Ottawa, Ottawa Hospital Research Institute, Ottawa, Ontario

Stephen Shafran MD
University of Alberta, Edmonton, Alberta

Susan Greenbloom MD
Toronto Digestive Disease Associates, Toronto, Ontario

Robert Enns MD
St Paul's Hospital, University of British Columbia

John Farley MD
Private Practice, Vancouver, British Columbia

Nir Hilzenrat MD
Jewish General Hospital and McGill University, Montreal, Quebec

Kurt Williams MD
Royal University Hospital, Saskatoon, Saskatchewan

Magdy Elkashab MD
Private practice, Toronto, Ontario

Nabil Abadir MD
Merck Canada Inc, Kirkland, Quebec

Manuela Neuman PhD
University of Toronto, Toronto, Ontario

Alan Hoi Lun Yau MD and Eric M Yoshida MD MHSc FRCPC
Department of Medicine, Division of Gastroenterology, University of British Columbia, Vancouver, British Columbia

Pranavi Ravichandran MD
Department of Surgery, Division of General Surgery, University of Western Ontario

Kris P Croome MD MS and Roberto Hernandez-Alejandro MD
Department of Surgery, Division of General Surgery, University of Western Ontario
Multi-Organ Transplant Program, London Health Sciences Centre

Michael J Kovacs MD FRCPC
Department of Medicine, Division of Hematology

Alejandro Lazo-Langner MD MSc
Department of Medicine, Division of Hematology
Department of Epidemiology and Biostatistics, University of Western Ontario, London, Ontario

Kathryn Martin MD, Catherine Deshaies MD CM and Sherif Emil MD CM
Division of Pediatric General and Thoracic Surgery, The Montreal Children's Hospital; McGill University Health Centre, Montreal, Quebec

Mahmoud Torabi PhD and Christopher Green PhD
Department of Community Health Sciences

Zoann Nugent PhD
Department of Community Health Sciences
University of Manitoba IBD Clinical and Research Centre,
University of Manitoba
Department of Epidemiology and Cancer Registry

**Salaheddin M Mahmud PhD, Alain A Demers PhD and
Jane Griffith PhD**
Department of Community Health Sciences
Department of Epidemiology and Cancer Registry

Harminder Singh MD MPH FACG
Department of Community Health Sciences
University of Manitoba IBD Clinical and Research Centre,
University of Manitoba
Department of Hematology and Oncology, CancerCare
Manitoba
Department of Internal Medicine, University of Manitoba,
Winnipeg, Manitoba

Mary Anne Cooper MSc MD MEd FRCPC
RNFS Program, Cancer Care Ontario
Department of Gastroenterology, Sunnybrook Health
Sciences Centre
Department of Medicine, University of Toronto

Jill Margaret Tinmouth MD PhD FRCPC
Department of Gastroenterology, Sunnybrook Health
Sciences Centre
Department of Medicine, University of Toronto
ColonCancerCheck Program, Cancer Care Ontario

Linda Rabeneck MD MPH FRCPC
Department of Medicine, University of Toronto
Cancer Care Ontario and the University of Toronto,
Toronto, Ontario

**Korosh Khalili MD, Ravi Menezes PhD, Leyla Kochak
Yazdi MD, Hyun-Jung Jang MD and Tae Kyoung Kim
MD**
Department of Medical Imaging

**Suraj Sharma MD, Jordan Feld MD and Morris
Sherman MD**
Department of Gastroenterology, University of Toronto,
Toronto, Ontario

**Christopher Skappak PhD, Kris Chadee PhD and
Deirdre Church MD PhD FRCPC**
Department of Medicine

Sarah Akierman BSc BA
Department of Biological Sciences, University of Calgary,
Calgary

Sara Belga MD
Department of Medicine, University of Alberta, Edmonton

**Kerri Novak MD FRCPC and Paul L Beck PhD MD
FRCPC**
Department of Medicine
Department of Medicine, Division of Gastroenterology

Stefan J Urbanski MD FRCPC
Department of Pathology, University of Calgary, Calgary,
Alberta

Mayur Brahmania MD and Charles N Bernstein MD
Department of Internal Medicine, Division of
Gastroenterology, University of Manitoba Inflammatory
Bowel Disease Clinical and Research Centre, Winnipeg,
Manitoba

**VGR Gangireddy MBBS and S Sridhar MBBS MPH
FRCP FACP**
Georgia Regents University, Augusta, Georgia

PC Kanneganti MBBS
Helena Regional Medical Center, Helena, Arkansas, USA

S Talla MBBS
Luzhou Medical College, Luzhou, China

T Coleman MD FACP
Archbold Medical Center, Thomasville, Georgia, USA

**Yvette PY Leung MD FRCPC, Remo Panaccione MD
FRCPC, Subrata Ghosh MBBS MD FRCPC FRCPE**
Department of Medicine

Cynthia H Seow MBBS MSc FRACP
Department of Medicine
Department of Community Health Sciences, University
of Calgary, Calgary, Alberta

Mohammad Bashashati MD
Gastrointestinal Research Group, University of Calgary,
Calgary, Alberta

Reza A Hejazi MD
Department of Internal Medicine, Texas Tech University
Health Sciences Center, Paul L Foster School of Medicine,
El Paso, Texas, USA

Christopher N Andrews MD
Division of Gastroenterology, Department of Medicine,
University of Calgary, Calgary, Alberta

Martin A Storr MD
Gastrointestinal Research Group, University of Calgary,
Calgary, Alberta
Division of Gastroenterology, Ludwig Maximilians
University of Munich, Munich, Germany

**Rachid Mohamed MD FRCPC, Maitreyi Raman MD
FRCPC MSc, Alaa Rostom MD FRCPC MSc and Sylvain
Coderre MD FRCPC MSc**
Department of Medicine (Division Gastroenterology),
University of Calgary, Calgary, Alberta

John Anderson BSc FRCP(Edin) MD
Department of Gastroenterology, Gloucestershire Hospitals NHS Foundation Trust Hospital, United Kingdom

Kevin McLaughlin MD MRCP PhD
Office of Undergraduate Medical Education, University of Calgary, Calgary, Alberta

Faruq Pradhan, Pam Crotty MSc, Jenna Tracey BSc, Christopher Schneider MD and Mark G Swain MD MSc
Liver Unit, Division of Gastroenterology and Hepatology, Department of Medicine

Scott Zimmer BA and Sophia Niu BSc MSc
Medical Services, Alberta Health Services, Calgary, Alberta

Jack XQ Pang MD, Steven J Heitman MD MSc, Gilaad G Kaplan MD MPH and Robert P Myers MD MSc
Liver Unit, Division of Gastroenterology and Hepatology, Department of Medicine
Department of Community Health Sciences, University of Calgary

Matthew S Chang MD, Sravanya Gavini MD and Julia McNabb-Baltar MD
Division of Gastroenterology, Hepatology, and Endoscopy, Brigham and Women's Hospital

Priscila C Andrade PharmD
Laboratory of Neuromodulation & Center for Clinical Research Learning, Spaulding Rehabilitation Hospital, Harvard Medical School, Boston, Massachusetts, USA

Marietta Iacucci MD PhD, Cesare Hassan MD, Miriam Fort Gasia MD, Bertus Eksteen MD, Gregory Eustace MD, Gilaad G Kaplan MD and Remo Panaccione MD
IBD Clinic, Division of Gastroenterology

Stefan Urbanski MD and Xianyong Gui MD
Department of Pathology, University of Calgary, Calgary, Alberta

Malcolm Wells MD MSc and Natasha Chandok MD MPH
Department of Medicine

Kris Croome MD MS and Roberto Hernandez-Alejandro MD
Department of Surgery, Schulich School of Medicine and Dentistry, Western University, London;

Toni Janik MLIS AHIP
Hotel Dieu Grace Hospital, Windsor, Ontario

Zane Gallinger MD BSc(H) and Geoffrey C Nguyen MD PhD
Mount Sinai Hospital Centre for Inflammatory Bowel Disease, University of Toronto, Toronto, Ontario

Brian Bressler MD MS
Division of Gastroenterology, University of British Columbia, Vancouver, British Columbia

Shane M Devlin MD
Inflammatory Bowel Disease Clinic, Division of Gastroenterology and Hepatology, University of Calgary, Calgary, Alberta

Sophie Plamondon MD
Division of Gastroenterology, Centre Hospitalier Universitaire de Sherbrooke and Centre de Recherche Étienne-LeBel, Université de Sherbrooke, Sherbrooke, Québec

Jonathan S Zipursky MD
Faculty of Medicine, Geisel School of Medicine at Dartmouth, Hanover, New Hampshire

Tivon I Sidorsky MD MBA
Department of Dermatology, University of California, San Francisco, San Francisco, California, USA

Carolyn A Freedman MD
University of Toronto Faculty of Medicine, Toronto, Ontario

Misha N Sidorsky AB
Dartmouth College, Hanover

Kathryn B Kirkland MD
Section of Infectious Diseases and International Health, Dartmouth-Hitchcock Medical Center, Lebanon, New Hampshire, USA

Alan Hoi Lun Yau MD and George Ou MD
Department of Medicine

Cherry Galorport MD, Jack Amar MD FRCPC, Brian Bressler MD MS FRCPC, Fergal Donnellan MD FRCPC, Hin Hin Ko MD FRCPC, Eric Lam MD FRCPC and Robert Allan Enns MD FRCPC
Division of Gastroenterology, University of British Columbia, Vancouver, British Columbia

Vladimir Marquez Azalgara MDCM MSc
Division of Gastroenterology, Vancouver General Hospital, Vancouver, British Columbia

Maida J Sewitch PhD and Alan N Barkun MDCM FRCPC FACP FACG AGAF MSc
Department of Medicine

Lawrence Joseph PhD
Department of Epidemiology, Biostatistics and Occupational Health, McGill University, Montreal, Quebec

Giada Sebastiani MD, Peter Ghali MD FRCPC MSc, Philip Wong MD FRCPC MSc and Marc Deschenes MD
Division of Gastroenterology, Royal Victoria Hospital, McGill University Health Centre

Marina B Klein MD MSc
Department of Medicine, Division of Infectious Diseases/
Chronic Viral Illness Service, McGill University Health
Centre, Montreal, Quebec

Robert P Myers MD FRCPC
Liver Unit, Division of Gastroenterology and Hepatology,
Department of Medicine, University of Calgary, Alberta

Harminder Singh MD MPH
Internal Medicine, University of Manitoba
University of Manitoba IBD Clinical and Research Centre
Winnipeg Regional Health Authority
CancerCare Manitoba, Department of Hematology and
Oncology
Community Health Sciences, University of Manitoba

Lisa Kaita RN BN and Gerry Taylor MSc
Winnipeg Regional Health Authority

Zoann Nugent PhD
CancerCare Manitoba, Department of Epidemiology and
Cancer Registry, Winnipeg, Manitoba

Charles Bernstein MD
Internal Medicine, University of Manitoba
University of Manitoba IBD Clinical and Research Centre
Winnipeg Regional Health Authority

Ian Plener MD and Andrew Hayward MD
Department of Medicine, University of Toronto

Fred Saibil MD
Department of Medicine, University of Toronto
Division of Gastroenterology, Sunnybrook Health
Sciences Centre, Toronto, Ontario

Mélissa Ratelle B Pharm MSc
Department of Pharmacy, Centre Hospitalier de
l'Université de Montréal

Sylvie Perreault B Pharm PhD
Université de Montréal

Jean-Pierre Villeneuve MD
Division of Hepatology, Department of Medicine, Hôpital
St-Luc, Centre Hospitalier de l'Université de Montréal,
Montréal, Québec

Lydjie Tremblay B Pharm MSc
Department of Pharmacy, Centre Hospitalier de
l'Université de Montréal
Université de Montréal

**Matthew D Sadler MD, Nikila C Ravindran MD, James
Hubbard MSc, Robert P Myers MD MSc, Subrata Ghosh
MD, Paul L Beck MD PhD and Steven J Heitman MD
MSc**
Departments of Medicine

Elijah Dixon MD MSc and Chad Ball MD
Surgery

Chris Prusinkiewicz MD
Anesthesia, University of Calgary, Calgary, Alberta

Gilaad G Kaplan MD MPH
Departments of Medicine
Community Health Sciences

www.ingramcontent.com/pod-product-compliance
Lightning Source LLC
Chambersburg PA
CBHW080459200326

41458CB00012B/4022